APPROACH
TO THE
PSYCHIATRIC
PATIENT

Case-Based Essays

APPROACH TO THE PSYCHIATRIC PATIENT

Case-Based Essays

EDITED BY

John W. Barnhill, M.D.

Associate Professor of Clinical Psychiatry
and Public Health, Weill Cornell Medical College
Chief, Consultation-Liaison Psychiatry
New York-Presbyterian Hospital/Weill Cornell Medical Center
Faculty, Columbia University Center for
Psychoanalytic Training & Research

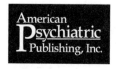

American Psychiatric Publishing, Inc.

Washington, DC
London, England

Books published by American Psychiatric Publishing, Inc., represent the views and opinions of the individual authors and do not necessarily represent the policies and opinions of APPI or the American Psychiatric Association.

If you would like to buy between 25 and 99 copies of this or any other APPI title, you are eligible for a 20% discount; please contact APPI Customer Service at appi@psych.org or 800-368-5777. If you wish to buy 100 or more copies of the same title, please e-mail us at bulksales@psych.org for a price quote.

Copyright © 2009 American Psychiatric Publishing, Inc.
ALL RIGHTS RESERVED

Manufactured in the United States of America on acid-free paper
12   11   10   09   08   5   4   3   2   1
First Edition

Typeset in Adobe's Berkeley and Kabel

American Psychiatric Publishing, Inc.
1000 Wilson Boulevard
Arlington, VA 22209-3901
www.appi.org

Library of Congress Cataloging-in-Publication Data
Approach to the psychiatric patient : case-based essays / edited by John W. Barnhill.
  — 1st ed.
    p. ; cm.
  Includes bibliographical references and index.
  ISBN 978-1-58562-300-6 (alk. paper)
  1. Psychiatry—Case studies. 2. Mental illness—Diagnosis—Case studies.
3. Mental illness—Treatment—Case studies. I. Barnhill, John W. (John Warren), 1959–
[DNLM: 1. Mental Disorders—diagnosis—Case Reports. 2. Mental Disorders—therapy—Case Reports. 3. Psychiatry—methods—Case Reports. 4. Psychotherapy—methods—Case Reports. 5. Treatment Outcome—Case Reports. WM 140 A652 2009]
  RC465.A67 2009
  616.89—dc22

                                                                        2008016939

British Library Cataloguing in Publication Data
A CIP record is available from the British Library.

CONTENTS

Contributors xv

Foreword xxxi
Jack D. Barchas, M.D.

Preface xxxv
Jeffrey A. Lieberman, M.D.

Introduction xxxvii
John W. Barnhill, M.D.

How to Use This Book .xli

1 Double Depression and James Avery . . . 1

DEPRESSION 5
David Kahn, M.D.

SUICIDE 9
Peter M. Marzuk, M.D.

THE PSYCHODYNAMIC FORMULATION 14
Elizabeth L. Auchincloss, M.D.

THE INTERVIEW OF THE DEPRESSED PATIENT 18
Gurmeet S. Kanwal, M.D.

THE AFRICAN AMERICAN PATIENT 21
Dionne R. Powell, M.D.

NEUROBIOLOGY OF STRESS 24
Bruce S. McEwen, Ph.D.

WHAT IS PSYCHIATRY? 29
George J. Makari, M.D.

INPATIENT PSYCHIATRY 32
Alfredo Nudman, M.D.

Psychopharmacology of Depression 34
  Richard A. Friedman, M.D.

Pharmacogenomics 38
  Charles Glatt, M.D., Ph.D.

Brain Stimulation and Neuromodulation 40
  Alexandra L. Sporn, M.D., and
  Sarah H. Lisanby, M.D.

Supportive Psychotherapy 45
  David J. Hellerstein, M.D.

Couples Therapy 49
  Phillip Lee, M.D., and Diane Rudolph, M.D.

Overview of Double Depression 53
  James H. Kocsis, M.D.

Summary Points 56

**2 Geriatric Depression and
Peter Burke 59**

Capacity 63
  John W. Barnhill, M.D.

The Psychiatric Attitude 67
  Kevin V. Kelly, M.D.

Depression and Medical Illness 70
  Peter A. Shapiro, M.D.

Neurotrophins 73
  Francis Lee, M.D., Ph.D.

Testing at the Bedside. 76
  Marianne N. Findler, Ph.D.

Interpersonal Psychotherapy 81
  John C. Markowitz, M.D.

Service Delivery.......................85
  Martha Bruce, Ph.D.

Overview of Geriatric Depression 88
  George S. Alexopoulos, M.D.

Summary Points 91

3 Mood Instability and Amy Cahill......93

Mood Instability......................96
  Michael F. Grunebaum, M.D.

Borderline Personality Organization........99
  *Frank Yeomans, M.D., Ph.D., and
  Otto F. Kernberg, M.D.*

Axis I and Axis II....................106
  John F. Clarkin, Ph.D.

Eating Disorders.....................108
  *Andrew Bennett, M.D., and
  Katherine A. Halmi, M.D.*

Dialectical Behavior Therapy 113
  *Beth S. Brodsky, Ph.D., and
  Barbara H. Stanley, Ph.D.*

Risk Management.....................118
  Marlin R.A. Mattson, M.D.

Pharmacology of Mood Instability........121
  David W. Galarneau, M.D.

Overview of Mood Instability 124
  Janis L. Cutler, M.D.

Summary Points 127

4 Schizophrenia and Anthony Da Piazza 129

SCHIZOPHRENIA. 133
Adam Savitz, M.D., Ph.D.

VIOLENCE AND SCHIZOPHRENIA 137
Zachary Freyberg, M.D., Ph.D.

SCHIZOPHRENIA AND BRAIN CIRCUITRY:
A NEUROIMAGING PERSPECTIVE 141
Daniel Weisholtz, M.D., Jane Epstein, M.D.,
and David Silbersweig, M.D.

PSYCHODYNAMICS OF PSYCHOSIS. 146
Eric R. Marcus, M.D.

OUTSIDER ART 149
Aaron Esman, M.D.

PHARMACOLOGY OF SCHIZOPHRENIA 151
Donna T. Anthony, M.D., Ph.D.

COGNITIVE-BEHAVIORAL THERAPY 156
Yulia Landa, Psy.D.

COMPREHENSIVE HEALTHCARE. 159
Steven P. Levine, M.D.

RECOVERY 162
David W. Schab, M.D.

HOMELESSNESS AND SOCIAL HISTORY 165
Kim Hopper, Ph.D.

OVERVIEW OF SCHIZOPHRENIA 168
Roberto Gil, M.D.

SUMMARY POINTS 172

5 Terminal Illness and Dorothy Ewing . . 173

Part A

DELIRIUM 175
John W. Barnhill, M.D.

Part B

PAIN AND SUBSTANCE ABUSE 181
Steven D. Passik, Ph.D., and
Kenneth L. Kirsh, Ph.D.

THE PSYCHODYNAMIC CONSULTATION 183
Milton Viederman, M.D.

WORKING WITH THE FAMILY 186
David W. Kissane, M.D.

THE DIFFICULT PATIENT 190
Sharon Alspector Mozian, M.D., and
Philip R. Muskin, M.D.

GENETIC COUNSELING 194
Mary Jane Massie, M.D.

SPIRITUALITY 197
Colleen Jacobson, Ph.D.

MEANING-CENTERED THERAPY 200
Shannon R. Poppito, Ph.D., and
William Breitbart, M.D.

THE DOCTOR–PATIENT RELATIONSHIP 204
John W. Barnhill, M.D., and
Joseph J. Fins, M.D.

OVERVIEW OF HOSPITAL PSYCHODYNAMICS 207
John W. Barnhill, M.D.

SUMMARY POINTS 211

6 Agitation and Stephen Franken 213

Part A

MANAGING MULTIPLE PATIENTS IN THE
    EMERGENCY DEPARTMENT 215
    Peter J. Freed, M.D., and John W. Barnhill, M.D.

EVALUATING AN EMERGENCY PATIENT 219
    Peter J. Freed, M.D., and John W. Barnhill, M.D.

STIMULANT ABUSE 225
    Petros Levounis, M.D., M.A.

Part B

CONSULTATION-LIAISON PSYCHIATRY 233
    John W. Barnhill, M.D.

INFORMED CONSENT 235
    Charles P. Stowell, M.D.

HIV AND AIDS 239
    Stephen J. Ferrando, M.D.

INTERNALIZED HOMOPHOBIA 243
    Richard C. Friedman, M.D.

SEXUALITY AND SEXUAL DYSFUNCTION 246
    Robert Kertzner, M.D.

JEKYLL AND HYDE 249
    Hilary J. Beattie, Ph.D.

PSYCHOTHERAPY SELECTION 251
    Carolyn J. Douglas, M.D.

OVERVIEW OF CONNECTION 254
    Francine Cournos, M.D.

SUMMARY POINTS 256

7 Adolescent Bereavement and
Amelia Gutierrez **257**

AN ETHICAL DILEMMA 261
  Paul S. Appelbaum, M.D.

ADOLESCENT BEREAVEMENT 264
  Cynthia R. Pfeffer, M.D.

SUICIDE. 267
  J. John Mann, M.D.

INTERVIEW OF THE ADOLESCENT 269
  Ayame Takahashi, M.D.

PSYCHOLOGICAL IMPACT OF DISLOCATION 273
  Mindy Thompson Fullilove, M.D.

THE DOMINICAN PATIENT 276
  Ian Canino, M.D.

VIRGINIA WOOLF: ON BEING ILL 280
  Katherine Dalsimer, Ph.D.

NEUROBIOLOGY OF ATTACHMENT 283
  H. Jonathan Polan, M.D.

PHARMACOLOGY OF ADOLESCENT DEPRESSION 286
  P. Anne McBride, M.D.

INTERPERSONAL PSYCHOTHERAPY 289
  Laura Mufson, Ph.D.

PSYCHODYNAMICS OF DEPRESSION 292
  Fredric N. Busch, M.D.

OVERVIEW OF ADOLESCENT BEREAVEMENT 296
  Theodore Shapiro, M.D.

SUMMARY POINTS 298

8 **Anxiety and Sophia Hastings 299**

Part A

ANXIETY DISORDERS 302
  Laszlo A. Papp, M.D.

ALCOHOL ABUSE. 305
  Bruce Phariss, M.D., and
  Jennifer Cooper Stelwagon, M.D.

NEUROBIOLOGY OF ALCOHOL 310
  Daniel Herrera, M.D., Ph.D.

PHARMACOLOGY OF ANXIETY. 313
  Smit S. Sinha, M.D., and Franklin Schneier, M.D.

COGNITIVE-BEHAVIORAL THERAPY 315
  Susan Evans, Ph.D.

PANIC-FOCUSED PSYCHODYNAMIC PSYCHOTHERAPY . . 319
  Fredric N. Busch, M.D.

Part B

AFTER EFFECTS OF SEXUAL ABUSE 328
  Daniel S. Schechter, M.D., and
  Erica Willheim, Ph.D.

OVERVIEW OF COUNTERTRANSFERENCE. 332
  John W. Barnhill, M.D.

SUMMARY POINTS 336

9 **Hypomania and Jennifer Ingram 337**

ATTENTION DEFICIT. 341
  James L. Rebeta, Ph.D.

BIPOLAR DISORDER. 345
  Marina Benaur, M.D.

Bipolar Spectrum Disorder. 348
  Sibel Klimstra, M.D., and Robert C. Young, M.D.

Premenstrual Dysphoria 352
  Margaret Altemus, M.D.

Sleep. 354
  Michael Terman, Ph.D.

Autism's Effect on the Family. 357
  Margaret E. Hertzig, M.D.

Creativity and Mental Illness 360
  William Frosch, M.D.

Being Lesbian 362
  Susan C. Vaughan, M.D.

Love 366
  Ethel S. Person, M.D.

Psychodynamic Psychotherapy 369
  Deborah L. Cabaniss, M.D.

Overview of Hypomania 373
  Cathryn A. Galanter, M.D.

Summary Points 378

10 Exam Failure and Grace Jin. 379

Part A

Interview of the Medical Student 382
  Scott J. Goldsmith, M.D.

Somatoform Disorders and Obsessionality. . . 387
  Brian A. Fallon, M.D.

Neurobiology of Obsessions 389
  Helen Blair Simpson, M.D., Ph.D.

NARCISSISTIC INJURY AND NARCISSISTIC DEFENSES . . 393
Nathan Kravis, M.D.

THE FIRST-GENERATION ASIAN AMERICAN 398
Sandra Park, M.D.

COMPLEMENTARY MEDICINE AND
   INTEGRATIVE PHARMACOLOGY 402
Richard P. Brown, M.D., and
Patricia L. Gerbarg, M.D.

MINDFULNESS MEDITATION 405
Susan Evans, Ph.D.

Part B

THERAPEUTIC ZEAL 410
Roy Schafer, Ph.D.

EMPATHY 413
Eve Leeman, M.D.

SELF PSYCHOLOGY 416
Jeffrey K. Halpern, M.D., and
Sharone Ornstein, M.D.

THE KOHUT/KERNBERG CONTROVERSY 421
Nathan Kravis, M.D.

EVIDENCE-BASED PSYCHOTHERAPY 426
Andrew J. Gerber, M.D., Ph.D.

THE SELF-DEFEATING PATIENT 431
Arnold M. Cooper, M.D.

OVERVIEW OF AN EVALUATION 434
Robert Michels, M.D.

SUMMARY POINTS 437

Bibliography 439

Subject Index 497

Index of Cases by Diagnostic Concepts 521

CONTRIBUTORS

Unless another hospital is indicated, all contributors are affiliated with New York-Presbyterian Hospital through one of its campuses: Columbia University Medical Center (New York City) or Weill Cornell Medical Center (either Payne Whitney Manhattan or Payne Whitney Westchester).

George S. Alexopoulos, M.D.
Professor of Psychiatry, Vice Chairman for Geriatric Psychiatry, Weill Cornell Medical College

Margaret Altemus, M.D.
Associate Professor of Psychiatry, Weill Cornell Medical College; Director, Women's Health Program, New York-Presbyterian Hospital/Weill Cornell Medical Center

Donna T. Anthony, M.D., Ph.D.
Associate Professor of Clinical Psychiatry, Weill Cornell Medical College ; Program Director for the Psychotic Disorders Continuum, New York-Presbyterian Hospital/Weill Cornell Medical Center (Payne Whitney Westchester)

Paul S. Appelbaum, M.D.
Elizabeth K. Dollard Professor of Psychiatry, Medicine & Law, Columbia University College of Physicians and Surgeons; Director, Division of Psychiatry, Law, and Ethics, New York State Psychiatric Institute

Elizabeth L. Auchincloss, M.D.
Professor of Clinical Psychiatry, Weill Cornell Medical College; Vice Chair for Education and Director of Residency Training in Psychiatry, New York-Presbyterian Hospital/Weill Cornell Medical Center; Senior Associate Director, Columbia University Center for Psychoanalytic Training & Research

Jack D. Barchas, M.D.
Barklie McKee Henry Professor and Chairman of Psychiatry, Weill Cornell Medical College; Psychiatrist in Chief, New York-Presbyterian Hospital/Weill Cornell Medical Center

John W. Barnhill, M.D.
Associate Professor of Clinical Psychiatry and Public Health, Weill Cornell
Medical College; Chief, Consultation-Liaison Psychiatry, New York-Presbyterian Hospital/Weill Cornell Medical Center; Faculty, Columbia University
Center for Psychoanalytic Training & Research

Hilary J. Beattie, Ph.D.
Assistant Clinical Professor of Medical Psychology in Psychiatry, Columbia
University College of Physicians and Surgeons; Faculty, Columbia University Center for Psychoanalytic Training & Research

Marina Benaur, M.D.
Instructor in Clinical Psychiatry, Columbia University College of Physicians
and Surgeons

Andrew Bennett, M.D.
Clinical Assistant Professor of Psychiatry, Weill Cornell Medical College

William Breitbart, M.D.
Professor of Clinical Psychiatry, Weill Cornell Medical College; Chief, Psychiatry Service, Memorial Sloan-Kettering Cancer Center

Beth S. Brodsky, Ph.D.
Assistant Clinical Professor of Medical Psychology in Psychiatry, Columbia
University College of Physicians and Surgeons; Research Scientist, New York
State Psychiatric Institute (Molecular Imaging and Neuropathology)

Richard P. Brown, M.D.
Associate Clinical Professor of Psychiatry, Columbia University College of
Physicians and Surgeons; Visiting Associate Professor of Clinical Psychiatry,
New York University

Martha Bruce, Ph.D.
Professor of Sociology in Psychiatry and Associate Vice Chair for Research
in Psychiatry, Weill Cornell Medical College

Fredric N. Busch, M.D.
Clinical Associate Professor of Psychiatry, Weill Cornell Medical College; Faculty, Columbia University Center for Psychoanalytic Training & Research

Deborah L. Cabaniss, M.D.
Associate Clinical Professor of Psychiatry and Director, Psychotherapy Training, Columbia University College of Physicians and Surgeons; Faculty, Columbia University Center for Psychoanalytic Training & Research

Ian Canino, M.D.
Clinical Professor of Psychiatry, Columbia University College of Physicians and Surgeons; Clinical Director, Alicia Koplowitz Fellowship Program at New York State Psychiatric Institute and New York-Presbyterian Hospital/Columbia University Medical Center

John F. Clarkin, Ph.D.
Clinical Professor of Psychology in Psychiatry, Weill Cornell Medical College; Co-Director, Personality Disorders Institute, New York-Presbyterian Hospital/Weill Cornell Medical Center; Research Faculty, Columbia University Center for Psychoanalytic Training & Research

Arnold M. Cooper, M.D.
Stephen P. Tobin-Arnold M. Cooper Professor Emeritus of Consultation-Liaison Psychiatry, Weill Cornell Medical College; Faculty, Columbia University Center for Psychoanalytic Training & Research

Francine Cournos, M.D.
Professor of Clinical Psychiatry, Columbia University College of Physicians and Surgeons; Director, Washington Heights Community Service, New York State Psychiatric Institute; Principal Investigator, New York/New Jersey AIDS Education and Training Center; Research Faculty, Columbia University Center for Psychoanalytic Training & Research

Janis L. Cutler, M.D.
Professor of Clinical Psychiatry, Columbia University College of Physicians and Surgeons; Director, Medical Student Education in Psychiatry, New York State Psychiatric Institute; Faculty, Columbia University Center for Psychoanalytic Training & Research

Katherine Dalsimer, Ph.D.
Clinical Associate Professor of Psychology in Psychiatry, Weill Cornell Medical College; Faculty, Columbia University Center for Psychoanalytic Training & Research

Carolyn J. Douglas, M.D.
Associate Clinical Professor of Psychiatry, Columbia University College of Physicians and Surgeons; Adjunct Associate Professor of Clinical Psychiatry, Weill Cornell Medical College; Faculty, Columbia University Center for Psychoanalytic Training & Research

Jane Epstein, M.D.
Associate Professor of Clinical Psychiatry, Weill Cornell Medical College; Director, Neuropsychiatry Clinical Services and Curriculum and Associate Director, Division of Neuropsychiatry, New York-Presbyterian Hospital/ Weill Cornell Medical Center

Aaron Esman, M.D.
Professor Emeritus of Clinical Psychiatry, Weill Cornell Medical College; Faculty, New York Psychoanalytic Institute; Faculty, Columbia University Center for Psychoanalytic Training & Research

Susan Evans, Ph.D.
Professor of Psychology in Clinical Psychiatry and Acting Vice Chair for Psychology, Weill Cornell Medical College

Brian A. Fallon, M.D.
Associate Professor of Clinical Psychiatry, Columbia University College of Physicians and Surgeons; Director, Center for Neuroinflammatory Disorders and Biobehavioral Medicine; Director, Lyme and Tick-Borne Diseases Research Center, Columbia University

Stephen J. Ferrando, M.D.
Professor of Clinical Psychiatry and Public Health and Vice Chair for Psychosomatic Medicine, Weill Cornell Medical College

Marianne N. Findler, Ph.D.
Assistant Professor of Psychology in Psychiatry, Weill Cornell Medical College

Joseph J. Fins, M.D.
Professor of Medicine, Public Health, and Medicine in Psychiatry, Weill Cornell Medical College; Chief, Division of Medical Ethics, New York-Presbyterian Hospital/Weill Cornell Medical Center; Adjunct Faculty, Rockefeller University

Peter J. Freed, M.D.
Assistant Professor of Clinical Psychiatry, Columbia University College of Physicians and Surgeons; Assistant Research Scientist, New York State Psychiatric Institute

Zachary Freyberg, M.D., Ph.D.
Postdoctoral Clinical Fellow, Department of Psychiatry, Columbia University College of Physicians and Surgeons

Richard A. Friedman, M.D.
Professor of Clinical Psychiatry and Director of Psychopharmacology, Weill Cornell Medical College

Richard C. Friedman, M.D.
Clinical Professor of Psychiatry, Weill Cornell Medical College; Faculty, Columbia University Center for Psychoanalytic Training & Research

William Frosch, M.D.
Professor Emeritus of Psychiatry, Weill Cornell Medical College; Research Faculty, Columbia University Center for Psychoanalytic Training & Research

Mindy Thompson Fullilove, M.D.
Professor of Clinical Psychiatry and Sociomedical Sciences, Columbia University College of Physicians and Surgeons; Co-Director, Sociomedical Sciences MPH Track in Urbanism and the Built Environment, Mailman School of Public Health of Columbia University; Co-Director, Community Research Group, New York State Psychiatric Institute and Mailman School of Public Health

Cathryn A. Galanter, M.D.
Assistant Professor of Clinical Psychiatry, Division of Child and Adolescent Psychiatry, Columbia University College of Physicians and Surgeons, New York State Psychiatric Institute

David W. Galarneau, M.D.
Assistant Professor of Psychiatry, Louisiana State University; Attending Psychiatrist and Medical Director of Inpatient Services, Ochsner Clinic, New Orleans, Louisiana

Patricia L. Gerbarg, M.D.
Clinical Assistant Professor of Psychiatry, New York Medical College

Andrew J. Gerber, M.D., Ph.D.
Fellow in Child and Adolescent Psychiatry, New York-Presbyterian Hospital/
Weill Cornell Medical Center

Roberto Gil, M.D.
Assistant Clinical Professor of Psychiatry, Columbia University College of
Physicians and Surgeons; Head of the Schizophrenia Research Unit, New
York-Presbyterian Hospital/Columbia University Medical Center

Charles Glatt, M.D., Ph.D.
Assistant Professor of Psychiatry, Weill Cornell Medical College

Robert A. Glick, M.D.
Clinical Professor of Psychiatry, Columbia University College of Physicians
and Surgeons; Former Director, Columbia University Center for Psychoanalytic Training & Research

Scott J. Goldsmith, M.D.
Clinical Assistant Professor of Psychiatry and Associate Dean for Continuing
Medical Education, Weill Cornell Medical College; Director, House Staff Mental
Health Services, New York-Presbyterian Hospital/Weill Cornell Medical Center

Michael F. Grunebaum, M.D.
Assistant Professor of Clinical Psychiatry, Columbia University College of
Physicians and Surgeons; Research Psychiatrist, New York State Psychiatric
Institute (Molecular Imaging and Neuropathology)

Katherine A. Halmi, M.D.
Professor of Psychiatry and Director, Division of Eating Disorders, Weill
Cornell Medical College

Jeffrey K. Halpern, M.D.
Clinical Assistant Professor of Psychiatry, Columbia University College of
Physicians and Surgeons; Faculty, Columbia University Center for Psycho-
analytic Training & Research

David J. Hellerstein, M.D.
Associate Professor of Clinical Psychiatry and Director of Medical Commu-
nications, Department of Psychiatry, Columbia University College of Physicians and Surgeons; Research Psychiatrist, New York State Psychiatric
Institute

Daniel Herrera, M.D., Ph.D.
Associate Professor of Psychiatry, Weill Cornell Medical College

Margaret E. Hertzig, M.D.
Professor of Psychiatry and Acting Vice-Chair for Child Psychiatry, Weill Cornell Medical College

Kim Hopper, Ph.D.
Professor of Clinical Sociomedical Sciences, Mailman School of Public Health, Columbia University; Research Scientist and Co-director, Center for the Study of Recovery in Social Contexts, Nathan S. Kline Institute for Psychiatric Research

Colleen Jacobson, Ph.D.
Postdoctoral Research Fellow, Columbia University College of Physicians and Surgeons and New York State Psychiatric Institute

David Kahn, M.D.
Clinical Professor and Vice Chair for Clinical Affairs, Department of Psychiatry, Columbia University College of Physicians and Surgeons

Gurmeet S. Kanwal, M.D.
Clinical Assistant Professor of Psychiatry, Weill Cornell Medical College; Faculty, William Alanson White Institute of Psychiatry, Psychoanalysis, and Psychology

Kevin V. Kelly, M.D.
Clinical Associate Professor of Psychiatry, Weill Cornell Medical College; Faculty, Columbia University Center for Psychoanalytic Training & Research

Otto F. Kernberg, M.D.
Professor of Psychiatry, Weill Cornell Medical College; Director, Personality Disorders Institute, New York-Presbyterian Hospital/Weill Cornell Medical Center; Faculty, Columbia University Center for Psychoanalytic Training & Research

Robert Kertzner, M.D.
Associate Clinical Professor of Psychiatry, University of California, San Francisco; Adjunct Associate Research Scientist, Columbia University College of Physicians and Surgeons

Kenneth L. Kirsh, Ph.D.
Assistant Professor of Pharmacy Practice and Science, University of Kentucky; Research Associate, Memorial Sloan-Kettering Cancer Center

David W. Kissane, M.D.
Professor of Psychiatry, Weill Cornell Medical College; Alfred P. Sloan Chair of Psychiatry, Memorial Sloan-Kettering Cancer Center

Sibel Klimstra, M.D.
Associate Professor of Clinical Psychiatry, Weill Cornell Medical College; Associate Vice Chair for Education and Associate Director of Residency Training, New York-Presbyterian Hospital–Weill Cornell Medical Center

James H. Kocsis, M.D.
Professor of Psychiatry, Weill Cornell Medical College; Director, Affective Disorders Research Program, New York-Presbyterian Hospital/Weill Cornell Medical Center; Adjunct Professor of Psychiatry, Rockefeller University

Nathan Kravis, M.D.
Clinical Associate Professor of Psychiatry, Weill Cornell Medical College; Faculty, Columbia University Center for Psychoanalytic Training & Research

Yulia Landa, Psy.D.
Assistant Professor of Psychology in Psychiatry, Weill Cornell Medical College

Francis Lee, M.D., Ph.D.
Associate Professor of Psychiatry, Weill Cornell Medical College

Phillip Lee, M.D.
Clinical Assistant Professor of Psychiatry, Weill Cornell Medical College

Eve Leeman, M.D.
Clinical Assistant Professor of Psychiatry, Columbia University College of Physicians and Surgeons

Steven P. Levine, M.D.
Fellow, New York-Presbyterian Hospital/Weill Cornell Medical Center/ Memorial Sloan-Kettering Cancer Center Combined Program in Psychosomatic Medicine

Peter A. Shapiro, M.D.
Associate Professor of Clinical Psychiatry, Columbia University College of Physicians and Surgeons; Director, Transplant Psychiatry Programs, New York-Presbyterian Hospital/Columbia University Medical Center; Associate Director, Consultation-Liaison Psychiatry and Director, Fellowship Training Program in Psychosomatic Medicine, New York-Presbyterian Hospital/Columbia University Medical Center

Theodore Shapiro, M.D.
Professor Emeritus of Psychiatry, Weill Cornell Medical Center; Faculty, New York Psychoanalytic Institute and Columbia University Center for Psychoanalytic Training & Research

David Silbersweig, M.D.
Stephen P. Tobin and Arnold M. Cooper Professor in Consultation-Liaison Psychiatry, Vice Chair for Research in Psychiatry, and Director, Division of Neuropsychiatry, Weill Cornell Medical College

Helen Blair Simpson, M.D., Ph.D.
Associate Professor of Clinical Psychiatry, Columbia University College of Physicians and Surgeons; Director of the Anxiety Disorders Clinic, New York State Psychiatric Institute

Smit S. Sinha, M.D.
Assistant Professor of Clinical Psychiatry, Columbia University College of Physicians and Surgeons

Alexandra L. Sporn, M.D.
Assistant Professor of Clinical Psychiatry (Neuroscience), Columbia University College of Physicians and Surgeons

Barbara H. Stanley, Ph.D.
Assistant Professor of Psychology in Psychiatry (Neuroscience), Columbia University College of Physicians and Surgeons and New York State Psychiatric Institute (Molecular Imaging and Neuropathology)

Jennifer Cooper Stelwagon, M.D.
Clinical Instructor of Psychiatry, Weill Cornell Medical College

Charles P. Stowell, M.D.
Clinical Instructor of Psychiatry, Weill Cornell Medical College

Ayame Takahashi, M.D.
Assistant Professor of Psychiatry and Training Director of Child and Adolescent Psychiatry, Southern Illinois University School of Medicine, Springfield, Illinois

Michael Terman, Ph.D.
Professor of Clinical Psychology in Psychiatry, Columbia University College of Physicians and Surgeons; Director, Center for Light Treatment and Biological Rhythms, New York State Psychiatric Institute

Susan C. Vaughan, M.D.
Assistant Professor of Clinical Psychiatry, Columbia University College of Physicians and Surgeons; Faculty, Columbia University Center for Psychoanalytic Training & Research

Milton Viederman, M.D.
Professor Emeritus of Psychiatry, Weill Cornell Medical College; Faculty, Columbia University Center for Psychoanalytic Training & Research

Daniel Weisholtz, M.D.
Neurology Resident, Massachusetts General Hospital/Brigham and Women's Hospital/Harvard Medical School Neurology Residency Program

Erica Willheim, Ph.D.
Instructor in Clinical Psychology in Psychiatry, Columbia University College of Physicians and Surgeons; Faculty, Parent-Infant Psychotherapy Program, Columbia University Center for Psychoanalytic Training & Research; Psychologist, Manhattan Center for Early Learning

Frank Yeomans, M.D., Ph.D.
Clinical Associate Professor of Psychiatry, Weill Cornell Medical College; Director of Training, Personality Disorders Institute, New York-Presbyterian Hospital/Weill Cornell Medical Center; Lecturer, Columbia University Center for Psychoanalytic Training & Research

Robert C. Young, M.D.
Professor of Psychiatry, Weill Cornell Medical College

Disclosure of Competing Interests

The following contributors to this book have indicated a financial interest in or other affiliation with a commercial supporter, a manufacturer of a commercial product, a provider of a commercial service, a nongovernmental organization, and/or a government agency, as listed below:

George S. Alexopoulos, M.D.—*Grant support:* Cephalon, Forest; *Scientific advisory board:* Forest, Sanofi-Aventis, Novartis; *Speaker's bureau:* Cephalon, Forest, Eli Lilly, Bristol-Myers Squibb, GlaxoSmithKline, Pfizer, Janssen

Margaret Altemus, M.D.—*Clinical trial:* Wyeth; *Consultant:* Merck

Stephen J. Ferrando, M.D.—*Speaker's bureau:* Pfizer, AstraZeneca, Forest; *Consultant:* AstraZeneca, Boehringer-Ingelheim

Cathryn A. Galanter, M.D.—*Grant support:* American Psychiatric Institute for Research and Education (sponsored by AstraZeneca)

David W. Galarneau, M.D.—*Speaker's bureau:* Janssen

Jeffrey A. Lieberman, M.D.—*Grant support:* Acadia, Bristol-Myers Squibb, GlaxoSmithKline, Janssen, Merck, Organon, Pfizer; *Consultant:* Eli Lilly, Pfizer; *Advisory board:* AstraZeneca, Eli Lilly, GlaxoSmithKline, Lundbeck, Organon, Pfizer; *Patent:* Repligen

Sarah H. Lisanby, M.D.—*Grant support:* NIH, DARPA, NYSTAR, NYS Office of Mental Health, Stanley Medical Research Foundation, American Federation for Aging Research/Beeson Scholars Program, NARSAD, Neuronetics, *Cyberonics; Equipment support:* Magstim Company; *Consultant:* Science and Technology Policy Institute/Institute for Defense Analysis; *Honorarium/travel reimbursement:* NIH, Northstar Neuroscience, Kinetics Foundation, MITRE, CENTRA, Magstim Company

John C. Markowitz, M.D.—*Book royalties:* American Psychiatric Press, Basic Books, Oxford University Press, Franco Angeli

Laura Mufson, Ph.D.—*Book royalties:* Guilford Publications

Philip R. Muskin, M.D.—*Speaker's bureau:* AstraZeneca, Bristol-Meyers Squibb, Cephalon, Forest Laboratories, Eli Lilly and Company, Pfizer, Takeda, Wyeth

Steven D. Passik, Ph.D.—*Grant/research support:* Cephalon, Ligand; *Consultant:* Cephalon, Ligand, Eli Lilly and Company, Pricara, King; *Speaker's Bureau:* Cephalon, Ligand, Eli Lilly and Company, Pricara, King

Franklin Schneier, M.D.—*Research support:* Forest Labs; *Scientific advisory board:* Jazz Pharmaceuticals

Helen Blair Simpson, M.D., Ph.D.—*Research support:* NIMH, OC Foundation, NARSAD, Janssen Pharmaceuticals; *Scientific advisory board:* Jazz Pharmaceuticals, Anxiety Disorders Association of America

The following authors have no competing interests to report:

Donna T. Anthony, M.D., Ph.D.
Paul S. Appelbaum, M.D.
Jack D. Barchas, M.D.
John W. Barnhill, M.D.
Hilary J. Beattie, Ph.D.
Andrew Bennett, M.D.
William Breitbart, M.D.
Beth S. Brodsky, Ph.D.
Richard P. Brown, M.D.
Martha Bruce, Ph.D.
Fredric N. Busch, M.D.
Deborah L. Cabaniss, M.D.
Ian Canino, M.D.
John F. Clarkin, Ph.D.
Arnold M. Cooper, M.D.
Francine Cournos, M.D.
Janis L. Cutler, M.D.
Carolyn J. Douglas, M.D.
Jane Epstein, M.D.
Aaron Esman, M.D.
Susan Evans, Ph.D.
Brian A. Fallon, M.D.
Joseph J. Fins, M.D.
Richard C. Friedman, M.D.
Mindy Thompson Fullilove, M.D.
Andrew J. Gerber, M.D., Ph.D.
Katherine A. Halmi, M.D.
David J. Hellerstein, M.D.
Margaret E. Hertzig, M.D.
David Kahn, M.D.
Gurmeet S. Kanwal, M.D.
Kevin V. Kelly, M.D.
Kenneth L. Kirsh, Ph.D.
David W. Kissane, M.D.
James H. Kocsis, M.D.

Nathan Kravis, M.D.
Yulia Landa, Psy.D.
Francis Lee, M.D., Ph.D.
Eve Leeman, M.D.
George J. Makari, M.D.
Eric R. Marcus, M.D.
Mary Jane Massie, M.D.
P. Anne McBride, M.D.
Bruce S. McEwen, Ph.D.
Robert Michels, M.D.
Sharon Alspector Mozian, M.D.
Alfredo Nudman, M.D.
Laszlo A. Papp, M.D.
Sandra Park, M.D.
Cynthia R. Pfeffer, M.D.
Bruce Phariss, M.D.
H. Jonathan Polan, M.D.
Shannon R. Poppito, Ph.D.
Dionne R. Powell, M.D.
James L. Rebeta, Ph.D.
David W. Schab, M.D.
Roy Schafer, Ph.D.
Daniel S. Schechter, M.D.
Peter A. Shapiro, M.D.
Theodore Shapiro, M.D.
David Silbersweig, M.D.
Barbara H. Stanley, Ph.D.
Ayame Takahashi, M.D.
Michael Terman, Ph.D.
Susan C. Vaughan, M.D.
Milton Viederman, M.D.
Daniel Weisholtz, M.D.
Erica Willheim, Ph.D.
Frank Yeomans, M.D., Ph.D.

FOREWORD

THE compelling stories and discussions that lie at the heart of *Approach to the Psychiatric Patient* reflect a current reality in which we can reliably diagnose and successfully treat a remarkable range of psychiatric problems. A few decades ago, we would have been far less sanguine in regard to both reliability and efficacy. Also inherent in this book is the acceptance of the usefulness of multiple approaches to a particular patient. Such a viewpoint would have been unthinkable 50 years ago.

If there is progress, there is also intense confusion. Where once we had only a few disorders in the classification system and few approaches to treatment, we have expanded the classification system and have developed a vast number of approaches to treatment, many untested. And while millions of people are improved, often dramatically, many people with severe mental illness continue to have troubled and difficult lives. As a field, then, we have promised much, delivered some, largely emptied asylums, and brought much relief, but we remain incompletely capable of treating the people who come to us for help. Given these strengths and limitations, how should our field approach science, significant clinical realities, public policy, and training the psychiatrists of the future?

The Knowledge Base

One of the great strengths of psychiatry is the remarkable range of primary disciplines that it incorporates. That breadth affords psychiatrists the opportunity to function in many different capacities with many different intellectual, service, and administrative foci. Even in fields where we think we know a lot, however, we actually know only a bit. For example, we know of hundreds of substances that serve as regulators, transmitters, or modulators of neuronal function. At the same time, it is likely that not all have been identified, only a few have been intensively studied, and much remains to be understood in regard to their relationships with each other and to normal or abnormal behavior. As they learn more, experts in all of the subspecialties become similarly aware of the limitations and possibilities of their respective fields. In addition, we find increasingly fruitful overlaps between fields that might be thought to be separate. For example, neuroimaging and genetics are incomplete without contributions from cognitive and social neuroscience.

Funding is critical for the development of all aspects of medicine, but for findings to be effectively translated into patient care, innovative cross-discipline collaborations must be created and developed.

The Diagnostic System

Our current diagnostic system is based on clinical description and psychosocial history. While important and useful, such a system has limitations. There appear to be multiple forms of many psychiatric illnesses, and we have no current way to know whether there are, for example, three types of depression, or six, or twenty. In addition, treatments are based on this flawed diagnostic system, and so we are unable to confidently know what treatments work best with which types of patients at which particular stages of their disorders.

We are in the early phase of a brave attempt to expand our classification system to include advances in genetics, neurobiology, and functional brain imaging. While the new information would still require a clinician to listen to and think about the individual patient, a more nuanced diagnostic system would provide that clinician with the tools to better understand and treat patients. Such a classification system would also allow for increasingly sophisticated systems research that could include important variables that tend to be systematically excluded from current research, such as comorbidities, chronic illnesses, and long-term treatments.

Public Policy

Too often, the field has acceded to rules and regulations that may be well intentioned but that are harmful in their overall impact. For example, reimbursement mechanisms have introduced an enormous burden on mental health practitioners as they try to gain approval for necessary psychiatric services. Often demoralizing and arbitrarily complex, these approval procedures serve a de facto gate-keeping function that often reduces care to the people who need it most. Limitations on yearly or lifetime psychiatric visits is a second way in which insurance companies inappropriately restrict care, limitations that are not shared by the rest of medicine despite the reality that psychiatric treatments are generally as successful as other medical treatments.

As is the case in the rest of medicine, patient records should be complete and quickly accessible to other clinicians. The stigma of mental illness makes privacy especially important within psychiatry, but the rest of medicine has become increasingly concerned about privacy in light of financial and insurance issues, genetic advances, and the rapidity with which documents can be disseminated via the Internet. As information systems become more sophisticated, they should be able to make record keeping both more efficient and more secure.

Training and Treatment Programs

It is critical that psychiatrists receive training that encompasses the field as a whole. While psychiatrists should have experience working in teams that include other mental health professionals, effective treatment of complex patients often depends on successful integration of psychosocial, pharmacologic, and medical issues. Organizations outside of medicine may prefer that clinical psychiatrists focus on medication management, for example, but the field need not cede its long-standing role as the medical specialty most devoted to the biopsychosocial model of illness and health. In addition to retaining their three-dimensional interest in the person, psychiatrists must also retain ties with the rest of medicine, both through an ongoing identification as physicians and through subspecialties such as consultation-liaison psychiatry and psychosomatic medicine. Psychiatrists also need to be trained to critique research. Translation of both basic and clinical studies into the diagnosis and treatment of patients depends on clinical psychiatrists being able to read the literature. In other words, all psychiatric training programs should expose its trainees to the breadth of psychiatry, ranging from the variety of psychotherapies to the ability to critically read a research paper.

Approach to the Psychiatric Patient reflects much of what is best in modern psychiatry. As intended, it presents the current status of much of our knowledge, highlights controversies, and demonstrates that psychiatry boasts a broad tent that includes all manner of clinicians and researchers. The ongoing success of these efforts can be assured through a creative development of knowledge; participation in the public policy arenas that guide psychiatric funding and structure; and vigorous, exciting training programs that appeal to the next generation of psychiatrists.

Jack D. Barchas, M.D.
Barklie McKee Henry Professor and Chairman of Psychiatry,
Weill Cornell Medical College; Psychiatrist in Chief,
New York-Presbyterian Hospital–Weill Cornell Medical Center

PREFACE

A multidisciplinary approach has always been a part of medicine. Given its breadth of responsibility, however, psychiatry may be the most multidisciplinary specialty in all of medicine. Psychiatry's purview includes children and the elderly; psychodynamics, physiology, and neurobiology; the idiopathic and the self-induced; the primary and the comorbid. In addition to psychiatric expertise, the field requires a working knowledge of medicine, forensics, culture, neuroscience, and health systems. Treatment modalities may focus on individuals, groups, or families and include psychotherapy, pharmacology, brain stimulation, and even surgery.

Approach to the Psychiatric Patient explicitly addresses this multidisciplinary approach. Since coordination and integration are vital to such complexity, it is fitting that the book has been edited by John Barnhill, a consultation-liaison psychiatrist. As Chief of the Consultation-Liaison service at one of the largest and most prestigious health care institutions in the world, he witnesses daily and helps to orchestrate an intricate dance of trainees, general clinicians, and subspecialists who assemble in teams to provide health care to a diverse and clinically complex patient population. Seasoned from years of experience in this challenging and rewarding process—and from years as a psychoanalyst—he has enlisted an army of his colleagues to write focused essays on one of ten clinical cases.

The result, as displayed in this volume, is a rich tapestry of clinical and scientific experience. The 10 cases have been carefully selected to represent the multidimensional clinical challenges that confront the twenty-first century psychiatrist. To compile the more than 100 essays, Dr. Barnhill has drawn from the faculty of the Columbia University College of Physicians and Surgeons and the Weill Cornell Medical College. Almost all of the authors are also affiliated with New York-Presbyterian Hospital through either the Columbia University Medical Center or the Weill Cornell Medical Center. These institutions provided a vast assemblage of talented clinicians, researchers, and scientists for the book, and their expertise illuminates each of these 10 very interesting cases. Although multiauthored, this book is a rewarding series of clinical stories that retains a consistent point of view and a distinct institutional identity.

Psychiatry is a field with a growing knowledge base and a broad clinical responsibility. Already a discipline with numerous subspecialties, psychiatry may yet develop additional new specialized expertise as it grows and matures. But for the present, *Approach to the Psychiatric Patient* depicts the clinical and scientific architecture of the field in its current state of the art.

Jeffrey A. Lieberman, M.D.
Lieber Professor and Lawrence E. Kolb Chairman of Psychiatry,
Columbia University; Director, New York State Psychiatric Institute

INTRODUCTION

THE practice of psychiatry consists of approaching the patient. The approach consists of getting information, developing theories about causation, formulating diagnoses, and providing treatment. Perhaps the most exciting aspect of psychiatry is that each of these processes is enriched and complicated by the vagaries of the human condition. Most obviously, psychiatry depends on the personal characteristics and symptoms of the patient. Less obviously, and to varying degrees, psychiatry depends upon the training of the individual psychiatrist, the era, the social context, and the degree of political, social, and financial support of the surrounding community, as well as such variables as the ethnic, cultural, family, and personal backgrounds of both the patient and the psychiatrist.

Approach to the Psychiatric Patient is organized around 10 cases that span the diagnostic spectrum. Each of the cases is followed by 8–14 essays, each of which focuses on one aspect of the case. Biological issues might be discussed from the points of view of a basic scientist and a pharmacologist, psychological issues might be addressed by a psychoanalyst and a clinical researcher, and social issues might be discussed by an anthropologist and a clinician interested in culture. Each case includes discussions of specific interview techniques, diagnostic dilemmas, and treatment possibilities. The discussions try to be clear when clarity is possible, but psychiatry is difficult and complicated.

Psychiatrists do many things to reduce the complexity and ambiguity of the humanness of their endeavor. Psychoanalysis is, for example, known best for the couch, daily sessions, free association, and rules for the analyst that include relative anonymity, neutrality, and abstinence. By reducing the daily hubbub, customs, niceties, persuasions, and self-interest that are typical in the world, the psychoanalyst and patient try to gain clearer access to the patient's unconscious patterns that are causing psychological suffering.

Researchers do much the same thing when they select unusually "pure" patients for their clinical studies. For example, the decision to exclude people with comorbidities allows for a relatively clear field on which to define a disorder or to test a therapeutic intervention, but it leads to research findings that are not directly applicable to many or most of the people with the putative disorder. Similarly, a basic science researcher might focus on a single neurotransmitter, while being well aware that dozens of other transmitters are affecting the system.

Textbooks tend to deal with the complexity in one of three ways. The first is to focus tightly on one aspect of psychiatry, thereby limiting the book's mandate and target audience. The second is to deal broadly with psychiatry, often in such a way that few people will read the book straight through but will instead read sections in order to study or to answer a specific clinical question. The third way of dealing with the complexity is to take a broad view of psychiatry, but in a fashion and length such that the material can be digested and memorized by a student on a 6-week rotation. All three types of books are important, of course, particularly in presenting the state of the science/art and in providing cognitive hooks upon which to hang unsettling and confusing experiences. On the other hand, the clarity of most texts suggests that psychiatric disorders can be neatly delineated, and since texts boast well-defined sections on treatment, they can imply a therapeutic efficacy that for some illnesses is overly optimistic. Texts tend to undervalue observation and independent thought, and they primarily emphasize recall. Of course, psychiatric education (and continuing education) consists largely of apprenticeship, face-to-face contact with patients, and curbside conversations, and texts are meant to supplement these other experiences. The psychiatric oral board examination does require the ability to successfully approach the psychiatric patient, but it is a stress laden and routinized rite of passage that is hardly an opportunity to explore the many possibilities within psychiatry.

It seemed an interesting challenge, therefore, to create a text that would aim to more accurately portray how psychiatrists approach patients, how they ask questions, and how they resolve—and sometimes simply accept—ambiguity. The book is intended to demonstrate that the process of diagnosing a patient is not the end of the inquiry. The book is also intended to show that the approach to the psychiatric patient includes not only a multifaceted, three-dimensional, biopsychosocial approach but also opportunities for much specialization for those who are interested.

A few explanations are in order. All of the authors are affiliated with one—or, in many cases, more than one—of the following interconnected institutions: Columbia University College of Physicians and Surgeons, Columbia University Center for Psychoanalytic Training & Research, Memorial Sloan-Kettering Cancer Center, New York-Presbyterian Hospital, Rockefeller University, and Weill Cornell Medical College of Cornell University. The institutions are legally joined in various ways, the faculties collaborate, and many of the trainees are in joint programs, but the history of these connections is beyond the scope of this book.

All of the authors were asked to provide a brief discussion of one angle on the case, as if they were giving a brief talk. They were asked not to take the broad view, and if it seems that individual authors did not notice or comment on something that seems obvious and important, it is likely that another author was intended to write on the subject. Many authors pointed out that the task was not possible in regard to their particular field of expertise, specifically pointing out that they would be unable to provide a meticulously documented review in under 1,500 words. But all of the authors were able to adapt to the unusual format and length restriction. References and suggested readings are provided, but statements in the text are often not individually referenced. In general, this book should be viewed as an accompaniment to a standard text rather than a replacement. Of course, if there are errors, particularly of omission, the fault would lie with me rather than with the author of the piece.

We use the terms *psychiatrist, clinician,* and *therapist* interchangeably. The book is written about psychiatric patients, and written primarily by psychiatrists, but the approach to psychiatric patients should vary less on one's educational background than on the patient, the circumstances, and the goals of the intervention. Each of the 10 clinical cases features a composite figure drawn from clinical experience. Composite cases run the risk of being unrealistic, but the cases were reviewed for authenticity by several dozen experts, and the use of composites guaranteed patient confidentiality and maximized flexibility in regard to pertinent historical information.

I am grateful to the members of the editorial board who reviewed individual essays and helped plan *Approach to the Psychiatric Patient.* Among them, Steve Ferrando deserves special mention for his daily involvement and calming sense of humor. I have worked for two remarkable chairmen—Jack Barchas and Bob Michels—since 1986, and both have offered counsel well beyond the necessities of their job description. Bob Hales has been wonderfully supportive from the day that I submitted the book proposal, as have been his colleagues at American Psychiatric Publishing Inc., particularly John McDuffie, Greg Kuny, Bob Pursell, and the strikingly perceptive anonymous reviewers. From among many colleagues who helped out with this book, I would specifically like to thank Lisa Dixon, Julia Golier, Dagmar Herzog, Jim Levenson, Jeff Lieberman, Costas Lyketsos, Hari Sampath, Herb Schlesinger, and Kerry Sulkowicz. A different sort of support came from friends and family who offered shelter at such places as Halcott, Nag's Head, Shingle Springs, Three Mile Harbor, West Tisbury, and Williamsburg; they didn't have much to do with the writing or editing of *Approach to the Psychiatric Patient,* but they helped give meaning to the effort. The book itself is dedicated to the people who suffer from psychiatric illness, with the hope that the text helps improve their care.

John W. Barnhill, M.D.

Associate Professor of Clinical Psychiatry and Public Health, Weill Cornell Medical College; Chief, Consultation-Liaison Psychiatry, New York-Presbyterian Hospital/Weill Cornell Medical Center; Faculty, Columbia University Center for Psychoanalytic Training & Research

HOW TO USE THIS BOOK

YOU have options in reading *Approach to the Psychiatric Patient*. You can read the 10 cases and more than 100 essays straight through. The cases do not depend upon one another, however, and so you might start with a case that sounds interesting or about which you have a specific interest. You can also pick and choose among the essay topics. Since each of the essays focuses on its case, however, you should probably read its case first. You can also read the book basically in order but skip the essay sections that don't interest you (yet). Finally, four of the cases involve treatment progression and are therefore split into two parts. If you are the sort of person who likes to read the last page of a novel first, then you should feel free to read immediately from the second half of the case. If you prefer to see how the case evolves—and perhaps be surprised—you might want to read the first half first.

Try to read with a curious but skeptical eye. In the 10 cases, for example, some of the hypothetical therapists make mistakes of commission and/or omission, and in the discussions, authors sometimes disagree with one another. In all situations, the specific author was asked to comment on one particular aspect of the case, but not all patients meshed perfectly with the assigned topic. In those—and most other—instances, the book emphasizes a multifaceted approach to the patient as much as it does the growing body of knowledge within psychiatry. In other words, process is valued in this book as highly as is content.

Not all of the essays will be equally comprehensible to you. We made an effort to present the most complicated and sophisticated of concepts with clarity. At the same time, some psychiatric subspecialties have evolved to a point that their basic vocabulary and body of knowledge will not be readily obvious to nonspecialists. Instead of deleting these important areas within psychiatry, we elected to include some of them with the caveat that if the essay seems beyond you, it probably is. Don't worry about the confusion, but rather let it wash over you and head to the next essay. Or read about the topic and come back and see if the essay has become more clear while you were away. Your choice.

In fact, choice is one of the cardinal aspects of the book. Psychiatry is about compassion, healing, and science, but it should also aim toward curiosity and the reality that in any psychiatric evaluation and treatment, there are choices. For example, all of the authors were asked to focus on only one aspect of the case, to limit comments to 1,500 words, to present opinions when warranted, and to act as if they were doing 10-minute "curbside consults" for colleagues. Such instructions left all of them with the choice of not just what to include but also what to leave out. No essay should be considered the "final word" on a particular subject, and if puzzled or interested, or both, you should explore the references, suggested readings, standard texts, subspecialty texts, and journals. If the essay does not answer your questions, you may find that the answer does not, as yet, exist.

At the same time that there is uncertainty, the book is intended to demonstrate a clear framework for exploration into the people who come to us for help. This framework has traditionally been learned through apprenticeship and personal experience (i.e., trial and error), while texts tend to supply the information which we hang on that framework. Central to the development of that framework is an assertive curiosity, and we encourage you to argue with what is written. Would you pursue the information differently? Would you devise a different diagnosis or treatment plan? In introducing a particular topic, did the authors over- or underemphasize anything? Did the editors skew the cases toward specific subspecialties and give short shrift to others? If some essays appear obvious while others appear inscrutable, to what extent does that reflect your own biases and imbalanced experience, and should you consider "rebalancing your portfolio"? Do you particularly like or dislike certain of the patients who are presented in the cases? If so, why? Are the patients intrinsically likable or unlikable or is there something about the match between the two of you that could interfere with or inform your own work? In other words, this is not a book to be read passively but rather with a questioning attitude and a pen in hand.

An aggressive reading of the book may leave you with more questions than when you started. Such a result would be gratifying to the authors if it also meant that you came away with less confusion and more coherence and with an appreciation of the complexity and richness of modern psychiatry.

Chapter 1

DOUBLE DEPRESSION AND JAMES AVERY

AN inpatient psychiatrist was called to see James Avery, a 57-year-old man who had just been hospitalized after he took an overdose with the intention of killing himself. He said he was depressed, hopeless, and ready to die. His wife was threatening divorce, his employer had put him on probation, both of his children had left home, and he had poorly controlled diabetes and hypertension. He believed he was at the end of his rope.

Mr. Avery had considered suicide for many years, but the possibility had become a plan only in recent months. He chose a combination of 120 mg of diazepam, 8 grams of acetaminophen, and alcohol after doing Internet research. Soon after his wife had gone to spend the weekend with her family in order to "clear her head" about their marriage, the patient had methodically begun to swallow pills. He had intended to die but had been interrupted by the arrival of his son, who had unexpectedly returned home from college to do laundry. The son had taken away the pills and called an ambulance. Mr. Avery was stabilized and evaluated in the emergency room and then transferred to the psychiatric unit.

The patient said he had gradually gotten more stressed during his lifetime and had never felt really happy. He described long-standing disturbances of sleep (early and middle insomnia) and appetite (nothing tasted good, but he overate anyway). His energy was generally poor, and he felt chronically worthless. He tended to get some pleasure from fishing and playing with his granddaughter, but everything had become dark and flat in recent months.

Mr. Avery had no history of suicide attempts, hospitalizations, or substance abuse. He said he had sought psychiatric help twice. Twenty years

1

earlier, he had seen a psychotherapist weekly for 5 months but had discontinued treatment because "all the guy wanted to talk about was my mother." He had tried an unknown antidepressant at that time but had discontinued it after 1 week because it made him sedated and dizzy.

During the year prior to hospitalization, Mr. Avery had met monthly with a psychiatrist for 20-minute sessions. He had tried 12 weeks of fluoxetine (Prozac) at a maximum dosage of 40 mg/day and 6 weeks of sertraline (Zoloft) at a maximum dosage of 100 mg/day. He said these medications had had no effect, and so he had quit the treatment. He expressed skepticism that psychiatry had anything to offer him and had agreed to sign in to the hospital only after his wife had applied pressure.

Mr. Avery said that no one in his family had psychiatric illness except his mother, who had killed herself while he was in college.

The history was elicited from the patient, the wife, and the medical records.

Personal History

Mr. Avery was a married, African American man with two children, ages 20 and 29, and one granddaughter. He was the eldest of three children born to parents who had owned and operated a small business in South Carolina; the business had failed just prior to his mother's suicide, when the patient was 21. After graduating from a well-known, historically black university, the patient moved to New York with the intention of using his engineering degree. He had been unable to find work in his field, a failure that he attributed to racism. Instead of engineering, he began work as a post office clerk, a job for which he felt overqualified but which he had maintained for 30 years. For much of that time, he said that his brain felt like it was in molasses and that he alternated between passive helplessness and irritability. An argument with a supervisor had led to the probation, but his wife was confident that it would not cost him his job.

Mr. Avery had met his wife, Martha, soon after moving to New York, and they married the following year. They had two children and a 7-year-old granddaughter. He said the relationship had been ruined by his depression and minimal success as a provider, but added that he was also convinced that his wife had always had one foot out the door and had never loved him very much. He rarely visited his father and two younger siblings, because "they lived a long ways away." Unlike his parents and wife, he was not religious.

Personal Psychiatric History

The patient described a lifelong history of depression along with failed medication trials. He was unable to characterize his efforts at psychotherapy, though the first appeared to be an exploratory psychotherapy.

His most recent treatment had been in the hospital's outpatient psychiatric clinic. He had been offered several choices, including cognitive-behavioral therapy (CBT), interpersonal therapy, and psychodynamic therapy, but he had chosen to enter the psychopharmacology clinic. The trials of fluoxetine and sertraline seemed to have had no effect. The patient said he discontinued treatment because the medication did not work and the psychiatrist "didn't understand my situation and background." The psychiatrist had noted that Mr. Avery appeared mistrustful and seemed to lack curiosity into his own problems. His wife said that her husband had been depressed "for at least 20 years" and that his blue moods were often caused by a real or imagined rejection.

Family Psychiatric History

The patient's mother had killed herself by barbiturate overdose. The patient said his mother had been a chronic worrier but had had no specific psychiatric diagnosis; he believed she had killed herself because of the bankruptcy. He denied illness in other family members.

Medical History

Mr. Avery's hypertension and diabetes were poorly controlled, primarily because of nonadherence to his regimen. His prescriptions included a beta-blocker, a diuretic, and insulin. He had no drug allergies.

Mental Status Exam

The patient was a stocky, tired-appearing African American man who appeared somewhat older than his stated age. Dressed in a hospital gown, he had no tremors and his gait was steady. He tended to avert his bloodshot eyes. His speech was slow and marked by a southern accent. His thought process was goal directed but without spontaneity. He said he felt "stressed," and his affect was constricted and appropriate to stated mood. He did not smile at references to fishing or his granddaughter. He said he wished he had died but denied intending to kill himself while in the hospital. He denied homicidality and all psychotic symptoms. He specifically denied believing that anyone was "out to get him," but he did feel that no one cared. He was oriented times three but inattentive and with reduced concentration. His score on the Mini-Mental State Examination (MMSE) was 24/30. His clock drawing test (CDT) was poorly planned and yielded a score of 2/4. His insight and judgment were thought to be impaired on the basis of his having overdosed and his insistence that his life had no meaning.

Summary

Mr. Avery was admitted to an inpatient psychiatric unit after he had made a serious suicide attempt in the context of an acute exacerbation of a chronic depression. The discussants in the following sections 1) explore the biological, psychological, and sociocultural issues that might have contributed to Mr. Avery's depression and 2) review interview techniques and treatments that might help him begin to recover.

Discussions of the Case of James Avery

Depression 5
  David Kahn, M.D.

Suicide 9
  Peter M. Marzuk, M.D.

The Psychodynamic Formulation .14
  Elizabeth L. Auchincloss, M.D.

The Interview of the Depressed Patient 18
  Gurmeet S. Kanwal, M.D.

The African American Patient 21
  Dionne R. Powell, M.D.

Neurobiology of Stress 24
  Bruce S. McEwen, Ph.D.

What Is Psychiatry? 29
  George J. Makari, M.D.

Inpatient Psychiatry 32
  Alfredo Nudman, M.D.

Psychopharmacology of Depression. 34
  Richard A. Friedman, M.D.

Pharmacogenomics 38
  Charles Glatt, M.D., Ph.D.

Brain Stimulation and Neuromodulation 40
  Alexandra L. Sporn, M.D., and Sarah H. Lisanby, M.D.

Supportive Psychotherapy 45
  David J. Hellerstein, M.D.

Couples Therapy. 49
  Phillip Lee, M.D., and Diane Rudolph, M.D.

Overview of Double Depression 53
  James H. Kocsis, M.D.

Summary Points 56

Depression

David Kahn, M.D.

DEPRESSION refers to a symptom as well as a cluster of syndromes. As a symptom, depression is generally equated with sadness, a feeling state that is protean in its manifestations, ranging from mild, transient disappointment to severe, confusing, enduring melancholy. Brief episodes of sadness are normal and can even be adaptive by encouraging us to connect with people and compensate for important losses. We have a complex relationship to the feeling of depression, however, since most of us "enjoy" sad books and movies, and many of us reexperience difficult events by rehashing them with friends and through rumination in solitude. One of the most important and ubiquitous of human emotions, depression remains normal as long as it does not interfere with our ability to work, connect with others, and experience pleasure.

James Avery's symptoms are consistent with a syndrome called *major depressive disorder*, an affective illness marked by feelings of sadness and/or an inability to feel pleasure or interest. He describes his moods in ways that are characteristic of severe depression (e.g., "dark and flat"). Nothing brings him pleasure, a state known as *anhedonia*. Other people may also have a major depression but lack the ability to understand and describe their inner worlds, a condition called *alexithymia*. While depression is generally viewed as a subjective experience, an objective observer is likely to notice dysfunction in one or more of the following areas:

- *Thinking:* Poor concentration, worthlessness, hopelessness, and sometimes delusions and hallucinations
- *Behavior:* Crying, psychomotor retardation or agitation, and suicidality
- *Physical functioning:* Alterations of sleep, appetite, libido, and/or energy

Major depressions persist at least 2 weeks but can last for months or years. Some patients recover fully from each episode, particularly with treatment, and may remain well for years; others recover only partially or endure frequent relapses despite treatments with medication and psychotherapy. Up to 13% of people with major depression remain in a chronic, severe state of illness (Kennedy et al. 2004).

It seems that the initial years of Mr. Avery's depression had been marked by relatively mild symptoms that persisted and worsened over the ensuing decades, a syndrome known as *dysthymia*. Dysthymic disorder was once thought to be a mild form of major depression. As we see with Mr. Avery, however, most people with dysthymia go on to develop major depression—a state known as *double depression*. Even if it does not develop into a major depression, dysthymia alone can have devastating long-term psychosocial consequences. Severe depressions can start at any age, though they tend to begin in late adolescence and young adulthood. In the United States, 10%–20% of the population will develop a major depression during their lifetime, making it one of the most common of medical illnesses (Kessler et al. 1994; Weissman et al. 1991). The rates of depression do vary between subpopulations. For example, one recent community survey comparing whites, Caribbean blacks, and African Americans found that a greater percentage of whites had had an episode of major depression, while both the Caribbean blacks and African Americans tended to have been treated less often and to have had depressions that were more chronic and felt to be more severe (Williams et al. 2007).

Significant symptoms of depression do not necessarily indicate a primary diagnosis of major depression. Substance abuse could have led Mr. Avery to a similar symptom cluster, as could hypothyroidism, the depressed phase of bipolar disorder, and some personality disorders. In addition to identifying psychiatric and medical comorbidities, the clinician must explore the duration of the patient's symptoms. If Mr. Avery had presented with the exact same symptoms and suicide attempt but the duration of his symptoms had been less than 2 weeks, he would be better characterized as having an adjustment disorder with depressed mood. Clarifying the diagnosis is vital in the development of a useful treatment plan. Missing a bipolar diagnosis would likely lead to a treatment that would increase his risk for a manic episode, for example, while missing substance abuse or hypothyroidism would likely lead to a persistence of both his comorbid problem and his depressive symptoms.

Mr. Avery is on probation at work, and he neglects his medical problems. One of the strongest public health arguments for aggressive intervention in depression is the high level of functional impairment due to the disorder. Depressed patients spend as many or more days in bed than patients with conditions such as arthritis and diabetes (Wells et al. 1989). Mr. Avery's brain has long felt like "molasses," as he describes it, and depression frequently leads to cognitive impairments. Deficits in concentration and executive function are well documented in depression, as are abnormalities in brain imaging. Neuropsychological changes may be reversible, but only with resolution of the depression (Gualtieri et al. 2006).

We do not know what caused Mr. Avery's depression. The case report indicates that his chronic symptoms developed in the context of his mother's suicide, societal racism, underemployment, and marital difficulties, while his acute suicidal ideation was precipitated by a threatened divorce, work probation, and his youngest child's going off to college. These stressors correspond to Claudius's lament in *Hamlet,* "When sorrows come, they come not single spies/but in battalions." It may be that several stressors combined to overwhelm his ability to rebound from normal sadness. Regardless of the exact psychosocial details, it is likely that genetics played a role. We do not know his mother's diagnosis beyond the history that "she had been a chronic worrier," but her suicide following her bankruptcy implies some sort of mood disorder, and family history is a strong risk factor for depression. While there is no single "depression gene," significant strides are currently being made in regard to understanding genes that may contribute to the etiology of depression or to predictors of treatment response.

Genetic discoveries inform the nature/nurture debate, but it is likely that environment played a role in the development of Mr. Avery's depression. While Mr. Avery appears to dismiss the importance of his mother's suicide, such an event would likely have been shattering. Further, she may have had mood problems during his childhood that would have left her relatively unavailable to him. These experiences would have primed him to be unusually sensitive to the possibility of later losses. The history notes that he believed his wife had "always had one foot out the door and never loved him much." We might want to talk to his wife to determine the extent to which this might be true, but we do know that depression tends to lead to pessimistic distortions. Mr. Avery asserts that his marriage was ruined by his depression and underemployment, but it is not clear that he recognizes that his curmudgeonly view of the marriage might have led his wife to act distant and unloving. Similarly, while his views on racism have their basis in reality, his depression has likely contributed to a pessimistic, self-fulfilling prediction of job failure. His failure to maintain close ties with his family of origin and religious community might also be implicated in his depression. Indeed, lack of social support is a strong predictor of depressive symptoms among older African Americans (Miller et al. 2004).

Mr. Avery's isolation appears to have worsened in the context of a long-standing view that his mother, wife, and previous therapists had failed him. It would be surprising if these feelings were not to be transferred at some point onto the current treatment team. His feelings of inadequacy and self-blame are likely to have combined with his cognitive deficits to create an amotivational syndrome that would also have contributed to incomplete and unsatisfactory treatments.

As will be discussed in greater detail in the subsections that follow, Mr. Avery has just been admitted to an inpatient psychiatric unit after a suicide attempt. Members of the team will debate pharmacology and consider ways in which his prior response to medications may have been affected by the dosage and duration of the medication trials, the likelihood of noncompliance, and the ways in which genetic variability might impact on the medication's effectiveness and side effects. Treatment team members will talk to him in order to provide support, develop an alliance, understand him and his background, and gain greater insight into ways in which he contributes to his depression. To accomplish these goals, they will do individual psychotherapy and couples therapy, focusing to varying degrees on such factors as psychodynamic insight and support. Perhaps most importantly, the treatment team will maintain an explicit focus on safety, since the grim hopelessness of depression is often associated with suicide.

Suicide

Peter M. Marzuk, M.D.

THE assessment and management of suicide risk involves four related goals: 1) assurance of the patient's immediate safety, 2) assessment of suicide risk, 3) provision for longer-term management of suicidality, and 4) documentation of the risk profile and the rationale for clinical decisions. Because a thorough initial suicide assessment requires gathering and organizing a lot of clinical and historical data, and because patients may have ulterior motives for minimizing, denying, or even exaggerating suicidality, it is critical to obtain data from a variety of sources, including the patient, family members, treating therapists, and, if available, friends, police, or others who may be familiar with the patient or the immediate suicidal crisis. In addition, charts and other physicians' notes should be used but should never be used as a substitute for one's own first-hand inquiry.

Assurance of Safety

James Avery has already been admitted to an inpatient unit, which is presumably locked and environmentally secured. Ongoing evaluation might, however, lead to alterations in his observational status so that he is placed on "frequent checks" or "constant observation."

Assessment of Suicide Risk

Demographics and history are "relatively unchanging" and establish a general profile of suicide risk. Mr. Avery's risk for a completed suicide is increased by his gender and reduced by being African American. His social isolation is a risk factor, as are his job difficulties and chronic medical problems. These factors interact in complex ways, so that, for example, Mr. Avery's hypertensive medications could worsen his depression and lead to increased marital, social, and occupational stress, all of which could increase his risk for suicide.

The single most important risk factor for a future completed suicide attempt is, however, his current suicide attempt. An attempt increases the risk of completed suicide by about 38 times; 6%–27% of those who attempt suicide will ultimately die of suicide, and most suicides occur in the first year after the attempt (Harris and Barraclough 1997). Mr. Avery's mother's suicide is also a poor prognostic sign, particularly since his overdose mirrors his mother's self-inflicted poisoning.

Mr. Avery's clinical state and diagnosis are likely to fluctuate and deserve ongoing evaluation. His depression is a serious risk factor, since major depression confers a 20-fold increase in suicide risk, while dysthymia increases risk by 12-fold (Harris and Barraclough 1997). The lifetime rate of suicide for those whose admission was a result of suicidality is close to 8% (Bostwick and Pankratz 2000). The "deadly triad" or "Bermuda Triangle" of overlapping diagnoses is *major depression,* a *personality disorder* (especially of the cluster B type, such as borderline or antisocial personality disorder), and *substance abuse.* While he apparently lacks a history of substance abuse, Mr. Avery used alcohol in his suicide attempt, and substance abuse is notoriously underreported.

Mr. Avery's mental status exam is pertinent for shame, worthlessness, insomnia, anhedonia, and hopelessness, all of which increase suicide risk. Hopelessness is a particularly strong risk factor and has been shown to have both traitlike (chronic) and state-dependent elements; that is, some individuals are chronically pessimistic about the future but may experience intensified bouts of despair during major depressive episodes (Beck et al. 1985, 1990)—a situation that seems to describe Mr. Avery. Evidence is also accumulating that suicidality is related to dichotomous all-or-none thinking—a mental inflexibility that reflects an inability of suicidal people to see alternative solutions to their problems (Marzuk et al. 2005). Most of the research in this area has centered on specialized tests of executive functioning that suggest frontal lobe dysfunction (e.g., Wisconsin Card Sorting Test, verbal fluency, etc). These tests do not seem to have been performed, but Mr. Avery displays poor planning in the Clock Drawing Test (CDT) and does have a lower-than-normal Mini-Mental State Exam (MMSE) score.

Religious affiliation tends to protect against suicide (Neeleman et al. 1997). Most major world religions specifically prohibit suicide or consider it immoral, shameful, or sinful; they also offer a social organization and support system. Mr. Avery's lack of religiosity and his sense that life is "meaningless or useless" are poor prognostic signs.

Additional clinical information that might contribute to an assessment of Mr. Avery's level of risk includes an assessment of his anxiety, impulsivity, aggressivity, and violence (Fawcett et al. 1990; Marzuk et al. 1992). None of these factors are discussed in the history.

Suicidality should also be directly assessed as a symptom. Like physical pain, suicidality can be addressed by asking the patient about its intensity, duration, precipitating and mitigating factors, and fluctuations. The evaluation includes careful, skeptical questioning; the acquisition of details; and the uncovering of minimization, denial, and distortion—all of which can be produced consciously or unconsciously. Such an investigation must be done, however, in an empathic, caring manner so that the patient feels understood and not grilled or criticized. Because patients often deny suicidal ideation on first inquiry, I revisit this question several times during the interview. I often give the patient tacit permission to acknowledge suicide feelings: for example, "With all your problems and the way you're feeling, many people would have thought of suicide… it's hard to imagine you didn't think of it even briefly." Sometimes I'll ask, "With all your problems… what is keeping you alive?" The evaluation of the suicidal patient is a delicate dance around trust, and it may only be later in the evaluation that the patient entrusts sensitive information to the clinician.

Evaluation of actual attempts may be easier than assessment of "ideation," since in the former there are often "hard facts," external corroboration, and a window into the patient's actual level of intent at the time of the attempt. An important issue in the assessment of a suicide attempt is the risk/rescue ratio. Patients who intend to die usually try to maximize risk and minimize rescue, which can be best achieved with careful planning. The general rule is that the more detailed and specific the plan for suicide, the greater the risk of successful completion. Mr. Avery's suicidal ideation had apparently been persistent, vague, and nonfocused, and his plan had only recently crystallized. Careful research on the Internet led to his cocktail of diazepam, acetaminophen, and alcohol. In regard to risk assessment, Mr. Avery's own subjective perception of the lethality is more important than whether his planned method was actually pharmacologically lethal. It is also worrisome that Mr. Avery planned to reduce the possibility of rescue by overdosing while alone; the serendipitous return of his son probably saved his life. It would be useful to explore whether he had written a will or a suicide note, given away gifts, taken out insurance, or left other instructions about his death or the future. Any of these would be worrisome.

The immediate precipitant for a suicide attempt might be a specific event or an accumulation of events, but it is important to clarify particular contributing factors in order to plan treatment. Focused therapy—which might be aimed at work, relationships, money, or family—can help reduce the hopeless "tunnel vision" that often accompanies suicidality. Such information can also predict suicidality when that particular stressor is repeated.

After being admitted to the hospital, Mr. Avery says that he "wished he had died." His persistent suicidality is ominous and contrasts with the fact that many other people feel better after surviving a suicide attempt. Some such patients feel relieved that they are no longer burdened by the stress of suicidality, while others are comforted by the psychosocial supports marshaled by the crisis. Still others are superstitious about a failed attempt, considering it a "divine sign" that they were meant to live longer. All of these feelings can be transient, however, and the clinician should not be lulled into thinking the patient will not return to a state of despair, hopelessness, and suicidality within hours or days.

In summary, Mr. Avery presents with a fairly high suicide risk profile. He has made a serious, well-planned suicide attempt and has a major depression and/or dysthymia with hopelessness and nihilism, insomnia, and anhedonia. He is on the brink of divorce, has chronic medical illnesses, and has a family history for suicide.

Management

Safety is a fundamental principle of management of the suicidal patient. Contemporaneous with Mr. Avery's clinical evaluation should be a careful observation for immediate and delayed effects of his overdose and for the likelihood of a possibly fatal second suicide attempt. These observations help the evaluating clinician decide on admission, observational status, medical interventions, and treatment regimes. Generally speaking, the best treatment setting is the one that is least restrictive and yet likely to be safe and effective. While usually safe, hospitalization is not risk free. There are about 1,500 inpatient suicides in the United States each year, with a third of them involving patients who were on one-to-one observation or frequent checks (Busch et al. 2003). Moreover, the benefits must be weighed against the negatives: disruption of employment and social/family relationships, financial stresses, and behavioral regression.

Another important management principle relates to the doctor–patient relationship. Suicidal patients can induce feelings of anger, helplessness, and mystical power in the clinician, and such countertransference can lead the psychiatrist to abandoning or arguing with the patient or being drawn into becoming "the savior." A reasonable working rapport is based on trust, mutual respect, empathy, and consideration of the patient's and family members' wishes for treatment. While the patient may pull for certain reactions, the clinician's ongoing professionalism can lead to a productive therapeutic alliance that can be the basis for recovery and the avoidance of another suicide attempt. Such a relationship is far more useful than "no-suicide contracts" or "contracting for safety." These so-called contracts have no legal standing, are no substitute for a careful suicidal evaluation, and are more intended to allay the clinician's fears than address the patient's needs. Few patients will feel beholden to a contract if they become desperately suicidal.

The "treatment" of suicidality largely consists of supportive psychotherapy and psychotropic medications. With the possible exception of lithium in bipolar disorder, there are no specific "anti-suicidal medications." Instead, almost all psychopharmacology is intended to treat specific disorders, such as depression, anxiety, or psychoses. Treatment-emergent suicidality should always be watched for carefully. The current controversy about the pharmacological propensity of some antidepressants to "cause" increased suicidality notwithstanding, the main point to remember is that a suicidal crisis will have "ups and downs," and suicidal ideation and intent need to be evaluated with regular frequency during the days following the immediate suicide crisis.

Mr. Avery has a history of discontinuing treatments, and the clinician should carefully explore his reasons for nonadherence. Treatment is often discontinued because of medication side effects, inconvenience (of either dosing schedules or therapy appointments), cost, or a poor therapeutic alliance. Treatment is also discontinued because of discouragement and anger as well as delays in symptom relief and misunderstandings about the need to continue treatment after the onset of initial improvement.

While challenging, the suicidal crisis can become an important therapeutic watershed. Acute management will generally include a multidisciplinary treatment team that features differing perspectives and types of expertise. The evaluating psychiatrist should discuss the situation in detail with the clinician who will be following the patient. With the patient's permission, the family can be instructed to observe the patient, remove dangerous methods from the home (e.g., guns, medications), facilitate and encourage outpatient treatment, and watch for warning signs of recurrent psychiatric illness or suicidality. Moreover, the family should also have a plan to obtain emergency services should a suicidal crisis recur. Mr. Avery's marital difficulties complicate the development of psychosocial supports, and it may be more useful to involve his children in treatment planning. At times, family members may impede treatment goals and need to be excluded, though this is unlikely to be the case with Mr. Avery.

Documentation

From a legal vantage point, the most brilliant assessment and treatment plan "never happened" if it was not documented. Documentation should include a brief summary of the risk evaluation (described in the previous section); the precautions taken, observations made, and treatments prescribed; and their rationale. The records should mention all the people involved in the decision-making process as well as the sources of additional information (e.g., medical records). It is helpful to document that the patient and the family were counseled about outpatient treatment, plans for obtaining emergency care, warning signs of suicidal crises, and removal of lethal medications and weapons from the home. In addition to written documentation at admission and discharge, such documentation is critical at other key points, including when there has been a change in clinical status, a new stressor, or an alteration in observational status.

The Psychodynamic Formulation

Elizabeth L. Auchincloss, M.D.

THE psychodynamic formulation is an important part of the evaluation and treatment of every psychiatric patient (Lister et al. 1995). Even for psychiatric disorders that have a clear biological basis, psychological factors contribute to their onset, worsening, and expression. Further, research has shown that treatments that focus solely on symptoms to the exclusion of emotional and interpersonal patterns are not effective in sustaining change (Westen et al. 2004). As we shall see when we explore the story of James Avery, the precipitating events for a major depressive episode vary from patient to patient, and the illness itself means different things to different people.

Psychological factors also have a profound impact on how a patient engages in treatment. Repeated studies have shown that quality of the treatment alliance is the strongest predictor of outcome for all psychiatric illnesses in all treatment modalities (Krupnick et al. 1996). A strong treatment alliance depends on understanding both the patient as a person and the transference and countertransference reactions that might disrupt or strengthen the doctor–patient bond. For example, if we are to engage Mr. Avery in treatment, we need to understand that he may experience even our best efforts to be supportive as intrusive, controlling, or demeaning. He may also reject treatment because he feels undeserving of attention and care. He may not adhere to his medication regimen because he is afraid to trust anyone or anything.

The psychodynamic formulation helps the psychiatrist organize the data of the clinical interaction into a working model of the patient's inner life. Without such a model, even the best clinician would quickly become lost and overwhelmed in a sea of experiential data. By contrast, a clinician equipped with a sophisticated model of the patient's mind is able to find his or her bearings in the doctor–patient interaction, organize clinical material, and chart a course for potential change. The formulation includes a picture of the patient's predominant representations of himself and of significant others, both conscious and unconscious. It also includes an understanding of his most important conflicts, his dominant wishes and fears, and his major defensive strategies. Finally, it includes an understanding of the organizing narrative themes that shape his behavior and his experience of himself in the world.

What do we listen for when we are with a patient in order to construct our psychodynamic formulation? In addition to the history and the mental status exam, the patient imparts a great deal of information about his psychological life through his verbal and nonverbal behaviors, in the stories he chooses to tell (as well as those he does not tell), in his choice of words, in his subtle and overt bodily language, and in his manner of relating. As clinicians, we also have valuable information available through self-observation. If we pay attention to our emotional responses to the patient, we will learn much about how he interacts with others. Turning now to the story of Mr. Avery, let's see how making sense of his inner life may help us to better help him.

Mr. Avery is a 57-year-old African American man who has made a serious suicide attempt in the context of long-standing feelings of sadness and hopelessness, chronic medical problems, and multiple stresses including work probation, separations, and marital conflict. His history is marked by his mother having killed herself when he was in college. A prior psychiatrist noted that Mr. Avery appeared mistrustful and lacked curiosity about himself. His wife stated that he became depressed after real or imagined rejection. His mental status examination was notable for poor eye contact, slow speech, minimal spontaneity, and a sense that no one cares about him or can help him.

As we look further at this story, patterns emerge. We can see that Mr. Avery's self image is characterized by a lack of autonomy in the form of feelings of weakness, passivity, and helplessness. He struggles with feelings of inferiority made worse by his failure to provide well for his family. His interactions with others seem to be few and far between. The only pleasurable activity we have heard of so far is fishing, which he pursues alone. He limits his interactions with others, most likely to protect himself from being controlled and abandoned and, perhaps, to protect them from his warded-off feelings of anger. Even his most intimate attachments are characterized by disappointment and feelings of not being loved. He is most comfortable playing with his 7-year-old granddaughter, who does not present a threat or a challenge. It is only in the interaction with this little girl that he is able to express his capacities for nurturing and his longings for attachment.

Let's turn to the *Psychodynamic Diagnostic Manual* (PDM; Alliance of Psychoanalytic Organizations 2006) for help making a psychodynamic/personality diagnosis. Using observable criteria to make diagnoses in much the same way as the *Diagnostic and Statistical Manual of Mental Disorders,* the PDM describes personality as "relatively stable ways of thinking, feeling, behaving, and relating to others." Mr. Avery's long history of sadness, guilt, hopelessness, and sensitivity to rejection fulfill the PDM criteria for depressive personality disorder. In addition, he has features of other personality diagnoses that often cluster with depressive personality. For example, his feelings of emptiness, inferiority, and shame suggest narcissistic features; his intense self-criticism, inhibition of anger, and self-defeating behavior suggest masochistic features; and his feelings of weakness, passivity, and mistrust of others are evidence of paranoid traits.

As with all personality traits, Mr. Avery's lifelong sadness, poor self-image, and difficulty trusting others are multiply determined. Although we know little about his childhood, his mother's suicide when Mr. Avery was in college leads us to suspect that she had suffered from severe depression during his early years and may have had difficulty meeting his emotional needs. The poor quality of his current relationship with his father leads us to imagine that his father had not been a source of emotional support. Loneliness and neglect in childhood were most likely aggravated by Mr. Avery's own tendency toward affective instability and depression. Indeed, it is important to note that a diagnosis of depressive personality disorder does not preclude a diagnosis of major depressive disorder and/or dysthymia, which should be made if the patient's symptoms meet the criteria described in DSM-IV (American Psychiatric Association 1994). Many patients will meet the criteria for major depression, dysthymia, and depressive personality.

In any case, Mr. Avery's mother's suicide, precipitated by the failure of the family business, was traumatic, as it would be for anyone. Prior to this catastrophe, Mr. Avery appears to have excelled academically. After his mother's death, he seems never to have recovered his previously high level of functioning, working at a job far below his educational level. While Mr. Avery managed to "escape" from the scene of the family disaster by detaching himself from his father and younger siblings, he was never able to escape from lifelong feelings of loss and despair. These feelings represent both an identification with his depressed and dead mother, and his guilty need for self-punishment. For years, Mr. Avery has likely harbored suicidal ideation as a way to reunite with his mother, to express his rage at her and others, and to escape from the pain and disappointment of his life. Again, it is important to note that exploring links between Mr. Avery's experience of his mother's suicide and his own depression and suicidal behavior does not imply that either his depression or his suicidality is *caused* by psychological factors, or that affective illness is not the main cause of his symptoms. Biological and psychological factors always work together to create each patient's unique experience.

Mr. Avery's worsening depression and recent serious suicidal behavior were likely precipitated by the double threat of losing his job and his wife. These potential losses came on the heels of his younger son having left home for college. It would be important to know more about the fight Mr. Avery had with his boss that led to his being placed on probation. Overt expression of anger seems not to be part of his usual behavior. We do not know what might have initiated the cascade of events, which includes his angry altercation at work, his probation, and his marital problems, but we wonder if Mr. Avery might not be unconsciously enacting a scene of professional and marital disaster at a time when his son is the same age as Mr. Avery was when his own family's business failed and his mother committed suicide. It may not be an accident that his son was the one who discovered Mr. Avery in the act of attempting suicide. In this repetition of painful events, so common in those who have experienced trauma (Westen et al. 2004), Mr. Avery is both identifying with his suicidal mother and arranging for new losses and abandonments for himself.

Mr. Avery's previous treatment relationships, like all his relationships, have been characterized by disappointment and mistrust. He has rejected offers of psychotherapy and neglected his serious medical problems. He is reported to have "lacked curiosity" and to have fled treatment when a previous therapist wanted to talk "too much about his mother." The inpatient treatment team will face challenges that range from prevention of suicide to vigorous pharmacology, but perhaps their greatest challenge will be to develop an alliance with a man who is isolated, pessimistic, uncommunicative, and mistrustful. Such an alliance is made more likely by an interview that is tailored to the individual patient while taking advantage of our experience working with depressed people.

The Interview of
the Depressed Patient

Gurmeet S. Kanwal, M.D.

As the interviewer, I meet James Avery with the intention of formulating a diagnosis, assessing dangerousness and prognosis, and beginning to think about a treatment plan. Additionally, I must try to establish an alliance and—through the interview itself—have a therapeutic effect. The process becomes even more complicated in that I must elicit detailed information and make an empathic connection simultaneously. How do we accomplish these complex tasks with a depressed patient like Mr. Avery? What should we focus on first? When do we push for information, and when do we back off? How do we manage our own feelings?

The psychiatric interview begins with observation. From the case write-up, we know that Mr. Avery presents with downcast eyes, nonspontaneous speech, and a sad, constricted affect. Like many people with depression, our patient appears to have difficulty expressing himself. As we talk, we are likely to notice more global impairments, and we would want to explore his feelings that he failed in his effort to work as an engineer, to provide for his family, and to maintain his relationship with his wife. The patient's withdrawal is likely to make such exploration difficult, however, and depressed patients can frequently frustrate interviewers who try to connect and elicit information. One-word, uninformative responses can lead the interviewer to feel disinterested, detached, and even bored, leading to an inadequate interview. Such an interview can exacerbate Mr. Avery's sense of isolation and failure, especially since he is someone whose depression seems to worsen because of "real or imagined rejection." To prevent such a reaction, the interviewer might make a particular effort to maintain eye contact, to sit close to the patient, and to make use of structured questions that can be successfully answered (e.g., "How old are you?") rather than open-ended questions that are likely to lead to mutual frustration (e.g., "Tell me something about yourself").

One of Mr. Avery's previous therapists noted that he was "mistrustful," and the interviewer might notice mistrust on the patient's face or in his preoccupation with such topics as safety, injustice, and exploitation. In such circumstances, the interviewer may need to sit further away from the patient; ask clear, unambiguous questions in a matter-of-fact tone; and avoid too much eye contact. Suspicious patients can also be dangerous, especially if they feel threatened or trapped, and the interviewer should not neglect risks if Mr. Avery becomes increasingly paranoid or agitated. In such circumstances, the interviewer should ensure a safe exit, the physical presence of another staff member, availability of sedative medications, and any other interventions that can make the interview feel safe.

Anxiety frequently coexists with depression, whether the patient is paranoid or not. Mr. Avery might verbally inform the interviewer of his main preoccupations, but it is more likely that he will demonstrate his anxiety through appearance, physical restlessness, obsessive concerns, and/or repeated demands for reassurance. These manifestations of anxiety can frustrate the interviewer, since they distract from the alliance and the interviewer's agenda to obtain information. A common therapeutic stalemate occurs when the patient demands reassurance and the clinician refuses to provide it in an attempt to remain "neutral." It may be preferable to allow such patients to talk about their fears for a while or to alternate between a reassuring comment and a question (e.g., "No, I'm quite certain that you are not having a heart attack, but tell me when did you first begin to feel so terrified?").

Mr. Avery's symptoms include hopelessness, worthlessness, pessimism, lifelong sadness, anergia, anhedonia, passivity, and rejection sensitivity. Perhaps related to the pain of these difficult emotions, Mr. Avery manifests emotional isolation, intellectualization, and lack of curiosity about himself—a common cluster of symptoms that not only complicate interpersonal connection but also worsen his depression. The interviewer might be reassured that Mr. Avery talks at length, for example, but might gradually become aware that he is saying little about his inner state. In such a situation, the interviewer should be active and alert in identifying the affect beneath the words. This can be done tactfully and without overt confrontation. For example, instead of saying, "You have difficulty expressing emotions," the interviewer might say, "That was a clear description of what happened. What would you say you felt—sad, irritated, or something else?"

Regardless of his specific personality style, Mr. Avery appears helpless, help rejecting, and hopeless—states that are common enough in depressed patients that Aaron Beck called them "the depressive triad" (Beck 1967). Identification of this triad is the basis for cognitive-behavioral treatments that try to alter thinking patterns that prolong and worsen depressive feelings. This triad can also be projected into the interviewer, who can begin to feel the same helpless and hopeless alienation already present in Mr. Avery's colleagues and family members. Failures to acquire meaningful information and deepen the therapeutic alliance can lead the interviewer to feelings of futility and pessimism. In approaching Mr. Avery, then, the interviewer may need to work hard to maintain a tactful curiosity that can support a connection to the patient. For instance, it might be useful to make an effort to talk about Mr. Avery's pain, suffering, and sense of failure prior to acquiring a lot of historical details. Such an effort is especially important in someone who quit a previous treatment because that therapist "only wanted to talk about [his] mother." Obvious distress does not always imply that the patient is unwilling to discuss painful issues, however, and in fact the patient may withdraw if the interviewer shies away from emotional content in order to pursue historical information. For example, the experience of Mr. Avery's suicide attempt may be more immediately important to him than details surrounding his mother's suicide attempt.

Timing and tactfulness are important in any interview, and it is generally useful to try to frame comments and questions so that the patient feels supported. For example, Mr. Avery may be offended if the interviewer bluntly asks, "Have you had difficulty with sex lately?" Instead, it might be more useful to say, "Depression is an illness that can cause a chemical change that can make it difficult to experience sexual desire. Do you think that you have had that experience?" In obtaining a detailed history in a depressed person, it is important to remember that many people view depression as a weakness. African American men appear to be especially unlikely to spontaneously discuss feelings of depression, and it would be important to remain sensitive to Mr. Avery's reactions to exploration of symptoms that he might feel are shameful.

Throughout the interview, the interviewer attempts to establish empathy, which implies getting as close as possible to the patient's state of mind. This process requires an ongoing inquiry into meanings, affects, and interests and is likely to be frustrated by Mr. Avery's bland façade and lack of curiosity. These defensive maneuvers are likely to become more active if he feels threatened or criticized, and so it may be useful for the interviewer to explore some of Mr. Avery's strengths. We know, for example, that he likes to fish, that he loves his family, and that he has maintained both his marriage and his job for decades. A brief detour into fishing or family may strengthen Mr. Avery's sense of self and allow him to more honestly look at difficult feelings that he had previously blocked from his awareness. At the same time that it is useful to set the stage for difficult questions, it is also important for the interviewer to actually explore difficult issues. How did he plan the suicide? Had he considered its effect on his family? Would he miss them? Does he still want to die? Does he have a plan to kill himself in the hospital? Did he have thoughts of hurting someone, perhaps thinking it was necessary in order to protect himself? Has he considered revenge against his supervisor or someone in his family? Does he own a weapon? Throughout these crucial inquiries into suicidality and violence, the interviewer's attitude should be less like an interrogator and more like an author working out the details of a story he or she is intensely interested in. As the interview evolves, empathy can allow the interviewer to hear the associated feelings as well as the words.

Teaching interviewing techniques can include a lot of bland generalizations. Every interview is unique, however, and a successful intervention with someone like Mr. Avery draws upon our knowledge of depression as an illness and the social skills that we develop during a lifetime, as well as skills specific to psychiatric interviewing.

The African American Patient

Dionne R. Powell, M.D.

A three-dimensional view of James Avery must take into account his experience as an African American, but it also must take into account his age, gender, sexual orientation, religion, and socioeconomic status. Each of these biopsychosocial variables should then be personalized, so that Mr. Avery is not simply a 57-year-old African American man, but a man who grew up in the segregated American South, where his parents owned a small business, and who attended an elite college that was likely to attract many members of the growing African American middle class. Mr. Avery is heterosexual, has two children, has been married for over 30 years, and does not go to church or maintain close ties with his family of origin. His mother killed herself, and he has just made a suicide attempt in the context of his youngest child going off to college, work probation, problems with his wife, and a chronic depression. He apparently believes racism is behind his long-standing inability to get a job as an engineer. We know a few things about Mr. Avery, but in the evaluation and treatment of him, we will need to know more.

This pursuit is stymied by a central dilemma: cultural generalizations may inform our understanding of an individual patient, and every patient is unique. In other words, as soon as we believe we "know" Mr. Avery because we can pigeonhole him into a stereotype, we do him a disservice. At the same time, our evaluation is likely to fail unless we have some understanding of typical experiences and common perspectives and recognize that there are multiple determinants to any situation or problem. Such a dilemma is not unusual. Within psychotherapy, we often try to understand the patient's point of view—for example, that Mr. Avery's work problems are secondary to racism—while also assessing the extent to which his work problems are related to a host of other problems that might include depression, a personality disorder, or low self-esteem contributing to his belief that he can't be an engineer.

We might, however, start with Mr. Avery's perspective on racism. Having been raised in the American South of the 1950s and 1960s, Mr. Avery would have experienced racism of many sorts. Some racism is relatively subtle and includes verbal and nonverbal slights, prejudices, and misunderstandings. Other racist experiences are more dramatic. For example, Mr. Avery's mother committed suicide 1 year before the Tuskegee Syphilis Experiment was disbanded. In that experiment, 399 poor, generally illiterate African American men were provided with "free health care" for their "bad blood" between 1932 and 1972. The "treatment" was essentially an observation of the natural course of syphilis that led not only to many of their deaths but also to the infection of many of their wives and children. Because of the study, Tuskegee is widely known not just as home to a prominent African American college, the name of an elite African American World War II air squadron, and the birthplace of Rosa Parks, but as a site of institutionalized American racism. Mr. Avery's reluctance to seek treatment for his depression could, therefore, be related to his skepticism about American institutions such as medicine. His hesitation may be labeled "paranoia," but our society has created real barriers to trust.

At the same time, the therapist should not simply accept Mr. Avery's explanation of "racism." The therapist may assume that the patient is an expert on the African American experience, but there are many African American experiences, and all of them are influenced by a host of cultural, demographic, and personal variables. We need to know Mr. Avery's individual story and not accept bland generalizations. While racism is real, Mr. Avery's report that racism has kept him from using his engineering degree could, for example, be a defense against neurotic conflicts. A therapist from a non–African American background may be tentative about exploring such issues for fear of insulting Mr. Avery or being considered a racist, and as such, racial differences can be a barrier to understanding. A different problem can occur when the therapist and patient are from the same cultural background. An African American therapist may be more aware of African American cultures, but familiarity can lead to racial assumptions being taken at face value instead of explored, which can lead to a problematic perpetuation of racial stereotypes and biases.

While racism might have influenced Mr. Avery's career choice, the therapist should feel free to consider alternative explanations. Perhaps Mr. Avery chose to work in the post office because it was considered a safe job and he unconsciously wanted to avoid the risks and pitfalls of a failed family business. Perhaps his disparaging comments about his job reflect the pessimism of depression, since many people consider the post office a fine place to work. Perhaps when he is not depressed, he enjoys the job and does well at it. The important point is that we do not know much about Mr. Avery, and we should not accept stereotypes and truisms when we are exploring possibilities.

Mr. Avery's walled-off isolation likely reflects his chronic depression and contributes to it. It may, however, be particularly difficult for him to discuss such issues with a therapist. African American men tend to not speak about their feelings with anyone, much less to someone who is likely to be from outside of his cultural group. The reasons for this tendency are complex but are likely fed by media stereotypes in which African American men are rarely viewed as sensitive or introspective. Further, as a relatively disenfranchised minority, African American patients are often experienced as "the other," an experience that may feel isolating and degrading.

The experience of being different is one factor in the underdiagnosis of depression and anxiety within the African American community. Mr. Avery recognizes that he is depressed, and he is now on the psychiatric unit and has long been in the psychiatric clinic. Depression is not, however, always obvious. Mr. Avery uses the word "stressed" to describe his feelings, for example, and under different circumstances, he might have presented to his internist with fatigue and insomnia and received refills on his hypertension and diabetes medications, accompanied by a brief reminder that he should take his pills. The underdiagnosis of depression within minority groups reflects, in part, the internists' limited time and psychiatric training, but it also reflects the reality that physicians are more likely to take physical complaints at face value when they are being expressed by people from unfamiliar subcultures. Untreated depression can lead to noncompliance with medical treatment and other destructive behaviors, such as abuse of drugs and alcohol.

Many African Americans adapt to difficult cultural conditions through their bonds within church and family. While Mr. Avery is married and has children, he has not maintained many ties, specifically saying he does not attend church or keep up with his family of origin. Such isolation may indicate early interpersonal problems, a chronic depression, and/or a powerful reaction to his mother's suicide. Whatever the causes, he has become very much alone.

The therapy would be an important opportunity for Mr. Avery to be heard; to explore his feelings of depression, anger, and guilt; to complain about his prior therapists; and to help him become curious about himself. Such an effort is not inherently different from that of other patients who are striving to adapt and succeed in their environments. It is important to recognize some differences, including the legacy of slavery and the persistent—if often subtle—signs of racial injustice that create an especially harsh environment for African Americans, regardless of their level of success or income. Environmental difficulties lead to elevated rates of depression and reduced amounts of mental health care, and, in a sense, Mr. Avery is a casualty of these demographic facts. In order to successfully treat him, the clinician needs to perform twin tasks that may or may not be explicitly stated: the first is to deeply appreciate that racial differences in the American environment are real and substantial, while the second is to recognize that Mr. Avery requires an individual understanding of his particular situation. If the therapist can openly and nondefensively explore both sets of these issues, reparative work can occur.

Neurobiology of Stress

Bruce S. McEwen, Ph.D.

STRESSFUL life events can precipitate depression. While the stress is experienced subjectively, depressed patients—like James Avery—demonstrate increasingly understood biological changes that can be both acutely adaptive and chronically problematic. The best-publicized changes occur in the monoamine system, which includes serotonin, norepinephrine, and dopamine. The malfunctioning monoamine system is not only scientifically interesting but also the basis for the effectiveness of virtually all of the currently available antidepressant medications. Adaptation to stress is more complex than the monoamine system, however, and involves a host of other neurochemicals as well as the brain regions heavily involved in mood, anxiety, and memory, such as the hippocampus, amygdala, and prefrontal cortex.

His mother's suicide was Mr. Avery's first reported stress. Her suicide hints at genetic loading for a mood disorder, suggests that his childhood might have been marred by neglect and/or uncertainty, and primed him to be especially sensitive to later loss and suggestions of loss. How can we understand Mr. Avery's initial biologic response to such a stress, and how might a chronic biologic response become pervasively maladaptive?

One immediate response to almost any stressful situation is the release of chemical mediators that increase heart rate and blood pressure and help the body prepare for action. If the body does not regulate itself back to its normal state, however, these same mediators lead to chronically elevated heart rate and blood pressure and an increased risk of such illnesses as strokes and heart attacks. The process of maintaining an active homeostasis is known as *allostasis,* a term that means to achieve stability through change (Sterling and Eyer 1988). Because chronically increased allostasis can lead to disease, we introduced the term *allostatic load* or *overload* to refer to the wear and tear that results either from too much stress or from the response not being turned off when it is no longer needed (McEwen 1998; McEwen and Stellar 1993; McEwen and Wingfield 2003).

Protection and damage are, therefore, the two contrasting sides of the physiology involved in defending the body against the challenges of daily life, whether or not we call them "stressors." There are many mediators that participate in allostasis, and they are linked together in a complex network in which each mediator can regulate the activity of the others.

Catecholamines (such as adrenalin) and glucocorticoids (such as cortisol) are the two major groups of stress hormones. Pro- and anti-inflammatory cytokines are produced by many cells in the body, and they regulate one another and are in turn regulated by the catecholamines and glucocorticoids. Whereas catecholamines can increase pro-inflammatory cytokine production, glucocorticoids generally—though not always—inhibit the production of cytokines (Sapolsky et al. 2000). The parasympathetic nervous system also plays an important regulatory role in allostasis, since it generally opposes the sympathetic nervous system by slowing the heart and inducing anti-inflammatory effects. In other words, when any one mediator is increased or decreased, there are compensatory changes in the other mediators.

This complex web of interactions ensures much "adaptive plasticity," so that in most situations, stress induces brain changes that are transient and routinely normalized. At other times, through interactions among genetics, the intensity and duration of stress, and previous life experiences, the changes lead to dysfunction and depression. Three regions figure prominently in this plasticity: hippocampus, amygdala, and prefrontal cortex. Mediated by neurochemicals that include adrenal steroids, serotonin, gamma-aminobutyric acid (GABA), and excitatory amino acids, these brain regions are exquisitely sensitive to remodeling.

What Are the Primary Brain Regions Involved in Adaptive Plasticity?

HIPPOCAMPUS

The *hippocampus* is vital to cognition and memory, and its dysfunction is believed to play a vital role in the development of depression. Within the hippocampus, the *dentate gyrus–CA3 system* is centrally involved in the memory of sequences of events and is therefore postulated to be importantly involved in how expectations and memories can contribute to depression. The connections between the dentate gyrus and CA3 pyramidal neurons are extraordinarily complex. One granule neuron in the dentate gyrus innervates, on average, 12 CA3 neurons, and each CA3 neuron innervates, on average, 50 other CA3 neurons as well as 25 inhibitory cells. The net result is a 600-fold amplification of excitation, as well as a 300-fold amplification of inhibition, that provides some degree of control of the system. This balance is made even more complex by the reversible removal of CA3 pyramidal cells during stress and by the constant production of new neurons in the dentate gyrus. For example, in the adult rat, 9,000 new neurons are born per day and survive, with a half-life of 28 days (Cameron and McKay 2001).

The hormonal, neurochemical, and behavioral modulators of neurogenesis and cell survival in the dentate gyrus include estradiol, cytokines, antidepressant medication, voluntary exercise, excitatory amino acids, endogenous opioids, and hippocampal-dependent learning; each of these also affects mood. Adrenal steroids play a particularly crucial role in the brain changes that occur during repeated stress, interacting with a such neurochemical systems as those involving serotonin, GABA, and glutamate to help mediate hippocampal remodeling.

Reorganization of the hippocampus is rapid and reversible and is generally not "damage" but a form of structural plasticity. For example, dendritic remodeling occurs within hours of the onset of hibernation in European hamsters and ground squirrels, and it is also reversible within hours of wakening of the animals from torpor (Arendt et al. 2003; Popov et al. 1992). With debilitating stress or an ongoing depression, however, the hippocampal changes lead to dysfunction.

AMYGDALA AND PREFRONTAL CORTEX

Adjacent to the hippocampus is the *amygdala,* which is thought to help synthesize internal information, such as hunger or thirst, with external sensations and, in so doing, create a sense of emotional significance. In rating the emotional importance of an experience, the amygdala activates the hippocampus to consign the experience to memory. It can exert a powerful effect on cognition and is likely to be central to the development of depression.

The *prefrontal cortex* is intimately involved in all other brain regions and is crucial to personality, emotion, and executive functioning. The *orbitofrontal cortex* is one of the three prefrontal regions. While incompletely understood, it seems to be involved in decision making and expectation as well as in sensitivity to reward and punishment. Another region in the prefrontal cortex, the *medial prefrontal cortex,* appears to play a role in a variety of social-cultural tasks.

In animal models, both chronic and acute stress cause substantial changes throughout these interrelated areas. For example, repeated stress causes dendritic shortening in medial prefrontal cortex (Radley et al. 2005) but produces dendritic growth in neurons in the amygdala as well as in the orbitofrontal cortex (Liston et al. 2006). Acute stress induces spine synapses in the CA1 region of the hippocampus, whereas chronic stress decreases hippocampal synapse formation (Pawlak et al. 2005). In contrast, both acute and chronic stress increase spine synapse formation in the amygdala (Vyas et al. 2002).

The fact that acute and chronic stress have different effects on the amygdala and hippocampus fits well with behavioral research. Chronic stress for 21 days or longer has been found to impair cognitive function that is linked to the hippocampus (McEwen 1999), while chronic stress enhances unlearned fear and fear conditioning, both of which are linked to the amygdala (Conrad et al. 1999).

How Do the Animal Findings on the Neurobiology of Stress Relate to Humans?

While limited, brain research in humans echoes the animal experimental models in regard to both brain imaging and neurophysiology. For example, during depression, human brain regions such as the hippocampus, amygdala, and prefrontal cortex show altered patterns of activity in positron emission tomography (PET) and functional magnetic resonance imaging (fMRI). In addition, recurrent depression has been found to lead to decreased volume in the hippocampus, prefrontal cortex, and amygdala (Sheline et al. 2003). Atrophy of the hippocampus has also been found in other disorders marked by chronic stress and anxiety, such as posttraumatic stress disorder (Pitman 2001) and borderline personality disorder (Driessen et al. 2000). And similar to the animal model, amygdala volume has been reported to increase in the first episode of depression, whereas hippocampal volume is not decreased (Frodl et al. 2003; MacQueen et al. 2003).

The neurophysiologic stress response is extraordinarily complex in both animals and humans. In looking at someone like Mr. Avery, it is likely that his ongoing depression would cause elevated levels of the stress hormone cortisol, which would induce emotional arousal and nonspecific psychic disorganization. Such a finding is substantiated by the fact that a disease of excess cortisol—Cushing's syndrome—is associated with both depressive and cognitive difficulties that can be significantly relieved by the surgical correction of the excess cortisol.

Glucose regulation is another important factor in hippocampal volume and function. Diabetes (both types 1 and 2) is recognized as a risk factor for chronic memory loss (dementia), while poor glucose regulation has been associated with smaller hippocampal volume and poorer memory function in the normal elderly (Convit et al. 2003). Further, diabetes and depression are frequently comorbid.

While links between basic science and clinical situations should always be tentative, it is interesting to note that Mr. Avery not only is chronically depressed and repeatedly stressed but demonstrates poor glucose regulation (diabetes) and diminished cognition (below-average scores on his Mini-Mental Status Exam and his Clock Drawing Test). This cluster of findings is not unusual and prompts the very interesting question of how these factors interact.

How Do These Neurobiological Findings Help Us Treat Depression?

Depressive mood and behavior may be an adaptive, normal response to a severe stressor (Nesse 2000), but when spontaneous recovery does not occur, we would like to be able to treat not only the mood, cognitive, and behavioral symptoms but also the underlying brain abnormalities. There is some limited evidence that antidepressant medications can reverse hippocampal changes (Vermetten et al. 2003). Brain changes may become permanent, however, and prompt treatment of depression may be crucial. There is also evidence that indicates that antidepressant medications may provide a protective role against hippocampal volume loss (Sheline et al. 2003).

Chronic depression affects not only the brain but also the body (e.g., abdominal obesity, bone mineral loss, cardiovascular disease). As is the case with brain changes, body abnormalities are the result of multiple interacting factors, including lifestyle changes that accompany depression (i.e., altered sleep, diet, alcohol use, lack of physical activity, isolation from social contacts). In turn, these behavioral changes affect multiple neurochemical mediators of allostasis that contribute to allostatic load or overload. Complicating the system is the fact that any one biological and psychosocial change impacts on other elements of the system, so that a reduction in alcohol, for example, may lead to changes in food intake, brain physiology, exercise, and medication compliance. The system's efforts at maintaining homeostasis in the face of change are, then, one complicating factor in the study of depression, even though it is just that complexity that is both highly adaptive and the cause of the depression itself.

What Is Psychiatry?

George J. Makari, M.D.

As any medical student knows, psychiatry is different. After rotating through medicine, gynecology, pediatrics, surgery, and neurology, the doctor-in-training stumbles into a strange world where the rules of biomedicine do not seem to apply. Subsequent confusion is understandable, for at its core, psychiatry makes demands—epistemological, clinical, and scientific— that are unknown in other medical specialties. Often these differences are not addressed or, worse, glossed over as if they are embarrassments. But these unique qualities go back to the origins of the field and give psychiatry its identity and its richness, as well as some of its daunting troubles.

Since time immemorial, shamans, priests, philosophers, educators, and quacks have tried to heal, treat, or control the possessed, the strange, the deviant, and the mentally ill; these efforts make up the *prehistory* of psychiatry. After the Enlightenment, the term *psychiatry* was coined to denote medical healing of the "psyche," that richly textured Greek word that initially meant life and spirit but then took on the connotation of mind. Two physicians first promulgated the term *psychiatry*: the German Johann Christian Reil, who coined the term in 1808, and his contemporary Johann Christian August Heinroth (Shorter 2005). Representatives of "Romantic medicine," both were committed to Friedrich Schelling's nature philosophy. According to Schelling, nature and spirit cannot be separated, for they are part of the same whole. Similarly, mind and matter are two aspects of the same unity, and as such, neither can be reduced to the terms of the other and each can be affected by the other. For Reil and Heinroth, doctors of the psyche should master therapies for both the mind and the body, both psychic and somatic treatments that cross over from one to the other.

Despite being derided by the next generation of psychiatrists for a tendency toward metaphysics and theism, the approach that Reil and Heinroth pioneered, with its balance between psyche and soma, has remained at the heart of psychiatry's promise and its perils. From this start, the field has contained a great conundrum, the mind–body problem, at its core. As patients like Mr. Avery have presented themselves, psychiatrists have had to ask whether the relevant object of focus is the mind and its meanings (loss of wife, job, character, inner conflict), the brain and body (genetic endowment, medical illness, neurobiology), or somehow both (heredity/exciting influence, stress/diathesis)? Overwhelmed by such complexity, psychiatry has been prone to convulsions in which some advance, real or imagined, has led to attempts to radically simplify the field into a purely somatic or mentalist one. Inevitably, the limitations of these partial theories of mind–brain have been exposed and new partial theories have developed. Late nineteenth-century psychiatrists committed to a view of the mind as an energy-processing machine could not account for human intention or even a modicum of free will. Their failings gave rise to, among other things, psychoanalysis, which in postwar America found adherents who made mentalist claims about illnesses like autism and schizophrenia, claims that were ultimately discredited. And so, over the past 200 years, psychiatry has veered from body to mind and back again.

In contrast, competing disciplines opted out of this vicious cycle around 1900 by simply narrowing their focus. Under the influence of the British physician John Hughlings Jackson, neurologists gave up efforts to model complex psychic phenomena alongside brain functioning by asserting that mind and brain run on separate, parallel tracks. This allowed neurological researchers and clinicians to bracket off mental events, as well as possible causal interactions between mind to brain, and focus their study on the brain alone. At the same time, academic psychologists, under the guidance of Wilhelm Wundt, began to insist on the autonomous study of psychic phenomena shorn of any reference to brain, thereby backing off from psychophysics, a nineteenth-century attempt to track the interactions between mental and physical phenomena.

Clinical psychiatry however, could not afford such clarifying reductions. For better or worse, this medical specialty, which began in asylums, found itself stuck with the whole patient, and hence the entire problematic of body, brain *and* mind. It had to somehow account for mental causes, brain causes, and interactions that seemed to cross the mind–body barrier. And, as if that were not enough, psychiatrists inevitably encountered another riddle that has troubled thinkers for ages, the nature–nurture question. The case of Mr. Avery, depressed "forever," with a family history of suicide, on the verge of losing his wife and job, forces any good psychiatrist to wonder about the roles of heredity and environment.

Leading research psychiatrists often split before these philosophical riddles, but over the last century, many clinicians have adopted a working solution. While keeping a foot in both the neurosciences and scientific psychology, these psychiatrists have taken a stubbornly pragmatic approach to their patients. In the last decades of the nineteenth century, this approach was codified by Emil Kraepelin, who, in the wake of the crushing failure of pathological anatomy to locate psychiatric illnesses in brain regions, sought to give some stability and uniformity to clinical work. Following Kraepelin's lead, clinical psychiatrists retreated from grand claims about etiology and relied on close phenomenological observation and description, a study of individual course and history, and therapeutic pragmatism. Adolph Meyer's "psychobiology" and George Engel's "biopsychosocial" model both embody a rejection of etiologic speculation in favor of close clinical engagement with the individual patient.

Psychiatrists are asked to take in mind and brain; they are asked to discover relevant causal determinants from an array of biological, developmental, psychological, and sociological factors. As such, psychiatry transgresses the boundaries of what we think of as "science." The field spans protein chemistry, genetics, microanatomy, electrophysiology, brain localization, affect regulation, inner thoughts and experience, identity, character, relationships, family, and social milieu. While psychiatric researchers may limit themselves to the examination of one of these domains, psychiatry as a whole must embrace them all. In sum, psychiatry becomes a cross between biography and chemistry, or to use old German words, a mix of *Naturwissenschaft* (natural science) and *Geisteswissenschaft* (human science). This has consequences for the science of psychiatry, for the field of study is so vast that it is often not reducible to one independent variable that can be studied according to the laws of reductionism and experimentation. Often, the mind's troubles seem to be a web of interdependent variables, not reducible to any one. There is no controlled, double-blind study for 57-year-old depressed men, threatened with divorce, on probation at their job, with poorly controlled diabetes and hypertension and a family history of suicide. There is much profitable research on each of these variables, as well as some clinical research that tries to pool risk factors, but nothing that truly synthesizes all that in a person, a life.

In these ways, psychiatry is a fascinating, demanding discipline and a vexing one. What other medical specialty requires its practitioners to think in so many registers at the same time? Contemporary psychiatrists attend to mind and brain, nature and nurture, neuroscience and psychoanalysis, serotonin and social life. Faced with a suicidal patient like Mr. Avery, the psychiatrist's thought spans genes, neurochemistry, neuroanatomy, physiology, mind and psychology, as well as behavior and social ties. Faced with overwhelming complexity, the psychiatrist must consider all these levels of possible cause and, working with limited scientific knowledge, decide what to do to be most effective. This overwhelming complexity and uncertainty is what the medical student encounters on the psychiatry wards. The "soft," "less than scientific" aspects of psychiatry are the result of very hard questions about what it is to have a mind and be human. We hope that science will someday give us more precise ways of understanding such dense networks of causality. Until then, psychiatry will have to play by slightly different rules.

Inpatient Psychiatry

Alfredo Nudman, M.D.

JAMES Avery has been admitted to the psychiatric inpatient unit for several related reasons. He made a serious suicide attempt. He remains hopeless and depressed. As indicated by his failing marriage and probation from work, his support system is in tatters. Finally, outpatient treatments have failed, at least partly because of his noncompliance and social isolation. Although specific to Mr. Avery, these factors conform to three general indications for an inpatient admission: *severity of illness*, as indicated by dangerousness, impairment of social functioning, and degree of relevant comorbidity such as substance abuse or delirium; *environmental factors*, including adequacy of the support and family systems and relevant psychosocial stressors; and *treatment factors*, including prior admissions, treatment history, anticipated treatment modality (e.g., electroconvulsive therapy [ECT]), and therapeutic goals (Munich and Gabbard 1992).

All of these variables require clinical judgment, since none is an absolute indication for or contraindication to admission. Further, clinical evaluations must be balanced against ethical, legal, financial, and practical concerns that have led to increasingly short lengths of stay, a reduction in long-term state hospitalization, and an increase in the severity and acuity of illness on inpatient psychiatric units.

During Mr. Avery's admission, we would focus on multiple issues, but our most pressing concern is safety. Upon admission, he would likely be observed every 15 minutes. If there were a significant risk of self harm, a staff member would be constantly present, observing and providing support (i.e., one-to-one observation). If Mr. Avery were to become intensely anxious or agitated, antipsychotic medications and benzodiazepines would be considered, as would seclusion and physical restraints. At the time of admission, none of these intrusive interventions appear warranted. While the suicide evaluation is crucial, it is also important to assess for signs and symptoms of substance abuse and dependence, since these tend to be denied by patients and can be lethal.

Around-the-clock interaction with the multidisciplinary team allows for a rapid and accurate diagnosis of acute pathology. In Mr. Avery's case, for example, we would be able to evaluate the extent to which his diagnostic symptoms fluctuate during the day, whether he experiences withdrawal phenomena, and the nature of his relationships with his family, co-patients, and staff. These observations enhance our ability to assess his mood, personality, and the possibility of covert substance abuse. The hospitalization would also afford the opportunity to more fully assess his depression and mild to moderate cognitive decline with further tests (e.g., thyroid function tests, B_{12}, folate, rapid plasma regain [RPR], brain imaging, and neuropsychological testing).

Inpatient treatments tend to be more intensive and interdisciplinary than outpatient psychotherapy. Since Mr. Avery would be observed 24/7, undetected medication noncompliance is unlikely, side effects would be quickly noticed, and dosages can be more quickly titrated upward. A variety of psychotherapies might be helpful, while psychosocial rehabilitation might help him learn new social and vocational skills. Finally, the structure and dynamics of the unit itself—the inpatient milieu—might help him internalize an organized and structured way of functioning as well as curiosity into the meaning of his own behavior.

This inpatient milieu can also address Mr. Avery's ambivalence and pessimism about treatment and improve his motivation and adherence. The doctors, nurses, social workers, psychosocial rehabilitation specialists, and mental health technicians are available throughout the day to help educate about illness and treatment, and they are often joined by psychologists, substance abuse counselors, and trainees from a variety of disciplines. Even though he has a clear history of isolation and mistrust, it is likely that Mr. Avery would connect with some members of this diverse group.

Regardless of the amount of offered support, however, psychiatric admission is stressful. Not only is Mr. Avery feeling depressed and hopeless, he has entered a locked unit surrounded by strangers. While possibly a relief, admission is more likely a serious narcissistic injury that can intensify depression and suicidality. A variety of supportive psychotherapies can help him regain his psychological footing and begin to actively address his problems.

The timing of discharge is based upon safety, self care, and the adequacy of an outpatient treatment structure. In Mr. Avery's case, we would aim for an absence of active suicidal ideation, increased hopefulness, psychosocial support, and likely adherence to an outpatient therapy. Twenty years ago, he would likely have been hospitalized for 1–3 months while his treatment and safety were solidified. As a result of deinstitutionalization and cost containment, Mr. Avery is now likely to be hospitalized for 1–3 weeks, which is likely to leave him with an incompletely treated depression and a tenuous connection with both his family and outpatient therapist. As a transition, then, he might require a partial hospitalization or continuous day treatment program, though both require insurance and motivation. A more likely plan is a referral to an outpatient psychiatrist, who will try to solidify and deepen the gains begun in the hospital.

Psychopharmacology of Depression

Richard A. Friedman, M.D.

THERE is little doubt that James Avery, who has a lifelong history of depression, is currently suffering from major depression; he has nearly every affective and neurovegetative symptom that characterizes major depression, and he has just made a serious suicide attempt.

There are a few clinical red flags that we need to keep in the back of our mind as we think about Mr. Avery's pharmacologic treatment: his prior treatment history of nonresponse with antidepressants; his medical comorbidity;

and his history of noncompliance. And while his cognitive dysfunction is probably the result of the benzodiazepine overdose, I would want to see his cognition improve as the diazepam clears from his system; if not, I would entertain other possible causes.

The first issue confronting the clinician in thinking about treating Mr. Avery with medication is the selection of the antidepressant. There are several classes of antidepressants from which to choose, including tricyclic antidepressants (TCAs), monoamine oxidase inhibitors (MAOIs), selective serotonin reuptake inhibitors (SSRIs), serotonin-norepinephrine reuptake inhibitors (SNRIs), and so-called atypical antidepressants. The current consensus is that the newer antidepressants—SSRIs, SNRIs, and the atypical antidepressants such as bupropion (Wellbutrin)—are the drugs of first choice because they are just as effective as the older antidepressants while being better tolerated at therapeutic doses and safer in an overdose.

Regardless of class, one expects a *response rate* to an antidepressant drug in the range of 50%–60%. *Response* is usually defined as a clinically meaningful change in depressive severity, meaning at least 50% improvement, while full *remission* occurs in only about 30%–35% of patients with the first antidepressant treatment; the other 30%–35% of patients experience a partial response (Agency for Health Care Policy and Research 1993).

Although the situation is going to change in the near future, we don't yet have a scientifically rigorous way of selecting an antidepressant for a depressed patient. Instead, we tend to pick medications based on past treatment response and side-effect profile. For example, if the patient had symptoms of atypical depression—mood reactivity, rejection sensitivity, hypersomnia, and hyperphagia—there is good evidence that an MAOI will be more effective than a TCA, even though neither of these would be a first-line choice because of factors like dietary restrictions and side-effect profiles (Quitkin 2002).

Prior response to antidepressant medication is a good predictor of future response, so that if Mr. Avery had responded to fluoxetine (Prozac) during a prior depressive episode, re-treating him with fluoxetine would be reasonable. Many clinicians also believe that it would make sense to use an antidepressant that had been effective for a patient's first-degree relative.

Pharmacogenomics will almost certainly take a lot of the current guess work out of the selection of antidepressant medication. We already know, for example, that there are polymorphisms of the serotonin transporter gene that knock out 90% of its function, making it unlikely that a carrier would respond to an SSRI (Malhotra et al. 2004). Stay tuned.

But in today's clinical practice, side-effect profiles and certain comorbid medical illnesses are the major considerations in choosing an antidepressant in someone without a history of therapeutic success. For example, bupropion is the antidepressant most likely to lower the seizure threshold and should generally be avoided in patients with seizure disorders. TCAs slow cardiac conduction and should not be used in patients with cardiac disease or in post–myocardial infarction patients because they increase cardiac morbidity and mortality. These are just a few examples of how certain medical illnesses would steer a clinician away from particular antidepressants.

In the meantime, which antidepressant should we select for Mr. Avery?

We know that Mr. Avery has been treated on three occasions in the past with antidepressants: once, many years ago, with an unknown medication for about 1 week; a second trial with fluoxetine at a maximum daily dose of 40 mg for 12 weeks; and a third trial with sertraline at a maximum daily dose of 100 mg for 6 weeks.

Antidepressants are effective only if given at a therapeutic dose over a period of at least 4–6 weeks. This constitutes a therapeutic trial and is the key concept in the pharmacologic management of depression, as it is in other psychiatric disorders. Each antidepressant has a different therapeutic dose range. In the absence of a clinical response or intolerable adverse effects, the dose of the antidepressant should be titrated aggressively to the upper limit of the therapeutic range. The most common reason why depressed patients in the community do not get better with treatment is not because their depression is truly "refractory;" but because they do not receive therapeutic trials of antidepressants—either the dose is too low or treatment is too short (Trivedi et al. 2006). Mr. Avery clearly did not respond to a therapeutic trial of fluoxetine. The dosage of sertraline was never rigorously pushed to the upper therapeutic limit (200 mg/day), however, and so one could argue that this was not a full therapeutic trial of sertraline. The trial of a second SSRI was reasonable since failure to respond to one SSRI does not predict failure to respond to a different one. Nevertheless, the patient's complete lack of response to sertraline, albeit not at the highest dosage, would weigh against a third trial of an SSRI.

If I were treating Mr. Avery, I would now consider a different class of antidepressant. My first choice would be either bupropion or the SNRI duloxetine (Cymbalta). The other available SNRI, venlafaxine (Effexor), is associated with the risk of increased blood pressure, and Mr. Avery has a history of poorly controlled hypertension. If his blood pressure were under control, however, I would certainly consider it.

Before putting my pen to a prescription pad, I would spend some time with Mr. Avery, particularly since he has a history of noncompliance with medication. I would want to know more about why he quit taking medications and would look specifically for such common reasons as worries about side effects, a denial of illness, a view that depression is a moral failing rather than a medical illness, or an incomplete understanding of the rationale for treatment. I would then explain how antidepressants work and emphasize that a therapeutic trial of antidepressant requires that he take the prescribed dose for at least 4–6 weeks. I would also explain that while he might not feel better for a few weeks, side effects like dry mouth, restlessness, and decreased appetite could occur immediately.

The role of psychoeducation and the therapeutic alliance cannot be stressed enough in successful pharmacotherapy. If the patient does not feel understood by his psychiatrist and understand what is wrong with him and what the treatment entails, the cleverest and most sophisticated medication treatment will be a useless exercise.

For argument's sake, let's start with bupropion, an activating antidepressant that increases noradrenergic and dopaminergic neurotransmission. After discussing the above issues, I would review Mr. Avery's medications to see if there might be any drug–drug interactions between bupropion and either this patient's beta-blocker or diuretic. Bupropion is metabolized in the liver by cytochrome P450 2B6 enzyme and can inhibit the 2D6 isoform, which means that it could potentially increase the level of any drug that is a substrate of 2D6.

I would start the bupropion at a dosage of 100 mg twice daily. If he tolerates the medication at that dosage but remains depressed, I would increase the dosage to 300 mg/day by the second week. One should not give more than 200 mg in one dose with the SR form of Wellbutrin; with the XL form, the entire daily dose (maximum=450 mg) can be given in one dose. I would continue to push the dose up to a daily maximum of 400 mg of the SR or 450 mg of the XL. Beyond this maximum daily dose, there is a substantially increased risk of seizure.

If Mr. Avery is in the lucky 30%–35% of patients, he will have a complete remission at the end of the acute treatment phase, which generally takes 8–12 weeks. If he has a partial response, one could consider either augmentation or a switch to a different type of antidepressant altogether. Augmentation often leads to a faster response and avoids discontinuation effects of the first agent. On the other hand, augmentation may lead to drug–drug interactions and more side effects.

Possible augmentation strategies with bupropion include an SSRI, lithium, thyroid hormone, buspirone, or an atypical antipsychotic medication. I would switch to a different antidepressant if Mr. Avery has either an absent or a minimal response to bupropion. In that case, I would consider an SNRI like duloxetine, which blocks reuptake of both norepinephrine and serotonin. There is a debate in the literature about whether so-called broad-spectrum antidepressants such as TCAs and SNRIs might be more effective than SSRIs. For example, one meta-analysis showed higher rates of complete remission with venlafaxine than with SSRIs (Thase et al. 2001).

Given Mr. Avery's skepticism about psychiatry and his history of non-compliance, I would frequently review with him whether he is taking the medication as directed and would aggressively address any adverse side effects or psychological resistances to medication adherence. Even assuming perfect compliance, I would not be surprised if Mr. Avery requires several more antidepressant trials, both monotherapy and in combination, before he has an adequate treatment response.

Pharmacogenomics

Charles Glatt, M.D., Ph.D.

JAMES Avery has been unresponsive to a series of antidepressant medications. He is likely to be wary of starting another medication trial, is at high risk for continued nonadherence, and will likely remain a significant suicide risk during the 4- to 8-week lag before a new drug begins to work. At this critical juncture, selection of the wrong medication could have grim consequences.

There are empiric, practical methods for medication selection (Kirchheiner et al. 2004), but there is much current interest in the possibility that drug selection could be guided by genetic testing that would be based on the heritable differences in drug response. This field—*pharmacogenomics*—holds particular promise within psychiatry, where there are clusters of drugs that are moderately effective at treating most diagnoses but little understanding of how to select a particular drug for a particular patient. Pharmacogenomics has the potential, therefore, of improving recovery rates, thereby reducing psychiatric suffering. By identifying the likelihood of various side effects, genetic testing could guide dosing, improve adherence, and further reduce morbidity. While its current clinical applicability is limited, pharmacogenomics has the potential to significantly change the way that psychiatry is practiced.

There are two ways that genetic differences between individuals can contribute to differences in drug response. *Pharmacokinetics* refers to the ways in which the body affects the drug, while *pharmacodynamics* refers to the ways in which the drug affects the body.

Pharmacokinetics can include the absorption, distribution, metabolism, and excretion of drugs. Within psychiatry, the most useful genetic variations currently revolve around *cytochrome P450* (CYP), a family of metabolic liver enzymes that serve as the first step in the inactivation and excretion of a large number of drugs, including almost all psychiatric medications. Of the greatest relevance to pharmacogenomics is the fact that many of the CYP enzymes contain common genetic variants, or *polymorphisms,* that affect enzyme activity. These variants determine the amount of drug—and in some cases, the amount of active metabolites—that reach the brain and other organs. These enzyme systems are an important cause of inter-individual differences regarding both therapeutic and side effects. In individuals with decreased enzyme activity, for example, drugs can accumulate to levels that lead to side effects or frank toxicity. Conversely, increased enzyme activity can prevent a drug from reaching therapeutic levels at a standard dose. Pharmacogenomics should eventually reveal which patients have liver enzymes that have mutated to be unusually active or inactive; these advances would allow for a more sophisticated dosing and selection of drugs. Until that time, however, it is useful for the clinician to be attentive to the fact that some patients will have side effects to low doses of medication, while others will require quite high doses in order to be effective.

Pharmacodynamics refers to all biochemical and physiologic effects of drugs, but genetic studies of the pharmacodynamics of psychiatric drugs have focused on variations in the *serotonin transporter.* A common polymorphism has been identified in the regulatory region for the serotonin transporter gene that has been associated with its level of expression (Lesch et al. 1996). This polymorphism consists of a variable number of a repeated DNA sequence motif. There are two common forms of this polymorphism, consisting of 14 or 16 of these sequence repeats, that are usually referred to as "short" and "long," respectively. The short allele is associated with lower expression of the serotonin transporter compared with the long form. In Caucasian populations, depressed people with the long form of this polymorphism seem to have a better response to SSRIs than do carriers of the short form (Glatt and Reus 2003). This finding has not been consistently replicated in Caucasians, however, and studies of East Asians indicate better clinical response in carriers of the short form. Such uncertainties are inevitable when using ethnic groups as an approximation of genotype status. Nevertheless, identifiable subgroups do possess clinically relevant polymorphisms.

How might Mr. Avery's treatment be informed by pharmacogenomics? We know that he has demonstrated nonresponsiveness to two or three different SSRIs. It is unlikely that this is due to genetic alterations in the CYPs, as there is no major isoform of the CYPs that metabolizes all three compounds that Mr. Avery has failed. It is possible that he possesses a serotonin transporter polymorphism that renders him less likely to respond to SSRIs, but there have not yet been pertinent studies on patients of African descent.

Pharmacogenomics does point to one concern if Mr. Avery begins to take bupropion (Wellbutrin), as proposed in the preceding section on the psychopharmacology of depression. Bupropion is converted by CYP2B6 into an active metabolite, hydroxybupropion, which is considered responsible for the majority of bupropion's side effects that range from anxiety to seizures. Thirty percent of the African American population possesses a variant form of CYP2B6 that is especially active, which leads to enhanced metabolism of the drug and, in turn, accumulation of hydroxybupropion (Kirchheiner et al. 2003). These elevated levels of hydroxybuproprion might cause side effects in Mr. Avery. Knowing this, the clinician might use relatively low doses of bupropion in people of African descent. Alternatively, the patient could combine bupropion with grapefruit juice, which contains bergamottin, an inhibitor of CYP2B6.

There is no genetic test in psychiatry with adequate predictive value to justify the effort and cost. As described above, however, ethnicity can be used as an approximation of genotype status since markedly different distributions of genetic variants and allele frequencies are known for many clinically relevant polymorphisms. In addition, the recognition of genetic variability can help the clinician attend more sensitively to the pharmacokinetic and pharmacodynamic differences between patients as we await more definitive genetic tests in psychiatry.

Brain Stimulation and Neuromodulation

Alexandra L. Sporn, M.D.
Sarah H. Lisanby, M.D.

JAMES Avery presents with a case of treatment-resistant depression in the context of a chronic mood disorder. When less invasive treatments such as psychotherapy and antidepressant medications fail to be effective, or when illness is so severe or acute that a quick response is needed, we turn to non-pharmacological means of modulating brain function. The most widely known form of nonpharmacological neuromodulation, ECT, is one of the oldest biological treatments in psychiatry. There are, however, a growing number of tools that use electrical or magnetic stimulation to modulate brain function in increasingly more precise and focal ways. These new tools represent an emerging family of interventions that may be referred to as *brain stimulation* and *neuromodulation* techniques. Focal brain stimulation opens for the first time the potential to target the neural circuitry underlying depression and other psychiatric disorders, thereby offering the promise of effectively treating patients for whom medications are ineffective. Likewise, they represent tools with unparalleled abilities to advance our understanding of the neural circuitry underlying psychiatric disorders by noninvasively probing that circuitry, either alone or in combination with functional neuroimaging.

In this portion of the chapter we introduce each of the brain stimulation techniques in use or under study in psychiatry and then discuss their potential relevance to the case of Mr. Avery. The only treatments discussed here that are presently approved by the U.S. Food and Drug Administration (FDA) for a psychiatric indication are ECT and VNS (vagal nerve stimulation).

Overview of Brain Stimulation Techniques

ELECTROCONVULSIVE THERAPY

ECT has been modernized substantially since it was first introduced some 70 years ago. ECT remains the most effective and rapidly acting treatment for severe medication-resistant depression and other disorders. ECT involves the induction of a generalized seizure under anesthesia. A muscle relaxant protects the body by blocking the motor convulsion. Recent modifications in treatment technique, including right unilateral electrode placement, seizure threshold titration, and ultrabrief pulse width, have significantly reduced the risks of amnesia.

ECT is appropriate to consider when several courses of antidepressant medications and augmentation strategies have failed to be effective or when there is an urgent need for rapid response (e.g., catatonia or cachexia). ECT is often used when the medical risks of antidepressant medications are high, such as in the elderly, who may not tolerate cardiovascular side effects, or during pregnancy, when transplacental delivery of antidepressants poses teratogenic risks. ECT can be expected to have an approximately 70%–80% response rate in major depression, with an onset of action that can be as fast as 1–2 weeks.

Vagal Nerve Stimulation

In VNS, an electrical device like a pacemaker is implanted in the chest. Electrical leads are sutured onto the vagus nerve in the neck. VNS was originally FDA approved for the treatment of resistant epilepsy, and in 2005 it was approved for the adjunctive treatment of chronic, treatment-resistant depression. Success rates with VNS are considerably lower than with ECT, and onset of action is comparatively slow (e.g., approximately 30% response rate after 1 year). If VNS fails to be effective, the device can be removed, but the electrodes are left on the vagus nerve, since removal carries more risks than leaving the electrodes permanently in place.

The FDA label states that VNS is indicated for the adjunctive long-term treatment of chronic or recurrent depression in patients 18 years or older who are experiencing a major depressive episode (unipolar or bipolar) and have not had an adequate response to four or more adequate antidepressant treatments. Consultation with another clinician experienced with treatment-resistant depression and VNS is recommended.

Contraindications to VNS include a history of bilateral or left cervical vagotomy and use of short-wave diathermy, microwave diathermy, or therapeutic ultrasound diathermy. Patients with VNS implanted cannot receive routine magnetic resonance imaging (MRI) scans, but can receive MRI with a special "send/receive" coil. Postmarketing studies under way now will yield important information on proper dosing strategies for this treatment.

Generally, VNS may be worth considering after patients have failed to respond to medications, psychotherapy, and ECT, or after it becomes clear that ECT relapse cannot be prevented with less invasive means. There is hope that VNS might be helpful with longer-term relapse prevention, but results of controlled trials would be useful to guide practice.

Transcranial Magnetic Stimulation

Transcranial magnetic stimulation (TMS) uses magnetic fields that are applied to the head with a compact and portable electromagnetic coil. These magnetic fields are turned on and off very rapidly, and this fluctuation in the field induces a small electrical stimulation that triggers frequency-dependent alterations in neuronal excitability. TMS can be focused on small regions of the brain (0.5 cm), allowing us to target specific brain structures. More than 30 published controlled trials support efficacy of TMS in depression, and TMS is approved in Canada. Studies are also beginning to find positive results in schizophrenia and in neurorehabilitation following stroke.

Magnetic Seizure Therapy

Magnetic seizure therapy (MST) uses TMS to perform a convulsive therapy that is more focused than ECT, which is highly effective but carries the risk of memory loss. By targeting the prefrontal cortex, MST limits the impact on the hippocampus, the region most implicated in the construction of memory. Initial studies suggest that MST may retain efficacy with a significantly reduced side-effect burden compared with ECT.

Transcranial Direct Current Stimulation

Transcranial direct current stimulation (tDCS) uses very weak electrical fields applied to the scalp to polarize the brain. Polarization changes the firing rate of neurons. Depending on the direction of current flow, this polarization can either inhibit or facilitate function. tDCS may enhance certain brain functions, and current research is focusing on its potential effectiveness in facilitating recovery from stroke and from certain forms of dementia. Work with this technology is at the very early stages. One study has been published on depression with encouraging results, but it awaits replication. If successful, tDCS could represent a safe and cheap alternative that could reach communities with less access to technological advancements.

Deep Brain Stimulation

Small electrodes are implanted into the brain to stimulate regions that are too deep to reach by stimulating the scalp. Deep brain stimulation (DBS) is already approved for the treatment of Parkinson's disease and is under study for the treatment of severe and treatment-resistant obsessive-compulsive disorder and major depression. Recently published work supported antidepressant efficacy of DBS. More controlled work in larger sample sizes will be important to establishing the potential clinical role of DBS, but early results are quite encouraging.

Implications for James Avery

Mr. Avery presents with a major depression in the context of a more chronic depression. The leading indication for ECT is major depression. Other indications are a major depressive episode in the context of bipolar disorder or schizoaffective disorder. Depression is also an indication for VNS, but it must be a chronic and resistant depression. TMS, MST, tDCS, and DBS are all under study for depression. Among these four experimental treatments, the one with the most published evidence for antidepressant efficacy is TMS. TMS has been tested in moderately severe, moderately chronic depression. MST is designed for more severely ill patients who would otherwise receive ECT. DBS, due to its invasiveness, would be reserved for those patients who were resistant to all less-invasive forms of treatment, include ECT.

The acuity of Mr. Avery's illness and the seriousness of his suicide risk call for the selection of a treatment that is rapidly effective, works in severe cases, acutely reduces suicidal impulses, and is not lethal in overdose. Among all of the available forms of antidepressant treatment, ECT is the one with the best evidence for efficacy in depressed, suicidal patients. In addition, it is the most rapidly acting.

Mr. Avery has only received two reasonable trials of antidepressant medications, and they were both SSRIs. Before recommending ECT, we would typically recommend patients be treated with several medications from different classes, such as TCAs and MAOIs, and we would also suggest augmentation strategies. Certain clinical scenarios justify using ECT earlier in the course. These include acute, serious suicidality as well as psychosis and catatonia. VNS would be indicated only after further medication trials and ECT. Mr. Avery's clinical presentation is similar to the depressions that were studied in the TMS trials, but he is far from being considered for more invasive treatments like DBS.

Relapse prevention is an important aspect of treatment planning, particularly for patients like Mr. Avery whose depression has had a chronic, recurrent clinical course. While it is recommended that antidepressant medications be maintained at their effective dosage for up to a year or more following remission from depression, ECT is stopped when patients respond. Without maintenance treatment following discontinuation of ECT, about 80% of patients will relapse within the first 6 months. It is recommended that patients begin maintenance medications immediately after an effective course of ECT, or even have them started during the course of ECT. For some patients, medications alone are insufficient and ECT needs to be continued on a maintenance basis, at decreasing frequency, over the months following the acute course. If Mr. Avery had not responded to ECT, or if he had responded to ECT but failed to maintain remission with combination pharmacotherapy or maintenance ECT, VNS could be considered.

Concomitant medical illnesses are an important factor in treatment selection. Poorly controlled hypertension or diabetes places this patient at risk for heart disease, which would need to be evaluated prior to ECT. Cardiac complications are the most frequent cause of medical morbidity from ECT. Hypertension and diabetes are also risk factors for cerebrovascular disease, which, even when clinically silent but apparent on MRI in the form of white matter hyperintensities, can predispose to increased post-ECT delirium. While transient memory difficulties are common during ECT, Mr. Avery's Mini-Mental State Exam score of 24/30 suggests the possibility of cognitive disorder, which would put him at an elevated risk for post-ECT cognitive impairments.

Suggestions

As long as Mr. Avery is stable, not psychotic, and denying active suicidal intent while in the hospital, I would suggest that he receive a well-controlled medication trial with another class of medications (e.g., an SNRI, TCA, or MAOI). If he remains severely depressed following that trial, ECT could be considered. VNS would not be appropriate at this time, given the inadequate number of failed medication trials and the urgent need for rapid response. In the future, if TMS or MST becomes approved, they might be considered before a trial of ECT. DBS would only be considered after all other options had failed.

New developments in brain stimulation are beginning to increase the available treatment options for resistant depression. While none of these novel treatments are likely to replace ECT, they represent new tools for use at different stages of the illness, and they stand to increase the available options for patients who fail to respond to less invasive interventions.

Supportive Psychotherapy

David J. Hellerstein, M.D.

SUPPORTIVE psychotherapy (SPT) has traditionally been seen as an ineffective treatment, synonymous with "hand-holding." In recent years, SPT has been redefined as a disciplined and change-oriented approach to psychotherapy that uses specific techniques and approaches and requires a good deal of sophistication by its practitioners. Rather than a last resort, we have described it as a "treatment of choice" that may benefit a wide range of patients. Nevertheless, patients are often referred for SPT after it is determined that they are "not good candidates" for other forms of psychotherapy, such as psychodynamic or cognitive-behavioral therapies. As a result, SPT therapists often work with patients who are more resistant or treatment-nonresponsive.

James Avery is in many ways typical of such patients, in that he has had several failed treatments that included both pharmacotherapy and psychotherapy. His therapist will have to work creatively to apply SPT interventions to engage Mr. Avery in a treatment process with the hope of alleviating his suffering. SPT focuses on improving self-esteem, adaptive skills, and psychological functions (or defense mechanisms). The SPT therapist uses techniques such as clarification, reframing, anticipatory guidance, education, and cognitive restructuring. Confrontation is used in a limited way, and the therapeutic relationship (or transference) is addressed only when the treatment is threatened. SPT psychotherapists have a conversationally responsive style, avoiding long silences and respecting the patient's adaptive defenses. The goal is to decrease the patient's level of anxiety and to enhance the therapeutic alliance.

Mr. Avery will present significant challenges to the SPT therapist. Not only has he had negative experiences (and results) from previous treatments, but he is mistrustful of clinicians and is reported to lack "curiosity into his own problems." It is doubtful that he is interested in "being in psychotherapy." His family seems estranged from him. He is also severely depressed and hopeless, which no doubt exacerbates these issues.

The initial (and ongoing) goal will be to develop a therapeutic alliance with Mr. Avery. The SPT therapist will look for aspects of Mr. Avery that are admirable and adaptive. Initially, this may appear to be difficult, since Mr. Avery very convincingly portrays himself as a failure. However, it is clear that Mr. Avery has many admirable qualities. He is an intelligent man with strong beliefs and opinions. He appears to have a high level of integrity. He has a strong work ethic, having kept his job for 30 years. Family is central to him. He has persevered through much adversity, including his experiences with a racist society. He has made a valiant effort to cope with a biologically based mood disorder, trying a number of treatments even though they have caused side effects or been ineffective.

The SPT therapist can use some of these adaptive characteristics to develop—and maintain—an alliance with Mr. Avery, the caveat being that Mr. Avery is likely to be exquisitely aware of any sign of insincerity or condescension. The therapist should also make honest acknowledgments or clarifications of Mr. Avery's doubts about the possible benefits of treatment (e.g., "It may be hard for me as a white person to understand your experiences as an African American"). It is clearly important for Mr. Avery to feel "understood," since he quit therapies when therapists did not understand his situation and background. Clarifications (e.g., "Very few people have been able to understand your suffering") or reframing (e.g., "You are a man of strong principles and passions") may be helpful. These should be used tactfully, since some comments may be true but likely to reduce the alliance (e.g., "You are a very angry person").

Enhancing Mr. Avery's adaptive skills and strengths is likely to be an ongoing process. In particular, it would be helpful to know how he has overcome adversity in the past. Has he recovered from previous depressive episodes? How has he managed previous life crises? Whom has he been closest to during his life—who has understood him best—and whom is he closest to now? What have been his greatest accomplishments? What kinds of things does he enjoy doing or get satisfaction from? These are themes that can be evaluated and developed over the course of treatment; the timing of the inquiry depends more on tactful curiosity than on a standardized checklist. The SPT therapist will use his/her understanding of these skills and strengths in order to provide interventions that highlight or strengthen his coping abilities.

Similarly, the SPT therapist will find ways to strengthen Mr. Avery's self-esteem as well as the positive aspects of his psychological functions (or defense mechanisms). Mr. Avery's self-esteem appears very low at present, which most likely reflects the severity of his depression, as well as the numerous losses and setbacks he has experienced. The SPT therapist would be alert to positive aspects of self-esteem as well—his pride in his own integrity, his sense of justice and honesty, and his need to speak his own mind.

The SPT therapist rarely asks "Why?" It is more useful to offer observations to which the patient may or may not respond. For example, the SPT therapist would avoid asking Mr. Avery, "Why do you think you are depressed?" or "Why don't your kids call you?" Instead, the therapist might say, "Sounds like you really wish you weren't depressed so much of your life" or "You wish you heard from the kids more often." Such comments reduce the likelihood that Mr. Avery might feel pressured, and yet they still provide an opportunity for exploration. A related tenet of SPT is to "strike while the iron is cold"— returning to issues when a person is calm rather than attempting to "explore" them in the heat of the moment. This may occur later in a session or during a subsequent session, often weeks or months later.

Identifying Mr. Avery's goals for treatment is a collaborative process, requiring ongoing revision. Goals of SPT are generally explicit, and the SPT therapist checks periodically with the patient regarding how well they are being accomplished. In general, the SPT therapist is present oriented; exploration of the past is done only to the degree of illuminating the patient's present situation. Mr. Avery's initial goals may be to feel better—or to tidy up his affairs so he can end his life. Therapist and patient may "agree to disagree" in this instance. Later on, his goals may be to leave the hospital, to get back to his own home, to get back to work, and to sort out his relationships with his wife and kids.

The word *and* has central importance in SPT. The SPT therapist may say to Mr. Avery, "You feel like you have failed in life *and* you are a person who has accomplished a lot." Or, "You feel like you want to die *and* you still yearn for better relationships with your kids and grandkids." The implication is that seemingly paradoxical things can both be true. *And* recognizes the central importance of hope, which is crucial for the treatment of depression. "You didn't want to talk to anyone *and* you ended up having a nice conversation with your neighbor." "There is a lot of hypocrisy and hatred in this world, *and* you still hope that people will be treated fairly." It can also be used to enhance the therapeutic relationship: "You feel absolutely hopeless *and* you brighten up when I say there is hope in treating your depression."

The goal of *and* is to allow Mr. A. to broaden his outlook and to add other options to his coping abilities, while not dismissing the validity of his own perspectives and feelings. To this end, "anticipatory guidance" may also be useful—"It sounds like you really spoke your mind to your boss. Are there other things you might consider doing if this situation came up again?" Mr. Avery's maladaptive patterns of behavior and interactions can be examined while trying to avoid criticizing him.

Aggressive pharmacotherapy (or ECT) may be very likely to help Mr. Avery's double depression. If this is the case, and if Mr. Avery's depressive symptoms improve over the coming weeks to months, then Mr. Avery may face a postdisorder state that is novel to him: euthymia. Such an improvement would necessitate an evolution of treatment goals. During recovery, SPT focuses not only on "slips" of mood that might indicate depressive relapses but also on issues that emerge as life becomes more enjoyable. He may find it necessary to start repairing damage at home and work, for example, and to reestablish meaningful connections to others. In the long term, if Mr. Avery's mood disorder enters a prolonged remission, goals may include developing new interpersonal skills, making the most of new opportunities and interests, and working on developing more intimacy in relationships.

The practice of SPT is consistent with current ideas of brain plasticity, in which the aberrant neurocircuitry in depression can be controlled with proper antidepressant pharmacotherapy (or CBT-related treatments). After depression remits, there may be hippocampal neurogenesis and reconnection and reintegration of adaptive brain connections in the higher brain. The SPT therapist would be alert for behavioral manifestations of these neurological changes, such as spontaneous positive activities or improved connections with others. The SPT goal of improving adaptive behaviors and linking them to pleasure can be seen, therefore, as a way of "rewiring" the brain.

It is important to note that SPT is not done in isolation—it is well suited for combining with other treatment approaches. For Mr. Avery, these are likely to include psychopharmacological interventions; case management and crisis management; psychoeducation about depression; family or couples therapy; group therapy or partial hospitalization programs; and participation in self-help groups, such as The Mood Disorders Support Group of New York City (http://mdsg.org). SPT may or may not be a specific antidepression psychotherapy (it has not been well studied as a depression treatment), but it can be an essential component of a treatment intervention that makes more specific treatments possible.

Couples Therapy

Phillip Lee, M.D.
Diane Rudolph, M.D.

WHILE not the first priority upon admission, meeting with James Avery and his wife and family might improve his mood, shore up the interpersonal infrastructure that is crumbling around him, and help the team assess how he and his family are dealing with the ramifications of the suicide attempt. Even if the hospital-based intervention uncovers that Mrs. Avery is pursuing a divorce and will not be a supportive presence, the meeting(s) would help clarify the resources that will be available to Mr. Avery following discharge. Such family interventions are often a vital part of an inpatient treatment.

For the sake of this discussion, however, let's assume that we saw Mr. and Mrs. Avery after discharge, after the lifting of his acute suicidality, and after he and his wife agreed to work to improve their marriage.

We would begin our work with them with the recognition that there are two basic tasks in couples therapy. The first is to eliminate repetitive negative interactions. The second is to rekindle the joy, affection, and respect that once infused the relationship. The one great truth about couples therapy is that no matter how poisonous the atmosphere may be, these two people once got along. And not just got along, but got along so well that they were willing—even eager—to commit for a lifetime. In most cases, the sourest of relationships can be improved through therapy.

Our initial session would focus on eliciting a history of the marriage, including both problems and pleasures. We would make explicit that we would not focus on individual issues but would instead be working toward building a happier, healthier relationship. From this perspective, "the marriage is the patient," an emphasis that can reduce the tendency to blame one member of the couple for all of the relationship problems. This tendency toward blame is likely to already exist between them, and the therapist should try not to let the therapy simply re-create destructive aspects of the relationship.

In regard to the problems within the relationship, we first try to clearly understand the arguments, and there are always arguments. We would start by asking Mr. and Mrs. Avery for a verbatim record of an argument. How does it start? Who says what? How does the other person reply? What happens then? These arguments will repeat themselves. Every couple has a limited number of such arguments, and a particular dispute repeats itself over and over, much like a boilerplate legal document purchased at a stationery store. In the blanks, the couple will fill in the details necessary to make any particular argument fit the pattern.

We don't know much about this particular relationship, but we do know a few things about Mr. Avery's depression that are likely to have had an impact on the relationship. He describes chronic depression, diminished energy, hopelessness, poor compliance with his medications for diabetes and hypertension, sensitivity to rejection, isolation from his family of origin, and a belief that his wife had long kept one foot out the door. From these details, we can hypothesize some possible arguments:

Martha: You never want to do anything with the family.
James: You always complain. Nothing I ever do is good enough. I went with our granddaughter to the park, and you were all over me because I didn't stay long enough.
Martha: You can't ever do anything on your own—you only went because I asked you to…

or

Martha: You don't do things that are healthy. You need to exercise and take your medications. I shouldn't have to be on your case all the time.
James: It's impossible to remember all the medications, but I think I do pretty well at it. Quit riding me all the time, and maybe I'd do better.
Martha: I've tried riding you, and I've tried leaving you alone. It doesn't matter what I do.

In these scenarios, James does too little, then feels unappreciated and does less. Martha is frustrated by James's apparently stubborn refusal to participate, then criticizes any effort he does make, increasing the likelihood that he will do even less in the future.

While the individual therapist might focus on Mr. Avery's depression, the couples therapist recognizes a two-person, cyclical problem in which James is discouraged and withdrawn, leading Martha to get frustrated and critical, which exacerbates James's initial discouragement and anger. Recognition of these cycles and patterns will be a central goal throughout the couples therapy.

In addition to problems, we would explore during this first session the overall history of their relationship. We would want to know how they met, what they liked about each other, how things progressed, how they decided to get married, what they used to do for fun, how things were after the marriage, and how things changed after the children were born. We would be curious about when the marriage started to slide but also about the qualities that attracted each of them to the other. It might turn out, for example, that James and Martha shared a love of music and had gone on many dates to concerts and clubs.

During this first session, we could generally elicit characteristic problems and pleasures, and we might then give two sets of suggestions for the following week. The first relates to the problems. We would describe the characteristic, boilerplate form of the argument: Martha gets upset that James doesn't do enough. James gets hurt and angry and does less. Martha gets angrier. Describing the standard arguments evenly and without blame, we might remind them that every conflicted relationship has a set of such arguments that serve to destroy the marriage. We might then suggest one activity for the week that addresses this pattern. For example, we might ask that James take the granddaughter to the park and ask Martha to verbally appreciate his effort.

In regard to positive aspects of their relationship, we might send them on an activity that resembles a previously fun activity. In their case, we might send them on a date to hear music. If they pretend they don't already know each other while on the date, they would be subtly encouraged not to continue their stereotyped arguments. If they do persist in their arguments, we might specifically ask that they not bicker using their traditional patterns; if they need to fight, they should find a new form for their complaints.

Underlying these therapeutic interventions is the idea that troubled relationships develop negative behaviors that become stereotyped. The intervention is to recognize the pattern and create bits of positive behavior that can seem simplistic and superfluous but which can contribute to fundamental change in a matter of weeks to months.

Between the first and second meeting with the couple, we would meet individually with each partner. We would ask each if there is any reason why the marriage shouldn't continue, which is, among other things, a tactful inquiry about affairs. Evasiveness prompts a more direct inquiry about outside relationships. Experts disagree about whether to allow these disclosures to be confidential. We take a middle ground in that we are willing to keep a confidence but refuse to treat the couple if there are undisclosed, important secrets. If, for instance, Martha had developed a "platonic" but intimate relationship over e-mail with a potential romantic partner, we would insist on discontinuation of contact for the duration of the therapy. The secret could relate to a different sort of problem, such as furtive alcohol abuse, which we would address the same way: the therapy can't progress unless the alcohol abuse is addressed. In addition to addressing hidden issues, we would pursue each person's history of previous serious relationships, looking for patterns and leverage in changing current behaviors.

When we meet with the couple together for the second time, we would review the suggested activities. We would ask whether James took his granddaughter to the park and, if he did, whether Martha was appreciative. We would also explore whether James and Martha had gone on a date, whether they had argued, and the extent to which each had noticed any tendency to resume a stereotyped conflict.

During the second and later sessions, we would try to deepen our understanding of the couple in a variety of ways. This might lead us to comment specifically on one person's family of origin:

> **Therapist to Martha:** So it seems like your mother used to attack your father for all the things he didn't do. This upset you as a child, and now you find yourself stuck in the same position with James.

We might also comment on the personal meaning of the argument:

> **Therapist to James:** It seems as though whenever Martha suggests you do something, you feel criticized with the same sort of intensity that you feel when you have a conflict at work. Do you think you might transfer some of your work resentments into your relationship with your wife?

These interventions are potentially problematic in that they can imply that one person is at fault. When the therapist is suggesting individual tendencies, it is generally useful to tactfully balance such suggestions so that one person isn't scapegoated within the relationship.

During this second meeting, we would also take a careful sexual history. What was it like at first? What did you enjoy about your partner? Who initiated sex? How often did you have sex? Has this pattern changed? How is it now? As problems emerge over the course of therapy, assignments expand. If it turns out that sexual relations have essentially stopped, for example, we might ask that dating include some "making out," which might lead spontaneously to improved sexual relations. If it doesn't, then further activities could be suggested and the resultant resistances explored. Like individuals, couples tend to return to familiar, maladaptive patterns after a successful intervention, and so much of the treatment would consist of recognizing these resistances and slips and devising new ways to look and act on them.

Couples therapy arouses intense feelings in both people. Amid the swirl of emotion is the fear of being blamed and the desire to be favored by the therapist. Maintaining neutrality is difficult, and the therapist might easily side with Martha, who has been long suffering and supportive, or with James, who has been fighting depression for decades. The therapist might prefer one person's sense of humor or perspective or life situation. Possible countertransference issues abound, and these undigested issues within the therapist have an impact on his/her ability to remain nonjudgmental, particularly when the couple's issues bring up relationship issues from the therapist's current life or family of origin. As in individual therapy, the couples therapist should model an empathic, nonjudgmental curiosity. This attitude can encourage both members of the couple to notice defensive patterns and work to improve their relationship and the life of their partner.

The couples therapist must be creative in order to see the potential underneath the relationship wreckage. The art is to see how the relationship could have ever worked. Some people can look at fine furniture covered with varnish or cheap paint, visualize potential, and restore the piece to its best possible condition. Refurbished, it can be more beautiful than when it was first created. Throughout the treatment, it is important to look beneath the angry, disappointed façade of the squabbling couple and find the likable and lovable in both people and in the relationship. Through this ongoing, detailed effort, one of the most central of human experiences—the intimate relationship—can be brought back to life.

Overview of Double Depression

James H. Kocsis, M.D.

JAMES Avery has been hospitalized following a suicide attempt. The 15 discussants in this chapter have explored various ways to understand him, his situation, his illness, and his history, and they have discussed his management and treatment. While their essays appear to work well together, their differing perspectives have historically led to significant debate over the cause of his suicide attempt, the name of his illness, and optimal treatment strategies.

One approach to Mr. Avery would be to emphasize temperament, personality, early life experience, and interpersonal relationships. Such an approach might lead a clinician to focus on his mother's suicide and the likelihood that his childhood had been affected by her depression and "worry." If she had been relatively absent or dysfunctional, he might have become sensitized to later disappointments and separations, which could have led to deep sadness as well as a tendency to behavior that might cause people to back away, leading to a self-fulfilling prophecy of abandonment. Such an understanding makes sense, is frequently seen, and dovetails well with ongoing research into the neurobiology of stress. This perspective on Mr. Avery might lead the clinician to view him as having a personality disorder or "depressive neurosis," which would have been at least one of Mr. Avery's diagnoses in DSM-I and DSM-II. At that time, treatment for depressive neurosis was a nonspecific, nonmanualized psychotherapy for which there was no efficacy data.

Research over the last few decades has firmly demonstrated, however, that chronic depressive symptoms like those in Mr. Avery fit under the umbrella of major affective disorder. As evidence accumulated (e.g., positive family histories of depression; significant psychosocial impairments; response to medications), depressive neurosis was moved onto Axis I in DSM-III, where it was called *dysthymic disorder*.

There have been, therefore, two competing philosophical perspectives on patients with chronic depression. Often, these differences were based on differences in treatment, so that clinicians with a psychopharmacologic bent would emphasize DSM-III and DSM-IV, while psychodynamic psychotherapists would emphasize development and personality.

A psychopharmacologist might, therefore, diagnose Mr. Avery with both dysthymia and major depression and make use of the data that indicate that several antidepressant medications have been shown to be "efficacious" for double depression, meaning that they outperformed placebo in randomized clinical trials. Sadly, though, only half of the patients in these trials responded to an antidepressant medication, and only about 30% had a remission of symptoms. Mr. Avery has had at least one therapeutic failure with an SSRI (more than one if the sertraline trial is deemed adequate); he would, therefore, not have been eligible for the studies that were designed for patients who had not previously taken medications. A more pertinent study involves people with double depression who did not respond to a trial of sertraline. When a switch to imipramine was made, 44% of the patients responded, and 23% achieved remission (Thase et al. 2002). In other words, while DSM criteria allow for the reliable identification of a cluster of people with dysthymia and major depression, a medication-only approach would stand a good chance of leaving Mr. Avery no better off than he was before his suicide attempt. Critics of the pharmacologic approach could point at these less-than-ideal data and assert their preference for psychotherapy. Supporters of the concept of a more biologic approach could argue that medications do help many people and could ask their opponents for data that indicated the usefulness of psychotherapy in treating severe depression.

When these debates were at their peak, well-informed clinicians might have legitimately developed very different treatment strategies for the same patient. With time and an ongoing dialogue, however, the debates have largely dissipated. Few would disagree with the idea that Mr. Avery's depression has some roots in biology or with the need for pharmacotherapy. Similarly, few would argue with the idea that Mr. Avery's depression has led to pessimism, irritability, and alliance difficulties, all of which can exacerbate the depression and interfere with treatment. While medications are likely to be central to his treatment, so are psychoeducation to enhance compliance and the development of a therapeutic alliance that can lead to interventions that may reduce his self-destructive and isolating behavior.

The merging of perspectives can allow Mr. Avery to carry three diagnoses. From DSM-IV, he would be diagnosed with dysthymia and major depression. As described by Dr. Auchincloss ("The Psychodynamic Formulation"), a psychodynamic formulation might lead to a diagnosis of depressive personality disorder with narcissistic, masochistic, and probably some paranoid features. The view of Mr. Avery as having a major depression, dysthymia, and a depressive personality disorder is not a statement of causation (i.e., biological, psychological, or sociological) or permanency (i.e., transient, permanent, or changing with treatment), but rather a description that provides a three-dimensional description of the clinical presentation.

Making use of these three diagnoses, the psychiatrist would emphasize more than one mode of therapy. Intensive somatic treatment might include using antidepressant medications at maximum doses for at least 6–8 weeks, and if only partially effective, adjunctive medications would be considered; if the trial is unsuccessful, the medications would be changed. In other words, pharmacology would be emphasized. At the same time, psychotherapy researchers have increasingly focused their efforts on depression, by trying, in particular, to develop and manualize treatments that can be specifically effective for certain subsets of patients.

One example of a focused psychotherapy addresses the specific challenges of treating individuals with chronic depression. Developed by McCullough (2000), Cognitive Behavioral Analysis System of Psychotherapy (CBASP) incorporates both cognitive-behavioral and interpersonal features. One study of chronic depression reported a response rate of 57% and remission rate of 36% among nefazodone nonresponders when a switch was made to CBASP alone (Schatzberg et al. 2005). The combination of antidepressant medication and CBASP has also been reported to be particularly potent in this population (Keller et al. 2000). While many clinicians believe that combining medication and psychotherapy holds promise for individuals with treatment-resistant chronic depression, much work remains to determine whether specific forms of therapy are more effective than others or whether specific therapies can be targeted to specific symptoms or problem areas (e.g., cognitive distortions or interpersonal problems). Nonetheless, CBASP seems to hold particular promise and is currently being studied in a large National Institute of Mental Health–sponsored multi-site clinical trial for treatment-resistant, chronic depression.

If Mr. Avery's depression responds to medications, psychotherapy, or combination treatment, a good deal of improvement can be expected in his vocational and psychosocial functioning (Kocsis et al. 2002). Long-term maintenance treatment is likely to be indicated and to be effective in prevention of a recurrence of his depression and associated role impairments (Gelenberg et al. 2003; Klein et al. 2004; Kocsis et al. 1996). At this time, however, much remains to be understood about the diagnosis and treatment of double depression, a common psychiatric illness whose cardinal features (depressed mood, anhedonia, relationship problems) not only cause significant suffering but also may directly interfere with recovery.

Summary Points

- Depression reduces connection, compliance, and intellectual and emotional flexibility. Interview techniques and treatments must be adapted to these realities and to the patient's specific personality and culture.

- Assessment of suicide risk is critical but depends heavily on demographic information that can only be imperfectly applied to a specific patient.

- There has historically been a dispute over whether chronic depression should be seen as a purely biological phenomenon or as a "depressive neurosis" that is akin to a personality disorder. Such a conflict seems to have dissipated, and experts agree that successful treatment requires multiple perspectives.

- Basic science is yielding critical insights into ways the brain self regulates and into genetic variations that affect the efficacy and metabolism of medications.

- Biological treatments are vital to the treatment of a serious major depression.

- When used alone, biological treatments are likely to completely fail or provide incomplete relief.
- Psychotherapy and the therapeutic alliance can reduce medication noncompliance and suicide rates and improve functioning, relationships, and mood.
- The likelihood of complete recovery from depression is greatest when multiple treatment modalities are used in conjunction.

Chapter 2

GERIATRIC DEPRESSION AND PETER BURKE

A consultation-liaison psychiatrist was called to see Peter Burke, a 71-year-old man who was refusing a leg amputation. Antibiotics and surgical debridements had not successfully treated the gangrene that had developed in the context of diabetes and peripheral vascular disease. The vascular surgeons believed that postponement of the surgery would be fatal and wanted the psychiatrist to determine whether Mr. Burke had capacity to make such an important treatment decision; if he did not, they planned to pursue involuntary surgery.

After reading the chart and talking with a surgical intern, the psychiatrist entered Mr. Burke's room to see an alert, wiry man, lying in bed, wearing a hospital gown and an FDNY cap. He was reading a newspaper. He looked sad. The patient asked, "And which kind of doctor are you?" When the consultant provided a name and specialty, the patient shook his head and said, "Jesus Christ. Nobody said they were calling in a head shrinker. So now they think I'm crazy?" The psychiatrist said, "Nobody is saying—" Mr. Burke interrupted, "The surgeons and my sons have been yelling at me for days, and they even sent in my daughter to cry at me. After all that, you think *you're* going to convince me to cut off my leg?" The psychiatrist smiled and assured him that convincing could wait until they knew each other better. The patient said, "You have 2 minutes." The consultant explained that there were two purposes to the visit: one was to see whether Mr. Burke understood the medical situation, and the other was for the two of them to get a better understanding of how he had come to his decision. The patient agreed to talk but added, "Let's stick to business. I don't need a headshrinker."

Over the course of 10 minutes, Mr. Burke made his case: "The decision is simple. I won't live like a dependent cripple....I know I could die without the surgery....I know it's not a big deal as long as it's not your leg that's being cut off....All my kids are saying that I could go live with them, but I don't want to....All these doctors look like they're 14 years old. Let them get to be my age, and then they can know what it's like to be ready to go....And that is that. Nothing more to say." He picked up his newspaper.

The psychiatrist said, "I hear that you're a fireman." The patient glanced up and said, "So, you can read my chart. Congratulations." The psychiatrist pointed at Mr. Burke's FDNY cap and said, "The chart didn't tell me you were proud of being a fireman." The patient shook his head and said, "So now we get into the headshrinking." The psychiatrist smiled and said, "Well, I am interested in hearing about your career and especially how it might relate to your not wanting to be dependent on anybody." The patient said, "What the hell," and began to describe his 40-year career with the Fire Department of New York. Mr. Burke appeared to relax. At one point, the patient paused, became noticeably sad, and said, "It's all felt like nothing since my wife and son died. And it's all my fault." Mr. Burke's chart indicated that his wife had died of cancer 2 years earlier and that his fireman son had died on the job 6 years before. When asked what was his fault, Mr. Burke explained he should have gotten his wife's cancer treated more aggressively. He also believed that his own successful career in the FDNY had led his son to choose an ultimately lethal line of work.

When asked, Mr. Burke said he would give anything to have been the one who died of cancer or in the fire, and he believed that his current medical situation "would be a good way out." The only reason that he had not already killed himself, he said, was that "suicide is a sin." When asked when he had begun to feel down, Mr. Burke said he had felt "useless" since he retired 10 years before, and he admitted to having had problems with sleep, mood, and energy even before his wife had been diagnosed with cancer.

The psychiatrist glanced at the wall clock and said that they would need to stop. The patient smiled and asked, "Well, do I pass?" The psychiatrist responded, "Grades aren't in. How about if I come back tomorrow?" Mr. Burke agreed.

Personal History

Mr. Burke was born in County Cork, Ireland. His family immigrated to the U.S. in his infancy. After a tour in the Navy, he joined the New York Fire Department and rose to the rank of battalion chief. At the time of her death, he and his wife had been married for 47 years. One of his three surviving sons was a chief in the FDNY. Another was a lieutenant in the New York Police

Department. A third was a surgeon at a nearby hospital. Both his daughters were at home raising children at the time of his hospitalization; one had married a fireman on Long Island.

Personal Psychiatric History

The patient denied psychiatric problems and all substance abuse. On weekends, he drank "one or two beers" but denied any history of alcohol abuse, dependence, or treatment.

Family Psychiatric History

Mr. Burke's father and grandfather had developed Alzheimer's disease in their 70's. Multiple family members had had occasional interpersonal difficulties while intoxicated, but none had been treated for alcoholism.

Medical History

Mr. Burke had diabetes and peripheral vascular disease, as well as the gangrenous leg. He had had a myocardial infarction 6 months earlier.

Mental Status Exam

The patient was a thin, alert, ruddy-faced man who appeared his stated age. He was dressed neatly in a hospital gown. He made good eye contact with the examiner. Gait was not tested. He was generally cooperative. His speech was of normal rate and rhythm and was spontaneous. He said he felt "depressed." His affect was generally constricted and appropriate to mood, but he did smile occasionally. He denied intending to kill himself but said he would be better off dead. He denied hallucinations. In regard to possible delusions, his sense of responsibility for the deaths of his wife and son appeared to be excessive and fixed. Although the patient was fully oriented and verbally fluent, his score on the Mini-Mental State Examination (MMSE) was 23/30, with diminished short-term memory and attention. His Clock Drawing Test was poorly planned and yielded a score of 2/4. His insight and judgment were considered somewhat impaired on the basis of his inflexibility regarding his surgery and his insistence that he was responsible for the deaths of his wife and son.

Summary

Peter Burke was a 71-year-old man whose capacity to refuse a leg amputation was being questioned by the surgical team. The discussants in the following sections explore issues relevant to the evaluation and treatment of an elderly man with depression, medical problems, and possible cognitive deficits.

Discussions of the Case of Peter Burke

Capacity 63
John W. Barnhill, M.D.

The Psychiatric Attitude 67
Kevin V. Kelly, M.D.

Depression and Medical Illness. 70
Peter A. Shapiro, M.D.

Neurotrophins 73
Francis Lee, M.D., Ph.D.

Testing at the Bedside 76
Marianne N. Findler, Ph.D.

Interpersonal Psychotherapy .81
John C. Markowitz, M.D.

Service Delivery 85
Martha Bruce, Ph.D.

Overview of Geriatric Depression. 88
George S. Alexopoulos, M.D.

Summary Points 91

Capacity

John W. Barnhill, M.D.

DOES Peter Burke have the capacity to refuse the amputation, a decision that might cost him his life? What are the rules for a capacity decision? What does capacity mean? Can a capacity evaluation be therapeutic to the patient, and, if so, how is this done?

Within medicine, *capacity* refers to the ability to provide informed consent for a specific procedure or a posthospital placement. Underlying the capacity assessment is the belief that doctors and patients should work together to develop a treatment plan that balances the desire to do what is best for the patient—the principle of *beneficence*—with the desire to maximize the patient's degree of freedom—the principle of *autonomy.*

While the patient's level of capacity is an implicit or explicit part of every medical decision, there is no single, official definition for capacity. Perhaps the most widely used definition of capacity was outlined by Appelbaum and Grisso in 1988. They describe four standards that must be met in order for the patient to have capacity. The patient must be able to

1. Articulate a consistent choice.
2. Understand relevant information, including risks and benefits.
3. Appreciate one's own situation.
4. Rationally manipulate information.

Mr. Burke has consistently refused surgery, which conforms to the first principle. He is able to repeat relevant information: the surgery could save his life and that the risks are small. In regard to the third principle, he is refusing the amputation to avoid being a "dependent cripple," which appears to be a distortion. In regards to the final criterion—the ability to manipulate information—Mr. Burke lacks cognitive flexibility but instead simply repeats his decision without an apparent ability to discuss differing possibilities. His inflexibility could reflect one or more of the following: a longstanding personality trait; a regressive response to his illness; hopelessness secondary to grief and depression; a resolving delirium; or a chronic cognitive decline. Although his conversational skills appear intact, brief screening using the Mini-Mental State Examination (MMSE) and Clock Drawing Test (CDT) reveals cognitive deficits that could contribute to his rigidity. Like personality issues, cognition can be affected by illness and hospitalization, however, and so the capacity decision may require serial evaluations and ongoing psychiatric involvement.

Mr. Burke's limitations place him in a gray zone, and an immediate capacity determination would probably vary depending on the consultant's relative interest in beneficence versus autonomy. Some consultants might be swayed by the reality that few surgeons and family members would be enthusiastic about amputating the leg of an alert, verbal, protesting former battalion chief in the New York Fire Department. Such pressures should not, however, play a role in the capacity assessment. If the decision is that the patient lacks capacity, the next step would be for the proxy to make the decision. If the patient is incapacitated and has never expressed an opinion about the particular situation, the proxy would generally use a "best interests standard," in which the decision would be based on the standpoint of a "typical" person. In most cases, however, the proxy tries to decide what the patient would have done in this situation based on what the proxy knows about the patient. In other words, if the proxy is confident that Mr. Burke would never have allowed such an amputation, then the proxy can refuse to sign the consent for surgery. And, even when the proxy provides consent, surgeons not infrequently refuse to operate against the patient's wishes if they think that involuntary surgery would have risky long-term consequences. For example, even if Mr. Burke were found to be incapacitated, his surgeons might refuse to do the surgery out of concern that he would refuse the necessary physical rehabilitation. Further, depending on the procedure, jurisdiction, and degree of urgency, an intervention might require a judge's assessment of competency. In other words, the capacity decision is not the final word.

Mr. Burke's children should be involved but may have divided opinions. One of his children may try to help him understand that an amputation is not necessarily crippling. A second child may be swayed by his depressive pessimism and/or patriarchal authority. A third may want to keep him alive regardless of his preference. Mr. Burke will also likely have varied relationships with each of his children. For example, he may want to demonstrate bravery with his fireman son, negotiate with his surgeon son, and defer to a daughter. A family meeting may be crucial in the creation of a unified perspective and a resolution of conflict.

While the primary medical team would generally prefer that the capacity decision be clean and quick, ambiguous situations require that the treatment team clearly think through the situation. For example, the team must be able to estimate the risks and the benefits of the surgery before the patient should be expected to appreciate and understand these risks and benefits. Mr. Burke's team must also be agreed that the amputation is necessary and that the antibiotics have been given a full trial. At times, the strong opinions of the primary team evolve with either the clinical progression of the illness or a changeover of staff, so that a procedure that is considered lifesaving on Monday becomes optional on Tuesday and unnecessary by Wednesday.

An important, additional principle that comes into play is that of the *sliding scale of capacity*. It reflects the pragmatic concept that a more stringent standard for capacity is necessary when the patient either refuses a low-risk, high-benefit intervention (e.g., a routine blood draw) or accepts a high-risk, low-benefit intervention (e.g., a risky, experimental treatment). A less stringent standard for capacity would be necessary when the patient accepts a low-risk, high-benefit intervention (e.g., the blood draw) or refuses a high-risk, low-benefit intervention (e.g., the risky treatment).

In Mr. Burke's case, his decision involves a relatively low-risk, high-gain procedure, and so treatment refusal involves a fairly high standard of cognitive and emotional flexibility. As reflected in his modestly low scores on the MMSE and CDT, his rigidity during the capacity discussion, and his guilt-ridden hopelessness, Mr. Burke is somewhat impaired. Is he impaired enough to take away his right to choose? That is not yet clear.

At this point, one treatment team might emphasize beneficence and continue to try to convince Mr. Burke or begin the pursuit of involuntary surgery. Another team might emphasize autonomy and discontinue active medical treatment. When a solution appears unknowable, it is often wise to back away temporarily and try another approach. In this case, the consultant might step back from the traditional capacity guidelines that emphasize the patient's level of cognition and focus instead on developing a deeper understanding of the patient.

The initial step to understanding Mr. Burke is the creation of an alliance. By the time the psychiatric consultation has been called, the patient will have likely rejected the well-meaning advice from a stream of doctors, nurses, and loved ones. While it can be useful for the psychiatrist to offer up the same advice to see the patient's reaction, it is unlikely that a stranger will immediately succeed where loved ones have failed. Instead the psychiatrist's nonjudgmental stance and mention of the FDNY cap allowed Mr. Burke to discuss his career, guilt, and depressive feelings. While he was embarrassed to admit it, his grief and depression had led him to feeling estranged from his close-knit family, and he had begun to believe his life held no meaning.

With this understanding, the consultant might make a clarification that emphasizes Mr. Burke's point of view and tactfully highlights the conflict between the well-meaning patient and the well-meaning doctors. In other words, the consultant might try to ally with Mr. Burke's healthy ego, enhance his sense of autonomy, and lay out a framework from which the patient can make a more beneficent choice, one that more accurately reflects his lifelong attitudes toward his world and his own health. The way that this is phrased depends on a number of factors, including Mr. Burke's level of interest, energy, and physical discomfort.

The consultant might say, "It sounds like you've been a deeply successful man. You immigrated to this country, did well with your work, raised a family that you're proud of, and had a wonderful relationship with your wife. You accomplished all of the things that you ever wanted. You don't feel proud of those things anymore, nothing makes you happy, and now they're telling you that they need to take off your leg. It feels like the end of the line."

During this talk, the consultant would watch for inattention or fatigue and might rephrase his comments or change the subject or rework the material over several interviews. The consultant would also continue to use the language and tone of voice that seem most likely to connect to a man who would not appreciate jargon or intellectualized phrases. The consultant might then continue,

> And now that it's the end of the line, you want to go quietly without being dependent on your kids. That's an admirable thing. At the same time, your kids love you very much, your grandkids love you very much, and when you are less depressed, you enjoy them as well. The problem here isn't the leg, since lots of people do fine without a leg. The problem here is your sadness and your helplessness. These are things we can treat. I worry that your need to be tough and independent is going to deprive your grandchildren of a chance to get to know their grandpa and deprive your children the chance to help you out and repay you for all you've done for them over the years.

Depending on Mr. Burke's level of attention, the consultant might continue, "Seems like if you just let yourself die, you'd be going against one of your deepest-held beliefs, that everybody should try as hard as they can, and you've never been a guy to take the easy way out. Seems like you think you'd be helping them by dying, and at the same time, that you'd be hurting them deeply by giving up."

Mr. Burke's response to this sort of statement will help decide the capacity question. If he is unable to understand this comment, regardless of how many pieces it is broken into, it is likely that he does not adequately appreciate the benefits of this low-risk, high-benefit procedure. If he understands but his response indicates a depressed, even suicidal, attitude, then he may lack capacity because of depression. If he understands and is able to coherently discuss his reasons against an amputation, then he may well have capacity to make the decision. If he does have capacity and refuses the surgery, the consultation need not end with a capacity determination, and, depending on the situation, Mr. Burke might agree to psychiatric medications, psychotherapy, and family meetings, all of which might affect his decision. Perhaps most likely, however, is that Mr. Burke would respond to this therapeutic capacity evaluation with a changed perspective and a subdued optimism about his medical and personal future.

The Psychiatric Attitude

Kevin V. Kelly, M.D.

NEUTRALITY, abstinence, and anonymity are principles that have become as identified with psychoanalysis as the couch. They distinguish a psychoanalytic session from an ordinary human interaction and allow the well-inducted patient to become freer to associate and to examine transference. Peter Burke is not in the middle phase of a psychoanalysis, however, when such techniques become most useful. Not only are the goals of his treatment different, but Mr. Burke himself is not a typical analysand. Nevertheless, psychoanalytic theory informs much of the work with Mr. Burke.

The psychiatric consultant immediately faces a challenge that brings psychoanalytic principles into focus. The surgeons are likely to see Mr. Burke's situation in a relatively straightforward way—the patient is making an unreasonable decision to refuse a lifesaving procedure. They may have requested a "capacity consult," but their (probably unexpressed) hope is that the psychiatrist will "talk some sense" into the patient.

The psychiatrist's initial approach to Mr. Burke thus involves a tension between the administrative/forensic task (to determine the patient's capacity to make a decision) and the therapeutic task (to affect that decision in a particular direction). The skillful consultant can perform both functions. Central to this effort is an honest transparency, so that patient and psychiatrist both understand the purpose and goals of the intervention. Underlying honest transparency is the core concept of *neutrality,* a term with a long history in the psychoanalytic literature; it refers to the analyst's position equidistant from id, ego, and superego so that the analyst does not try to influence or coerce the patient in any particular direction. Neutrality is an essential principle in psychoanalysis, but *suggestion,* in the interest of promoting health, is a valuable tool in other psychotherapeutic and medical treatments. While the general medical hospital may seem an odd place to invoke psychoanalytic concepts, the principle of neutrality can help Mr. Burke receive a useful and ethically sound intervention, beginning with the idea that the ethical psychiatrist should refrain from using the therapeutic connection to manipulate the patient into simply doing what the medical team thinks best.

The psychiatrist can begin by explaining honestly that the goal of the consultation is to assess the patient's ability to make a decision about the amputation. People tend to appreciate honesty. The second step is for the psychiatrist to put aside personal convictions and to avoid the trap of becoming yet another doctor trying to coerce Mr. Burke into something he does not want. Technical neutrality allows the psychiatrist to explore how the patient has arrived at a particular position without trying to change that position. As more is known about Mr. Burke, some amount of benevolent manipulation may be indicated, but the initial capacity consultation should be done without such coercion.

While the capacity question might be most pressing, the clinician might defer questions that directly relate to capacity in order to gather a more complete history. An acutely ill man dressed in a hospital gown, Mr. Burke wears a cap from the New York Fire Department. Further, he had been a battalion chief, which is a very high rank within a very hierarchical organization. One of the interesting aspects of psychiatry is the opportunity to learn about many different types of people and different types of work, and the consultant's approach should be quickly informed by some tentative generalizations, which can be revised as more is learned about the patient.

In the case of Mr. Burke, we learn quickly that he is the patriarch of a traditional Irish American Catholic blue-collar family in New York City. Firefighting is a popular occupation in this demographic group, and the men tend to value both their physical vigor and their family connections. They also have a relatively high prevalence of alcohol abuse, and Mr. Burke hints that people close to him had developed difficulties with alcohol. Tact is as important as honesty in psychiatry; further exploration into possible alcohol abuse can be deferred if the patient says he rarely drinks. Nevertheless, it would be wise for the consultant to check other sources for information about alcohol abuse, since alcohol withdrawal could impair Mr. Burke's judgment. This might mean tactfully asking his children and checking lab values for abnormalities such as elevated liver enzymes and mean corpuscular volume.

The clinician might decide to deepen the relationship by asking about Mr. Burke's career. Firemen tend to love their work, and he might feel connected to the consultant through the recounting of stories. At the same time, his discouragement might preclude talking about the old days, especially since he is still grieving his son's death on the job. The patient might particularly enjoy being called "Chief" Burke, a title that would explicitly recognize his accomplishments and remind him of better days.

The consultant should also mull over psychological issues that are typically found in firefighters. These attributes include self-reliance, which might affect Chief Burke's antipathy toward being "a dependent cripple," and a keen sense of guilt and responsibility, which might feed his depressive preoccupation with having failed his wife and son. Another common trait of firefighters is a combination of physical courage and adaptive denial, which allows them to function effectively at times of great physical danger, and which might make Chief Burke relatively unconcerned about death, especially if the alternative is dependency and continued guilt.

Such generalizations may often be true of firemen, but approaching the psychiatric patient involves a more specific understanding that transcends stereotype. The interaction can feel like an enjoyable conversation to both the patient and the clinician, especially if the psychiatrist follows his or her own interest and curiosity about the patient. Psychoanalysts are justifiably wary of using a therapy session for the analyst's personal gratification; this caution is expressed in the principle of *abstinence*. Nevertheless, this patient, like many, will be more likely to interact meaningfully with a clinician who appears to enjoy the interaction.

The project of understanding Mr. Burke is complicated by the limited time available, by his illness, and by his own level of interest in such a process. These limits test other core psychoanalytic principles. One of these is the principle of *anonymity*, which refers to the analyst's resistance to the natural tendency to reveal personal facts and feelings in order to maximize the patient's freedom to fantasize. Patients in nonpsychoanalytic treatments tend not to understand such a concept. If the therapeutic goal includes the patient's honest self-revelation and the rapid creation of a therapeutic alliance, then it is acceptable, and even advisable, for the clinician to reveal some personal thoughts, experiences, and feelings. In so doing, the psychiatrist can indicate that much of what the patient is experiencing is normal and can also model for Mr. Burke a certain way of looking at problems. At the same time, the clinician should not expect Mr. Burke to value his own internal world to the same extent as does the typical therapist; many patients believe that behavior and personal responsibility are more important than feelings, and such a philosophical belief should be respected.

A final pertinent psychoanalytic concept relates to *irony*, which refers to the psychoanalyst's appreciation of the ability to look at a feeling, a memory, or an experience from multiple angles. Irony is generally treasured by analysts, but not by firemen. Through my work with the Fire Department of New York following 9/11, I learned that firemen do not want a clever, uninvolved approach, nor do they want a therapist who uses irony defensively to ward off his own discomfort. Firemen want a "real person" who appears to care about them. In the case of Mr. Burke, he is facing what may be the end of a long and successful life, and doing so without his beloved wife, son, or job. If he accepts the amputation, he will suffer not only a permanent reduction of mobility but also the loss of an important part of his body—a loss that is likely to incite narcissistic and castration fears. The psychiatrist who sits with Mr. Burke should not simply ask a series of cognitive questions but should appreciate the gravity of the situation, recognize that Chief Burke is doing the best he can, and try to understand him in a way that makes practical use of core psychoanalytic concepts.

Depression and Medical Illness

Peter A. Shapiro, M.D.

THE primary surgical team asked the psychiatrist to answer a narrow question: does Peter Burke have the capacity to refuse life-saving surgery? As it became clear that guilt and hopelessness were impeding Mr. Burke's ability to make a decision—and affecting the quality of his life—the psychiatrist rightly expanded the consultation's scope to include psychiatric diagnosis and treatment.

The core diagnostic issue revolves around whether or not Mr. Burke has a major depression. He has many symptoms of depression: depressed mood, guilt, psychomotor slowing, diminished self-esteem, thoughts of death and suicide, and difficulties with sleep, appetite, energy, and concentration. At first blush, he meets symptomatic DSM criteria for a major depressive episode.

The diagnosis of depression in the medically ill is complicated by the overlap between medical and psychiatric complaints. For example, Mr. Burke's lack of appetite, fatigue, and insomnia could reflect depression, but they are also common among sick, hospitalized patients. The problem of *symptom attribution* has led some psychiatrists to argue for exclusion of symptoms that could plausibly be attributed to the comorbid medical disorder. In place of physical complaints, they have suggested an emphasis on cognitive-affective symptoms such as guilt, suicidality, and hopelessness. Exclusion of insomnia as a criterion for depression would make sense if Mr. Burke's sleep were interrupted by leg pain or a noisy roommate. At other times, however, symptom inclusion is appropriate. For example, a study of patients with depressed mood after myocardial infarction found that persistent depressed mood and persistent loss of interest and pleasure rarely occurred in patients who did not also have sufficient other symptoms to make a diagnosis of depression (Lesperance et al. 1996).

Some patients appear depressed, anxious, or personality disordered during a hospitalization but return to a normal psychological state upon discharge. A single cross-sectional perspective is often inaccurate, therefore, especially if it excludes an evaluation of time course. For example, Mr. Burke's depression appears to have persisted for a decade, worsened by the losses of his wife, son, and job. It seems likely that he has developed a chronic major depression, and it seems unlikely that he will rebound into euthymia if his medical situation stabilizes.

Depressive disorder is common but not universal in patients with medical illnesses. While some physicians are prone to normalize depression as a concomitant of medical illness (e.g., "Of course he's depressed—he has to have his leg cut off"), the majority of medically ill patients are not seriously depressed. Prevalence estimates vary widely, but depression is found in about 10%–40% of patients with common, serious medical illnesses such as coronary artery disease, stroke, cancer, AIDS, and diabetes, with the highest prevalence rates seen in more severely ill patients. Neurological disorders such as stroke, Alzheimer's disease, Parkinson's disease, and amyotrophic lateral sclerosis are associated with especially high rates of secondary depression (Rodin et al. 2005). Certain malignancies, such as pancreatic cancer, have a reputation for being associated with depression, but the strength of this association is uncertain. Mr. Burke should be specifically evaluated for medical conditions that are directly implicated in depression, including hypothyroidism and dementia.

While Mr. Burke's medical problems may have worsened his depression, his depression may have contributed to his medical problems. Depression increases the risk of coronary artery disease, for example, and for patients with heart disease, the presence of depression is associated with about a threefold increase in recurrent cardiac events and death. Similar associations have been observed in poststroke and diabetes populations. The triad of previous depression, current depression, and current medical illness has been associated with mortality in excess of that expected with the medical illness alone (Schulz et al. 2000). These negative medical outcomes have been associated with abnormalities of neuroendocrine and autonomic nervous system output, platelet function, inflammatory and cytokine activation, and patient behaviors such as adherence to medication.

Although Mr. Burke may quickly recover from his depression, there is a significant chance that if untreated, he will remain depressed for the rest of his life. An observational study in patients with newly diagnosed coronary artery disease found that 80% of patients with major depression had persistence of depression symptoms at 12-month follow-up. Treatment was associated with an increased likelihood of remission of symptoms (Hance et al. 1996). In a trial of depression treatment in patients with acute coronary syndromes, severity of symptoms in the current episode, onset of the current episode of depression before the acute medical event, and history of prior episodes of depression all predicted a better likelihood of response to antidepressant medication (sertraline) than to placebo (Glassman et al. 2006). While limited, the available data indicate that depression causes suffering, worsens medical outcome, and is not normal or typical. Attempts at treatment are warranted.

Psychotherapy interventions in the medically ill depressed patient have a time-honored place in the literature of psychosomatic medicine, beginning with psychodynamic approaches to understanding and supporting patients through experiences of illness (Kahana and Bibring 1964) and including such specific techniques as the construction of a psychodynamic life narrative (Viederman and Perry 1980), meaning-centered psychotherapy for the terminally ill patient (Breitbart and Heller 2003), and the psychodynamically informed capacity consultation, as well as educational, behavioral, and group-supportive interventions. Few of these interventions have been studied in controlled fashion. Interpersonal psychotherapy (IPT) has been shown to ease the role transitions that are common in patients with depression and medical illness (see Dr. Markowitz's discussion of IPT in the context of Mr. Burke's treatment later in this chapter). For example, studies of IPT in depression associated with HIV/AIDS and with pre- and postpartum depression have had modestly encouraging outcomes (Weissman and Markowitz 2000). Similarly, cognitive-behavioral treatment has improved depression in patients with coronary artery disease (Writing Committee for the ENRICHD Investigators 2003). Pharmacotherapy can be very useful but is complicated by the usual side effects as well as common pharmacokinetic issues and drug interactions. Electroconvulsive therapy and other brain stimulation techniques can be life-saving in the treatment-resistant patient.

It is not clear whether psychiatric treatment improves morbidity and mortality in the depressed medically ill. In the largest studies to date, which involved post–myocardial infarction patients, cognitive therapy did not reduce the rate of recurrent myocardial infarction or death, and a possible beneficial effect of sertraline was suggested but not established (Glassman et al. 2002; Writing Committee for the ENRICHD Investigators 2003). Nevertheless, clinical experience amply supports the view that when depression is successfully treated, medically ill patients feel better, function more effectively, and are more able to participate in their medical treatment. And, in regard to Mr. Burke, an improvement in mood might lead to acceptance of life-saving treatment and a renewed interest in life.

Neurotrophins

Francis Lee, M.D., Ph.D.

NEUROTROPHINS are a unique family of growth factors that influence the proliferation, differentiation, survival, and death of neuronal and non-neuronal cells. Particularly relevant to psychiatry, they mediate learning, memory, and behavior. Alterations in neurotrophin activity have been implicated in psychiatric disorders such as depression, bipolar disorder, and substance abuse, as well as in neurodegenerative disorders such as Alzheimer's disease and Huntington's disease. Although not directly related to the clinical care of Peter Burke, an understanding of neurotrophins can lead to a deeper understanding of his psychiatric illness and may pave the way for a new generation of antidepressant treatments.

Clinical Relevance

The strongest evidence for a role for neurotrophins has been in the pathophysiology of depression, especially depression associated with stress. Underlying this research is the hypothesis that depression causes a dysregulation of synaptic plasticity and neuronal survival in regions of the brain such as the hippocampus. This hypothesis has been strengthened by several lines of evidence that involve one of the major neurotrophins, *brain-derived neurotrophic factor* (BDNF). In animal models, restraint stress has been shown to lead to decreased expression of BDNF in the hippocampus, while chronic physical or psychosocial stress leads to atrophy and death of hippocampal neurons. In humans, neuroimaging has demonstrated a small decrease in hippocampal volume in both depression and posttraumatic stress disorder.

In the case of Mr. Burke, then, it could be hypothesized that decreased or pathological neurotrophin expression could contribute not only to depressive symptoms but to hippocampal atrophy with resultant cognitive decline as detected in his testing.

While its role in mediating these processes has not been entirely clarified, BDNF is an especially attractive candidate molecule in the search for both etiologies and treatments for depression. For example, exogenously administered BDNF in the midbrain or hippocampus has been shown to produce antidepressant effects in two animal models of depression (forced swim and learned helplessness paradigms). These effects were comparable to those of chronic treatment with antidepressant medications. In addition, BDNF has been shown to have trophic effects on serotonergic and noradrenergic neurons in vitro and in vivo. Mutant mice with decreased levels of BDNF have been shown to have a selective decrement in serotonergic neuronal function with behavioral dysfunction consistent with serotonergic abnormalities.

It has long been unclear why antidepressant medications affect serotonin and norepinephrine within hours but do not have a clinical effect for several weeks. Interestingly, selective serotonin reuptake inhibitor (SSRI) and serotonin-norepinephrine reuptake inhibitor (SNRI) antidepressants upregulate BDNF, its receptors in the hippocampus, and c-AMP response element binding factor (CREB), a transcription factor that further upregulates BDNF. These upregulations take 10–20 days, a time course that corresponds to onset of therapeutic action of the antidepressants. Monoamine oxidase inhibitor (MAOI) antidepressants and electroconvulsive therapy (ECT) have also been shown to upregulate BDNF transcription. Finally, in rodent models, ECT has been shown to elicit sprouting of hippocampal neurons.

The Neurotrophin Family

The neurotrophins are the best understood growth factors in the nervous system. Examples include BDNF and *nerve growth factor* (NGF), which was the first identified neurotrophic factor. In the peripheral nervous system, NGF acts on sympathetic neurons, as well as on sensory neurons involved in nociception and temperature sensation. In the central nervous system, NGF promotes the survival and functioning of cholinergic neurons in the basal forebrain. These neurons project to the hippocampus and are believed to be important for the memory processes affected in Alzheimer's disease.

Neurotrophins are unique in exerting their cellular effects through the actions of two different receptors, the Trk receptor tyrosine kinase and the p75 neurotrophin receptor (p75^{NTR}), a member of the tumor necrosis factor (TNF) receptor superfamily (Chao 2003; Huang and Reichardt 2003). NGF binds most specifically to TrkA, while BDNF binds more specifically to TrkB. The p75^{NTR} receptor can bind to each neurotrophin but has the additional capability of regulating Trk's affinity for its cognate ligand.

Neurotrophins promote cell survival and differentiation during neural development (Huang and Reichardt 2003). Paradoxically, they can also induce cell death. p75^{NTR} serves as a pro-apoptotic receptor during developmental cell death and after injury to the nervous system (Roux and Barker 2002). In the context of neurotrophin processing, pro-neurotrophins are more effective than mature NGF in inducing p75^{NTR}-dependent apoptosis (Lee et al. 2001). These results suggest that the biological action of the neurotrophins can be regulated by proteolytic cleavage, with pro-forms preferentially activating p75^{NTR} to mediate apoptosis and mature forms selectively activating Trk receptors to promote survival.

What are the reasons for having a Trk receptor that mediates neuronal survival and a p75^{NTR} receptor that mediates apoptosis, or cell death? Neurotrophins may use a death receptor to prune neurons efficiently during periods of development. In the event that neurons establish connections to the incorrect target, for example, the appropriate set of trophic factors may not be encountered, and this can trigger the release of neurotrophins that fail to activate TrK receptors (failing to trigger growth) but do bind to p75^{NTR} (triggering apoptosis and cell death). Cell death mediated by p75^{NTR} may be important not only for the refinement of correct target innervation during development but also during inflammation, injuries, and nerve lesions.

Genetics

A recent series of studies have linked a single-nucleotide polymorphism (SNP) in the BDNF gene with depression, bipolar disorder, and schizophrenia. The polymorphism involves a single amino acid change (from valine [Val] to methionine [Met]) at position 66 in the pro region of the BDNF protein. Humans with this SNP have reliably been shown to have altered hippocampal memory, as well as decreased hippocampal volume (Egan et al. 2003). In genetic association studies, this SNP appears to confer altered risk for bipolar disorder and depression, as well as higher levels of what researchers call *neuroticism*. In contrast, schizophrenia patients with the Met allele have relatively impaired cortical memory functions. Recently, a mouse model for BDNF SNP was developed; this genetic alteration was demonstrated to lead to increased anxiety-related behaviors during exposure to stressful situations (Chen et al. 2006). The demonstration of the link between psychiatric illness and a polymorphism in the BDNF gene further substantiates the potential importance of BDNF.

Conclusion

Crucial to cell survival, maintenance of differentiated neuronal phenotypes, and the regulation of synaptic connections, synaptic plasticity, and neurotransmission, neurotrophins are increasingly being shown to play a role in the development of such psychiatric illnesses as depression, bipolar illness, and schizophrenia. Neurotrophic factors may also help explain the several-week delay in the efficacy of antidepressant medications—a delay that may be attributable to the delay in upregulation of BDNF after the initiation of medications. Perhaps most importantly, the use of neurotrophins may prove to be an important way to treat the sorts of psychiatric disorders that prevent patients like Mr. Burke from living full lives.

Testing at the Bedside

Marianne N. Findler, Ph.D.

BEDSIDE testing is used to clarify and enrich the clinical impression and is especially useful for patients—like Peter Burke—who manifest overlapping symptoms of depression and cognitive decline. Mr. Burke's evaluation would begin during the initial clinical interview, and observations guide the use of more formal testing. When tactfully confronted with questions that assess memory, for example, depressed patients tend to answer questions with, "I don't know," while cognitively impaired patients tend to perseverate and to try to conceal their memory loss with superficially believable but inaccurate answers. In other words, depressed patients tend to complain of a memory loss, whereas patients with dementia tend to deny the memory loss that objectively exists. Further, in contrast to depressed patients, cognitively impaired patients forget more quickly, fail to make use of memory prompts, and have diminished recognition memory. Evaluation begins, therefore, before the examiner pulls out a scale or worksheet.

Tests for Cognitive Decline

More formal testing can help clarify both the depression and the cognitive decline, and some of these tests are brief and easily administered. Mr. Burke has already had two such tests, both of which were intended to assess cognitive status. Mr. Burke appears to have mild cognitive decline as indicated by both the Mini-Mental State Examination (MMSE) and the Clock Drawing Test (CDT). The MMSE is an observer-rated questionnaire that focuses on distinct but related domains: orientation, attention and concentration, language and praxis, and memory (see Table 2–1). Mr. Burke's score of 23/30 is at the cut-off typically used for identifying cognitive impairment. Advanced age, below-average education or intelligence, poor effort, and coexisting psychiatric or medical illness may lead to a low MMSE and overdiagnosis of impairment. In the case of Mr. Burke, for example, he is 71, depressed, and sick, all of which are likely to lower his score. On the other hand, his professional success indicates a baseline intelligence that may lead to a relatively intact exam, which can, in turn, mask a cognitive decline.

On the second cognitive test, the CDT, Mr. Burke scored a 2 out of 4. The CDT is administered by asking the patient to draw the face of a clock and then to place the hands to indicate 10 minutes past 10 o'clock. The patient receives one point each for drawing a closed circle, for placing numbers in the correct position, for including all 12 numbers, and for placing the hands in the correct position. This task requires executive control, planning and organization, ability to perform in a novel situation, and visuoperceptual and graphomotor skills; these are not evaluated by the MMSE. While results on the MMSE and CDT tend to be at least moderately correlated, the CDT screens especially well for subcortical pathology and deficiencies in executive functioning that are important for assessing functional status. A low CDT score with a grossly normal MMSE can indicate, for example, a person who may have trouble living independently despite reasonably intact memory and verbal skills (Samton et al. 2005).

TABLE 2–1.   DOMAINS ASSESSED BY THE MINI-MENTAL STATE EXAM

Domain	Assessment question	Scoring	Points
Time orientation	Ask for the date, day of the week, and season.	One point each for year, season, date, day of week, and month	5
Place orientation	Ask the patient where he is and then ask specifically for omitted items.	One point each for state, county, town, building, and floor or room	5
Registration	Name three objects and ask the patient to repeat them.	One point for each repeated item	3
Attention	Ask the patient to count backward from 100 by 7. Stop after five answers. (Or ask him to spell "world" backwards.)	One point for each correct answer	5
Recall	Ask the patient to recall the three objects mentioned above.	One point for each	3
Naming	Point to your watch and ask the patient, "What is this?" Repeat with a pencil.	One point for each	2
Repetition	Ask the patient to say "no ifs, ands, or buts."	One point if successful on first try	1
Comprehension	Give the patient a plain piece of paper and say, "Take this paper in your right hand, fold it in half, and put it on the floor."	One point for each correct action	3
Reading	Show the patient a piece of paper with "CLOSE YOUR EYES" printed on it, and ask patient to do what it says.	One point if the patient's eyes close	1

TABLE 2–1. DOMAINS ASSESSED BY THE MINI-MENTAL STATE EXAM *(continued)*

Domain	Assessment question	Scoring	Points
Writing	Ask the patient to write a sentence.	One point if sentence has a subject, has a verb, and makes sense	1
Drawing	Show the patient a pair of intersecting pentagons and ask him to copy the drawing.	One point if the figure has 10 corners and two intersecting lines	1
Total score		Total possible points	30

Source. Adapted from Folstein et al. 2001.

Mr. Burke's results indicate a possible decline in both memory and executive functioning, though it is certainly possible that his MMSE and CDT scores will improve as he recovers medically. Other tests can be used to assess for cognitive decline. The Dementia Rating Scale–2 (DRS-2), a widely used screen for dementia, is especially sensitive to behavioral changes that most often occur in dementia of the Alzheimer's type (Jurica et al. 2002). The DRS-2 can identify differing levels of dementia and can differentiate between Alzheimer's disease, Parkinson's disease, and Huntington's disease. Other useful screening batteries include the Cognistat (Kiernan et al. 1995) and the Repeatable Battery for the Assessment of Neuropsychological Status (RBANS; Randolph et al. 1998). Another well-known screening measure, the Alzheimer Disease Assessment Scale (ADAS; Rosen et al. 1984), combines brief cognitive testing and direct behavioral observation. The Blessed Dementia Scale (Blessed et al. 1968) relies solely on a diagnostic interview with a caregiver.

The Wechsler Adult Intelligence Scale–III (WAIS-III; Wechsler 1997) is more comprehensive and measures general intelligence on the basis of subtests assessing verbal and visual-spatial problem-solving and reasoning abilities. Since language-based functions are relatively resistant to age-related decline, the WAIS-III can offer an estimate of premorbid functioning. The WAIS-III also measures attention and concentration, verbal conceptual thinking and expression, visuospatial skills, and psychomotor speed and coordination. Few psychiatrists are trained in its use, however, and Mr. Burke would likely be administered the WAIS-III only after a referral to a psychologist with expertise in testing.

Tests for Depression and Personality

Mood and personality variables are important components of neuropsychiatric assessment. Two widely used depression scales are the Beck Depression Inventory–II (BDI-II; Beck et al. 1996) and the Hamilton Rating Scale for Depression (Ham-D; Hamilton et al. 1967). While somewhat different from each other (e.g., the BDI is self-report and the Ham-D is observer rated), they have been extensively used in research and clinical practice. Both tests rely heavily on physical complaints, however, that are common in hospitalized patients. For example, Mr. Burke may complain about insomnia, bodily aches, and deficits of energy, sexual interest, and appetite, but these are just as likely to derive from his medical illnesses and prolonged hospitalization as from a depression. In screening Mr. Burke, therefore, it may be useful to deemphasize somatic complaints and focus more sharply on the guilt, pessimism, and wish to die that are more typically found in depressed people. Nevertheless, the Ham-D is the depression scale best known to psychiatrists, and, like the BDI, readily lends itself to serial measurements to assess clinical change. Other scales—including the Cornell Dysthymia Rating Scale (Mason et al. 1993), Geriatric Depression Scale (Yesavage et al. 1982–1983), and Zung Self-Rating Depression Scale (Zung 1967)—assess depression in specific populations.

Efforts are recurrently made to simplify such bedside tests. In their study of a terminally ill population, Chochinov and colleagues (1997) used a variety of brief screening measures and found that none was as valid as a single-item interview that asks, in effect, "Are you depressed?"

Among "personality" tests, the Minnesota Multiphasic Personality Inventory (Butcher et al. 1989) is best known, but it is long (567 true-false questions) and has no age-controlled norms. It is credited in hospital-based psychiatry for its ability to identify patients with factitious disorder and malingering. The Personality Assessment Inventory (Morey 1991) does provide age-stratified norms, but its length (344 questions) precludes its use by the typical sick, depressed patient.

Bedside cognitive tests can be an important adjunct to the clinical interview, particularly when they measure otherwise-overlooked deficits and concerns. Clear delineation of neuropsychiatric disorders can critically inform treatment and planning and allow for a more objective longitudinal assessment of decline and recovery. Just as important as accuracy, however, is the increasing effectiveness of shorter, more accessible tests for the bedside clinician.

Interpersonal Psychotherapy

John C. Markowitz, M.D.

LIFE events can be traumatic, especially if they change self-perception. This link between stressors and emotion is the basis for interpersonal psychotherapy (IPT), a time-limited psychotherapy that has been empirically validated for several psychiatric disorders. In IPT for depression, the therapist and patient link life events and role changes and then work toward transitioning the patient to a more competent, hopeful sense of himself (Weissman et al. 2000).

Mr. Burke is a promising candidate from an IPT perspective, since a confluence of sad events has rendered him depressed. IPT divides such events into several categories, and the initial evaluation would assign Mr. Burke to two such categories. First, his depression began, and never fully resolved, in the wake of two deaths in his family—life events defined by the IPT problem area of *grief (complicated bereavement)*. Second, this former fireman is facing the loss of his physical integrity and competence. IPT therapists define such a life change as a *role transition*. Other interpersonal foci are *role disputes*, which might be pertinent if Mr. Burke's struggles with his children are deemed to be contributing to his depression, and *interpersonal deficits*, a category used primarily for people without significant life events (and hence not applicable here). The goal in treating a role transition is to help the patient mourn the loss of the old role and come to terms with the positive and negative aspects of the new role. For Mr. Burke, IPT might include helping him mourn the loss of his wife and son, mourn the loss of his leg, and come to terms with the roles of widower and amputee. This may seem a daunting task, but the approach works well for many depressed patients and can lead to dramatic changes in outlook and functioning.

The chronicity of Mr. Burke's symptoms raises the question of dysthymic disorder and chronic major depression (Markowitz 1998). In this instance, the crisis of amputation, which presumably coincides with a worsening of depressive symptoms, provides an acute fulcrum for treatment. The IPT therapist, while acknowledging the past events and lengthy duration of Mr. Burke's symptoms, would probably use the acute IPT model to organize the treatment narrative.

One reason that the IPT approach works is that people naturally link depression to upsetting life events. Instead of a weakness, defect, or flaw, IPT therapists view depression as a medical illness that results from life stressors interacting with underlying biological vulnerability. This pragmatic explanation helps define depression as a treatable medical illness rather than a hopeless situation that is the patient's fault. IPT emphasizes that depressive hopelessness and guilt are powerful but misleading symptoms. By working to solve a focal interpersonal crisis, the patient may improve his or her life and simultaneously alleviate the symptoms of the depressive episode. Its medical model makes IPT a good complement to antidepressant pharmacotherapy and also provides a good fit for depressed patients who have comorbid medical illness, like Mr. Burke (Koszycki et al. 2004; Markowitz et al. 1998; Schulberg et al. 1996).

An IPT therapist would use the first 1–3 treatment sessions to accomplish several goals:

1. *Diagnose depression,* using the DSM-IV and a rating scale such as the Hamilton Depression Rating Scale (Ham-D; Hamilton 1960) to assess the depressive syndrome and its severity. It would be important to rule out alcohol abuse as a factor in Mr. Burke's presentation in addition to thyroid and other potential medical confounds. It is also important to determine whether his cognitive difficulties preclude a sustained psychotherapeutic intervention.

2. *Take an interpersonal inventory.* Evaluate the interpersonal context of the depression, including the patient's relationship history and interpersonal strengths and weakness. Who are key social connections, and what sorts of relationships does the patient have with them? Underlying this interpersonal inventory is the idea that social supports protect against depression and that losses increase vulnerability.

3. *Assign the sick role.* Assigning the sick role encourages Mr. Burke to excuse himself for and to accept the acute limitations of his medical illnesses (the depression as well as the diabetes and vascular disease), while underscoring his responsibility to work to maximize his health (Parsons 1951).

4. *Formulate a story that links the depression diagnosis with the interpersonal inventory* (Markowitz and Swartz 2007).

In the case of Mr. Burke, these steps might lead to the following summary:

> Mr. Burke, you've already given me a lot of information, and I want to make sure I understand you. As we've reviewed, you're suffering from major depression. According to your Hamilton score, it is pretty severe. But it's a treatable illness, and it's not your fault. From what you've said, your depression seems connected to what's been going on in your life: it started when you lost your son and then your wife, and it's worse now that your diabetes has gotten worse and you're facing the loss of your leg. Those are terrible losses for anyone to deal with, and they often bring on depression in vulnerable individuals. No wonder you feel like your life has turned upside down and everything's out of control. "I suggest that we spend the next 12 weeks working on all you're going through, which we call a *role transition.* You need to mourn what you've lost or are losing, and see what you can do to make the best of your situation. If you can solve this dilemma, it should not only make your life better, but you'll feel better, too. Does that make sense to you?

Setting a time limit encourages the patient that quick change is possible while pressuring both patient and therapist to proceed apace. When agreement on this formulation has been reached, IPT moves into the middle phase, during which the therapist links the patient's mood to ongoing life events: upsetting events worsen mood, whereas good events improve it. Patients learn to see this connection and to undertake activities that increase their social supports, further their goals, and resolve their life crisis. An IPT therapist might help Mr. Burke to mourn his wife, his son, and his own lost health by exploring his feelings and experiences. For example, did his wife help with his diet and diabetes care? Did she die in the same hospital where he is being treated? How does he feel about losing a leg, and what are his current physical limitations? How has he handled physical injury in the past? These discussions could then explore ways in which this senior fireman could regain as much independence and self-sufficiency as possible. His self-sufficiency may be increased if he can enlist the support of his five remaining children and his friends from his career with New York's Bravest.

Once engaged in his own rehabilitation, Mr. Burke is likely to be a good patient; treating his depression is likely to improve his diabetic care. The therapist would re-administer the Ham-D sequentially so that therapist and patient could mark his progress. Mr. Burke might emerge from treatment thinking of himself as a battered but still proud and active survivor of his diabetes and surgery, sad about his losses but no longer depressed. Sadness per se is a normal affective response to separation and loss; guilt and hopelessness are not.

The final few sessions constitute a termination phase that is used to bolster the patient's sense of competence, anticipate potential problems, and acknowledge sadness over separation from the therapist.

IPT may be an excellent choice for Mr. Burke's treatment, and IPT has been validated as a maintenance treatment of geriatric depression (Reynolds et al. 1999). At the same time, IPT recently appeared ineffective against relapse for depressed patients over the age of 70. This may reflect age-related cognitive deterioration interfering with psychotherapy (Reynolds et al. 2006). Hence Mr. Burke's compromised mental status, diabetes, possible alcohol abuse (given his family history), and family history of Alzheimer's disease might weigh against treating him with IPT. Nevertheless, IPT has been validated as an efficacious antidepressant treatment in randomized controlled trials and may be an especially important treatment for him, especially in conjunction with antidepressant medications (Weissman et al. 2007).

Service Delivery

Martha Bruce, Ph.D.

PETER Burke's situation highlights the complexity of providing appropriate mental health services to community-dwelling, frail older adults. His depression coexists with social losses, medical illness, cognitive decline, physical disability, and social isolation, and these conditions tend to reinforce one another and diminish quality of life. So, while the consultation psychiatrist may successfully help Mr. Burke agree to the amputation, his mental health, medical, and social service needs are far from over.

If Mr. Burke does have the surgery and it is successful, he will need physical and occupational therapy upon discharge. He may be admitted to a rehabilitation hospital. From there, he may be discharged to home (or to the home of an adult child), perhaps receiving home health care services from a nurse to help with medication management and wound care. He will likely qualify for home-based physical therapy. A personal care attendant may come for an hour daily for several weeks. If all goes well, he will become increasingly independent. If all does not go well, Mr. Burke may need additional services, such as home-delivered meals from a social service agency or relocation to residential care. Whether or not "all goes well" for Mr. Burke will depend on many factors—including his mental health—but from a services delivery point of view, the success of his treatment will significantly depend on whether he can access quality, coordinated care that is continuous over time.

Access to Quality Care

Mr. Burke is fortunate to have received a psychiatric assessment during his hospitalization, since mental health problems are typically unrecognized in health care and social service settings. Even in Mr. Burke's case, the consultation question referred to capacity rather than mood, implying that the team's primary concern was efficient medical care rather than the patient's psychiatric issues. When depression is detected by the medical and surgical teams, it is often considered a natural response to stressful events and losses.

Indeed, many people without expertise in mental health would view Mr. Burke's depression as an understandable response to his social losses, medical illness, and disabilities. Sympathy and understanding can serve as barriers to care, however, to the extent that they normalize Mr. Burke's condition as something that does not warrant treatment.

Psychiatry has made significant advances in recent years, but research findings do not immediately reach the clinicians who treat most of the patients. The time lag between the development of a diagnostic or therapeutic finding and its use in community-based practices results in what is known as the "gap" between science and service. This problem is especially true for primary care clinicians, who receive minimal psychiatric training and tend to inconsistently use evidence-based treatments but who provide the majority of depression care. Since their training and focus is elsewhere, the primary care physicians who are most likely to treat Mr. Burke upon discharge will be unlikely to have the time or expertise to adequately monitor treatment side effects, adherence, symptom response, and adequacy of dosage. Mr. Burke's cognitive deficits and inflexibility suggest that his depression may not respond well to typical antidepressant treatment and that his treatment would ideally be performed by a specialist. Such a specialist is likely, however, to not be available.

Access to home health care may help Mr. Burke avoid institutionalization, but most agencies have too few mental health specialists to meet the needs of their medical patients. If Mr. Burke's primary diagnosis were "depression," compensation would likely drop to a point that he would be unable to find a home health care agency that would be able to afford to work with him. Similarly, most health insurers do not provide as much coverage for inpatient psychiatric treatment as they do for nonpsychiatric medical care. Mr. Burke's outpatient psychiatric insurance is presumably covered by Medicare, but it is still common for psychiatrists to avoid geriatric patients because of medical complexity and fee restrictions.

Continuity of Care

Mr. Burke's anticipated travel across health care settings—the hospital, rehabilitation center, home care services, outpatient primary care, residential care—is not unusual among older hospitalized patients. The major health services challenge with every new admission is ensuring that essential health information is transferred with the individual patient. Transferral of information across providers and institutions is notoriously poor, and each step in Mr. Burke's care will lead him further away from the psychiatric consultation in the medical hospital.

If the surgery goes well, Mr. Burke will remain in the hospital only a few days before being transferred for rehabilitation, at which point he will likely still be depressed. Successful rehabilitation may depend upon resolution of depression symptoms such as hopelessness, fatigue, and inattention. Information about his depression and treatment may be critical to the initial success of Mr. Burke's physical therapy, and early progress may be vital to his self esteem and optimism. In addition, successful pharmacotherapy requires that physicians at the rehabilitation center not only know he is taking medications but be willing to reassess dosages and choice of medication. If the rehabilitation hospital and/or homecare physical therapist are adequately informed of Mr. Burke's depression and its treatment, they can adjust their interventions, help monitor his depression, and reduce the likelihood that his depression will undermine his ability to become independent.

Even if information is transferred efficiently, moves are difficult for frail older adults, often leading to heightened anxiety and cognitive difficulties. Stressful life events such as discharge and admission require emotional and logistic adjustments to people who may be experiencing a cognitive decline and may not have spent the night in unfamiliar surroundings in decades. Good continuity of care includes monitoring the well-being of patients as they make transitions, even when the new situation reflects medical improvement.

Coordination of Care

Given the complexity of Mr. Burke's medical and psychiatric conditions, he would ideally be receiving care from a variety of specialists. The challenge is, however, to ensure that their different recommendations and treatments complement rather than conflict with one another. For example, medically ill geriatric patients are frequently prescribed 10 or more medicines. At least one of Mr. Burke's physicians should check for nonadherence to medications, a behavior that may stem from a misunderstanding, a belief that a lack of symptoms means that the drug can be stopped, or cost cutting by the patient. In addition, Mr. Burke is liable to develop serious drug–drug interactions, many of which are psychiatric in nature; his physicians should be prepared to assess medications in regards to their possible contribution to depression, anxiety, psychosis, dementia, and disruptive behaviors.

Electronic medical records are often used successfully within hospitals and provider networks, but such systems are not coordinated between organizations, and, even within organizations, records may be incomplete or inaccessible. Individual pharmacy records tend to be more complete and available. Coordination may be effectively organized around the patient's condition. For example, a chronic disease manager could monitor treatment adherence, side effects, and symptoms related to Mr. Burke's depression, diabetes, and vascular disease. Alternatively, a case manager could focus on his multidisciplinary needs and arrange for services like home-delivered meals. Some of this management could be done by telephone. Mr. Burke is a good example of the efficiencies (from the service perspective) and kindness (from the patient perspective) of integrating these functions into one person.

Family members can play a critical role in ensuring that care is coordinated across providers and over time. They often serve as caregivers and sometimes as health care advocates. Mr. Burke does not want to be a burden to his family, a desire that is laudable in many ways. Given his growing medical needs, physical disability, and cognitive impairment, however, his relationship with his family members is changing. The psychiatrist might introduce the possibility that family involvement could lead to a more-rapid recovery, which would decrease the degree to which he is a burden and increase the possibility that he might eventually return to his own home.

In summary, this case highlights the challenges of providing ongoing, quality care for frail, community-dwelling older adults like Mr. Burke. The current American system does not function well for many of our elderly, and the demand for psychiatric and social services will continue to increase as the population ages. In order to assess the issues and to document the efficacy of treatments, it is vital that geriatric mental health services research grows. As evidence accumulates, it is equally important to diminish the gap between the science and the clinicians who serve our elderly.

Overview of Geriatric Depression

George S. Alexopoulos, M.D.

PETER Burke's case illustrates many of the challenges that face the consultation psychiatrist. The first task for the psychiatrist is to understand the context of the consultation. Clearly, Mr. Burke's physicians are convinced that amputation will be life-saving and that other action is irrational. In their view, the best outcome of the consultation would be for Mr. Burke either to accept their recommendation or, if he is lacking capacity to consent, to have a proxy assigned so that he can have the procedure. The consultant knows that Mr. Burke believes amputation will lead him to becoming a "dependent cripple," but the origins of his fear are unclear. Is he unaware of the support structures now available that increase independence in amputees? Does the state of dependency have an overwhelming personal meaning that interferes with rational thinking? Does his depression lead to unreasonable hopelessness? These questions can be answered only if the psychiatrist develops an alliance with Mr. Burke, clarifies his clinical state, understands the origins of his concerns, initiates treatment for his psychiatric disorder, engages his family and other persons important to him, and participates in the planning of his aftercare.

On a diagnostic level, Mr. Burke has symptoms and signs that are consistent with a major depression. His mood problems occur in the context of personal crises, so the clinician should also consider adjustment disorder with depressed mood. The severity and duration of Mr. Burke's depression are, however, beyond the level of an adjustment disorder. Misdiagnosis of adjustment disorder is common in older adults who face adversity and leads to undertreatment of depression.

Mr. Burke's medical burden, cognitive impairment, and depression have a complex relationship with one another. Vascular disease predisposes to depression and cognitive impairment (Alexopoulos et al. 1997). Moreover, depression itself worsens the outcomes of cardiovascular and cerebrovascular diseases (Davidson et al. 2006; Peterson et al. 2002). These relationships suggest that Mr. Burke would require aggressive antidepressant treatment and careful evaluation of the trajectory and stability of treatment response.

While there is little doubt about the diagnosis of major depression, several diagnostic questions remain (Alexopoulos 2005; Alexopoulos et al. 2002). For example, Mr. Burke is convinced that he has contributed to the death of his son and his wife. Does this belief reach the intensity of a delusion? If so, delusions would indicate a psychotic depression, a disorder that requires a different pharmacological approach than nonpsychotic depression. A delusional belief has personal meaning, is idiosyncratic, is not shared by the patient's culture, and does not yield to reason. Mr. Burke is wracked by guilt; he believes that his own career as a firefighter led his son to the job that caused his death. This belief certainly has personal meaning, the first criterion for a delusion. One can argue that Mr. Burke's thought is idiosyncratic both because its logic is loose and because its content would not be shared by the typical firefighter. It would be important for the psychiatrist to assess the flexibility of Mr. Burke's beliefs. If Mr. Burke's thinking is fixed and false, then Mr. Burke might have a psychotic depression that would require either a combination of an antidepressant and an atypical antipsychotic agent or the use of electroconvulsive therapy (Alexopoulos et al. 2001).

This diagnostic assessment would require a tactful exploration of his relationship with his children and their families. For example, why might Mr. Burke be especially concerned about being dependent upon his children? His son, who is a surgeon, must have discussed the merits of amputation with Mr. Burke. Why did Mr. Burke not respond to his message? Does he want to maintain the proud image of the brave firefighter or does he have a competitive relationship with his sons that make the dependent position unbearable? A dialogue based on such understanding can help Mr. Burke make a rational decision, unless he has psychotic depression, and in that case, his delusions may only respond to antipsychotic agents.

The chronicity of Mr. Burke's depression also raises concern. Was his depression unrecognized by his physician, his family, and himself as often is the case in late life depression? Did his physician or someone in his family identify the symptoms of depression but thought that it was an expected consequence of his circumstances and decided not to intervene? Does he have a "double depression" with major depressive episodes superimposed on a chronic dysthymic state? If so, one should anticipate many relapses and recurrences and plan intense and long preventive treatment.

Characterizing the type of Mr. Burke's cognitive impairment is important because it may influence treatment decisions. Impairment in executive functions, and in its underlying brain abnormalities, predicts poor or slow response to serotonin reuptake inhibitors (Alexopoulos et al. 2005). This effect is rather specific because overall cognitive impairment or memory impairment may not influence the response of depression to antidepressants. While many test batteries for executive functions are available, the Stroop Color-Word Test (Golden 1978) and the Initiation-Perseveration Domain of the Dementia Rating Scale (Mattis 1989) each can be administered at the bedside in less than 5 minutes and predicts response to antidepressants. In depressed patients with abnormal IP or Stroop tests, *problem-solving therapy*—a type of cognitive-behavioral therapy that requires minimal ability to abstract and can be administered to patients with mild cognitive impairment—has been found to be effective (Alexopoulos et al. 2003). If Mr. Burke has abnormal executive functions, a behavioral intervention like problem-solving therapy might be added to the antidepressant medication.

The history of Mr. Burke's cognitive impairment has implications for long-term planning. Vascular disease and depression each can contribute to cognitive impairment and eventually to dementia. While pure vascular dementia is a rather rare disorder, cerebrovascular lesions accelerate the development of dementia in patients with an underlying Alzheimer's process.

Chronic depression with onset in early life may be a risk factor for Alzheimer's disease; inhibition of neurogenesis in the dentate nucleus of the hippocampus is one of the hypothesized mechanisms (Duman et al. 1997). Late-onset depression is often a prodrome of Alzheimer's disease. The syndrome of "pseudodementia" (dementia occurring in the context of major depression, which improves after remission of depression) is no longer viewed as benign. About 40% of patients with depressive "pseudodementia" are diagnosed either with Alzheimer's disease or with vascular dementia 2 years after the identification of pseudodementia (Alexopoulos et al. 1993). If Mr. Burke's signs and symptoms meet the criteria for dementia while depressed or after improvement of depression, cholinesterase inhibitors should be considered, because these drugs may slow down the course of dementia.

The clinical science of psychiatry is much like that of the rest of medicine. The art of psychiatry is the ability to articulate its message in a meaningful way to the patient. To do that in Mr. Burke's case, the psychiatrist needs to understand Mr. Burke's values, long-held views, relationships with his family and friends, and aspirations for the future. Developing a shared vision might be the crucial factor in helping Mr. Burke accept the amputation.

In this case, the evaluation of capacity is less important than the task of understanding Mr. Burke and establishing a dialogue with him that addresses his human needs. The complexity of this dialogue begs the question whether nonspecialized physicians have the training, time, and inclination to engage in such a process. Many difficult clinical decisions are negotiated between patients and nonpsychiatric physicians. Complicated cases such as Mr. Burke's require, however, precise diagnostic thinking, an awareness of the complexities of late-life depression, and a working knowledge of the usefulness and limitations of psychotropic agents. Most importantly, Mr. Burke's complex situation demands a clinician who is able to connect with him and demonstrate that he is understood and has a competent ally who will help him make an important decision and develop a vision about the rest of his life. And that is what a consultant psychiatrist should be especially able to offer.

Summary Points

- Capacity consultations should be ethical and should try to be therapeutic.
- Psychoanalytic principles are useful in the hospital.
- Diagnosis of mood disorders can be complicated by overlapping medical symptoms.
- Depression involves more than serotonin, norepinephrine, and dopamine.

- Assessment of mood and cognition assists with diagnosis and treatment planning.
- Community mental health care often is fragmented, inadequate, and not based on the latest scientific evidence.
- Stressful life events can cause depression in vulnerable individuals.
- Depression can be treated by focusing on stressful life events.

Chapter 3

MOOD INSTABILITY
AND
AMY CAHILL

AMY Cahill, a 30-year-old woman, was brought to the emergency room (ER) by ambulance after she threatened suicide during an argument with her boyfriend. Ms. Cahill had a history of mood instability and tumultuous relationships and had recently been discharged from the hospital's psychiatric unit. The discharge note from that hospitalization concluded:

> It would be difficult to overstate the extent to which Ms. Cahill disrupted the unit. From the time of admission, she split staff, was sexually provocative with male and female patients, and alternated between episodes of tearful hopelessness and superficial levels of cooperation. She became a leader on the unit, but her version of "leading" led to widespread noncompliance with medications and unit activities, complaints to Patient Services, and a flurry of bulimia among several of the adolescent patients. Although she frequently threatens suicide and has a chronically elevated risk of self-destructive behavior, we do not believe she should be readmitted. We say this with the understanding that this hospitalization was precipitated by an overdose of 20 mg of clonazepam and that a similar overdose is likely in the future. Further, since she has been tried on multiple medications without success, we recommend that medications be deemphasized and that treatment should focus on intensive psychotherapy aimed at her borderline personality disorder.

Armed with this information, the psychiatrist approached Ms. Cahill with trepidation but was surprised to find a composed and articulate young woman who, with a smile and moderately pressured speech, described how she was "fine" and did not need to be admitted. With little prompting, she explained that her boyfriend had overreacted during an argument but that she had been doing well since beginning work with an outpatient psychiatrist who understood her. He had diagnosed her with an atypical bipolar disorder with rejection sensitivity and had specifically criticized the earlier diagnosis of borderline personality disorder.

At the time of discharge from the hospital, Ms. Cahill was taking fluoxetine (Prozac) 20 mg/day. To that, her current psychiatrist added valproic acid (Depakote) 500 mg q 12 hours and risperidone (Risperdal) 0.5 mg q 12 hours. He also prescribed three medications to be used as needed: clonazepam (Klonopin) 0.5 mg q 12 hours prn for anxiety, zolpidem (Ambien) 10 mg prn for insomnia, and dextroamphetamine (Dexedrine) 5 mg prn for daytime fatigue. She said this was an optimal combination.

Physical exam revealed a well-groomed, right-handed woman with superficial healed and healing cuts on her left arm. While thin, she had a round face and significantly worn teeth. Labs included a positive toxicology screen for benzodiazepines, elevated amylase level, and a low-normal level of potassium. Her valproic acid level was zero, and her electrocardiogram (ECG) was normal. She denied any substance abuse or bulimia and insisted that her cuts were obtained while she was playing with her cat. She complained of occasional dizziness but denied other medical problems.

Ms. Cahill's boyfriend said he worried for her safety. He said that she had periods of intense energy characterized by a reduced need for sleep, overspending, hypersexuality, irritability, and rapid speech. These symptoms usually lasted a few days. He said that a small disappointment would often send her into a psychological tailspin and she would become desperate. During these periods, she would cut herself and threaten suicide. He was also certain she used laxatives and frequently vomited. He wanted her admitted so that he could safely break up with her.

Personal History

The patient was born and raised in nearby suburbs and had no particular problems until, at age 14, she began to date much older boys and men and disappear for days at a time. These activities troubled her parents, and they frequently fought. Episodes of reckless behavior alternated with an almost symbiotic relationship with her mother, marked by an inability to make independent decisions. Her first psychotherapy began at age 15.

She seemed to manage fairly well in school because of her skills, which included photography and art, and a charismatic interpersonal style that intrigued her classmates and teachers. Since graduating from an elite arts college, she had held no jobs but had sold some of her paintings. She had been supported by her parents and a series of boyfriends.

Personal Psychiatric History

The patient had been hospitalized six times following suicide threats or impulsive, low-lethality drug overdoses. She had tried multiple psychotherapies and medications without noticeable success.

Family Psychiatric History

No family members have been in treatment, but the mother was noted to be "moody and nervous."

Medical History

Noncontributory.

Mental Status Exam

The patient was a thin, round-faced, well-groomed young woman who appeared younger than her stated age. Her speech was of normal rate and rhythm, and she was goal directed and spontaneous in her responses. There were no abnormalities of gait or movement. She said her mood was "fine," and her affect was full range with appropriate smiles. She was not emotionally labile. She denied suicidality, homicidality, and psychotic symptoms. She was cognitively intact, with a Mini-Mental State Exam (MMSE) of 30/30 and a Clock Drawing Test (CDT) score of 4/4. Her insight and judgment were, by history, impaired.

Summary

Amy Cahill was a 30-year-old woman who was brought to the ER by her boyfriend after she threatened to kill herself. The immediate cause of the suicide threat was an argument, while the more chronic psychiatric issues appear to include rejection sensitivity, an eating disorder, and mood instability. The discussions in this chapter explore approaches to Ms. Cahill's diagnoses, the usefulness of a psychiatric hospitalization, and treatment options.

Discussions of the Case of Amy Cahill

Mood Instability 96
  Michael F. Grunebaum, M.D.

Borderline Personality Organization 99
  Frank Yeomans, M.D., Ph.D., and Otto F. Kernberg, M.D.

Axis I and Axis II 106
  John F. Clarkin, Ph.D.

Eating Disorders 108
  Andrew Bennett, M.D., and Katherine A. Halmi, M.D.

Dialectical Behavior Therapy 113
  Beth S. Brodsky, Ph.D., and Barbara H. Stanley, Ph.D.

Risk Management 118
  Marlin R.A. Mattson, M.D.

Pharmacology of Mood Instability 121
  David W. Galarneau, M.D.

Overview of Mood Instability 124
  Janis L. Cutler, M.D.

Summary Points 127

Mood Instability

Michael F. Grunebaum, M.D.

AMY Cahill's unstable moods have left her psychiatrists in conflict over whether she has a bipolar disorder or borderline personality disorder (BPD). The debate is complex, not only because of overlapping symptoms but also because of frequent comorbidity. Understanding the similarities and differences between bipolar disorder and BPD is not merely a matter of academic or philosophical importance, but an issue that may have a significant impact on Ms. Cahill's treatment and ultimate outcome.

As is often the case, the diagnostic "answer" will depend on the quality and reliability of the information as well as on the manner in which this information is organized. For example, Ms. Cahill's discharge note emphasizes her disruption of the unit, sexual provocativeness, emotional lability, sublethal overdose following a fight with her boyfriend, failure of multiple medications, and splitting of staff. Each of these is a description of behavior, but lying beneath these apparently objective descriptions are code words for BPD. Especially telling is the use of the phrase "split staff," a term that refers to an immature coping style in which the patient inappropriately idealizes or devalues different staff members or the same staff member at different times. Not only does this style of relating lead to conflict; the use of the term on an inpatient psychiatric unit is tantamount to a BPD diagnosis.

The current diagnostic system recognizes, however, the frequency of psychiatric comorbidity and—except when specifically noted—demands the recognition of all diagnoses rather than simply the most obvious or dramatic. According to DSM-IV-TR (American Psychiatric Association 2000), a manic episode is diagnosed if the person fulfills several criteria: first, the patient must have experienced a period of elevated, expansive, or irritable mood that persists for greater than 1 week or that leads to a hospitalization. We do not know the exact duration of Ms. Cahill's mood symptoms, but mood problems did lead to the recent hospitalization. Second, the diagnostic manual insists that she demonstrate three of seven specific symptoms. According to the discharge note and her boyfriend, Ms. Cahill has as many as five of these seven criteria: reduced need for sleep, rapid speech, possibly racing thoughts, increased goal-directed activity (sexuality and disruption of the unit), and increased risky, pleasurable behavior (overspending, hypersexuality).

In comparing the two diagnoses with each other, there are many overlapping symptoms. Both illnesses are marked by problematic behavior, particularly high rates of suicide and suicide attempts. People from both groups manifest affective instability, irritability, dysphoria, and anxiety. While DSM-IV-TR notes that BPD is often characterized by "affective instability due to a marked reactivity of mood," it is not uncommon for bipolar disorder to be characterized by "rejection sensitivity." Both groups are frequently noted to be impulsive.

Cognitive symptoms are an important way of differentiating the two disorders. Unlike individuals with bipolar disorder, people with BPD tend to be plagued by chronic emptiness and fears of abandonment. While we do not have direct information regarding either of these, Ms. Cahill's superficial cutting (which she denies) and her apparent desperation do point to the possibility of BPD. Other aspects of the history are nonspecific. The onset of symptoms during adolescence can relate to either disorder. The apparent failure of medications might point toward the personality disorder, but her Depakote level of zero hints at a common problem in patients with bipolar disorder: noncompliance that is often attributable to some combination of side effects and a desire to maintain hypomania. Overall, then, it seems that neither diagnosis can be excluded and that there are multiple preliminary indications that both diagnoses may be accurate.

Ms. Cahill seems to prefer the bipolar disorder diagnosis, presumably because it lacks the stigma of BPD. The inpatient medical team emphasized BPD, possibly because it reduces the blame that they might feel for the messiness of the hospitalization. A particular diagnosis might reassure one or another person, then, but how does a diagnosis actually impact treatment?

It might appear that BPD would lead to a predominant focus on psychotherapy, while bipolar disorder would lead to a focus on medications. There is some truth to this point of view, but psychiatry is rarely an either/or enterprise. It has been widely shown that many psychiatric disorders respond best to a combination of therapy and medications (Rucci et al. 2002), and this is likely the case with Ms. Cahill. She has not responded to multiple medication trials, for example, but these prior failed trials should prompt further inquiry rather than pharmacologic hopelessness.

It is not clear which of the two diagnoses is more likely to create complicated medication regimens, but polypharmacy is especially common in the large cluster of patients with symptoms of both bipolar disorder and BPD. The decision to treat Ms. Cahill with six different psychiatric medications is likely to be well intentioned but is liable to create a host of iatrogenic problems and to distract the patient and therapist from the hard work of psychotherapy. In other words, although there is some evidence for the usefulness of "polypharmacy" (Trivedi et al. 2006), many such efforts are doomed to failure.

Ms. Cahill has not been helped by the psychotherapies that she has tried since the age of 15, but this information should not inevitably point to a BPD diagnosis or to therapeutic nihilism. Patients with either BPD or bipolar disorder are often a psychotherapeutic challenge, and it would be inaccurate to conclude that she has BPD just because she has not been successfully treated by combinations of medication and psychotherapy.

While much has been written about both of these disorders, there remains significant controversy over their pathogenesis. While BPD is often thought of as an interpersonal illness, and bipolar disorder as a primary mood disorder, there is significant overlap. For example, many of the symptoms of BPD seem related to mood unpredictability and instability. Similarly, people with manic-depressive illness have debilitating problems with mood, behavior, and cognition that are likely to lead to interpersonal problems.

A definitive diagnosis may not be possible in the emergency setting. Given her cluster of symptoms, however, Ms. Cahill is likely to profit from conservative, targeted pharmacologic management regardless of the diagnosis. In addition, her lability and interpersonal instability warrant an intensive, well-structured psychotherapy. At the least, a therapeutic alliance could help diminish her chronic noncompliance (Berk et al. 2006; Colom et al. 2005). Further, an ongoing treatment could help teach her ways to control her feelings of desperation, deal more effectively with her relationship problems, and improve her ability to cope with stress.

Borderline Personality Organization

Frank Yeomans, M.D., Ph.D.
Otto F. Kernberg, M.D.

AMY Cahill is in the sort of psychological chaos that is consistent with borderline personality disorder (BPD), though it is also important to evaluate her carefully for bipolar disorder. Misdiagnosing BPD as bipolar disorder is currently common in clinical practice. This may stem from a tendency to interpret the affective lability of BPD as mania and depression. In addition, some clinicians and patients may avoid a BPD diagnosis because of unwarranted stigma and a misperception that treatment is futile. If Ms. Cahill does suffer from bipolar illness, the treatment should, of course, include adequate medication trials. But this case provides ample evidence of borderline personality. In regard to DSM-IV-TR criteria for BPD, Ms. Cahill is noted to demonstrate self-damaging impulsivity (bingeing and purging), recurrent suicidal and self-mutilating behavior, and affective instability. In addition, there is evidence for unstable relationships, a tendency toward idealization, and identity disturbance. Ms. Cahill also demonstrates rapidly shifting self states, as evidenced by her shift from threatening suicide to being "composed" and "fine" in the emergency room.

While DSM-IV emphasizes overt behaviors, it is helpful to consider a model of psychological structure that may underlie and explain this chaos. Borderline personality organization (BPO) is a non–*Diagnostic and Statistical Manual of Mental Disorders* (DSM) diagnostic category based on the concept of a split psychological structure, or structure of the mind (Kernberg 1967). The specific DSM symptoms of BPD can be understood as the external manifestation of this underlying personality structure that determines the individual's experience of self and other. To effectively treat the personality disorder, one must address the structure. Personality—an individual's habitual and automatic way of experiencing self, others, and the world—is the result of the interaction of biological factors, emerging as temperament, and environmental factors. On the psychological level, we can understand the mind as structured around internalized images or representations of the self and of others that are associated with strong affects. This model of the mind derives from object relations theory in which representations of self and other become organized as units, called *dyads*, which link a specific image of the self with a specific image of the other linked by an associated affect (Jacobson 1964; Kernberg 1980; Klein 1957) (see Figure 3–1).

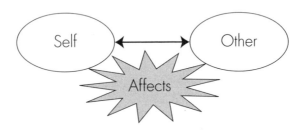

Object Relations Dyad

FIGURE 3–1.   Theoretical underpinnings of transference-focused psychotherapy: objects relations theory.

It is theorized that in early development, the infant is aware of only one state of being at a time: he may experience himself as a satisfied and nurtured infant experiencing loving attachment to a caring and nurturing caretaker, or during moments of discomfort, he may experience himself as unloved, neglected, and abandoned, experiencing fear, anxiety, or rage in relation to an unavailable caretaker who is perceived as cruel and harmful. The dependent state of the infant adds to the intensity of the affects, since survival depends on the other. In the course of development, other basic experiences are internalized in the form of paradigmatic dyads. These experiences of self and other are internalized as memory traces that begin to organize the developing child's experience of himself and the world. In day-to-day life, a particular stimulus can provoke the activation of a dyad, resulting in the imposition of an internal sense of self and other onto the external, real-life situation. In the course of normal human development, narrow and extreme self states (one is *all* angry or *all* loving; the other is *totally* depriving or *totally* giving) become integrated into a more nuanced sense of self and other (e.g., one is angry for a specific disappointment but recalls that the other person has also been generous at times) (see Figure 3–2).

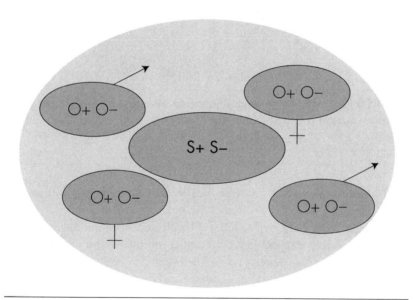

FIGURE 3–2. Normal psychological organization: integration of a complex sense of self and others.

O=object representation; S=self representation; + and − indicate positive and negative affect, respectively.

Why are we speaking of developmental theory when asked to discuss a clinical case? This model of understanding borderline pathology posits that the borderline individual does not achieve the integration of the separate self states into a nuanced and complex sense of self. This situation of *unintegrated and extreme representations of self in relation to other* is the psychological structure we refer to as the *split internal world,* where distinct and disconnected senses of self and other coexist, with one of them determining the patient's sense of self in any given moment (see Figure 3–3).

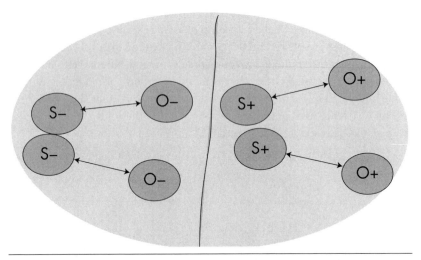

FIGURE 3–3.   Split psychological organization: splitting off and segregating of representations of good and bad self and other.

O=object representation; S=self representation; + and – indicate positive and negative affect, respectively.

This internal structure results in the clinical state of identity diffusion, in which there is a lack of definition of the self, a lack of clear objectives and goals, and a shifting sense of self that is highly dependent on the immediate context. With this split internal structure, a stimulus, especially the action of another person, can activate one of the internal dyads so that the individual's experience of, and reaction to, the situation does not correspond to the complex reality of most interactions, but instead is based on simplified, narrow, and extreme views determined by the internal representations that are imposed, or projected onto the external reality. This way of experiencing life, through the limiting lenses of the internal dyads (representations), can explain the borderline patient's rapidly shifting emotions. A minor stimulus can activate a "total" reaction (a good moment, and the world is perfect; a slight disappointment, and the life is empty and hopeless). It can also explain the chaotic interpersonal relations and sense of emptiness in which there is no continuous sense of self, or "ballast," that carries the person through experiences of different emotional coloring.

This structure can also explain the tendency to experience self and others in terms of idealization and devaluation. If all seems well, the other is experienced as perfect, and perfectly caring. If a problem arises, the other becomes worthless or, perhaps, evil. The same is true of the experience of the self. The sense of self can abruptly shift from grandiose to worthless. In fact, the sense of self is determined by both "poles" of the dyad. The dyad—each whole relationship paradigm—is internalized and becomes part of the self. The sense of self is made up of parts that interact, often in conflict, within the mind. For example, a critical part of the self might attack the rest of the self. In terms of traditional ego psychology, this judging part would be considered the "superego." In terms of object relations, the superego is composed of object relations dyads that come together through the individual's modes of self-evaluation and judgment. In the borderline individual, these judging parts are not integrated with more moderating parts and exist not as a consistent superego but as fragments, or superego precursors.

From a psychodynamic view, we all live in a state of internal conflict between our wishes/impulses, our internal prohibitions, and the constraints of external reality. Borderline patients are particularly prone to experience these conflicts not as internal or intrapsychic but as occurring between themselves and others. This is accomplished through the process of projection of one part of the conflict. For example, if a part of the mind is harshly criticizing the self, that part may be projected and experienced as coming from someone else. One complicating feature of the disorder is that the individual may induce in others precisely the response they both expect and fear.

Turning to Amy Cahill, she sits in the emergency room, contented and composed. For the moment, she experiences herself in a positive state. She feels understood by her idealized new psychiatrist in contrast to his now-devalued predecessors. Shortly before, however, she had threatened suicide when fighting with her boyfriend. At that moment, her subjective experience was probably governed by a sense of her boyfriend as a malevolent, rejecting person in relation to her helpless, hurt self. At that time, she may also have been disturbed by a less-conscious sense of her own intense aggressive feelings and capacity for destructive action. The hospital discharge note adds to the impression of a split structure and identity diffusion. Her sexually provocative behavior with both men and women suggests an unclear sense of self. The leadership role that she used in the service of provoking rebellion on the unit suggests a polarized attitude between the "oppressors" and the "oppressed" in which she consciously identifies with the latter but acts as the former.

How might therapy help Ms. Cahill? *Transference-focused psychotherapy* (TFP) is a psychodynamic therapy based on the object relations concepts described above. TFP focuses on shedding light on the internal structure and working of the patient's mind as they play out in immediate experience, in the here-and-now of the lived moment when feelings and thoughts are simultaneously present, especially in the relation between patient and therapist. We call the therapy "transference-focused" because the treatment centers around the relationship between the patient and therapist, an emphasis that derives from the concept that elements of the patient's internal world are transferred from within the mind and played out and experienced as the reality of the current moment. In other words, the person's experience of a given moment is a combination of perception of external stimuli and of internal images that are not fully conscious but which the patient "reads into" the current experience (see Figure 3–4).

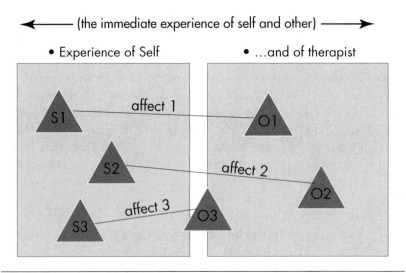

FIGURE 3–4.   Focus on transference in psychotherapy.

S1–affect 1–O1=a particular experience of self and other in the moment.

S2–affect 2–O2=a different experience of self and other in the moment.

S3–affect 3–O3=a third experience of self and other, in which the patient has some awareness that the representation of the other may come from the self.

An overview of the treatment is as follows: an initial assessment establishes the diagnosis *and* the specific problem areas that are relevant to the individual patient.[1] The therapist then proceeds to the discussion of the *treatment contract* (Yeomans et al. 1992), which establishes, in collaboration with the patient, the necessary conditions for treatment. Previous barriers to successful treatment

---

[1]The current diagnostic system leads to a diagnosis of BPD in patients who may present with different prominent features. Some borderline patients may be more externalizing and aggressive, some may be more regressive and withdrawn, and so on.

are identified and parameters to deal with them are agreed upon. For Ms. Cahill, it would be important to discuss her dishonest reporting of information, bulimic behavior, and suicidality, including the establishment of a plan for the patient to follow in the event she feels unable to control suicidal impulses. In this regard, TFP allows for adjunctive resources such as a nurse or internist to monitor amylase levels, electrolyte balances, and dental condition.

If the therapist and Ms. Cahill agree to the conditions of treatment, the therapy begins. The core of the therapy is to engage the patient in observing and becoming aware of the different representations of self and other that are activated in the relation between her and her therapist. Until these representations are observed and discussed, many of them are not in her conscious awareness, but rather are put into action (acted out) without awareness of the meaning and possible distortion that they represent. An example is the aggressive position that Ms. Cahill manifested in threatening her boyfriend with suicide while her conscious experience of herself was limited to feeling helpless and hurt. Judging from her experience on the inpatient unit and with the boyfriend, it can be assumed that such situations will arise in the patient's relation with her therapist. For example, Ms. Cahill might ask if her therapist could change the time of a session. If the therapist checks and says the change is not possible, Ms. Cahill might become enraged and start to yell that this was proof that no one cared. This might culminate in her pacing back and forth and shaking her fist at him in a menacing way. This would be an opportunity for the therapist to ask Ms. Cahill if she might join him in observing and reflecting on the situation. The therapist might then suggest that an observer might see her as treating him badly in much the same way as she accused him of treating her. The therapist might add that such feelings are part of the human repertoire and can be mastered and controlled, but that they pose a special problem if they are denied, because it is not possible to master something of which one is not aware.

As the patient gains awareness of the different images she has of self and others, she will be better able both to compare these images to the lived reality and to reflect upon the experience and intentions of the other (e.g., in the above example, Ms. Cahill might recall occasions when her therapist did change the session time for her). As patients come to have greater awareness of their shifting and contradictory mental states (all good/all bad self and other), they are able to begin to integrate these images into a more full-bodied, nuanced, and realistic sense of themselves and others. As the patient can begin to think, with the therapist, about herself and others in less rigid and dichotomous ways, there is a reduction in the need to keep good and bad aspects of self and others separate. This helps the patient achieve a sense of a more cohesive, intact self, reducing the need to project or act out painful emotions, with a concomitant reduction in the severe symptoms of BPD.

Axis I and Axis II

John F. Clarkin, Ph.D.

THE categorical approach of the *Diagnostic and Statistical Manual of Mental Disorders* (DSM) emphasizes psychopathology, bullet points, and behavioral criteria in an attempt to define subgroups of patients who are relatively homogeneous and who are different from people in other categories. In so doing, it allows for relatively straightforward diagnoses and conforms well to a medical model for both diagnosis and treatment. Critics of the categorical approach to diagnoses point out that behavior and psychology exist on a continuum and that it is not surprising that the current diagnostic system is rife with comorbidities, ambiguities, and controversies. The diagnostic situation is complicated further by the distinction in DSM between Axis II (which consists of personality disorders and mental retardation) and Axis I (which consists of all other psychiatric disturbances). All of these issues are pertinent to the case of Amy Cahill, whose psychiatric diagnoses may lie on Axis I (bipolar disorder and/or an eating disorder) and/or Axis II (borderline personality disorder [BPD]).

The DSM distinction between the two axes is not intended to allow one to make assumptions regarding pathogenesis and treatment, and the differences between the two categories are often uncertain. There is significant evidence that the personality disorders have biological and genetic components for example, and that experience and personality play important roles in the onset, intensity, and clinical characteristics of many of the Axis I disorders. Schizotypal personality disorder may not be fundamentally different from schizophrenia, for example, and Cluster C disorders (avoidant, dependent, and obsessive compulsive personality disorders) may be very similar to Axis I anxiety disorders.

Amy Cahill's clinical presentation lies at the heart of one such ambiguity, that between BPD and bipolar disorder. Both diagnoses are notable for mood fluctuations, for example, and the two diagnoses are sometimes comorbid. Delineating between the two disorders is important—particularly in regard to the creation of an optimal treatment plan—but DSM also makes it clear that if the patient meets criteria for both diagnosis, then both diagnoses should be given. BPD and bipolar disorder are common, severe, and require different (though sometimes overlapping) treatments, and so the diagnostic controversy has spawned a large psychiatric literature.

While there is controversy, clinical experience and research—including our work at Weill Cornell's Personality Disorders Institute—indicates that the key factor in differentiating between the two diagnoses lies in an exploration of Ms. Cahill's self-destructive behavior and interpersonal relationships. The view that these personality-related features should take precedence over the affective symptoms is controversial but supported by a recent multi-site investigation into the relationship between bipolar disorder and BPD (Gunderson et al. 2006). The investigators found that BPD was frequently comorbid with a variety of Axis I disorders, particularly major depression, substance abuse, and posttraumatic stress disorder. Bipolar disorder was less often comorbid with BPD, though comorbidity was still found in almost 20% of the sample. Particularly important in regard to Ms. Cahill is the finding that the presence of comorbid bipolar disorder had no impact on the course of patients with BPD, which underlines the principle that the treatment of borderline personality should take precedence when the two disorders appear comorbid. In other words, patients who meet criteria for both bipolar disorder and BPD and who engage in brief, repeated acts of self-harm and suicide attempts that occur in the context of interpersonal stress and disruption should receive treatment for BPD. Such a treatment may or may not include medications, but an overreliance on medication can lead to unrealistic expectations and neglect of a structured, therapeutic relationship that provides needed grounding for the impulsivity and rejection sensitivity (Stone 2006).

In addition to the important issue of distinguishing between two diagnoses is the larger decision for psychiatry to emphasize psychiatric categories rather than a dimensional perspective that recognizes that psychiatric disorders reflect behaviors, moods, thoughts, and personality traits that merge not only into normality but into each another. In regard to personality, many different dimensions have been proposed and researched. The *Five Factor Model* is perhaps the most widely used; it divides personality into five dimensions: neuroticism, extraversion, agreeableness, conscientiousness, and openness to experience. Everyone can be assigned a percentile score for every dimension, so that an 80th percentile score in conscientiousness indicates a relatively strong sense of orderliness and responsibility. Each of the five dimensions is further subdivided into related components. For example, "extraversion" includes such related qualities as sociability, excitement seeking, and positive emotions, while "neuroticism" reflects a tendency to experience unpleasant emotions easily (e.g., depression, anxiety, angry hostility, self consciousness, impulsiveness, and vulnerability).

In looking at Ms. Cahill, it is likely that her sensitivity to rejection, depression, anxiety, hostility, feelings of desperation, and suicidality would lead to a very high score on the neuroticism dimension. Her relationships seem marked by suspicion, antagonism, and interpersonal conflict, and so it is likely that her agreeableness score would be low. It has been hypothesized that the use of such dimensional scores would provide an important adjunctive source of information. Some researchers have noted, however, that the combination of high neuroticism and low agreeableness is common to many of the personality disorders, while others have proposed that DSM-IV criteria (American Psychiatric Association 1994) may be better predictors of functional impairment than Five Factor scores; these researchers propose the use of dimensional ratings of the DSM criteria that make up traditional diagnostic categories for personality disorders (Skodol et al. 2005). Looking more dimensionally at the criteria for BPD and bipolar disorder—the distinction between which is the diagnostic dilemma that bedevils Ms. Cahill and her therapists—another researcher (Benazzi 2006) found a useful difference in results from structured interviews: affective instability was found in individuals with BPD and those with bipolar II disorder, while "impulsivity" was found in persons with borderline personality but not in persons with primary bipolar illness. Benazzi asserted, in the conclusion to that study, that the DSM category of BPD leads to diagnostic confusion because there are many combinations of criteria that can lead to the same diagnosis.

In the midst of these classification controversies, it remains clinically important to distinguish between BPD and bipolar disorder. Such a distinction may seem academic, but the use of categories and/or dimensions guides the ways in which we think about psychiatric illness, personality, and treatment and, as such, is central to effectively working with people like Amy Cahill.

Eating Disorders

Andrew Bennett, M.D.
Katherine A. Halmi, M.D.

IN addition to problems with mood, impulsivity, and relationships, Amy Cahill has evidence of an eating disorder that may be as lethal as her suicidality. By the time Ms. Cahill leaves the emergency room (ER), the clinician should have assessed safety, made a tentative diagnosis, and devised a treatment plan that takes into account her particular symptoms, preferences, and motivation.

The psychiatrist was first alerted to the possibility of an eating disorder by the boyfriend, and there is abundant confirmatory evidence. The severe erosion of her teeth commonly reflects self-induced vomiting, for example, as do her low-normal potassium and modestly elevated serum amylase. Her dizziness may have been caused by some combination of vomiting, diuretics, and laxatives that would have contributed to volume depletion and electrolyte imbalance. She is described as "round faced," which may reflect the parotid gland enlargement that results from frequent vomiting. She is thin, though we are not given her weight, height, or weight history, all of which would be important in assessing whether she has anorexia and whether her thinness is, in itself, dangerous. Her electrocardiogram (ECG) was normal, which is an important finding since prolonged QTc intervals and arrhythmias are relatively common in people with eating disorders and can be fatal. Finally, we have heard nothing about prior treatment history.

We can assume from an initial glance at her records, then, that Ms. Cahill has an eating disorder. Nevertheless, Ms. Cahill calmly denies that she has a problem with eating, much as she denies that she cuts herself or has been suicidal. Denials can lead the interviewer to try to persuade, cajole, and insist. Such an attitude is likely to lead to frustration and the acquisition of inadequate information.

Instead, it is useful to remain focused on the immediate task, which is to decide whether or not she can be safely discharged or needs to be hospitalized. To make this decision, some definitions should be made clear. There are two primary eating disorders: anorexia nervosa and bulimia nervosa.

Anorexia nervosa is characterized by four related findings:

- Efforts to lose weight and to keep weight below what is considered minimally appropriate, generally below 85% of ideal body weight
- Irrational fears of getting fat
- Disturbance of body image
- In postmenarcheal females, amenorrhea

Bulimia nervosa is characterized by

- Binge eating
- A compensatory behavior(s), usually self-induced vomiting

Under the DSM-IV system, when bingeing and compensation occur in a normal-weight patient, bulimia nervosa is the correct diagnosis. When they occur in low-weight patients, the likely diagnosis is anorexia nervosa, binge-eating/purging type.

The evaluation of Ms. Cahill in the ER is complicated by the fact that she has not admitted to purging, fears of getting fat, disturbance of body image, or amenorrhea. Criteria for hospitalization do not, however, depend on such history. If Ms. Cahill has bulimia nervosa, admission would be recommended if her electrolyte imbalances or ECG were worrisome, if she were dangerously suicidal, or if she had failed multiple outpatient treatments. If she is determined to have anorexia nervosa, binge-eating/purging type, then reasons for admission would include the above criteria but would also include a body weight under 75% of the expected body weight with the need for hemodynamic stabilization, regardless of whether or not her electrolytes are abnormal. To make such a decision, the psychiatrist will need to calculate a body mass index (BMI), assess medical problems and suicidality, and obtain history from the patient, boyfriend, and outpatient psychiatrist.

While the admission decision is central to the job of the ER psychiatrist, Ms. Cahill's long-term treatment for her eating disorder should include many of the same goals and techniques regardless of where her treatment is administered. For the purpose of this discussion, we will assume that Ms. Cahill is diagnosed with anorexia nervosa, binge-eating/purging type and that she has been referred for an outpatient treatment that can be administered in conjunction with treatment for her comorbid psychiatric conditions. It may be difficult for Ms. Cahill to begin such a treatment, and she may fall into a group of patients who are impaired by an eating disorder but are inadequately ill to receive involuntary treatment. In such a case, pressure from family or friends may be useful, as can a straightforward therapeutic attitude that does not blame but rather points out the reality that her physical signs could only come from purging and that it is clear that her eating disorder has taken on a life of its own but can be treated.

The goals of Ms. Cahill's treatment—whether inpatient or outpatient—will include restoration of weight, reduction of efforts to lose weight, nutritional rehabilitation, and improvement in her mood, behavior, and sense of stability. In order to begin such a treatment, the clinician should understand more about Ms. Cahill's eating disorder. The evaluation can begin with a discussion of what she eats on a typical day, including foods that she commonly avoids. This discussion can lead to nonjudgmental inquiry about episodes of purging, including her preferred foods, triggering affective states, and frequency (e.g., after every meal, after some meals). It is also important to understand her pattern of "bingeing," which is the rapid ingestion of food that generally follows a period of fasting. As the eating pattern is clarified, the therapist can discuss and educate about the *bulimic cycle,* which is highly typical of people with Ms. Cahill's cluster of signs and symptom (see Figure 3–5).

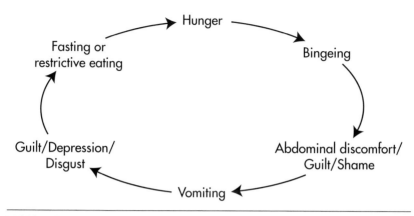

FIGURE 3–5. The bulimic cycle.

This cycle of guilt/fasting/bingeing/vomiting/guilt leads the patient with bulimia to the loss of both internal and external controls. Loss of these controls in turn leads patients like Ms. Cahill to eat irregularly, to fear not being able to stop eating, and to tend not to feel full at the end of a normal meal. While such behavior is intensely private, this cycle is almost universal in bulimic patients.

Treatment is based on the observations that cognitive-behavioral therapy (CBT) techniques can interrupt the binge–purge cycle that is precipitated by dieting and fasting. A first step is to understand and clarify the cycle by keeping a daily record of the times and duration of meals, of binge-eating and purging episodes, and of descriptions of moods and circumstances surrounding binge-purge episodes. Maintenance of a regular eating schedule and avoidance of prolonged periods of restriction is a goal, but at the onset of treatment, an equally important goal is the development of a therapeutic alliance that will allow the patient to discuss a behavior that often evokes shame and secrecy. As the treatment develops, the focus shifts to techniques such as avoidance of cues that trigger a binge-purge episode, development of alternative behaviors, and delay of the vomiting response. Self-monitoring is important, partly because it clarifies patterns to a patient who generally feels out of control. Over time, Ms. Cahill will be asked to develop a list of fear foods and slowly incorporate them into her diet.

It would probably be useful to incorporate CBT for anorexia nervosa in the treatment of Ms. Cahill. The core assumption in CBT is that anorexia nervosa has a significant positive role in the patient's life and develops as a way of coping with adverse experiences. Preoccupation with food and weight distracts her from anxiety and fear associated with difficult transitions and distressing life events. Behavioral methods such as monitoring food intake and the details surrounding food intake, along with techniques such as increasing exposure, are used to increase the patient's food intake gradually. She would be encouraged to challenge her distorted ideas about food and overvalued beliefs about thinness.

Family and significant others may ask about their roles. The general advice, at least regarding an adult patient, is that they should not become "the food police." Such attempts reinforce disputes over food and secrecy. If Ms. Cahill refuses to follow a regular diet, she must take responsibility for the consequences.

Pharmacotherapy will have a role, although a limited one, in treating Ms. Cahill's eating behavior. Antidepressant medications have consistently shown some efficacy in the treatment of bulimia nervosa and have been shown to improve mood and reduce preoccupation with shape and weight. Fluoxetine (Prozac) has been shown to be particularly helpful for treatment in high-normal doses, though any selective serotonin reuptake inhibitor (SSRI) or serotonin-norepinephrine reuptake inhibitor (SNRI), such as venlafaxine (Effexor), is likely to be efficacious. While they may help reduce purging, antidepressants tend not to help normalize weight in anorexia nervosa patients. In addition, even mildly underweight patients with anorexia are susceptible to agitation as a side effect of an SSRI or SNRI. If Ms. Cahill's response is poor, an atypical antipsychotic medication, such as olanzapine (Zyprexa), may be useful in treating the severe anxiety and ruminative, obsessional thinking about food and weight. Olanzapine's appetite stimulation may lead to significant weight restoration but may also exacerbate binge behavior.

Mood stabilizers have a limited role in the treatment of Ms. Cahill's eating disorder. Although there is some evidence that topiramate (Topamax) reduces bulimia nervosa, it would be a poor choice for Ms. Cahill, since it tends to cause weight loss. Purging would make her vulnerable to lithium toxicity, and she would be unlikely to accept the weight gain propensity of valproic acid. Further, it is not clear that mood-stabilizing medications would be justified. Her sleeplessness, irritability, and mood lability may have been caused not by a primary mood disorder but by recurrent episodes of binge eating and purging as well as by diet pills and excessive use of caffeine.

Ms. Cahill has calmly denied her eating disorder in the face of obvious evidence to the contrary. The ER clinician should recognize, however, that there is inevitable shame regarding food and weight among people with eating disorders. She may look calm, but her eating disorder has taken on a life of its own and is likely out of her control. There are a variety of psychological theories that attempt to explain anorexia and bulimia. These include a response to the sexual and social tensions caused by physical changes and maturity fears of puberty, as well as a means to maintain an enmeshed relationship with the mother. In the early stages of treatment, Ms. Cahill will be unlikely to be interested in such theories. Instead, she may be intrigued by a therapist who respects her efforts to maintain her equilibrium; shows tactful, non-judgmental interest; is clear and practical; and does not argue about beliefs that are likely to be firmly held and zealously defended.

Dialectical Behavior Therapy

Beth S. Brodsky, Ph.D.

Barbara H. Stanley, Ph.D.

AMY Cahill's presentation prompts debates about diagnosis, treatment, and hospitalization, but while there is uncertainty, some of Ms. Cahill's problems are clear. She is interpersonally ineffective; distress causes behavioral dysfunction; and she experiences emotional dysregulation. Since these three problems have repeatedly intruded upon her life, Ms. Cahill stands to benefit from dialectical behavior therapy (DBT), a cognitive-behavioral therapy that was designed for the outpatient treatment of self-destructive behavior in individuals with borderline personality disorder (BPD).

The "D" in DBT stands for a dialectic approach that informs the treatment stance. The main dialectic is between two opposing assertions: first, total acceptance of the patient's life by both the therapist and the patient, and, second, recognition of the need for drastic behavioral change. The emphasis on acceptance and validation encourages a nonjudgmental stance toward a population of patients who tend to evoke intense reactions (both positive and negative) from mental health providers. The behavioral perspective is addressed, in part, through the learning of new ways to cope and interact with other people, thereby reducing the perceived need for self-injurious and suicidal behavior. DBT also assumes that the patient is suffering and needs to create a life worth living. To increase personal responsibility and to enhance the potential for happiness, DBT aims for outpatient treatment; inpatient hospitalization is used only when all other means of support for safety are exhausted.

How can the DBT approach help the emergency room (ER) clinician who is trying to assess risk and make decisions regarding hospitalization and treatment recommendations? From a DBT perspective, Ms. Cahill's discharge note might have offered the same final recommendation—avoid hospitalization—but would have been written quite differently. According to that note, Ms. Cahill "disrupted the unit," "split staff," and "was sexually provocative." It is understandable that the psychiatrist "approached Ms. Cahill with trepidation." A stance informed by DBT would understand these behaviors as Ms. Cahill's best efforts to manage what must have felt like an unbearably out-of-control situation. To improve the quality of her life, Ms. Cahill needs to learn the interpersonal effectiveness, distress tolerance, and emotion-regulation skills that are taught in DBT (Linehan 1993a, 1993b), a treatment that could be done following discharge. Such a treatment would depend upon the therapist helping Ms. Cahill become more active regarding her treatment and more curious about her problems.

In the outpatient setting, DBT consists of both individual and group therapy modalities. In the individual session, therapist and patient identify concrete behavioral goals in which life-threatening behaviors (suicide attempts, threats and deliberate self-harm) are the number one target of treatment. Patients are taught how to record their thoughts, feelings, and emotions on a daily diary card, which is reviewed at each session. When self-destructive behaviors and significant suicidal ideation are present, they are the focus of the session. The therapist engages the patient in a detailed review of the self-injury episode, a *behavioral analysis* that helps to identify contributory thoughts and feelings as well as environmental triggers. The analysis also reviews the positive and negative consequences of such behaviors. At each step along the chain of the analysis, the therapist may weave in alternative, more skillful behaviors for the patient to employ in these situations. These behaviors are learned in the *skills training group,* in which emotion regulation, distress tolerance, interpersonal effectiveness, and Zen mindfulness skills are taught through didactics and homework assignments. Incorporating the general skills that are learned in a group setting, the individual therapist helps the patient develop an expanding behavioral repertoire.

In the ER, the DBT-informed clinician would initially focus on assessment of suicidality. Ms. Cahill appears to have become desperate soon after discharge, and while she denies any desire to kill herself, many people do commit suicide in the postdischarge period. While as lethal as those made by people with major depression, suicide attempts made by people with BPD are more likely to be triggered by interpersonal stressors (Brodsky et al. 2006). Such self-destructive behaviors may rally support and can be interpreted as interpersonally manipulative, but self-injury in BPD is often less a communication than an attempt to emotionally self-regulate. In other words, the interpersonal context of suicidal behavior in BPD does not make it less of a safety concern. Since suicide attempts and nonsuicidal self-injury—such as cutting—often serve to regulate emotions, it is not surprising that Ms. Cahill appears euthymic in the ER. Her good mood is also not necessarily reassuring, however, since her mood could quickly darken; in addition, people with BPD who hurt themselves tend to underestimate the lethality of their self-injury (Stanley et al. 2001). Even attempts of low intentionality to die may result in suicide.

At the same time that Ms. Cahill is at significant risk of suicide, an unnecessary hospitalization may deepen the patterns of ineffective behavior and increase the likelihood of unsuccessful treatment and eventual suicide. Psychiatrists charged with deciding whether to admit a patient like Ms. Cahill must skate, therefore, between underestimating the likelihood of suicide in a high-risk population—leading to an inadequate safety net and a potential suicide—and being overly sensitive to the chronic suicide risk—leading to a premature and potentially damaging hospitalization (Stanley and Brodsky 2005).

A DBT approach would expand the evaluation beyond an assessment of apparent suicidality and focus on her internal and external supports. Behavioral analysis focuses on life-threatening behaviors (e.g., eating disorders, unsafe/impulsive sex, reckless driving) as well as behaviors that threaten quality of life (e.g., gambling, overspending,). In the ER, a behavioral analysis assessment would evaluate these behaviors in regard to their precipitants, associated thoughts and feelings, and consequences.

Dysfunctional behaviors have positive as well as negative consequences, and it is important to appreciate the positive consequences without judgment. For example, Ms. Cahill's self-cutting might scar her arms and disturb her friends, but it is likely to contribute to intense emotional and physiologic relief. These behaviors also have an interpersonal context, and the cutting might make her boyfriend less critical and demanding and might temporarily keep them together. Such short-term positive consequences are extremely powerful. For Ms. Cahill to refrain from these behaviors would require tolerating intense amounts of distress. The primary reason to tolerate such distress is the awareness of long-term negative consequences, such as the possibility of losing her boyfriend. With an alliance that is based on understanding both positive and negative consequences to self injury, the outpatient therapist would work to validate the usefulness of tolerating such distress while helping her develop skills to tolerate the distress. In the ER, the evaluating psychiatrist might assess the tools that she already has to control distress, emotional dysregulation, and interpersonal problems, since these are the skills that can help her prevent another suicide attempt and improve the quality of her life. The following vignette illustrates how a (partial) behavioral analysis might proceed with Ms. Cahill:

> **Therapist:** I'd like to know a little more about the fight you had with your boyfriend and the thoughts and feelings that led up to you saying that you wanted to kill yourself.

Ms. Cahill: Oh, I didn't really mean that I would kill myself—I don't have any desire to kill myself now and I'm OK.

T: Well, I'm glad to hear that. I guess when you said that you were very up-set—a lot of people say things they don't mean when they're upset.

Ms. C: Yes, I was desperate—my boyfriend was angry with me and I was afraid that he might leave me. I guess I said whatever I thought would get him to stay.

T: What exactly was he saying to you?

Ms. C: He accused me of overreacting when he wanted to go out with his friends.

T: What happened next? What did you think or feel about that?

Ms. C: I was afraid that if he left, he wouldn't come back.

T: And then what happened?

Ms. C: I told him that if he left I would take Klonopin and die.

T: Did you mean it when you said you wanted to kill yourself?

Ms. C: I guess so—I really can't imagine living without my boyfriend. But I never take enough to die, just enough to calm down. I wouldn't have died.

T: Then what happened?

Ms. C: He called the ambulance to bring me here to the ER.

T: How did that make you feel?

Ms. C: Annoyed. Okay, it's nice that he cares, but I'm still stuck here waiting around and may even get locked up. It's ridiculous.

T: So let's take a look at the positive and negative effects of threatening to overdose.

Ms. C: Well, my boyfriend took care of me, which felt good. But now I'm in another ER, and he's probably running out of patience.

T: So, in the short-term, the threat led your boyfriend to take care of you, but in the long term, you're stuck in the hospital, and he's upset. We call those environmental consequences. How about consequences within yourself? How did you feel right after you threatened to over-dose?

Ms. C: When I first said it, I felt as if I were taking control of the situation, but now I'm embarrassed that I've ended up losing control by being here.

T: In order to hold back from making such a threat, you would have had to tolerate a lot of painful feelings.

Ms. C: That sounds fine now, but in the moment, it's impossible.

T: If I told you that it is possible to learn skills for tolerating distress and controlling your emotions, would you be willing to try?

In real life, of course, the interview may not proceed so smoothly, and Ms. Cahill may retain a tendency to externalize blame, behave impulsively, and refuse to engage in a dialogue. In the context of a nonjudgmental, curi-ous interview, however, it becomes more likely that she will be able to har-ness healthy aspects of herself and participate in a behavioral analysis that would explore the sequence of events, thoughts, feelings, and actions that lead to her self-injurious behavior. The interviewer can assist this process by validating her perspective through supportive comments (e.g., "You must have been upset," "A lot of people say things they don't mean when upset," "You would have to tolerate a lot of emotional pain"). A central goal of the intervention is the identification of consequences (positive and negative, short-and long-term) of the target behavior (suicide threat), consequences that occur both in the environment and in Ms. Cahill's subjective experience. Once these are clarified, changes can be considered. For example, in the dialogue above, the therapist might explore with Ms. Cahill some of her underlying beliefs regarding her boyfriend's motivation in going out with his friends and her own ability to tolerate his leaving.

In addition to working with Ms. Cahill, the therapist would try to change the environmental reaction to her self-destructive behavior. For example, suicidal threats and impulsive low-lethality drug overdoses have previously led to urgent involvement of her boyfriend and hospitalizations. A discharge from the ER would be a significant change in environmental response. If at all possible, a structured DBT day program and enhanced family supports would provide a less comfortable but more beneficial structure that might increase her sense of responsibility for skillful, safe behavior. Such a disposition would be an example of *contingency management,* a DBT technique aimed at modifying the positive consequences for unskillful behaviors.

On the other hand, a brief hospitalization might prevent suicidal behavior while Ms. Cahill regains perspective on her emotions and works toward a more active outpatient treatment program. The meaning of the hospitalization should, however, be redefined. Gunderson and Ridolfi (2001) describe the scenario in which multiple unnecessary hospitalizations create a patient who comes to view hospitalization as the only way her pain can be validated, and who presents herself as needing hospitalization even when the clinician does not believe it is necessary. While such patients may often tolerate discharge, others may benefit from *false submission,* in which the clinician agrees to hospitalize but works toward changing the meaning the patient ascribes to hospitalization. Such a redefinition could be the first step in reducing the positive consequences of hospitalization.

In summary, a DBT approach within the ER would assume that Ms. Cahill's distressing and dangerous behaviors represent her best efforts to regulate extremely painful emotional experiences and that her self-destructive actions are learned, reinforced behaviors that can be addressed in therapy. The goal of the evaluation would be the creation of a comprehensive outpatient treatment that would provide support, enhance safety, and allow for the development of more effective coping skills. If supports are readily available or if the patient is deemed to not be dangerously self-destructive, she should be discharged from the ER. If a discharge is too risky, the plan should be a short-term hospitalization aimed at containment and quick mobilization to an outpatient program.

Risk Management

Marlin R. A. Mattson, M.D.

AS is generally the case in the emergency room (ER), Amy Cahill's psychiatrist is trying to decide whether she can be safely discharged. She has apparently considered killing herself, has been noncompliant with medications, and has a boyfriend who is considering a break up. She denies an obvious eating disorder. She appears to have borderline personality disorder (BPD) or bipolar disorder, or both. The discharge summary from her recent hospitalization identified Ms. Cahill as exceptionally difficult. While the case may fill the ER psychiatrist "with trepidation," it provides an excellent opportunity to explore ways to provide quality care while managing risk.

Before seeing the patient, the psychiatrist read the recent discharge note that asserts that Ms. Cahill should not be readmitted regardless of her presentation. It might be a relief to follow the instructions of a previous psychiatric team, but failure to do an independent assessment would not only reflect poor clinical care but would put the psychiatrist at significant liability risk. Like other ancillary information, discharge notes and summaries should be integrated into a fresh evaluation of the patient.

While the hospital team may have known Ms. Cahill very well, much may have happened in the interval since discharge. As usual, the ER evaluating clinician will need to assess suicidality, outpatient supports (e.g., the boyfriend, the family, the psychiatrist), other potentially dangerous behaviors (e.g., the eating disorder), and the current diagnosis and outpatient treatment plan. Uncovering this information may not be easy, especially if Ms. Cahill is dishonest or if she requests "confidentiality" and asks the psychiatrist not to speak to anyone. In light of her history of overdoses and recent suicidality, however, the ER psychiatrist may determine that additional information is required in order to assess the risk of suicide. Under the circumstances, to *not* speak to important sources of history (e.g., the boyfriend, the psychiatrist) would open the psychiatrist to much more liability than speaking to people over her objection. The interview with the boyfriend may reveal whether or not he has a planned timetable for breaking up with her (i.e., whether he will be a source of support after discharge), as well as provide information regarding her reaction to stress and to prior ER visits. In addition to considering whether to contact family, roommates, and friends, the psychiatrist should be active in the pursuit of data that might not seem obvious, including reports from the police, ambulance, triage nurse, and ER staff members.

The outpatient psychiatrist may be especially important in the determination of disposition. While Ms. Cahill has portrayed him in a particular way, we do not actually know his assessment of her. In addition to understanding his working diagnosis and treatment plan, a safe discharge will likely depend on his assurance that he will treat her even though her suicidality has recurred and her boyfriend may leave. His point of view is likely to be important enough that should he be unavailable, Ms. Cahill may require an overnight stay in the ER until he can be reached.

While the specific criteria for admission are discussed elsewhere, it is important to remember that documentation is a vital part of the evaluation process. Not only is a well-written note helpful to other clinicians, documentation is the best way to demonstrate high quality care and to reduce the risk of legal liability. Further, the process of writing a note can help clarify the clinician's own thinking. In situations with unusual amounts of uncertainty and/or risk of suicide, it may feel safer to write minimally, but the more prudent course is to succinctly but thoroughly document the thought process that went into each of the significant decisions. In regard to Ms. Cahill, for example, the psychiatrist may elicit additional history and decide that it would be in her best interest to be discharged. In such a case, a note might conclude,

> While the chronic risk of suicide remains significant, Ms. Cahill's suicidal ideation has dissipated after each of her prior ER visits, and she is currently denying all suicidal ideation. She has an appointment with her psychiatrist tomorrow, and he has no intention to discontinue treatment. Further, she has an intake appointment with a day program for the end of the week. While her relationship with the boyfriend is tenuous, he denies an intention to immediately break up. An involuntary psychiatric hospitalization was considered, but we decided that it would be in her long-term interest to gain experience dealing with her difficult emotional states through outpatient work rather than through another admission. I do not believe that she is an acute risk for suicide at this time.

A thorough evaluation is important clinically, but it is the ensuing note that demonstrates that the clinician has met professional standards, a core element of medical malpractice. Even in the tragic event of a suicide, a well-documented note renders an adverse legal outcome unlikely. Malpractice does involve three other criteria: that the psychiatrist had a duty to the patient, that the patient was harmed, and that the breach of professional conduct was the direct cause of the harm to the patient. Nevertheless, it is important to recognize that the courts recognize that errors in judgment and bad outcomes are inevitable, but they are not considered malpractice if the physician has documented a thorough, reasonable process of decision making.

On the other hand, the psychiatrist may obtain a different history and decide that Ms. Cahill needs an admission against her will. Under these circumstances, the ER note might conclude,

> Ms. Cahill is being admitted because of a history of significant suicide attempts, and, despite a recent reported history of a suicidal threat, is refusing to reveal any such ideation. Further, her boyfriend has revealed he is leaving her, her outpatient psychiatrist has just begun a month-long vacation, she is estranged from all other family and friends, and she refuses outpatient referrals. While she insists that she will sue the hospital if she is admitted, and the prior discharge summary discourages admission, we have concluded that a brief hospitalization is warranted to reduce the immediate threat of suicide and to organize outpatient treatment. When admitted, she should be carefully observed and warrants constant observation.

Although the worst-case scenario would be the tragedy of a suicide, the more likely scenario would be a temporarily frustrated patient. In either case, a well-written note would likely avert legal consequences. In the above scenarios, it is likely that either ER note would be thorough enough that a malpractice attorney would decline to pursue the case.

In other words, when a physician supports clinical decision making with thorough documentation, the courts provide considerable protection even if errors are made. If the assessment and judgment are not documented, however, the most thorough and thoughtful evaluation may not be sufficient in court, and an attorney or jury may decide that the physician had not met professional standards. As implied in the discussion above, understanding risk management does not eliminate the possibility of a bad outcome, nor does it immediately simplify difficult clinical decisions. Understanding legalities and documentation can, however, reduce the "trepidation" elicited by patients like Ms. Cahill and allow the clinician to do the difficult work of psychiatry with less anxiety.

Pharmacology of Mood Instability

David W. Galarneau, M.D.

THE classic task of the psychopharmacologist is to make a diagnosis, identify target symptoms, select a medication that has been reliably tested for that diagnosis, prescribe, possibly add psychotherapy, wait, and assess the response. If the first medication does not work, then the pharmacologist either switches to or adds a second medication. All of the common Axis I disorders boast clearly defined first-line medications as well as algorithms for use when the first medication is ineffective.

Amy Cahill highlights the common problems of what to do if the diagnosis is unclear, if the symptoms fit best with a diagnosis that lacks an established algorithm, and if the target symptoms fluctuate without apparent regard to medication intervention. Underlying this difficulty is a philosophical one: should physicians aim their medications at diagnoses or at symptoms? This dilemma has been central since the time of Hippocrates, whose *Corpus* argued that treatments should be focused on the cause of the disease rather than the symptoms. This conservative approach helps to avoid treatment complications that were at least as common in ancient Greece as they are today. Such an approach has its limitations in modern psychiatry, however, not least because none of our pharmacologic interventions strike at the heart of the underlying disease. While psychiatric medications can lead to improvements in mood, cognition, and behavior for many patients, they do not change the underlying disease process. For most patients with serious psychiatric disorders, medications may be very helpful, but an optimal clinical outcome requires the addition of psychosocial interventions that help increase the patient's capacity to resiliently adapt.

The initial step in medication selection is identification of diagnoses for which there are reliable treatment algorithms, such as bipolar disorder or an eating disorder. If borderline personality disorder (BPD) is the primary diagnosis, however, treatment is more complicated and controversial. There are currently no medications approved by the U.S. Food and Drug Administration

(FDA) specifically for the treatment of BPD. Psychotherapy is the primary treatment, and medications are adjunctive. When used for BPD, pharmaco-therapy targets symptoms that can be subdivided into three clusters:

- *Affective dysregulation:* mood lability; rejection sensitivity; intense, explosive anger; and depressive symptoms
- *Impulsive-behavioral dyscontrol:* aggression, self-mutilation, and self-damaging behavior
- *Cognitive-perceptual symptoms:* referential thinking, paranoia, illusions, derealization, depersonalization, and hallucinations

How do Ms. Cahill's symptoms correlate with pharmacotherapy that includes fluoxetine (Prozac), valproic acid (Depakote), risperidone (Risperdal), clonazepam (Klonopin), zolpidem (Ambien), and D-amphetamine (Dexedrine)? While it would be useful to hear directly from the outpatient psychiatrist, it appears likely that the fluoxetine is intended to target her affective dysregulation and anxiety symptoms. There is good evidence that all of the antidepressants sometimes reduce BPD symptoms, but selective serotonin reuptake inhibitors (SSRIs) and serotonin-norepinephrine reuptake inhibitors (SNRIs) are most often used because of their relative safety. Fluoxetine may also have been chosen because it is the only FDA-approved drug for bulimia, though its efficacy appears to depend on dosages of 60–80 mg/day rather than the 20 mg/day that Ms. Cahill is being prescribed. Both tricyclic antidepressants (TCAs) and monoamine oxidase inhibitors (MAOIs) might be used instead of the fluoxetine, but they are potentially lethal in overdose, which is especially worrisome given Ms. Cahill's chronic suicidality. Further, her impulsivity and eating disorder reduce the likelihood that she would be able to maintain the low-tyramine diet that is required while taking an MAOI. A final antidepressant that should be avoided is bupropion (Wellbutrin), since it appears to occasionally induce seizures in people who purge.

Valproic acid might have been prescribed for the possible diagnosis of bipolar spectrum disorder, but there is little evidence for its usefulness in reducing impulsivity in BPD. The mood stabilizer may also have been prescribed to reduce the risk of a fluoxetine-induced manic episode. One useful aspect of the valproic acid prescription is that it is accompanied by a blood level of zero, providing us a window into her compliance and honesty.

Clonazepam may reduce anxiety, but Ms. Cahill is at risk for dependence and for misusing the drug in order to become sedated. She recently used her clonazepam in an overdose that may have been precipitated at least partly by the fact that, like all benzodiazepines, clonazepam can exacerbate disinhibition, desperation, and impulsivity in people with BPD. She may have started with 1 mg of clonazepam, for example, and as she became more morose, se-dated, and disinhibited, she might have begun to take more and more until she was eventually brought to the ER. The drug can contribute to memory problems and to daytime sedation that may have led her outpatient psychi-atrist to prescribe the D-amphetamine, a drug that is most indicated for at-tention-deficit/hyperactivity disorder (ADHD) but that may most intrigue Ms. Cahill because of its tendency to cause weight loss. Similarly, Ms. Cahill may have a sleep disorder that requires zolpidem, but it is more likely that she complains of nighttime insomnia because of some combination of poor sleep hygiene and daytime sedation secondary to her use of clonazepam, ris-peridone, valproic acid, and/or amphetamines. Further, sedating medica-tions tend to affect sleep architecture, so that even when medications induce sleep, patients often report not feeling rested the next day.

Like the antidepressants, the antipsychotic medications have been shown to reduce the impulsive–behavioral dyscontrol symptoms that are found in BPD. In addition, the second-generation antipsychotics (SGAs) have been shown to be primary mood stabilizers. Since we are still entertaining a possible diagnosis of bipolar disorder, an SGA, like risperidone, might be directly effec-tive and prevent exacerbation of manic symptoms. Further, the antipsychotic medications may reduce the cognitive-perceptual difficulties that are often found in people with BPD and that may episodically be seen in Ms. Cahill.

Given the many possible side effects and interactions, it seems reason-able to simplify Ms. Cahill's pharmacologic regimen, and I would aim toward using either an SSRI or a low dose of an SGA, or both. She is likely to resist such a reduction. If we are able to develop an alliance and an overall treat-ment plan, I would emphasize the usefulness of targeting our medications and the necessity of ongoing psychotherapy and proceed to work out a schedule for tapering most of her other medications, maintaining the ris-peridone and fluoxetine. If it turns out that she had been entirely noncom-pliant with medications, which seems possible given her valproic acid level of zero, I would probably begin fluoxetine and risperidone simultaneously, though I would consider delaying the SSRI for a few days to give the SGA sufficient time to reach a reasonable blood concentration; such a delay might reduce the likelihood of side effects and an exacerbation of her possible bi-polar illness. While the SGA would likely remain at a low dose, I would be prepared to steadily increase the SSRI, since a relatively high dose would be most likely to target both her depressive symptoms and her comorbid eating disorder.

The use of two medications for Ms. Cahill is not without controversy. Some psychiatrists would prefer to start with only one medication so as to more specifically target symptoms and more carefully assess adverse effects. Some psychiatrists would defer all medications, perhaps in an attempt to emphasize the importance of psychotherapy. Others might add medications from virtually every pharmacologic category to address each of her symptoms, as her current psychiatrist appears to have done. In general, however, the most important aspects of her treatment include a focus on psychotherapy, an effort to prudently make use of the limited evidence that is currently available, and observation of the ancient medical aphorism that suggests that we do no harm.

Overview of Mood Instability

Janis L. Cutler, M.D.

PUTTING oneself in the shoes of the psychiatrist assigned to evaluate Amy Cahill in the emergency room (ER), one can certainly understand approaching her with "trepidation." Given the circumstances, the image of a surprisingly "composed, articulate woman" does not assuage our anxiety. In fact, it is disconcerting. The picture then becomes murkier. We hear about an idealized new outpatient psychiatrist, but if things are going so well with him, and she is on an "optimal combination" of medications, why is she in the ER? We meet a boyfriend who appears to be guilt ridden and possibly on the verge of a breakup. The evaluating clinician's own anxiety and confusion in response to Ms. Cahill provide useful data in understanding this challenging patient and in developing a treatment plan.

It is reasonable to assume that patients who elicit intense feelings may be using primitive defense mechanisms such as splitting and projective identification (Gabbard 2005; MacKinnon et al. 2006). The unusually affect-laden discharge summary suggests that Ms. Cahill displayed emotional states and behaviors consistent with these primitive defense mechanisms during her most recent hospitalization. Furthermore, while the written description of her behavior may be accurate, the intensity of the descriptions suggests that there may be "unmetabolized" affect clouding the writer's judgment. The recommendations have an underlying tone of retribution for the apparent havoc wreaked by Ms. Cahill.

Ms. Cahill is probably inducing a similarly strong emotional reaction in the evaluating psychiatrist in the ER. One danger of such intense counter-transferential responses is that the evaluating clinician might unconsciously act upon those feelings. For example, a psychiatrist who is made uncomfortable by Ms. Cahill may be tempted to prematurely discharge Ms. Cahill from the ER without an adequate treatment plan or to quickly admit without considering ramifications and alternatives. Self-observation and awareness of one's feelings make such an outcome less likely.

Diagnostically, the presence of the primitive defense mechanisms displayed by Ms. Cahill, including splitting, projective identification, and denial, does not by definition mean that Ms. Cahill has a borderline personality disorder (BPD), but it is certainly consistent with that diagnosis. The hodge-podge of "optimal" medications, including three different as-needed ("prn") medications, is suggestive as well. Of particular concern is prescription of an amphetamine in a "thin" woman with a likely eating disorder. One could get mired in a number of differential diagnostic issues as one tries to make sense of Ms. Cahill's history and presentation. Possible diagnoses include bipolar disorder, depression, anorexia nervosa, bulimia, and BPD, as well as other personality disorders (perhaps antisocial, narcissistic, dependent) and even other categories of disorders, such as anxiety, psychosis, trauma, and substance abuse. A general rule of thumb is that one should try to explain as many aspects of a patient's problems with as few diagnoses as possible. How is that helpful in this situation? It may be that there is not one diagnosis that could explain everything, but it is reasonable to assume that the many problems presented here are related in some way. It does seem that at least a subgroup of patients with BPD have a high rate of other comorbid conditions (Zimmerman and Mattia 1999). Thus, the somewhat chaotic list of medications provides further support for the diagnosis with which she was most recently discharged, despite the reported criticism of that diagnosis by her current psychiatrist.

The differentiation between BPD and bipolar disorder remains an unresolved issue in the psychiatric literature (Magill 2004; Stone 2006). One can say with some certainty that Ms. Cahill's presentation in the ER does not seem consistent with a current episode of mania, hypomania, or depression. A definitive diagnosis is probably not possible at this time, at least partly because the patient is obscuring the clinical picture. Her denial of bulimia, insistence that her cuts are not self-inflicted, and valproic acid level of zero all suggest dishonesty. As is often the case, this diagnostic uncertainty may be partly resolved by collateral information such as other discharge summaries, as well as impressions of family members and other involved clinicians.

A definitive diagnosis is not, however, what is most essential at the moment. What is essential is an accurate assessment of Ms. Cahill's suicide risk.

Treatment planning in the ER turns on the following question: Does this patient at this time require hospitalization, or is it possible to provide sufficient outpatient services for safe treatment? (Cutler 1999; MacKinnon et al. 2006). Answering this question is not necessarily straightforward, but it does help to keep the clinician focused: What is Ms. Cahill's immediate suicide risk, and does she require hospitalization? Despite the heartfelt pleas of the discharge summary, hospitalization does need to be considered when thinking about the management of any recently suicidal patient in the ER (Feinstein 1999).

What are Ms. Cahill's risk factors for suicide? One of the strongest predictors of suicide risk is past history. In Ms. Cahill's case, her past history is significant for previous suicide attempts. Assessment of current and past impulse control is also important in considering suicide risk. Ms. Cahill apparently has a pattern of poor impulse control, including self-mutilation and sexual promiscuity. Finally, what is the quality and stability of Ms. Cahill's current support system? While we do not know the nature of her current relationship with her family, close friends are not mentioned, and it seems that she is very reliant on a boyfriend with whom she has been fighting and who wants to break up with her. Ms. Cahill's current suicide risk seems significant.

Does this current high suicide risk automatically necessitate hospitalization? No. But it does necessitate further evaluation in the ER. In particular, Ms. Cahill's composure should be challenged. First, she should be confronted with the inconsistencies in her history and presentation, including the fact that she recently threatened suicide. A modification of Kernberg's structural interview (Kernberg 1984) is a useful model, in that one wants to assess Ms. Cahill's ability to maintain psychological equilibrium in the face of mild stress. "Confrontation" in this case means not that the clinician should be hostile or threatening but that he or she should present a stance of curiosity accompanied by empathy, kindness, and concern. Continued lack of insight and denial on Ms. Cahill's part would suggest the need for at least a brief psychiatric admission, in consultation with her current psychiatrist.

Second, if Ms. Cahill is able to tolerate a more probing interview, the clinician should consider holding a joint meeting with her boyfriend in the ER. In preparation for such a meeting, the boyfriend should be interviewed by himself in more depth, exploring their recent interactions. Perhaps he has already made his dissatisfaction relatively clear to Ms. Cahill, in which case the final "breaking up" would not be a particular surprise. How intent is he for an immediate end to the relationship? It seems doubtful, on the basis of what we currently know, that he would be willing to serve as a stable support for any significant period of time. If he's not, that information may as well be put on the table while Ms. Cahill is in the ER. Thus, in the joint meeting, the boyfriend would be encouraged to present Ms. Cahill with his concerns about the future of their relationship. While such an intervention may seem counterintuitive, in that we are possibly provoking further "acting out" on Ms. Cahill's part, it is far better to observe that reaction in the safe setting of the ER, in which her response can be taken into account in assessing the need for hospitalization.

Finally, how can we consider disregarding the discharging psychiatrist's recommendations? As discussed earlier, they need to be considered, but within the context of possible countertransferential distortions. Certainly, if hospitalization is pursued, it should be brief and should be informed by the course of this recent admission, as well as other admissions. It is probably best for the hospitalization to take place on a different unit. An intensively supervised outpatient setting, perhaps even a day program, may be sufficient. Most importantly, the psychiatrist in the ER should avoid feeling that certain options, such as hospitalization, are a priori off limits, which would be succumbing to the black-and-white thinking that this patient needs help in overcoming.

Summary Points

- The goal of the emergency evaluation is generally the least-restrictive safe disposition.
- Cross-sectional symptom assessment may be misleading.
- Careful assessment of symptoms and history usually yields a reliable diagnosis.
- Psychiatric evaluation and treatment planning can be affected by the clinician's countertransference.
- Borderline personality disorder (BPD) and bipolar disorder have overlapping symptoms and are frequently comorbid but can usually be differentiated.
- In addition to DSM diagnoses, it is useful to assess levels of personality organization.
- The bulimia cycle generally begins with dieting, not overeating.
- Thoughtful risk assessment and documentation are clinically and legally important.
- A prominent treatment of people with BPD features a central dialectic: patients are doing the best they can and they need to change.
- Pharmacology that targets symptoms rather than syndromes can lead to unnecessary polypharmacy.

Chapter 4

SCHIZOPHRENIA AND ANTHONY DA PIAZZA

AN inpatient psychiatrist went to evaluate Anthony Da Piazza, a 54-year-old single man with schizophrenia. Mr. Da Piazza had just been admitted for his fourteenth psychiatric hospitalization after he decompensated in the context of his mother's hospitalization for recurrent cancer. Via telephone, the emergency room (ER) psychiatrist reported that Mr. Da Piazza lived with his 84-year-old mother and that her illness was terminal. That morning, during the third week of her own hospitalization, Mrs. Da Piazza became alarmed when it appeared that her son had neither showered nor eaten for days and had apparently begun to burn the artwork in his bedroom. She was specifically concerned because his previous auditory hallucinations had revolved around the imminent end of the world and because she was his only living support. Worried, she called her medical intern, who escorted Mr. Da Piazza to the ER.

Mrs. Da Piazza said that her son had been psychiatrically stable since moving in with her 9 years before. He had previously lived in a series of group homes and homeless shelters but returned home after his father had died. She explained that he had remained isolative and suspicious of strangers but had developed a routine that included spending many hours each day drawing highly detailed self-portraits, which he tacked neatly around his room. The walls and ceilings had become encrusted with several layers of art. She had arranged for his drawings to be shown in three art shows in the past 2 years, and several of them had been sold to collectors.

Personal History

Mr. Da Piazza was raised in Queens, New York, the only child of working-class parents. He had graduated as a below-average student from high school, where he had been an odd and isolative teenager. He attended some college and was a part-time student at the time of his first psychotic decompensation. He did not earn a degree and had never held a job. He learned to draw at Fountain House, a community center for the chronically mentally ill. He attended Fountain House several times per week, where he drew but made no friends. Mrs. Da Piazza noted that "being an artist" was the first thing that her son had said he wanted since childhood.

Personal Psychiatric History

The patient was first hospitalized after he attacked his father with a knife when he was 22 years old. On the day of the attack, he was noted to be agitated, paranoid, and hearing voices. The psychiatrists had initially considered the possibilities of drug intoxication and mania, but when his psychosis persisted for many weeks, he was diagnosed with schizophrenia. Records from his first hospitalization referred to a family "double bind," difficulty with his "schizophrenogenic mother," and the need for restraints and seclusion despite the use of "rapid neuroleptization." Ongoing conflicts led to frequent hospitalizations, noncompliance with treatment, and prolonged periods of homelessness and estrangement from his family. Mr. Da Piazza tended to gain weight when his illness was under control. When psychotic, he tended to quit eating and become very thin.

According to his mother, the patient had smoked marijuana frequently as a teenager and had experimented with LSD during college. At the time of his first psychotic break, he was enrolled in college but had made little progress toward a degree. She did not know about his history of substance abuse or violence during the time in which they were out of contact. At present, he was being treated in a community health clinic, where he saw a psychiatrist every 6 months and adhered to his medication regimen. He had passed multiple drug screens and had been psychiatrically stable during the 9 years that he had lived with his mother.

Medications

Haloperidol 10 mg daily and benztropine 1 mg twice per day. Uncertain recent adherence.

Family Psychiatric History

Mr. Da Piazza's maternal grandmother was institutionalized at a state hospital for the final 30 years of her life with an uncharacterized psychotic disorder.

Medical History

Noncontributory.

Mental Status Exam

The patient was disheveled, disorganized, and thin. His tongue darted repeatedly out of his mouth, and his jaw clenched rhythmically. His speech was slow and nonspontaneous. He said he was worried but denied a specific threat. His affect was sad and constricted. While he appeared to be responding to internal stimuli, he admitted only to hearing his father say, "Finish." He explained that he had created his intricately detailed drawings in an effort to "save his mom" but had begun to burn them because his plan had not been working. He was grossly inattentive but refused formal cognitive testing. His insight and judgment appeared poor.

Summary

Anthony Da Piazza was a 54-year-old man with schizophrenia who was hospitalized in the context of a psychotic decompensation that appears to have been triggered by his mother's terminal illness. The discussants in the following sections explore the nature of schizophrenia, its impact on patients and their families, and the various treatment modalities that can be used to improve the quality of life of those afflicted with this neuropsychiatric disorder.

Discussions of the Case of Anthony Da Piazza

Schizophrenia 133
  Adam Savitz, M.D., Ph.D.

Violence and Schizophrenia 137
  Zachary Freyberg, M.D., Ph.D.

Schizophrenia and Brain Circuitry:
A Neuroimaging Perspective 141
  *Daniel Weisholtz, M.D., Jane Epstein, M.D., and
  David Silbersweig, M.D.*

Psychodynamics of Psychosis .146
  Eric R. Marcus, M.D.

Outsider Art 149
  Aaron Esman, M.D.

Pharmacology of Schizophrenia 151
  Donna T. Anthony, M.D., Ph.D.

Cognitive-Behavioral Therapy .156
  Yulia Landa, Psy.D.

Comprehensive Healthcare 159
  Steven P. Levine, M.D.

Recovery 162
  David W. Schab, M.D.

Homelessness and Social History 165
  Kim Hopper, Ph.D.

Overview of Schizophrenia 168
  Roberto Gil, M.D.

Summary Points 172

Schizophrenia

Adam Savitz, M.D., Ph.D.

SCHIZOPHRENIA has caused Anthony Da Piazza enormous hardship. There is no way to know who he might have become, but it is clear that his illness threw him off a normal life trajectory and led to recurrent psychosis, relentless isolation, and profound psychosocial dysfunction. His long-suffering mother is now facing the possibility that her own death will lead him to further marginalization and a future that may include homelessness and institutionalization. Mr. Da Piazza's tragic situation not only is typical of schizophrenia but also reflects the varied ways in which schizophrenia has been conceptualized over the past century.

Emil Kraepelin first described *dementia praecox* in the late 1800s (Kraepelin 1919/1971). He focused on the early cognitive decline, odd behavior, lack of socialization, and deteriorating life course that separates these patients from those with manic-depressive illness. Eugen Bleuler coined the term *schizophrenia* in 1911. He emphasized the hallucinations, delusions, and disorganization that are common in schizophrenia, conceptualizing the central problem as a mind split off from reality (Bleuler 1911/1950). Unlike Kraepelin, Bleuler did not emphasize the deteriorating course of the illness. In the 1950s, Kurt Schneider focused on *first-rank symptoms* in an effort to identify psychotic symptoms that would differentiate schizophrenia from the psychotic mood disorders. These Schneiderian symptoms include audible thoughts, voices arguing and commenting on one's actions, thought broadcasting, delusional perceptions, and experiences of being controlled by others. Later work showed that these psychotic experiences are found in other psychoses and are not limited to those with schizophrenia (Carpenter et al. 1973). In the 1980s, researchers began to characterize schizophrenia by sets of symptom clusters that included *positive symptoms* (symptoms in excess of the average), *negative symptoms,* and *disorganized symptoms* (Andreasen and Olsen 1982; Buchanan and Carpenter 1994). Positive symptoms are hallucinations and delusions. Negative symptoms are often listed as the "5 A's": *anhedonia* (lack of interest or pleasure in things), flat *affect, alogia* (lack of or slow speech and thoughts), *avolition* or *apathy,* and poor *attention.* In the 1990s, Michael Green demonstrated the link between schizo-phrenia and cognitive impairment. Deficits in memory, concentration, and executive function (e.g., planning and shifting from one activity to another) contribute to much of the social and community dysfunction associated with the illness (Green et al. 2000).

All of these clinicians would have recognized Mr. Da Piazza as a person suffering from schizophrenia, but each would have emphasized a different aspect of the illness. Kraepelin would have noted the chronic course of Mr. Da Piazza's illness and emphasized his inability to hold a job as well as his odd, repetitive drawing of self-portraits. Bleuler would have focused on Mr. Da Piazza's auditory hallucinations, his delusion that his paintings might save his mother's life, and his lack of social interaction. Schneider might have emphasized the command auditory hallucinations and the special meaning of the paintings. Carpenter would have conceptualized the delu-sions and hallucinations as positive symptoms and the lack of socialization, poor grooming, and constricted affect as negative symptoms. Though not much is known about Mr. Da Piazza's cognitive functioning, Green might speculate that the patient's poor attention and likely poor memory and plan-ning led to his dependency and overall poor functioning. These differing viewpoints on schizophrenia may reflect differing theoretical backgrounds, but the varying emphases may reflect either that persons with schizophrenia present with varying symptoms or that there are multiple types of schizo-phrenia.

While there are disputes about the relative importance of the different symptoms, psychosis is one of the two central problems in schizophrenia. Broadly defined, psychosis is a distortion of reality testing. In other words, the person believes something to be true that is either known or believed to be false by an external consensus (or by the observing psychiatrist). Psycho-sis usually includes delusions (false, fixed beliefs) and/or hallucinations, which are false sensory perceptions that are usually auditory in schizophre-nia. Psychotic people often demonstrate disorganization of speech and behav-ior, such as nonsense talk, inappropriate use of language, and odd or repetitive actions. Psychosis can be caused by many different disorders including mood disorders such as depression and bipolar disorder, dementia, and per-vasive developmental disorders such as autism and severe mental retarda-tion. Psychosis can also be caused by intoxication with such substances as methamphetamine, cocaine, and angel dust (PCP; phencyclidine) and by med-ical problems such as infection, intracranial masses, and stroke. The quintes-sential psychotic disorder is, however, schizophrenia.

Mr. Da Piazza's psychosis may be obvious and dramatic, but his chronic disorganization and cognitive deficits may have been more incapacitating during the preceding decades. These symptoms are the ones that likely deprived him of the ability to function independently even in the absence of psychosis.

The debilitating effects of schizophrenia generally begin in early adulthood. As is typical, Mr. Da Piazza's first "psychotic break" occurred while he was in college. Other men first show signs of schizophrenia during military boot camp. The onset of schizophrenia tends to be a few years later in women, though the illness can begin anytime between childhood and middle age. Later onset tends to be associated with greater functionality.

As a teen, Mr. Da Piazza was odd, isolative, and a below-average student. This may reflect a schizophrenic *prodrome* during which he became less able to function at school or work, increasingly withdrew from society, became less able to groom and care for himself, and appeared increasingly odd. It is unclear what Mr. Da Piazza was like as a child. Some patients are entirely normal before the prodrome, while others are long noted to be isolative and unusual. Mr. Da Piazza's use of marijuana and LSD may reflect typical adolescent behavior of the early 1970s, but he may have used the marijuana to control anxiety and may have used the LSD as a way to give himself the impression that he was in control of his own psychosis. Mr. Da Piazza also has a history of violence as a young man. Violence is not uncommon in young men with schizophrenia, and it would be important to further explore this aspect of his history. As with many people with schizophrenia, Mr. Da Piazza's twenties and thirties were marked by recurrent hospitalizations, homelessness, deterioration of functioning, and noncompliance with antipsychotic medication.

Mr. Da Piazza found stability during his 40s, likely because of a stable home situation and compliance with medications. It appears that his relationship with his father had been stormy and that he returned home only after the father died. Environments that are critical and deprecating or are chaotic are said to be high in *negative expressed emotion*. Such environments tend to lead to relapse in patients with schizophrenia (Bebbington and Kuipers 1994). During this latter period, Mr. Da Piazza lived with his supportive mother, had few responsibilities, and participated in a social club—Fountain House—that was created for people with schizophrenia. Mr. Da Piazza's hobby of painting is unusual, since the negative symptoms of schizophrenia tend to create apathy.

Mr. Da Piazza is facing the loss of his mother, but he is also entering into a phase of illness that is unpredictable and less well studied. Some patients improve significantly during their fourth and fifth decades of having schizophrenia. People like John Nash, whose life was depicted in the film *A Beautiful Mind,* are, however, quite unusual. More common is a second phase of cognitive and functional deterioration. Much of this deterioration may be secondary to medical problems that cluster in people with schizophrenia.

People with schizophrenia smoke tobacco at very high rates, leading to increased cardiac, cerebrovascular, oncologic, and pulmonary diseases. In addition, the widely used atypical antipsychotic medications are associated with increased rates of obesity, diabetes, hyperlipidemia, and hypertension (Shirzadi and Ghaemi 2006). Mr. Da Piazza does not appear to have significant medical problems, but he has developed repetitive, abnormal movements of the tongue and jaw that indicate tardive dyskinesia (TD), a common side effect of long-term use of haloperidol. While not usually dangerous or uncomfortable, TD increases the oddity of his appearance and reduces his ability to fit comfortably into society.

Beginning with early observers like Kraepelin and Freud, most theories of causation have emphasized the biological underpinnings of schizophrenia rather than psychological or social causes. The precise origin of schizophrenia remains unknown, though genetics is clearly implicated. The risk for the disease is elevated for relatives of a patient with schizophrenia, but the risk is highest if the affected person is an identical twin. In that case, the other twin has a 50%–60% chance of also having schizophrenia. While Mr. Da Piazza had a grandparent with a psychotic illness, most patients do not have a close family member with schizophrenia. Unlike some illnesses that are caused by one abnormal gene, it appears schizophrenia may be caused by collections of multiple abnormal genes. The affected genes may differ from patient to patient, and this variation may partly explain the heterogeneity of symptoms and clinical course of schizophrenia. A number of other factors modestly increase the risk of schizophrenia. These include maternal viral infection during the second trimester, starvation conditions in utero, winter birth, birth trauma, and being raised in an urban setting (Mortensen et al. 1999).

Mr. Da Piazza and his family appear to have suffered from theories that have been disproved and/or purged from clinical practice but likely influenced his early treatment. For example, his old records mention terms that were developed during a period when psychoanalysts strayed from Freud's view of schizophrenia as a biologic illness. Theoreticians hypothesized that "schizophrenogenic mothers" contributed to the illness by being cold, distant, and controlling (Parker 1982), somewhat akin to the "refrigerator mothers" who supposedly caused autism. Other writers created the "double-bind theory," in which schizophrenia was more likely in homes where there was no possibility of a good outcome (i.e., "damned if you do, damned if you don't") (Bateson et al. 1956). Before these theories were disproved, family members had to struggle not only with an ill family member but also with unnecessary guilt. As is often the case in medicine, however, theories swing back and forth, and it is now recognized that stressful transitions can indeed precipitate the onset of schizophrenia, while criticism and stress can lead to a schizophrenic relapse. Further, it is now clear that having a psychotic child can lead reasonable parents to suboptimal behavior, so that parenting styles may be a response to the child's abnormalities rather than be the cause of a largely genetic illness. Psychosocial intervention becomes, then, less about criticism and more about understanding, counsel, and the creation of a supportive environment.

Mr. Da Piazza is at a crossroads. His life course is similar to many people with schizophrenia. He went from being an odd teenager to dropping out of college with full-blown illness. He has had many common symptoms of schizophrenia and an extended period of instability, with multiple hospitalizations and homelessness. He was able to find relative stability upon his return home to a stable, noncritical living situation and the structured, nonpressured activity at Fountain House, an organization that grew out of the highly influential Recovery movement. While he has found an activity—drawing—that occupies his time, he remains unable to work or function independently. Mr. Da Piazza's history is consistent, therefore, with the fact that while there have been great strides in the understanding of schizophrenia's underlying pathophysiology, its high rates of disability have not changed in the last century (Hegarty et al. 1994). While he and his mother have worked hard to help him develop his artistic talent and to achieve a stable home life, Mr. Da Piazza's future is uncertain. Neither society nor the scientific literature has much to say about middle-aged patients with schizophrenia who are no longer able to live with their families.

Violence and Schizophrenia

Zachary Freyberg, M.D., Ph.D.

ANTHONY Da Piazza threatened his father with a knife when he was 22 and now, at age 54, is burning his drawings. In addition to these documented episodes of violence, his history is marked by prolonged periods in which he was apparently homeless or living in shelters, group homes, or psychiatric hospitals—places in which violence is relatively common. Mr. Da Piazza's history bears upon the controversial link between schizophrenia and violence.

While most people with serious mental illness are not violent, one large schizophrenia study found a 19% prevalence rate of violence in a 6-month period (Soyka et al. 2007). Other studies have found that 5%–10% of severely mentally ill people commit acts of serious violence each year and that psychotic people are responsible for 9% of the homicides in Europe and 5% of the homicides in the United States (Torrey 2006).

In reviewing Mr. Da Piazza's history, he meets most of the general risk factors for violence. Specifically, he is a male with a history of violence who quit school relatively young, exists on the fringes of society, and has used illicit substances (Webster 2005). In addition, Mr. Da Piazza has had periods of medication noncompliance, with poor insight into his condition and need for treatment. His auditory hallucinations and delusional beliefs regarding the end of the world are schizophrenia-specific risk factors for violence (Soyka et al. 2007). While not noted in Mr. Da Piazza, antisocial behavior would also increase his risk (Torrey 2006).

Though difficult and imprecise, the assessment for future violence is critical, especially in people like Mr. Da Piazza who have a history of violence and are being evaluated in an acute care setting. Observation of affect and physical activity helps determine the risk for immediate violence, and many agitated or fearful people may need to be calmed by medication before the interview can proceed. During the actual interview, the interviewer should try to be straightforward and nonthreatening, avoiding prolonged eye contact and overly challenging questions. To minimize his or her own risk of being hurt, the psychiatrist should ensure a quick exit by sitting next to the door or by conducting the interview in a hallway. Security personnel and other staff members should also be available to help in case of attack. In other words, safety outweighs other important goals that range from the maintenance of absolute privacy to rapid, uninterrupted data acquisition.

In interviewing him about violence, it might be useful to ask whether anyone had ever started a fight with him. Such an approach might allow Mr. Da Piazza to provide justification for prior violence and/or allow him to report important but embarrassing aspects of his history. If some alliance is created, it would then be useful to directly ask whether he has been violent toward others. Throughout the evaluation, observation remains critical and if Mr. Da Piazza were to appear to become dangerously agitated or paranoid, the interviewer might tactfully defer questions, leave the room, and give Mr. Da Piazza a few minutes to cool down (Alpert and Spillmann 1997).

Since we lack a thorough history, we do not know the extent to which Mr. Da Piazza's illness and history of violence were affected by substance abuse.

Like half of all persons with schizophrenia (Gregg et al. 2007), Mr. Da Piazza has used illicit substances. A high rate of substance abuse has been attributed to the so-called self-medication hypothesis, which posits that persons with schizophrenia use drugs to treat their underlying positive and negative symptoms. Others have postulated that individuals with schizophrenia want to feel that they control their symptoms and so they take drugs that will induce psychotic symptoms so as to "normalize" their psychosis. Others have suggested that persons with schizophrenia are increasingly exposed to substance-abusing peers as they drop out of school and begin to occupy marginalized fringes of society. A more biologic model suggests that since schizophrenia and illicit substances share dopamine pathways, there may be a greater vulnerability toward addictive behaviors (Gregg et al. 2007). None of these observations has, however, been confirmed. Similarly, researchers have tried to clarify a possible link between substance abuse, schizophrenia, and violence, but results are mixed (Foley et al. 2005; Soyka et al. 2007; Vevera et al. 2005).

The neurobiological exploration of violent behavior in schizophrenia is in its infancy. Nevertheless, preliminary evidence suggests that persons with schizophrenia with a history of violence are more likely to have neurological soft signs than are nonviolent persons with schizophrenia. Imaging studies of individuals with schizophrenia with a history of violence have also found impaired connectivity between the orbitofrontal cortex and amygdala, as well as more frequent structural abnormalities in the amygdala, compared with individuals with schizophrenia without such history. Other studies found, however, that men with schizophrenia who have a history of violence did *better* on neuropsychological testing than those without a history of violence. Moreover, those with early-onset antisocial behaviors had fewer brain abnormalities than those without these behaviors (Naudts and Hodgins 2006). These results are as yet unexplained, and as is often the case, early research findings will have little impact on the evaluation and treatment of any one patient like Mr. Da Piazza.

How should we treat Mr. Da Piazza's agitation, portrait burning, and potential violence? The most important interventions center on returning him to his baseline level of health. As discussed elsewhere, such efforts will likely include restarting his medications and helping him deal psychologically with his mother's illness. In the acute setting of the emergency room, staff members should do several things, especially if Mr. Da Piazza is agitated and threatening. The first is to reduce external stimuli such as noise, crowds, and interpersonal conflicts, though such an intervention is often more easily done on an inpatient unit than in the typical hubbub of an emergency room. The second would be to acutely manage agitation pharmacologically (Citrome 2007a). Using medications early will decrease the likelihood of violence and may be therapeutic in treating underlying psychosis. Typically, an antipsychotic medication is administered either alone or in concert with a benzodiazepine such as lorazepam.

If Mr. Da Piazza remains agitated, paranoid, and (potentially) violent in the context of his mother's terminal illness, he will likely warrant a multimodal intervention that would include both medications and behavioral treatments. If Mr. Da Piazza fails two or three trials of a standard antipsychotic medication, he should be considered for clozapine, which appears to have an unusually positive antihostility effect that is independent of its effects in reducing positive and negative symptoms (Citrome 2007b). Mood-stabilizing medications have been used for treatment of aggressivity in schizophrenia, but without evidence of their efficacy. Benzodiazepines have also been used, and while they do acutely sedate, they can cause disinhibition and dependence, leading to possible exacerbation of agitation and violence.

Psychotherapy might help Mr. Da Piazza de-link his concern and love for his mother from the need to burn his drawings; his mother might be enlisted in this effort, and he might become able to recognize that his world will continue after she dies. Cognitive-behavioral treatments might include the creation of a token economy that would reinforce his saving his old portraits, while *activity programming* might include structured recreational activities such as a painting class (Alpert and Spillmann 1997). These activities could help him develop strategies to elicit positive feelings without the need to resort to fire and destruction. Therapists might also use *negative feedback* strategies that could reduce his destruction of his drawings through negative consequences. In the acute outpatient setting, it is difficult to see how these strategies might help someone as desperate and psychotic as is Mr. Da Piazza, which is one reason he required inpatient hospitalization.

Once an alliance is created, a variety of therapeutic techniques may be quite helpful, in regard to not only the reduction of violent behavior but also his compliance with medication and his willingness to enter a supportive setting. Perhaps more importantly, an ongoing therapeutic relationship (or cluster of relationships) may be critical in helping Mr. Da Piazza deal with the looming loss of his mother and develop techniques, connection, and hope that can provide him with the wherewithal to safely overcome his crisis.

Schizophrenia and Brain Circuitry: A Neuroimaging Perspective

Daniel Weisholtz, M.D.

Jane Epstein, M.D.

David Silbersweig, M.D.

STRUCTURAL and functional neuroimaging may be useful in the evaluation of new-onset or atypical psychotic symptoms, but they are unlikely to assist in the diagnosis of Anthony Da Piazza, whose history is typical of schizophrenia. In conjunction with advances in cognitive and affective neuroscience, however, research using neuroimaging techniques does provide considerable insight into the systems-level neuroscience that underlies many clinical features of schizophrenia.

In a classic study, Liddle and colleagues used positron emission tomography (PET) to investigate how regional neural activity correlated with three schizophrenia subsyndromes determined by factor analysis: disorganization, psychomotor poverty, and reality distortion (Liddle 1987; Liddle et al. 1992). The subsyndrome of disorganization subsumes the disorganization and gross inattentiveness displayed by Mr. Da Piazza on mental status exam. Psychomotor poverty incorporates many of schizophrenia's negative symptoms, such as the poverty of speech and constricted affect seen in Mr. Da Piazza. The reality distortion subsyndrome consists of delusions, such as Mr. Da Piazza's belief that his drawings could save his mother, and hallucinations, such as his history of auditory hallucinations concerning the end of the world. The investigators found that patients with prominent psychomotor poverty and disorganized symptoms demonstrated hypoactivity in distinct regions of the prefrontal cortex (PFC), while patients with prominent reality distortion symptoms demonstrated increased activity most strongly in regions of the temporal lobe (described below).

Prefrontal cortex has been one of the brain regions most consistently implicated by functional imaging studies in the pathophysiology of schizophrenia. Individuals with schizophrenia generally show reduced activity (hypofrontality) in PFC compared with control subjects. Much of this research has focused on the *dorsolateral prefrontal cortex* (DLPFC), a region of the PFC occupying the superior and lateral aspects of the cerebral convexity. The DLPFC is involved in retrieval of learned information, planning and strategy development, working memory, and maintenance of a set of abstract rules (Cummings and Mega 2003). Dysfunction in this system is therefore a likely substrate for many of the cognitive impairments seen in schizophrenia (see Figure 4–1A).

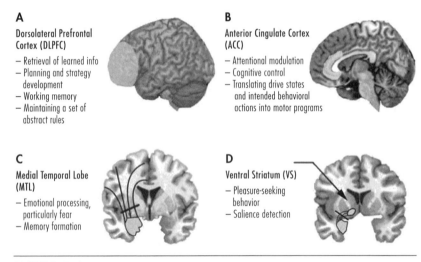

A

Dorsolateral Prefrontal Cortex (DLPFC)

– Retrieval of learned info
– Planning and strategy development
– Working memory
– Maintaining a set of abstract rules

B

Anterior Cingulate Cortex (ACC)

– Attentional modulation
– Cognitive control
– Translating drive states and intended behavioral actions into motor programs

C

Medial Temporal Lobe (MTL)

– Emotional processing, particularly fear
– Memory formation

D

Ventral Striatum (VS)

– Pleasure-seeking behavior
– Salience detection

FIGURE 4–1. Brain regions involved in schizophrenic psychopathology and some of their functions.

Dysfunction of particular frontal lobe regions (**A and B**) are likely to play a role in the cognitive disorganization and psychomotor poverty seen in schizophrenia. Dysfunction of medial temporal lobe structures and their interactions with other areas of the cortex, particularly in the frontal lobes (**C**), is implicated in the pathophysiology of schizophrenic hallucinations. Abnormal interactions between the ventral striatum and medial temporal lobe structures (**D**) may lead to an oversensitive salience-detection system that could lead to paranoid delusions. Hash marks through the lines that connect brain regions in C and D indicate dysfunctional interactions between the connected regions.

Cognitive tasks that activate the DLPFC in normal control subjects tend to do so to a lesser degree in schizophrenia patients. Interpretation of this finding is complicated by the fact that schizophrenia patients tend to perform more poorly on the tasks relative to psychiatrically healthy control sub-jects. Therefore, it is difficult to determine if the poor performance is a result of an intrinsic dysfunction in DLPFC circuitry or if the failure to activate DLPFC is simply a reflection of the patients' failure to perform the task prop-erly for other reasons (e.g., poor attention, distractability, low motivation). It has been shown that, like schizophrenia patients, normal control subjects who engage in a working memory task that is beyond their abilities demon-strate a decrease in activity in DLPFC commensurate with the decline in their performance (Weinberger et al. 2001). Conversely, studies of schizo-phrenia patients with normal or near-normal working memory performance tend to show increased rather than decreased activation of the DLPFC as com-pared with normal subjects (Callicott et al. 2000). Thus, DLPFC efficiency may be decreased in schizophrenia, such that a greater mobilization of DLPFC circuitry is necessary in schizophrenia patients than in healthy control sub-jects in order to achieve a given level of performance.

Abnormalities in the functioning of another region of PFC, the *anterior cingulate cortex* (ACC), have also been noted in schizophrenia. The ACC lies on the medial surface of the PFC and plays an important role in attentional modulation and cognitive control. Additionally, it serves an important role in translating drive states and intended behavioral actions into motor pro-grams. In schizophrenia, abnormalities of ACC function may contribute to both cognitive disorganization and psychomotor poverty (see Figure 4–1B).

Multiple methodologies have implicated medial temporal lobe structures in the pathophysiology of hallucinations and delusions. Both physiologic and structural abnormalities in this region have been identified in associa-tion with these features of schizophrenia. In patients with temporal lobe ep-ilepsy, the prevalence of psychoses (10%–19%) is nearly double that found in patients with generalized epilepsy (Gaitatzis et al. 2004). In the study of schizophrenia described above (Liddle et al. 1992), the severity of reality distortion (hallucinations and delusions) was found to correlate with in-creased resting activity in the left temporal lobe, particularly in the parahip-pocampal gyrus, a cortical gyrus on the medial surface of the temporal lobe overlying the hippocampus and amygdala. The hippocampus and parahip-pocampal gyri are also specifically activated during schizophrenic hallucina-tions, along with lateral temporal and parietal neocortices (Silbersweig et al. 1995).

Subtle structural abnormalities in the medial temporal lobe have been shown in schizophrenia both antemortem and postmortem. Pathology stud-ies have demonstrated smaller and disarrayed pyramidal neurons in the hip-pocampi of deceased patients with schizophrenia (Harrison 1999), and MRI studies of living patients have demonstrated modest decreases in the size of the hippocampi and parahippocampal gyri (Wright et al. 2000). In addition, focal lesions of the ventral hippocampus in rats during early development can lead to the emergence of schizophrenia-related behaviors in adolescence—an effect not seen if the lesion is made in adult animals (Lipska and Weinberger 2000). Therefore, hippocampal abnormalities present early in development may not manifest behaviorally until frontotemporal and subcortical circuits have reached a sufficient degree of maturation in late adolescence/early adulthood. This finding may help to reconcile the wealth of evidence implicating developmental and genetic factors in the etiology of schizophrenia with the observation that major symptoms of the disorder do not usually manifest themselves until late adolescence or early adulthood.

While the frontal and temporal lobe abnormalities described above may account for different aspects of schizophrenic psychopathology, they are not independent of each other. These lobes and their subregions are highly interconnected, and integrated *frontotemporal networks* mediate many important cognitive and emotional processes. In a study utilizing both PET imaging and structural magnetic resonance imaging, Weinberger and colleagues (1992) demonstrated that in subjects with schizophrenia, decreased left anterior hippocampal volume correlated with decreased activation of the DLPFC during a cognitive task. This suggests interdependence of medial temporal lobe pathology and functional abnormalities in the frontal lobe and highlights the significance of frontotemporal circuits in the pathophysiology of schizophrenia. Altered frontotemporal functional interactions have also been described in this population (Friston and Frith 1995), and structural imaging studies have demonstrated decreased integrity of the uncinate fasciculus, the cingulum bundle, and the arcuate fasciculus—white matter tracts connecting the frontal and temporal lobes (Kubicki et al. 2005). These findings support a model of disconnectivity of frontotemporal networks in schizophrenia (see Figure 4–1C).

One potential consequence of disrupted frontotemporal connectivity of relevance to psychosis concerns the disruption of what is known as *efference copy*. When a behavioral or mental activity is initiated in the frontal lobes, a signal is relayed to temporal or posterior cortices that helps these cortices to distinguish between self-initiated versus externally initiated perceptions. Disruption of such efference copy may result in the misinterpretation of self-initiated thoughts or actions as coming from an external source and may underlie the symptoms of auditory hallucinations and delusions of alien control commonly experienced by individuals with schizophrenia (Blakemore et al. 2002).

The delusions and hallucinations of patients with schizophrenia are most often experienced as personally relevant and emotionally charged, and frequently exert considerable influence on a patient's behavior and social interactions. These features likely reflect dysfunction of limbic networks involved in the evaluation of internal and external stimuli in terms of their significance to the well-being of the organism, and the subsequent guidance of motivated behavior. Key regions in these networks include medial temporal structures such as the amygdala and hippocampus, the ventral striatum, and paralimbic cortices such as the parahippocampal gyrus and orbitofrontal cortex.

Functional imaging studies of patients with schizophrenia have shown impaired responses to salient stimuli in the ventral striatum (Taylor et al. 2005) and abnormally elevated activity in the medial temporal lobe in response to non-emotional stimuli (Epstein et al. 1999; Holt et al. 2006), specific to patients with active paranoid delusions (Epstein et al. 1999). Psychosis has been proposed to reflect a state of aberrant attribution of salience, a processing bias associated with abnormal interactions between the ventral striatum and the medial temporal lobe, such that importance is excessively and inappropriately attributed to external or internal stimuli (Epstein et al. 1999; Kapur 2003) (see Figure 4–1D). Interactions of an abnormal "salience-detection" system with perceptual, cognitive, and behavioral systems can result in misinterpretations and maladaptive behaviors, particularly in the setting of impaired frontal executive function, with decreased top-down modulation of limbic circuitry.

The *ventral striatum* is of particular interest because it receives a robust dopaminergic projection from the midbrain. Medications that ameliorate hallucinations and delusions are believed to work by affecting this dopamine pathway, either by directly blocking dopamine receptors in the ventral striatum or by indirectly modulating the dopaminergic influence of the ventral striatum (Roth et al. 2003). Antipsychotic medications have also been shown to alter DNA transcription in this brain region (Heimer et al. 1997).

There is no doubt that functional neuroimaging methodologies, combined with allied methods of investigation, have advanced our understanding of the roles played by various brain circuits in mediating the symptoms of schizophrenia. This enhanced understanding can pave the way for the development of novel treatments involving direct brain stimulation and, together with a growing knowledge of the locations of specific receptor subtypes, will allow for rational drug design, such that future pharmacotherapies will target abnormal brain circuits with increasing sensitivity and specificity. This should lead to more effective treatment while minimizing the side effects that lead so many patients like Mr. Da Piazza to abandon their medications. The complexity of schizophrenia is immense, but a functional neuroanatomic approach to its understanding holds great promise for improving the lives of those afflicted by this devastating illness.

Psychodynamics of Psychosis

Eric R. Marcus, M.D.

PSYCHODYNAMIC psychotherapy helps psychotic patients improve their adaptation to reality and decrease their psychotic functioning. In addition, psychodynamic and psychoanalytic theory can help make sense of Anthony Da Piazza's emotional experience as well as the psychotic symbolic representations that stem from his abnormal ego functioning.

The word *ego* was originally used by Freud to mean a sense of self. As psychoanalytic theory evolved, ego came to mean a set of psychic functions that organize reality, including defenses, reality testing, cognition, memory, and the ability to synthesize information. All of these functions are likely to be impaired in a patient like Mr. Da Piazza. Such impairments do not mean, however, that Mr. Da Piazza lacks a sense of himself or that his experience is without meaning. Further, while antipsychotic medications are the mainstay of schizophrenia treatment and can help organize ego functions, the effects of these medications are modest, the side effects are many, and compliance tends to be fairly poor. Psychodynamic therapy can help Mr. Da Piazza become more able to work with his illness and find meaning in his life, and it can also help him develop insight into his need for the medications that can help reduce his symptoms.

There have been multiple psychoanalytic perspectives on psychosis. Melanie Klein focused on symbolic derivatives of aggression, especially feelings of envious hatred; according to Klein, the intensity of the aggression led to the ego dysfunction. Michael Balint theorized that severe mental illness was caused by a "basic fault" in the personality that led to the emptiness and terror of psychosis. The interpersonal approach emphasized the connection between the therapist and the patient and sought causes in the interpersonal relationships of the patient. In each of these theories, ego dysfunction was not primary but the result of a more fundamental problem. Modern theory is less interested in hypotheses as to psychological causality and is more comfortable with the reality that genetic and biologic processes play important roles in the causation of psychoses.

Instead of broad theorizing, modern ego psychologists would try to create an alliance with Mr. Da Piazza and work to explore the meaning of his hallucinations and delusions. For example, it appears that Mr. Da Piazza has developed a catastrophic emotional reaction to the terminal illness of his mother, on whom he has relied for structuring both his external life situation and his ego functioning. He experiences this impending loss symbolically as an "end of the world" psychotic catastrophe that includes both auditory hallucinations and delusions. While these psychotic phenomena can be viewed in multiple ways, they appear to be a condensation of his concern about his mother's terminal illness, the likely loss of his supportive home environment, and the end of his life as he knows it. In regards to ego dysfunction, the psychosis reflects a dissolution of the boundaries separating reality experience, emotional experience, and sensation/perception.

After gathering an initial history and creating a safe environment, a dynamically oriented therapist would begin an intervention that could go in a number of directions. Regardless of the details, the underlying goal would be the creation of an alliance that is based on the therapist's tactful recognition that Mr. Da Piazza is dealing with an overwhelming emotional experience and that he does, indeed, believe that his world is ending. The dialogue also provides an opportunity to fill in some of the gaps in Mr. Da Piazza's ability to make sense of his experience. It would be important to learn more about Mr. Da Piazza than is outlined in his history. In particular, we would want to know more about his strengths and worries. As is true in all therapies, a central skill is the use of tact and timing, both of which are especially important in patients who, like Mr. Da Piazza, are prone to ego dysfunction and an intensification of symptoms.

The therapist might begin by asking Mr. Da Piazza exactly what he hears when he hears the voices. The history indicates that he hears his father's voice muttering, "Finish." The therapist might then ask what this means. Schizophrenia tends to impair the ability to free associate, and it is likely that Mr. Da Piazza will not have a theory about the meaning of his words. Nevertheless, Mr. Da Piazza may be able to discuss the psychotic phenomena and is likely to feel comfort that someone is interested in his perspective. When asked to say what comes to mind when he hears the word "Finish," Mr. Da Piazza might respond, for example, by saying that his mother was born in Finland and that his father thought Italy was the center of civilization and that Finland was at the end of the world and that he loved his mother. The psychiatrist might then ask if his father's voice is saying that the two Finnish, he and his mother, are finished. Such an intervention would be likely to produce an emotional connection; it is also likely to induce anxiety.

If the anxiety is obvious and the therapist appears to be on the right track, the therapist might point out that Mr. Da Piazza's mother's illness is very frightening because it seems as though were she to die, his whole world would end. Mr. Da Piazza may be able to discuss such a possibility, but the fractured state of his ego functions may lead to a response that is mute or something simple, like "Finish." As the conversation proceeds, the therapist would provide reflections and suggestions that make use of the patient's specific symbolic representations; such an effort would be an attempt to provide support and increase Mr. Da Piazza's awareness of possibilities despite his mother's illness. The therapist might then explicitly suggest that Mr. Da Piazza needs to live with other people in a situation where mother's functions are provided; a warm, caring, motherly place—a clean, safe place with good food, a routine, and a place to do his art—and not a cold, uncaring Finland place.

Recognizing the importance of his mother and his mother's opinion, the therapist might point out that Mrs. Da Piazza always encouraged and valued his art. Even if the drawings had not prevented her illness, his art had made her feel good and was an important connection between the two of them; the therapist might then suggest that there is no reason for him to burn something that had been so helpful and important to her. The way in which this information is conveyed to Mr. Da Piazza will depend on multiple variables, including his level of paranoia, cognitive disorganization, and ability to create an alliance, but much of it will depend on the clinician's ability to creatively resonate with the patient. In maximizing the intervention's effectiveness, it is urgent to include the mother in the treatment so that she can help transition him into a new living situation and encourage him to continue his drawing. The psychiatrist might suggest that she reinforce that his drawings can be a continuing bond between the two of them and that he should stop burning them, that she loves his drawings and that, while *she* may be dying and may be finished, *he* isn't finished. Such a family meeting can provide the opportunity for them to say goodbye and for her to encourage him to be brave and to continue his work without her physical presence. Such an interaction can also help clarify to Mr. Da Piazza that he and his mother are not the same person and that he can live on after she dies (i.e., the family meeting can help strengthen the boundary between self and other).

Talking to the psychotic patient is important since there is no other way to understand that person's psychotic experience, and it is the emotional story that informs and reinforces the psychotic process. Working in conjunction with antipsychotic medications, family therapy, cognitive-behavioral therapy, and milieu therapy, individual psychodynamic psychotherapy can serve to strengthen such dysfunctional aspects of the ego as boundary dissolution, reality testing, and the synthesizing functions that organize the patient's relationship to the world around him.

Outsider Art

Aaron Esman, M.D.

THE term *outsider art* designates the artistic products of untrained, often eccentric persons who are outside the mainstream of the conventional art world (Cardinal 1972). The painter Jean Dubuffet (1949) termed such work "art brut" ("raw art") in contrast to "cultural art" or "the art of the museums." Many of the most creative "outsiders" have been persons suffering from mental illness; most of these have been diagnosed with schizophrenia and have been long-term—even lifetime—patients in psychiatric hospitals. Among the best known of these are the Swiss Adolf Wölfli and Aloïse Corbaz, the Mexican American Martin Ramirez, the Italian Carlo Zinelli, and, though never hospitalized, the Chicagoan Henry Darger, each of whom has by now been to some degree embraced by the "official" art world.

The formal study of the art of psychotic patients dates essentially from the work of the German psychiatrist Hans Prinzhorn, who while at the Department of Psychiatry at Heidelberg, collected works from hospitals all over Central Europe and in 1922 published his landmark book *The Artistry of the Mentally Ill.* Prinzhorn elaborated in great detail the influence of what he called the "schizophrenic process" on the formal aspects of creative efforts, and pursued provocative comparisons with the art works of children and of persons from "primitive" cultures. Though he denied that there were specific features that distinguished the art of the mentally ill from that of "normals," he did point to some typical characteristics such as "horror vacui" (the need to fill all available space), a quality of "playfulness," a powerful tendency to compulsive ordering, a preoccupation with symbolism, and, often, a divorce from the character of "reality." Others (e.g., Kris 1952) have pointed to a repetitiveness in subject matter and a lack of stylistic development over time. All agree that these persons are motivated to their creative efforts by intense inner needs rather than by a wish to make "art" in the conventional sense.

Prinzhorn's book had an enormous influence on the art world of his time. It was taken up by many artists of the avant garde, such as Max Ernst, Alfred Kubin and Paul Klee. In particular, the Dadaists amd Surrealists, despite Prinzhorn's disdain for psychoanalysis and depth interpretation, found his illustrations and his conceptualizations liberating in their efforts to reach to the wellsprings of the unconscious in their art. Even today a number of avant garde artists continue to be inspired by the work of such "outsiders," responding to what they see as their freedom from conventional constraints.

The present case appears to resonate with many of the issues raised by the "outsiders" in question. We are told little about the inner workings of Anthony Da Piazza's mind, but we understand that without formal artistic training, he is compulsively driven to create self-portraits—and only self-portraits—in endless profusion. Although his mother has contrived to have them exhibited, the patient does not appear to be so motivated. His work appears to show the characteristic patterns of repetitiveness, lack of stylistic development, and narcissistic concern that are, as Prinzhorn pointed out, usual in the productions of psychotic "outsiders." Lacking detailed description, however, we cannot say to what degree his paintings show the influence of "official" art, past or present. After all, we know that many great artists—Rembrandt, Munch, Beckmann, Picasso—have been the repeated subjects of their own artistry; not, however, as with our patient, to the exclusion of all other subject matter.

Above all, it seems clear that Mr. Da Piazza's artistry is the product of powerful and, almost certainly, unconscious impulses. Absent any opportunity to explore his inner world, we can only speculate about his motives, but the very nature of his monolithic subject matter offers us some clues. It seems safe to suggest that he is troubled by a profound sense of fragmentation, or at least uncertainty, of his identity such that he needs repeated and unremitting assurance of an intact self-representation. (World-destruction hallucinations such as his have long been understood as projected representations of the sensed danger of internal, psychic collapse.) He seeks to obtain this reassurance through an externalized, concrete, self-created image that, never fully convincing to him, requires endless repetitive re-creation. At the same time he would seem to be trying, by plastering the walls and ceiling with his images, to communicate something of his concerns and his attempted solutions to the world around him—his mother, at the very least.

Thus the patient appears to be impelled both by self-directed and by object-directed aims—on the one hand, to restore something of an integrated self-organization in the face of his disorganizing illness and, on the other, to establish or to maintain contact with the object world in the face of his regressive and introversive disorder. His recent threat to burn his paintings betokens the impending failure of these defensive and restitutive efforts, and would seem to constitute a danger signal, perhaps of suicidal or other self-destructive intentions.

Of course, many—indeed, most—psychotic patients live out similar internal struggles without expressing them artistically. Prinzhorn estimated that no more than 2% of hospitalized schizophrenia patients, in the absence of formal art therapy programs, undertook spontaneously to draw, paint, or sculpt; more recent commentators are in essential agreement. Indeed, in the current world of brief hospitalizations and ubiquitous chemotherapy, the number is probably even less. What has accounted for this infrequent activity remains a mystery. Innate talent? An unusually powerful drive for what Prinzhorn called "configuration"? Right-brain dominance? But then, it is probably no more or less mysterious than whatever directs a comparably small number of nonpsychotic persons to do similar things with similar materials and thus become the practitioners of the art we all know and admire—Dubuffet's "art of the museums."

Pharmacology of Schizophrenia

Donna T. Anthony, M.D., Ph.D.

THE inpatient psychiatric unit can keep Anthony Da Piazza safe, and its structure can help him reorganize, but a third important component of his hospitalization will be a reevaluation of his medication regimen. In order to choose one medication from among many, the inpatient psychiatric team will need to take into consideration three related issues—adherence, therapeutic effects, and adverse effects—all of which are directly pertinent to Mr. Da Piazza's situation.

We do not know why Mr. Da Piazza has stopped taking his antipsychotic medication. His mother has been out of the house for 3 weeks, and she may have been in charge of the purchase or the daily distribution of his haloperidol. He may be overwhelmed by the stress of his mother's terminal illness or has come to believe that the medication is poison or that it will limit his ability to save his mother. Perhaps he felt side effects or, like many persons with schizophrenia, he has *anosognosia,* a neurological condition in which insight is lost (Amador and David 1998). While the details are uncertain, it seems likely that Mrs. Da Piazza was the key factor in his medication compliance, and she is dying. Without ongoing dialogue and a therapeutic alliance, Mr. Da Piazza is likely to re-join the majority of people with schizophrenia who are chronically nonadherent with medications.

Given Mr. Da Piazza's history, resumption of his haloperidol is probably the most reliable way to control his psychotic decompensation. Not only has it worked for him in the past, it is available as an injection that lasts 2–4 weeks, a useful option in patients like Mr. Da Piazza who tend to be non-compliant with medications. The haloperidol is likely to calm him quickly and, over the course of weeks, should reduce his hallucinations and delusions. Like other antipsychotic medications, however, haloperidol is relatively ineffective in ameliorating other schizophrenia-related impairments, such as negative symptoms, cognitive deficits, social isolation, and family conflicts. As we see with Mr. Da Piazza, antipsychotic medications are often helpful, but they have not increased the overall likelihood that people with schizophrenia will be able to work or live independently.

The primary effect of all antipsychotic medications—including haloperidol— is the postsynaptic blockade of the dopamine D_2 receptor. In the mesolimbic pathway, such blockade helps reduce the dysregulation that contributes to hallucinations and delusions. With few exceptions, all of the antipsychotic medications are equivalently effective, and medication selection is based on the patient's history of response and the varying side-effect profiles of the different medications.

Many of these side effects are caused by the fact that blockade of D_2 receptors occurs not just in the mesolimbic pathway but in other parts of the brain and body. While Mr. Da Piazza has not spontaneously complained of side effects, he may have a limited ability to recognize and communicate his concerns unless someone specifically asks. Even without his complaints, his darting tongue and clenching jaw are signs of tardive dyskinesia (TD), a relatively permanent and disfiguring movement disorder. Like other syndromes involving extrapyramidal signs and symptoms (EPS), such as dystonia and pseudoparkinsonism, TD reflects blockade in the mesostriatal—also known as the *nigrostriatal*—pathway. More commonly associated with older antipsychotic medications like haloperidol, TD generally worsens when the medication is discontinued or lowered. The presence of TD indicates the need to consider a change to a newer medication. In addition to side effects that are commonly noticed by patients and their families, blockade of D_2 receptors in the hypothalamic–pituitary axis leads to hyperprolactinemia, sexual dysfunction, amenorrhea, galactorrhea, and osteoporosis. Akathisia—a very unpleasant below-the-neck jumpiness—is commonly misdiagnosed as agitation or anxiety and often leads to noncompliance and sometimes to suicide. Rare but serious risks of antipsychotic medications include seizures, neuroleptic malignant syndrome (NMS), and prolongation of the QT interval leading to the possibility of a fatal arrhythmia.

Given Mr. Da Piazza's TD and nonadherence, it is reasonable to consider other medications. One possibility would be chlorpromazine (Thorazine), which, like haloperidol, is a member of the group known as the first-generation antipsychotics (FGAs). Chlorpromazine is less tightly bound to the D_2 receptors and is therefore considered to be a "low potency" antipsychotic, while haloperidol is considered "high potency." Because they are less tightly bound, low-potency FGAs are associated with lower rates of EPS. At the same time, chlorpromazine has the potential to cause many side effects through its effects on a host of other receptors (e.g., serotonergic, histaminic, sympathomimetic, and muscarinic cholinergic receptors) and, like the other FGAs, is likely to worsen Mr. Da Piazza's TD. While chlorpromazine and haloperidol have been the standard pharmacological treatment for schizophrenia for over 50 years, they have been increasingly replaced by newer medications that have safer side-effect profiles.

The medications that have increasingly replaced the FGAs are called atypical, new, or second-generation antipsychotics (SGAs); these medications combine D_2 receptor and serotonin type-2a (5-HT_{2A}) receptor antagonism. The serotonin receptor antagonism modulates the blockade of dopamine and of other neurotransmitters, leading to reduced risk of EPS, noncompliance, and relapse (Lieberman et al. 2005; Robinson et al. 2005). While the atypical antipsychotics are generally better tolerated by patients, they do cause many of the same side effects as the FGAs. Some are fairly similar to high-potency FGAs in being potent D_2 receptor blockers with the resultant risk of EPS but with relatively little sedation (e.g., risperidone [Risperdal] and ziprasidone [Geodon]). Others are more similar to low-potency FGAs in binding to many different receptors throughout the brain, leading, for example, to significant sedation (e.g., clozapine [Clozaril], olanzapine [Zyprexa], and quetiapine [Seroquel]). These sedating SGAs are also among the most likely to cause the metabolic syndrome, which is marked by weight gain (sometimes over 50 pounds), hyperglycemia, hypertriglyceridemia, and an increased risk of diabetes. These side effects lead to increased risk of cardiovascular disease and discontinuation of the drug. The newest member of the SGAs is aripiprazole (Abilify), a mixed agonist-antagonist at the D_2 and serotonin 5-HT_{1A} receptors and, like the other SGAs, is a 5-HT_2 receptor antagonist. Being a mixed agonist-antagonist, aripiprazole only partially blocks D_2 receptors, leading to low rates of EPS, weight gain, the metabolic syndrome, and sedation.

Clozapine is not only the most effective antipsychotic medication for the positive symptoms of schizophrenia but also the only one that tends to improve negative symptoms (McEvoy et al. 2006). It also appears to reduce suicidality, which might be especially beneficial to Mr. Da Piazza given the looming loss of his mother. Clozapine carries almost no risk of EPS and TD and may even treat preexisting TD. Unfortunately, clozapine carries elevated risks of many side effects, most importantly agranulocytosis, a potentially catastrophic reaction that necessitates frequent blood monitoring. For that reason, the use of clozapine requires at least two or three failed antipsychotic trials.

In regard to Mr. Da Piazza, I would probably take this opportunity to switch his antipsychotic medication to one of the SGAs. If compliance is likely to be a problem, risperidone could be used in the now-available depot form. Given his TD while taking the high-potency FGA haloperidol, I might choose a low-potency SGA such as olanzapine. On the other hand, he has a history of weight fluctuations and so is at particular risk for weight gain and the metabolic syndrome. To make a medication decision, I would need more information and would want to explore his and his mother's preferences.

The dosage of antipsychotic medication is guided by a few basic principles. First, it is important to balance the desire to reach a therapeutic dose with the recognition that untoward side effects will reduce adherence. Mr. Da Piazza's lifelong struggle with taking his medications might well have stemmed from his early experience with "rapid neuroleptization," an outdated practice in which antipsychotic medications were aggressively pushed to high doses. Rapid neuroleptization led to diminished physical aggression but also to significant problems, including a particularly unpleasant combination of pseudoparkinsonism and akathisia as well as greatly increased rates of TD. It is now recognized that for all of the antipsychotic medications except clozapine and aripiprazole, antipsychotic effectiveness requires the blockade of 60%–80% of D_2 receptors. Positron emission tomography (PET) studies indicate that this level of blockade is reached, for example, by dosages of 2.5–6.0 mg/day of haloperidol, 10–20 mg/day of olanzapine, and 2–6 mg/day of risperidone. These data are supported by clinical research that indicates that there is no increase in efficacy of haloperidol at dosages greater than 8 mg/day. As with other classes of medication, real-life effective dosage must take into consideration inter-individual differences of metabolism and sensitivity to side effects. Management must also take into consideration the patient's preferences, which means that symptom control may need to be somewhat compromised in order to increase compliance. Dosage control is also important in regard to the many medications that are used to treat side effects to the antipsychotic medication. For example, if Mr. Da Piazza's antipsychotic medication is switched to an SGA, I would probably discontinue his benztropine. An anticholinergic medication that is commonly used to treat EPS, benztropine can also worsen cognition, negative symptoms, constipation, narrow angle glaucoma, and prostatic hypertrophy.

If two or three trials of SGAs were either ineffective or not tolerated, despite ongoing psychosocial interventions, I would then consider switching his antipsychotic medication back to haloperidol or to clozapine. If these efforts fail, some clinicians would then try a combination of antipsychotic medications, an effort that should generally be avoided because of the enhanced risk of side effects, particularly the potentially lethal neuroleptic malignant syndrome (NMS). Adjunctive mood stabilizers (valproate, lamotrigine, lithium) have been used for aggression and treatment-resistant schizophrenia, but there is little evidence of effectiveness.

Current challenges in the pharmacology of schizophrenia involve improvement of both efficacy and tolerability, initiation of medications early in the course of the disease, enhanced efficacy through combinations of pharmacology and psychosocial interventions, and greater effectiveness in the treatment of negative symptoms, cognitive deficits, and disorganization. Particularly intriguing research efforts include the development of medications that might affect neurotransmitter systems that are also implicated in schizophrenia, like the glutamate system. Another is pharmacogenomics, in which DNA testing would allow pharmacologists to tailor treatment regimens to the individual patient so that, for example, slow metabolizers would get lower doses of medication.

Mr. Da Piazza has a number of pharmacological options that may be able to help him survive the death of his mother and lead a relatively independent life. Further, research may soon bring advances in terms of both efficacy and side-effect reduction. At the same time, however, there remains the reality that Mr. Da Piazza has a chronic disease for which we have moderately effective medications that are associated with moderately toxic side effects.

Cognitive-Behavioral Therapy

Yulia Landa, Psy.D.

COGNITIVE-BEHAVIORAL therapy (CBT) for schizophrenia has been shown to reduce psychotic symptoms and be particularly effective for residual delusions. In addition, CBT has a low dropout rate, and its treatment effect is maintained after the end of therapy. The key elements of CBT include identification of target symptoms, a shared understanding of the illness between the patient and therapist, and development of specific cognitive and behavioral strategies to cope with symptoms (Landa et al. 2006).

The goal of Anthony Da Piazza's treatment would likely be to improve his functioning and overall life satisfaction by reducing the distress and disability caused by his delusions, hallucinations, and negative symptoms. This could be achieved by changing his beliefs about symptoms and improving coping. For example, Mr. Da Piazza is likely to be afraid of his auditory hallucinations if he believes that they are spoken by the Devil, and he is likely to hear them more when he is scared or worried. His distress might decline if he can explore alternative origins of his voices, particularly the possibility that, although the voices are not imaginary, they are created by his own mind, perhaps because his brain mistakes thoughts for voices. In CBT, a normalizing approach helps patients make sense of such experiences. For example, Mr. Da Piazza may be relieved to discover that most people have experienced hearing their name called when nobody was around and that hallucinations are common in people after they have been deprived of sleep for 2 days.

CBT does not require that a patient accept the diagnosis of schizophrenia or the biological model of symptom causation. Instead, the focus is on the role of stress in the development of symptoms and unusual experiences. According to this model, various genetic predispositions and life events make us vulnerable to developing symptoms when we are under stress.

What would CBT with Anthony Da Piazza involve? The first step would be to establish a *therapeutic alliance,* a task that is complicated by his isolation, mistrust, and experience of doctors dismissing his ideas as delusional. Alliance would be enhanced by letting Mr. Da Piazza lead the conversation, displaying an explicit interest in his words, thoughts, and feelings, and being empathic and reflective.

The next step is *assessment.* The therapist would try to understand Mr. Da Piazza's experiences, the meaning he applies to them, and his resulting feelings and behaviors. The therapist would also aim to understand Mr. Da Piazza's first psychotic episode in detail, which may hold the key to his current beliefs. For example, his mother is ill. The therapist might empathize with him first and then explore how Mr. Da Piazza has been dealing with it. What scares him most about his mom's illness? Is he worried about what might happen to him if she dies? Is he, for example, afraid that he could end up living on the street (like he has in the past) or in a state hospital (like his grandmother)? Is he scared or stressed by something else? For example, he used to hear voices warning him that the end of the world was coming. Does he still hear these voices? What are his beliefs about the origins of these voices? Does he think that the voices are there to help or harm him? Does he believe that the voices are powerful, or does he view himself as being more powerful than the voices? Does he think that his mother's death will usher in the end of the world, including his own demise?

During the evaluation, Mr. Da Piazza might say that he thought that his portraits would prevent his mother's illness and that he decided to burn his drawings because his efforts had failed. A CBT therapist might explicitly recognize Mr. Da Piazza's valiant attempt to help. The therapist might then ask if Mr. Da Piazza has tried anything else. Mr. Da Piazza may say that he believes there is nothing else he could do to help. To reduce his helplessness and promote hope, the therapist may then suggest they think collaboratively about possible ways to improve the situation ("two heads are better than one"). In contrast to some analytically oriented treatments, CBT welcomes the therapist's self-disclosure to help normalize the patient's experiences. This might lead the therapist to reveal, for example, that he felt stress during his own mother's illness, and how he made use of other people's advice and help during that difficult time. Such revelation can enhance the alliance and help normalize the patient's own reactions to stress.

The assessment stage results in the development of a *formulation,* which is a psychological model of symptom formation and maintenance created collaboratively with the patient. The formulation, which is constructed in a form of a narrative, guides the treatment. Every formulation has an *activating event* that triggers dysfunctional thoughts leading to distress. In Mr. Da Piazza's case, it appears that his mother's illness is the activating event. He may believe that he is not able to survive on his own, which makes him very worried. This worry sparks his auditory hallucinations concerning the end of the world. This seemingly omniscient and omnipotent voice scares Mr. Da Piazza into isolation and medication nonadherence, which intensifies the voices. While brooding on the end of the world, he sees no reason to eat or shower. He also sees no reason to do the one activity he enjoys—his art—

because the drawings have failed in their mission to control her illness. The destruction of his art continues this spiral of anxiety and demoralization. It may be very comforting to Mr. Da Piazza to realize that his symptoms follow a recognizable pattern that is amenable to change.

Once assessment has been completed and a formulation developed, the therapist and patient collaboratively establish *treatment goals*. Treatment goals are based on a *problem list* that stems from the formulation. The problem list is usually a set of general issues that concern the patient. The goals should be specific, positive, realistic, achievable, measurable, time limited, and based in the future. For Mr. Da Piazza, the problems and goals could be formulated as shown in Table 4–1. The problems are addressed in an order that corresponds to the level of urgency and to the likelihood that the problem can be quickly resolved.

TABLE 4–1.   PROBLEM LIST AND TREATMENT GOALS IN COGNITIVE-BEHAVIORAL THERAPY FOR ANTHONY DA PIAZZA

Problems	Goals
Worrying about not being able to function independently	To evaluate my fears about not being able to function without my mother. To reduce the stress associated with these thoughts from 100% to 80%.
A voice is telling me that the end of the world is coming	To find out more about the voice and either reduce the frequency of the voice (from every half hour to every few hours) or stop the voice from being so upsetting (from 90% to 70%).
Worrying about not being able to help my mother	To evaluate my belief that I am not able to help my mother. To develop a plan to help my mother through her illness and to reduce my belief that I am not able to help her from 70% to 40%.
Feeling depressed when thinking that my artwork has failed to save my mother	To evaluate my belief that my artwork is a failure and to reduce the depressed feelings associated with this thought from 100% to 70%.

A common goal is working with delusions. The initial step is to explore the evidence: how does the patient support his delusional beliefs? This exploration is an implicit challenge to the validity of unsustainable beliefs. The therapist might then encourage a patient to look for alternative explanations for the specific beliefs. For example, Mr. Da Piazza believes the voice when it says that the end of the world is near. The therapist might know that Mr. Da Piazza had the same hallucination in the past and so might ask him whether the voices had previously been accurate. Assuming an intact alliance, the therapist could ask Mr. Da Piazza to consider alternative explanations for the origins of the voice (e.g., "Perhaps your brain creates the voices when you are under a lot of stress").

Another important goal of treatment is to develop a sense of self-efficacy in patients suffering from hallucinations. Mr. Da Piazza might believe that he has no control over these voices. The therapist and patient might then be able to devise interventions that can reduce the voices. Mr. Da Piazza might, for example, be encouraged to talk to other people, read aloud, or listen to music. If successful—if even for a few minutes—the intervention can be used to demonstrate that the patient has some control and that, perhaps, the voices are not omnipotent.

When Mr. Da Piazza's treatment goals are reached, the therapy will focus on *relapse prevention,* which is an important aspect of CBT.

Cognitive-behavioral therapy for psychosis aims to improve the person's ability to function despite psychotic symptoms. Based on the general principles of CBT, this approach emphasizes the development of strong therapeutic alliance, normalization, interest in personal meaning of symptoms, self-regulation of psychotic experiences, and improvement in reality testing.

Comprehensive Healthcare

Steven P. Levine, M.D.

ANTHONY Da Piazza has reached a critical point in his life. Not only must he cope with the imminent loss of his most important stabilizing force and social connection—his decidedly nonschizophrenogenic mother—but he is also approaching a phase of life in which cognitive and functional decline is common among people with schizophrenia. Some decline may be directly attributable to progression of the psychiatric illness, but much of the debilitation is secondary to preventable medical illness.

While the psychiatric team does need to be attentive to the risk of suicide, of course, the greatest threat to Mr. Da Piazza's life expectancy and quality of life is his physical health. People with schizophrenia have elevated rates of cardiovascular disease, substance abuse, respiratory illnesses, infectious diseases, obesity, and diabetes mellitus. These illnesses lead men with schizophrenia to have life spans that are—on average—10 years less than those of average men. Of particular concern is the fact that people with schizophrenia have a 40% risk for the metabolic syndrome (Casey 2005; McEvoy et al. 2005), a condition marked by a cluster of related changes that include abdominal obesity, insulin resistance, and dyslipidemias (including low high-density lipoprotein [HDL] cholesterol levels, high triglyceride levels, and high low-density lipoprotein [LDL] cholesterol levels). Mr. Da Piazza is currently thin, but he apparently has a history of significant weight fluctuations. Lower-than-normal weight was common in patients with schizophrenia before the introduction of second-generation antipsychotic medications, and Mr. Da Piazza may not be suffering metabolic syndrome, because he is taking a relatively weight-sparing antipsychotic, haloperidol. His weight may change rapidly if he is put on a second-generation antipsychotic, particularly clozapine or olanzapine (Berkowitz and Fabricatore 2005). Though clozapine reduces the risk of suicide and death by violence, most of these benefits in mortality are lost by increases in death from cardiovascular and pulmonary disease.

While Mr. Da Piazza is at high risk for multiple medical disorders, he is likely to not follow up with primary care physicians and to be poorly compliant with recommendations for a healthier lifestyle. The lack of follow-up may be caused by a number of factors, including limited income and insurance, making it expensive to see doctors and buy medication; amotivation and negative symptoms, which may contribute to poor planning and missed appointments; and the discomfort of nonpsychiatrist physicians who have limited training about and exposure to people with psychotic disorders and a lack of understanding about the cognitive and emotional limitations in patients with schizophrenia. Such factors contribute to the fact that many people with schizophrenia rarely see a physician aside from a psychiatrist.

Given the frequency of the metabolic syndrome among persons with schizophrenia, the American Diabetes Association and American Psychiatric Association have issued guidelines for monitoring metabolic adverse effects (American Diabetes Association et al. 2004). Though the full impact of these recommendations remains to be seen, a large survey conducted shortly after their introduction revealed infrequent monitoring for hypertension, hyperglycemia, and dyslipidemia (Newcomer et al. 2004). A large, multi-site study recently indicated that 30% of persons with schizophrenia who had diabetes were not receiving any treatment to control blood glucose levels, almost 90% with hyperlipidemia were not taking a statin, and over 60% with hypertension were not receiving antihypertensive medication (Nasrallah et al. 2006).

The options for medical management are limited. Mr. Da Piazza's primary physician may be a psychiatrist, for example, who is far removed from medical school. One option might be for Mr. Da Piazza to be treated at a trainee-driven outpatient clinic; such a clinic would expose Mr. Da Piazza to psychiatrists who may be more current with the latest recommendations for care and would likely have easier access to hospital-based services such as laboratory tests and imaging. The frequency of resident turnover would not only affect the continuity of care, however, but also tax Mr. Da Piazza's limited capacity to form trusting relationships.

Perhaps Mr. Da Piazza would best be served by a group of affiliated clinicians who would monitor, diagnose, and treat his medical and psychiatric problems, all in one place. Consider the following scenario: One year after starting a second-generation antipsychotic, Mr. Da Piazza arrives for a scheduled visit. He is greeted by the familiar face of the nurse practitioner, who then measures his weight, blood pressure, pulse, and waist circumference and orders appropriate tests, such as a complete blood count, basic metabolic profile, liver function tests, fasting glucose, lipid profile, urinalysis, and any age-appropriate screening tests. The group's focus would be on preventative care (e.g., weight reduction, smoking cessation), but the nurse practitioner would also treat basic hypertension, hyperlipidemia, and diabetes. Therapeutic activities could be personalized to fit his specific needs and might include cognitive training, cognitive-behavioral therapy, supportive psychotherapy, and nutritional advice. Such therapy might be done by a psychiatrist or a nonphysician therapist and could be done individually or in groups. Medications would be prescribed in the context of a broader understanding of Mr. Da Piazza's needs and wishes and with the recognition that the key to improving his overall quality of life will not be found in selecting the "correct" medication from among a group of medications with strikingly similar rates of symptom reduction. Such a team might be more likely than an individual practitioner to remind him about an upcoming appointment and to call him if he missed a session. Further, the affiliated clinicians could serve to help Mr. Da Piazza connect with people in a world that is likely to be without his most supportive ally, his mother.

Such groups do not widely exist and may be seen as unlikely. Nevertheless, they seem best suited to improving the overall quality of life in people who suffer from a chronic, debilitating, isolating illness for which there exist only partially effective treatments. A recent, large randomized controlled trial found that collaborative care of comorbid depression and diabetes was clinically beneficial and no more costly (Katon et al. 2006). Ongoing service delivery research and political involvement may be the next steps toward creating the infrastructure and financial inducements that can make cost-effective multidisciplinary programs more widely available to the people who need it the most.

Recovery

David W. Schab, M.D.

PSYCHIATRISTS have traditionally focused on symptom response with a goal of remission. In the absence of completely effective treatments, however, the emphasis on remission of symptoms has contributed to a sense of hopelessness among generations of psychiatrists, patients, and their families. In the face of such futility, a different paradigm—that of *recovery*—was developed.

In its original formulation, recovery focused on restoration of function. Independent living and social engagement, for example, were typical benchmarks by which recovery could be measured. Recent work in recovery still emphasizes these functional benchmarks but sees three positive states of mind as paramount goals: 1) hopefulness despite setbacks; 2) self-empowerment; and 3) spirituality, which is defined as the expectation of inspiration and guidance beyond the world's immediate exigencies (Corrigan 2006). While these goals, as well as much of the passion and creativity in the recovery movement, originally stemmed from people with schizophrenia, their families, and organizations such as the National Alliance on Mental Illness (NAMI), recovery's goals are increasingly being adopted by clinicians and psychiatric researchers. There are multiple models for recovery, but all recognize that the focus of treatment should be on the growth of the individual, that the patient should participate actively, and that a good outcome does not necessarily mean an absence of symptoms.

Anthony Da Piazza's case summary emphasizes that he has been hospitalized because of delusions that developed in the context of his mother's illness, but is it absolutely mandatory that this delusion be treated? During acute presentations, such delusions may appear horrifying, but many delusions harbored by chronically psychotic patients do not noticeably or detrimentally influence behavior. Treating Mr. Da Piazza's delusion is not as important as addressing the stressors that kindled the delusion and caused him to withdraw from the world. Further, zealous pharmacology may lead to side effects that amplify withdrawal and diminish the likelihood of ongoing treatment acceptance. It would be necessary to help convince him of the danger of burning his drawings, but, afterward, the therapeutic priority should be on helping him develop an engaged and satisfying life in the context of a serious psychiatric illness.

Involving Mr. Da Piazza as early as possible in decisions about his care may reduce his paranoia and anxieties about passively submitting to treatment. Developed for use in people with substance abuse problems, *motivational interviewing* has taught us that simply asking patients to articulate *out loud* the advantages and disadvantages of adopting treatments is likely to both enhance their own sense of agency and resolve their ambivalence about undergoing those treatments.

Because the exact choice of antipsychotic is almost certainly less important than compliance with whatever is chosen, and because we hope to enhance Mr. Da Piazza's sense of personal agency, he should be invited to help choose his medication. This is especially true given his history with medication treatments that have been discredited because of their high likelihood of side effects (e.g., rapid neuroleptization). His clinical team should further explore with him the documented advantages of long-acting intramuscular depot medications over oral ones: they enhance compliance, reduce relapse, and are often preferred by patients (Nasrallah and Lasser 2006). Further, intramuscular medications would leave him less encumbered by daily pill-taking, less harried by other people's well-meaning reminders, and more likely to see himself as an autonomous person whose identity is not based solely on having schizophrenia.

Any efforts at recovery must acknowledge the negative impact of relapse and rehospitalization. As disruptive as rehospitalization is to the practical aspects of the patient's life, the psychological demoralization may be more debilitating. Further, in about one third of patients, each psychotic relapse is associated with worsened residual symptoms and impairment (Shepherd et al. 1989).

Because subthreshold symptoms often precede relapse and lead to rehospitalization, every patient should develop a personalized list of symptoms and behaviors that indicate an impending illness exacerbation. Mr. Da Piazza might be more likely to reveal these early symptoms if he understands that use of an early warning system can reduce hospitalization. Such a discussion should be part of each discharge plan.

During our inpatient and later outpatient care of Mr. Da Piazza, we must identify what he finds important: relationships, social causes, his body, minor enjoyments, and hobbies—any investment that might kindle his discovery of meaning and hope. Often a great deal of historical excavation is required to identify old sparks of passion that, buried under years of illness, are either forgotten or are transformed into symptoms or odd or obsessive behaviors.

In Mr. Da Piazza, however, we find in his drawing an overt investment that is likely an excellent prognostic factor. He is currently committed to his art and probably enjoys it. This is an important opportunity to understand him better and to gain a stronger alliance through demonstration of our interest. Why drawing? How did he start, and what was its role before his illness? Does he take hearty, ebullient enjoyment in his efforts? Does drawing serve a function that may not be obvious, like a psychological defense or a strategy to reduce discomfort? In some other patients, for example, television is a tool to dampen auditory hallucinations and a venue into which to channel fantasy.

Mr. Da Piazza's preoccupation with self-portraiture may suggest withdrawal from the outside world, or it may suggest a wandering search for identity. His mother mentioned that his drawings are "highly detailed," and so they may reflect compulsions, as counting tiles would be for a patient with obsessive-compulsive disorder. A deeper understanding of Mr. Da Piazza's experience with painting might help us channel his energy into an activity that might further his recovery, whether it be drawing classes in a therapeutic community or painting walls in a supported employment program. Such activities would enrich his life by enhancing his interaction with the outside world.

Cognitive-behavioral therapy and motivational interviewing have both been shown to reduce relapse. In addition, family therapy has been shown to reduce excessively expressed emotion and to heighten emotional warmth within the household. In addition, supportive employment, in which job coaches help patients with job-specific challenges, is more effective for people with severe mental illness than prevocational training, which is aimed more broadly at preparing patients for future employment. The effect may be larger when supportive employment is enhanced with cognitive training (McGurk et al. 2005).

Recovery can also be enhanced by *assertive community treatment* (ACT), an integrated team-based approach to treating heavy users of the mental health system in their communities. ACT is conducted by an integrated multidisciplinary team of nurses, physicians, pharmacists, social workers, and case managers who provide—on an around-the-clock basis—almost all the services that a patient needs to live independently. These might include assistance with or direct management of housing, finances, symptoms, and medication. Some ACT teams even have the milieu of a family. Although a large evidence base supports the effectiveness of ACT, the consumer movement has balked at what it sees as ACT's paternalism, especially when the treatment is court-mandated.

The consumer movement has very successfully advocated, however, for additional psychosocial treatments, whose rather plain names—such as psychoeducation, relapse prevention, and skills training—fail to capture their sophistication, rigor, and evidence base. Involvement in the consumer movement itself through such organizations as NAMI can be a liberating and hopeful experience for the person with schizophrenia as well as for the families and clinicians who seek creative interventions to help patients recover.

Homelessness and Social History

Kim Hopper, Ph.D.

PSYCHIATRY may make its own history, but it does not do so under circumstances of its own choosing. This hoary homespun truth becomes especially vivid in the lives of its protagonists—patients and providers alike—when they span periods of unusually disruptive change. Such is the case with Anthony Da Piazza: born in the era of secure confinement, suffering his first psychiatric crisis during the heyday of deinstitutionalization, and then settling into an extended period of residential and clinical instability (punctuated by bouts of outright homelessness) during a time when the mental health system itself was struggling to find its bearings, recoup public confidence, and establish a fresh set of ground rules.

Among the difficulties that complicate planning for Mr. Da Piazza at this stage in his psychiatric career is the fact that none of these projects—not the bearings, not the confidence, and not the ground rules—have achieved the clarity or consensus one might have hoped for. And so while recovery is being proclaimed as watchword and guiding principle of a new era, that claim must somehow take root and flourish in a public mental health system that—

for all the energy, innovation, evidence-based experimentation, and sheer commitment one can find in its interstices—has been characterized by one state mental health commissioner as "a shambles" (Hogan 2002). This means that merely stabilizing Mr. Da Piazza's clinical status (as though that weren't challenging enough) will not suffice. Any lasting intervention will have to deal not only with his pending displacement but also with what has been his existential homelessness all along. Whatever treatment complexities it may raise, Mr. Da Piazza's instability is also emblematic of a system still struggling to find/define its own place in the world.

An anthropological approach to Mr. Da Piazza's predicament is as much concerned about the changing configuration of the structural features of the relevant contexts of support and livelihood as it is with his treatment. The concept of *structure* takes in all the explicit programs and policies, local market realities, and shifting kin arrangements that make for a dynamic set of constraints and enablements. It also includes that collective, improvisational script of belief and custom bound under the name of *culture*. Together, these contextual realities, along with Mr. Da Piazza's own shaky clinical state and uneven (untried?) competencies, define the field of prospects and liabilities within which public psychiatry plies its trade. An aggressive case manager, lucky in her choice of an agency to work for and unflagging in her efforts, may be able to cobble together the full package: find an affordable, supported apartment; engage a dedicated clinician; and make arrangements to stick close by during what promises to be a tough transition. She may even locate (though this is even less likely) an appropriate job placement. (Fountain House, mentioned in passing in the case summary ["Schizophrenia"], is especially practiced at this.) Absent that, or banking on a resurgence of his interest in drawing, she may be able to renew his informal studio privileges.

But none of these is assured. Under present circumstances, they are not even good bets (hence the hedges: "aggressive...lucky...unflagging"). So it may be worthwhile to consider, for a moment, the genealogy of this predicament—the contingencies that have shaped, only to disappear from sight and memory, what present-day practitioners take for granted (like a de facto public mental health system that has come to include homeless shelters among its resources). It is also worth noting that Mr. Da Piazza's circumstances are replicated thousands of times over, in the unheralded labor of elderly parents like his, fretfully making possible a residential alternative to the streets for their middle-aged sons and daughters (at least for the near future). To see how things have arrived at this unhappy juncture, we rejoin the social history sketched above. In this way, illness narratives come to signify beyond the confines of personal stories—"small facts [contrive to] speak to large issues"— not because they bear legible traces of their origins, but because "they can be made to" (Geertz 1973) with the right interpretative tools.

To judge from the spare biographical details provided, Mr. Da Piazza belongs to the postwar baby boom, coming of age during a prolonged stretch of unprecedented security and growth, undercut by a gathering "cold war" anxiety. He was also an apparent (how avid?) recruit to its "flower power" brigades and a recreational drug user. Ironic echo of a troubled time, the double-bind theory of schizophrenia invoked in an early diagnostic note, was crucial to Laing's existential psychiatry (Laing 1959), which would morph into a widely denounced "psychedelic" model of madness (Laing 1967). Its fevered pronouncements, coupled with a wispy, empirically suspect promise of return and renewal through the ordeal of psychosis (if only society's keepers would hold confinement and medication at bay), provoked bitter censure in turn (Trilling 1972). Such outlandish cultural skirmishes not only tarred the cause of recovery with the phantasmagoric excesses of the drug scene but also effectively camouflaged what would eventually take shape as a disastrous failure to plan. While Haight-Ashbury throbbed, a mental health system fell apart.

New York State is a case in point. In the early 1970s, the director of Manhattan Psychiatric Institute refused to carry out mandated reductions in inpatient census that would have inevitably made public psychiatry party to "dumping, nursing home misuse and homelessness." (He resigned not long thereafter.) A decade later, according to an internal Office of Mental Health report, fully 59% of discharges from the same hospital were to "unknown" living arrangements. Clerical oversight, "elopements," and mishaps aside, many of these destinations were unknown because those leaving had no place to go. Fully 8,000 individuals each year were refused admission to state hospitals under tightened eligibility criteria (Hopper et al. 1982). The net effect was serious institutional displacement and haphazard accommodation elsewhere. By 1976, psychiatric disorders rivaled alcoholism as a presenting diagnosis at the Municipal Shelter for men in New York City. In the early 1980s, the American Psychiatric Association's own Task Force on the Homeless Mentally Ill documented the explosive increase of severe psychiatric disorders among street and shelter populations (Lamb 1984). The nascent effort to renew what had been a promising effort to make community integration a reality (Estroff 1981) effectively ground to a halt. The more pressing need was the aboriginal one of housing, and until that was met it made little sense to talk of "less-restrictive alternatives" where a community-embedded psychiatry might work.

Remarkable headway has since been made. Not that the work of ending homelessness is done, or that completing this process will be easy, but effective means of reaching and rehousing the street-dwelling homeless have been refined and patented as evidence-based practices. Adequate resources are needed to bring them to scale, but proven technologies are there (O'Hara 2007). Prospects for social recovery, symptom management, and employment have brightened, even if old awkward questions about the terms of belonging and full citizenship remain. We've relearned that solving homelessness—literal or, as in Mr. Da Piazza's case, pending—leads us back to first principles and long-shelved questions. What mediates social membership for persons denied the usual passports of worth? Is stigma alone sufficient to explain such denials? How can inclusion translate into practices that enhance valued capabilities rather than sanction convenient disqualifications? Answering these may require contesting the terms of durable patienthood, revisiting the terms of moral agency, and reexamining issues of coercion, autonomy, and the balance of power and respect in treatment decision making.

But for Mr. Da Piazza, the urgent issue is finding a place to call his own, along with world enough and time to make it so. He has a great deal of ground to make up, and some developmental milestones to finesse. In any given case—and this is what makes reading signifying value tricky—targeted resources, seasoned clinical expertise, and indefatigable case management can make the decisive difference. Whether they exist in sufficient stores to meet the looming crisis of displacement among similarly situated persons, struggling with their own problems, is another question entirely.

Overview of Schizophrenia

Roberto Gil, M.D.

One must on principle beware of attributing characteristic significance to a single morbid phenomenon. . . . [U]nfortunately, there is in the domain of psychic disorders no single morbid symptom which is thoroughly characteristic of a definite malady.

Emil Kraepelin (1919, p. 261)

THESE words, written almost a century ago, remain significant today. Although Anthony Da Piazza's symptoms are similar to those of many other patients with schizophrenia, the illness is complex. Within the current diagnostic boundaries of schizophrenia, we encounter patients with a broad array of symptoms, varying degrees of severity, and divergent clinical trajectories. The heterogeneity of schizophrenia challenges our diagnostic categories, highlights the limitations of our knowledge, and may explain the partial efficacy of our treatments

Let us first consider the heterogeneity of schizophrenia as it affects diagnosis. The contemporary diagnosis of schizophrenia relies on a description of psychopathology and the exclusion of other illnesses that might cause the symptoms of schizophrenia. There is, however, no single diagnostic indicator or symptom that is common to all forms of schizophrenia or that can reliably differentiate schizophrenia from other medical or psychiatric disorders. Exclusion of other disorders is further complicated by the fact that psychosis—a cardinal symptom of schizophrenia—may also be seen in severe forms of depression, mania, and substance abuse.

Without a defining pathognomonic symptom, the diagnosis of schizophrenia relies on diverse clinical features. Early descriptions of psychotic disorders separated the disorders according to the predominant symptoms. Kraepelin (1919) subdivided schizophrenia into the paranoid, catatonic, and hebephrenic types, corresponding to the predominance of psychotic, motor, and disorganized symptoms, respectively. Bleuler (1911/1950) added the "simple" subtype, recognizing the prominence of negative symptoms in some patients. It is a tribute to the excellence of these early observations that the subtypes of schizophrenia have changed little over the course of a century.

Dr. Savitz's review (see section "Schizophrenia") of the historical aspects of the diagnosis of schizophrenia helps us understand schizophrenia's variability. While Kraepelin emphasized schizophrenia's chronic and deteriorating course, Bleuler pointed out that some patients with schizophrenia have a chronic but nondeteriorating course that might include independence and self support, productive work, and the creation of a family. Follow-up studies indicated that 15%–20% of schizophrenia patients "recovered" prior to the introduction of antipsychotic medications (Winokur and Tsuang 1996), although it should be noted that the definitions of recovery were not uniform across studies. The introduction of antipsychotic medications led many schizophrenia patients to leave inpatient institutions, but the overall rate of significant recovery was increased to no more than 25% of patients.

Schizophrenic symptoms are as varied as the clinical course. Bleuler theorized that central to schizophrenia was the splitting of thought processes and affect, a mechanism that led to a cluster of problems: disturbed association, impaired attention, autism, ambivalence, affective blunting, and avolition. These symptoms are, however, notoriously absent in patients with paranoid-type schizophrenia. In fact, patients with paranoid-type schizophrenia tend to be diagnosed on the basis of having as little as one prominent positive symptom (i.e., hallucinations or delusions) in the presence of a characteristic course and the exclusion of other causes. Other people are diagnosed with schizophrenia based on negative symptoms in combination with a behavioral or thought disorder.

Cognitive deficits in schizophrenia are also variable. Although cognitive deficits are not formally included in the current diagnostic criteria for schizophrenia, neuropsychological testing detects cognitive difficulties in up to 85% of patients with schizophrenia. While some cognitive domains are affected in most patients (e.g., executive functioning, verbal memory and fluency, and working memory), there is significant inter-individual variability in regard to both severity and type of deficit. Recent recognition of the impact of cognition on long-term functioning has sparked research into the basic science of cognition and into possible treatments that have focused on the use of second-generation antipsychotic medications (Keefe et al. 1999).

It is clearly beyond the scope of this book to discuss the many theories that try to explain schizophrenia, but we do suspect that schizophrenia, as we define it today, is likely to include several disorders with different underlying etiologies and neurobiological abnormalities. From among these theories of schizophrenia, we review here only three pharmacologic models of psychosis as they relate to schizophrenia. These models are particularly helpful in understanding the pathophysiological mechanisms of symptoms of schizophrenia. In addition, they provide insight into the benefits and limitations of current pharmacotherapies.

Three pharmacological models have been proposed to explain psychotic symptoms, each one of them rooted in a different neurotransmitter (Krystal et al. 2004):

1. *The serotonergic model* is based on observations that serotonergic agents such as LSD cause positive psychotic symptoms (more hallucinations than delusions, and more visual hallucinations than auditory). These agents induce little thought disorder and few negative symptoms and so constitute a model best suited to symptoms primarily seen in first-break schizophrenia patients.
2. *The dopaminergic model* follows observations that dopaminergic agents (e.g., amphetamine and cocaine) cause predominant positive symptoms (e.g., hallucinations and delusions). This model seems applicable to paranoid type schizophrenia and also to some nonschizophrenic psychotic disorders (i.e., severe major depression with psychosis).
3. *The glutamatergic model* is based on observations that NMDA (N-methyl-D-aspartate) antagonists (e.g., phencyclidine [PCP] and ketamine) generate thought disorder, cognitive impairment, and negative symptoms rather than hallucinations or delusions. The disorganized and undifferentiated subtypes of schizophrenia seem to best fit this model of psychosis.

The dopaminergic and serotonergic models seem to apply to the paranoid subtype of schizophrenia, while the glutamatergic model appears more clearly relevant for the undifferentiated and disorganized subtypes. However, these models do not appear to completely define subtypes of schizophrenia and may instead be complementary rather than mutually exclusive. For example, people with schizophrenia often present with positive symptoms early in the illness but gradually manifest increasing numbers of cognitive and affective deficits.

The complementary relationship of these models extends to the pharmacological treatment of symptoms. As pointed out by Dr. Anthony in her section on the pharmacology of schizophrenia, all antipsychotic medications act on dopamine through blockade of D_2 receptors. Although the second-generation antipsychotic medications also act on serotonin receptors, there have been no effective antipsychotic treatments that target serotonin or glutamate receptors exclusively. Given the likelihood that schizophrenia reflects a disturbance of multiple transmitter systems and complex neurologic circuitry, it should not be surprising that the targeting of a single neurotransmitter has led to limited therapeutic efficacy. While current medications are not generally effective in regard to negative symptoms and cognitive deficits, they are moderately effective at reducing positive symptoms, most likely because of the relationship between positive symptoms and increased stimulation of D_2 receptors by dopamine. For example, in an imaging study by Abi-Dargham et al. (2000), elevated synaptic dopamine measurements in the striatum were predictive of a reduction of positive symptoms after 6 weeks of treatment with antipsychotic medications. In the same study, negative symptoms did not show any relationship to baseline dopamine measurements and were undiminished by treatment.

The limited efficacy of the currently available antipsychotic medications contributes significantly to the fact that a majority of patients with schizophrenia remain impaired over the long term. In the context of limited pharmacologic efficacy, psychotherapeutic efforts—such as cognitive-behavioral therapy—have become increasingly sophisticated. Similarly, the recovery movement has become vital to the lives of many people with severe mental illness and their families.

In summary, Anthony Da Piazza's longitudinal course, symptoms, and suboptimal treatment response are typical of schizophrenia, as is his ability to function best when compliant with medications and while psychologically and socially supported. He has benefited significantly from his participation in Fountain House, which lent him significant support through its emphasis on recovery. The recovery movement is also likely to have aided his mother as she tried to learn the best ways to help her son. This type of psychosocial effort would be enhanced by the increasingly sophisticated models of cognitive-behavioral therapy and psychiatric interviewing as described by Drs. Landa and Marcus, respectively. After an extended period of stability, however, the illness of his mother presents Mr. Da Piazza with a major crisis, and his future is uncertain. In our efforts to help people like Mr. Da Piazza, we must become increasingly adept at defining subtypes of schizophrenia, understanding the pertinent neurobiology, and creating more effective treatment options.

Summary Points

- Schizophrenia affects perception, cognition, behavior, relationships, and life span.
- Schizophrenia moderately increases the risk of violence and substance abuse.
- Schizophrenia is associated with abnormalities in the prefrontal cortex, temporal lobe, and frontotemporal networks.
- Without a therapeutic alliance, psychiatric interventions with persons with schizophrenia are likely to fail.
- Persons with schizophrenia stand to benefit from evaluations and interventions that include psychodynamics, cognitive-behavioral therapy, and other therapies.
- Antipsychotic medications are at the core of schizophrenia treatment.
- Antipsychotic medications have significant side effects, are frequently not taken by patients, and are generally ineffective against negative symptoms.
- Patients and their families have taken the lead in psychosocial recovery.
- Many people with schizophrenia have inadequate supports and are homeless.
- The use of multiple treatment modalities is most likely to benefit patients.

Chapter 5

TERMINAL ILLNESS AND DOROTHY EWING

Part A

A consultation-liaison psychiatrist was called to see Dorothy Ewing, a 60-year-old married woman, in order to assess her capacity to make medical decisions and to explore the possibility of substance abuse. Asymptomatic in the 2 years since she had been diagnosed with breast cancer, Mrs. Ewing had recently developed shortness of breath, fever, failure to thrive, and "pain throughout her body." The psychiatric consultant was called after the patient refused a chest X ray and all blood work. The psychiatrist's call to the medical intern revealed that the team was concerned that Mrs. Ewing had been medicating herself with her husband's opioids—which he had been prescribed for back pain—and that she appeared depressed and uncommunicative. They had started a long-acting pain medication, MS-Contin (morphine), which they felt should have led to reasonable pain control, and were concerned that she was depressed and drug addicted and lacked capacity to refuse important medical procedures.

Personal History

Mrs. Ewing lived in Queens with her husband. Her three daughters lived nearby. All of them were involved in her care, as was her sister, who was an executive vice president of the hospital. Mrs. Ewing was Catholic and attended Mass "fairly often."

Personal Psychiatric History

None known.

Family Psychiatric History

None known.

Family Medical History

Three relatives had died from cancer: Mrs. Ewing's mother was diagnosed with breast cancer at age 46; her aunt was diagnosed with ovarian cancer at age 49; and her uncle was diagnosed with prostate cancer at age 50.

Medical History

Breast cancer had been diagnosed 2 years earlier. After the tumor was surgically excised, Mrs. Ewing received chemotherapy and radiation therapy. She was seen regularly by her oncologist and had an upcoming appointment.

First Mental Status Exam

The patient was a thin woman who appeared older than her stated age. She was lying at a 45-degree angle in bed, and her hospital gown was carelessly askew. She answered questions with monosyllables and minimal spontaneity, all the while keeping her eyes shut. She agreed with the question "Does it feel like your mind is playing tricks on you?" When she did open her eyes, she stared fearfully at a nearby turned-off television and said that she saw bugs crawling on the screen. She thought she was at home and that the date was 1907. She refused further calculations.

Summary

Dorothy Ewing was a 60-year-old woman who was admitted for a medical evaluation. The first discussion, in Part A, focuses on her confusion, while the remainder of the discussions, in Part B, explore issues that developed in the course of the hospitalization.

Discussion of the Case of Dorothy Ewing, Part A

Delirium 175
   John W. Barnhill, M.D.

Part B 178

Delirium

John W. Barnhill, M.D.

THE treatment team has asked the consulting psychiatrist to evaluate Dorothy Ewing's capacity to refuse simple medical procedures and to assess possible substance abuse and depression. Most urgently, the medical team is eager to do its job, which the team is likely to define as the rapid identification of the cause of Mrs. Ewing's increasing pain, particularly in light of her cancer history. As is often the case, the psychiatric consultant is called not so much to treat an underlying psychiatric disorder or to ameliorate psychosocial distress—though these may be desirable—but rather to help the medical team get to work.

While reading the chart and talking to the medical team, the psychiatrist should quickly develop a tentative differential diagnosis. Few people become dramatically noncompliant because of a sudden onset of sadness, and so depression is unlikely to be the lone problem. Similarly, "drug seeking" might lead to a refusal of blood draws and X rays, but such refusals do not usually occur in 60-year-old married women on the first hospital day, especially when they lack psychiatric and substance abuse histories.

Before seeing the patient, the psychiatrist is likely to have one primary diagnosis in mind, and it is confirmed almost immediately. Mrs. Ewing is disheveled and lying sideways across her bed. She speaks minimally, and when she does say anything, she keeps her eyes shut, as if the world were too much for her. She sees bugs crawling on the turned-off television. She is oriented only to self and appears worried, confused, and constricted. She presents with classic features of a delirium.

The primary team might have missed the delirium diagnosis because fluctuating symptoms are a hallmark of delirium, and her mind may have been relatively clear when she was evaluated. A more likely possibility is that the treating team saw a dysphoric, irritable, noncompliant patient and simply assumed that she was depressed, difficult, and drug addicted.

Missed or delayed diagnoses are a problem for several reasons. First, the delirium will typically not resolve until the cause has resolved; more so than in almost any psychiatric disorder, the diagnosis should prompt a search for an underlying etiology. Second, an accurate diagnosis allows for temporizing psychosocial and pharmacologic interventions. Finally, the patient, family, and staff will be relieved to know that this sort of mental status change is common in hospitals and is likely to be temporary. Even in situations in which the delirium may not resolve—as in some cases of terminal cancer—it can be reassuring for the patient and family to at least know that there is a name for a confusing clinical condition.

Since delirium can be regarded as a failure of brain metabolism, common precipitants can include anything that increases metabolic need, decreases oxygenation, or disrupts neurocircuitry. The case summary features multiple potential causes for Mrs. Ewing's delirium. Her fever increases the brain's metabolic need, while her shortness of breath indicates suboptimal oxygenation. She has a recent history of cancer, which can not only directly cause delirium but also contribute to the delirium through intercurrent infections, electrolyte abnormalities, and/or medications. Her weight loss and failure to thrive underline the importance of a careful search for electrolyte abnormalities, anemia, fluid imbalances, renal or liver failure, acid–base disturbances, thyroid storm, and hyper- or hypoglycemia—all of which can contribute to delirium. Many types of medications are often implicated in delirium, but Mrs. Ewing's opioids are an especially common cause, during either intoxication or withdrawal. Although not applicable to this particular case but of particular note to psychiatrists, medications such as selective serotonin reuptake inhibitor (SSRI) antidepressants and antipsychotics can cause a potentially catastrophic delirium through serotonin syndrome and neuroleptic malignant syndrome, respectively. The hospital-based psychiatrist should pay close attention to all psychiatric medications, especially in cases of polypharmacy and/or higher-than-recommended dosages. In addition to the risk factors of a history of cancer and opioid use, Mrs. Ewing's age puts her at a modestly increased risk for delirium. If she were much older than 60, age-related brain changes would markedly increase her risk; relatively minor infections like pneumonia and urinary tract infections are common precipitants of delirium in the elderly.

As we see with Mrs. Ewing, *hypoactive* delirium is often mistaken for depression. *Hyperactive* delirium—most frequently found during a drug intoxication or withdrawal—is less commonly missed since it causes obvious management problems. Dementia can also appear similar to a delirium, and the two are also often found together. With these distinguishing details firmly in hand, the clinician can immediately diagnose most cases of delirium by glancing at the patient and hearing that the patient has become suddenly "confused." A diagnosis can be made in most of the remaining cases by asking a few cognitive questions. While the Mini-Mental State Examination (MMSE) is probably the most widely used bedside test (Folstein et al. 1975), the Clock Drawing Test is quicker and may be as valid an indicator of cognitive and executive dysfunction (Samton et al. 2005). In the rare case of diagnostic uncertainty, delirium may manifest as slowing on an electroencephalogram (EEG), except in cases of alcohol and benzodiazepine withdrawal, where the EEG tends to show normal or fast waves.

The diagnosis of delirium should prompt the psychiatrist to focus on safety. For example, Mrs. Ewing is at risk for falling and should be assessed for a 1:1 companion. If she is suspected of either using significant doses of pain medications or abusing other substances such as alcohol or benzodiazepines, vital signs should be checked frequently for signs of withdrawal. Her irritable dysphoria may put her at risk for hurting herself or others, and the psychiatrist must evaluate and document the patient's stated intentions and recent history of dangerousness.

Mrs. Ewing's medication regimen should be carefully assessed for contributors to her confusion. Typical culprits are pain and anxiety medications, both of which are often used by primary medical teams to treat worry and irritability. In at-risk patients, however, both opioids and benzodiazepines can exacerbate confusion, even if the immediate effect is sedation. Psychiatric consultations for delirium commonly discontinue or taper such medications. In Mrs. Ewing's case, the psychiatrist would try to help balance her pain complaints with regulated dosages of both short and long-acting opioids.

Patients with delirium do tend to have an impaired sleep-wake cycle, fearfulness, and episodic aggression. To help with these—and to possibly improve cognition—antipsychotic medications are generally used. The choice of antipsychotic is guided by potential side effects and hospital custom, but the antipsychotic is generally used at low dosages at night and during periods of agitation. Recent studies suggest that antipsychotic medications may be associated with a small increase in sudden deaths in the elderly. These studies are not definitive, however, and theoretical medication risks must be weighed against the risks of falls, insomnia, agitation, and noncompliance, all of which can significantly increase morbidity and mortality.

Psychosocial interventions may seem obvious but are appreciated by both the patient and family. Most prominent is helping Mrs. Ewing and her family understand that delirium is common and that it is likely to be of short duration. Psychoeducation can help reduce a variety of problems, including the sort of hostility that is seen in Mrs. Ewing's family (see Part B), and it may also reduce the fear and anxiety that are often a consequence of delirium (Breitbart et al. 2002). It is also useful to reduce sensory deprivation by ensuring that Mrs. Ewing has her glasses and hearing aids, reducing disorientation by encouraging a windowed room and the use of calendars and photographs of relatives, and frequently reorienting her to date, place, and situation. Such psychosocial interventions probably do not shorten the duration of delirium, though they can improve subjective distress and, if used prophylactically, can decrease the incidence of delirium and shorten the hospital length of stay (Inouye et al. 1999).

Delirium is so commonly found that each hospital service has its own name for the same condition. Whether called *ICU psychosis, acute brain syndrome,* or *metabolic encephalopathy,* however, delirium remains one of the most underdiagnosed and dangerous of the conditions that lie on the border between psychiatry, neurology, and medicine. As the specialists who focus on comorbid behavioral, psychological, and cognitive problems, hospital-based psychiatrists are uniquely positioned to diagnose and treat this potentially fatal disorder.

Part B

THE initial medical and psychiatric evaluations revealed a delirium and a lack of capacity. With consent of the husband, noninvasive tests were done, and Mrs. Ewing was found to have an elevated white blood cell count and an infiltrate on her chest X ray. Low-dose antipsychotic medication was prescribed for the delirium and her pneumonia was treated, and over the ensuing 4 days, Mrs. Ewing's cognitive status improved. She became alert, clear, and coherent, and her family believed that she was 85% of her usual self.

Despite her improving cognition, she often refused tests because of pain. When staff acceded to her requests for increased pain medication, she would go to the test but would then be asleep upon her return. Staff members believed that she wanted to be "gorked out" all the time and worried that opioids could cause a recurrence of her delirium, while Mrs. Ewing complained that staff members alternated between being withholding and punishing her by knocking her out with excess medication. The psychiatrist suggested that she be maintained with a moderate dosage of a long-acting opioid (e.g., MS-Contin) in conjunction with a short-acting opioid (e.g., Actiq [oral transmucosal fentanyl citrate]) that she would use as needed for severe pain and procedures.

The adjusted regimen of pain medication led to her acceptance of several important tests over the ensuing several days. She was found to have lesions on her pelvis, lungs, and liver that indicated cancer metastases. Her oncologist told her that her prognosis was poor but that they would work together to develop treatment options. Almost immediately, Mrs. Ewing's shortness of breath worsened, and she began to make increasing use of the short-acting opioid. During brief supportive therapy sessions with the psychiatrist, Mrs. Ewing described the wrenching experience of watching her own mother die of breast cancer. She denied ever having had much anxiety in the past, but she was now terrified of developing the kind of pain that her mother had experienced. It appeared that she was using pain medication to treat anxiety. The psychiatrist met with her daily and continued the low-dose antipsychotic medication, and Mrs. Ewing modestly improved. Staff members grew reluctant to provide her with as-needed opioid medications and so reduced the total amount that she received each day. Mrs. Ewing's anxiety and anger mounted until she became convinced that the staff was composed of mean-spirited technicians who simply wanted to do tests without regard to her well-being. The medical and nursing staffs were convinced that the patient was a complainer and probably a drug addict. The patient's sister, an administrative vice president of the hospital, began to check in on her frequently, often suggesting ways in which the team could improve.

During therapy sessions, Mrs. Ewing explained that she still enjoyed the company of loved ones but was angry that she was going to be unable to watch her grandchildren grow up. While she appreciated the consultant's suggestions for pain medications, she was skeptical that talking would do anything to help the fact that she was being robbed of all that she valued. She had "always believed in God" but now feared that her illness resulted from His wrath. If she had done nothing wrong, why was He punishing her now? Her husband and daughters agreed with the idea that the cancer was being inflicted upon her, but they tended to blame the doctors rather than God. They stared angrily at the medical staff and threatened lawsuits. Mr. Ewing was specifically angry that doctors had not predicted that his wife would inherit the cancer from her mother and wanted to know what they were going to do to prevent breast cancer from occurring in his three daughters.

Additional meetings clarified some historical points. Mrs. Ewing had helped run the family's taxi service, a field in which women were a rarity. She had long been hard-edged and mistrustful, attributes that she believed were essential to success. She and her husband had not been affectionate for years.

Second Mental Status Exam

The patient was a thin, alert, well-groomed, and attentive woman who was wary but cooperative with the interview. She was edgy and fiddled frequently with items on her tray. No tremor or gait abnormality was noted. She described herself as worried and sad but was able to smile when recounting events in her life about which she was proud. She denied suicidality, homicidality, and psychosis. She denied confusion and was fully oriented. Her MMSE score was 26/30, with deficits in attention and concentration.

Summary

After her delirium cleared, Mrs. Ewing was still in significant pain. In addition, she was told that she had terminal cancer. Some of the following discussions explore psychiatric issues related to Mrs. Ewing's medical illness, while the others focus on characteristic responses experienced by the patient, the family, and the medical staff.

Discussions of the Case of Dorothy Ewing, Part B

Pain and Substance Abuse 181
    Steven D. Passik, Ph.D., and Kenneth L. Kirsh, Ph.D.

The Psychodynamic Consultation .183
    Milton Viederman, M.D.

Working With the Family 186
    David W. Kissane, M.D.

The Difficult Patient 190
    Sharon Alspector Mozian, M.D., and Philip R. Muskin, M.D.

Genetic Counseling 194
    Mary Jane Massie, M.D.

Spirituality 197
    Colleen Jacobson, Ph.D.

Meaning-Centered Therapy 200
  Shannon R. Poppito, Ph.D., and William Breitbart, M.D.

The Doctor–Patient Relationship 204
  John W. Barnhill, M.D., and Joseph J. Fins, M.D.

Overview of Hospital Psychodynamics 207
  John W. Barnhill, M.D.

Summary Points 211

Pain and Substance Abuse

Steven D. Passik, Ph.D.
Kenneth L. Kirsh, Ph.D.

DOROTHY Ewing and her medical team face a dilemma regarding control of her severe pain, especially in light of her frequent demands for more opioids than the medical team thinks is wise. Her situation is common among the severely ill, and it reflects some important misconceptions regarding pain, drug-seeking behavior, and addiction.

This 60-year-old woman with bony cancer pain had no prior history of alcohol or drug abuse, and so we would consider it unlikely that she is suffering from opioid addiction. Instead, we would be concerned about undertreatment of cancer pain, especially since Mrs. Ewing has some of the characteristics that have been repeatedly identified as increasing the likelihood of undertreatment, including being an older female. We do not know Mrs. Ewing's ethnicity, but her risk would be even higher if she were nonwhite.

We would anticipate, therefore, that Mrs. Ewing's central problem relates to undertreatment rather than drug abuse and assume the staff misconceptions reflect a "personality clash." We have found, for example, that pain and delirium are often missed in gruff and demanding patients, because their baseline moodiness obscures the changes caused by the organic mental state.

The staff's view of Mrs. Ewing as "difficult" probably began during her initial delirium. Delirium is found in as many as 85% of patients with advanced cancer (Massie and Holland 1992), and delirium can lead to a cluster of symptoms—including irritability, dysphoria, and noncompliance—that are also found in substance abusers. The attentive psychiatrist will try to treat the delirium with support, antipsychotic medications, and the discontinuation of unnecessary centrally acting medications (e.g., benzodiazepines). Particular attention should be paid to the opioids, which are well known to increase the likelihood of delirium. If Mrs. Ewing has impaired renal function—from chemotherapy, for example—it might have been useful to rotate to an opioid(s) with a shorter half-life, fewer active metabolites, or reduced renal metabolism (generally fentanyl or hydromorphone).

Regardless of the exact origin of the problem with her pain management, Mrs. Ewing is facing the very difficult problem of *incident pain*, which is a rapid crescendo of pain caused by movement. Common among people with bony metastases, incident pain refers to a situation in which adequate pain treatment during movement usually causes sedation at rest. Like other patients with incident pain, Mrs. Ewing faces a difficult clinical dilemma: mental clarity with residual pain or relative comfort with excess sleepiness. While sedation may be preferred by patients who are nearing death, are exhausted, and have said their goodbyes, the outspoken Mrs. Ewing would likely want to remain alert. If undermedicated, Mrs. Ewing complains and is seen as drug seeking. If receiving adequate medication for a procedure, Mrs. Ewing is likely to doze when in bed and to then be seen as overmedicated. One common consequence to treatment of incident pain is *pseudo-addiction* (Weissman and Haddox 1989). Pseudo-addiction is defined as poor pain control that creates desperate behavior that is confused with addiction. Incident pain and pseudo-addiction are the likely reasons that Mrs. Ewing used her husband's pain medication in the weeks prior to hospitalization, a behavior that is considered aberrant and worthy of discussion. A the same time, her behavior is understandable and is one reason that as many as 60% of cancer pain patients engage in at least one aberrant behavior (Passik et al. 2000, 2006). Given their frequency and legitimate rationale, such aberrant behaviors are not necessarily a sign of addiction.

In the case of Mrs. Ewing, two medications were combined to successfully treat her incident pain and reduce her "drug seeking." First, she needed a standing dose of an opioid with a moderate half-life in order to cover most of her pain that she felt at rest. In addition, she needed an opioid that would begin to work within 15 minutes so that she could reliably agree to tests and procedures. That same opioid should also have a short half-life to reduce accumulation and intoxication. In many cases, such patients are offered a medication such as oxycodone tablets or immediate-release morphine, but if given on the way to a procedure, neither of these medications is likely to provide symptomatic relief until the end of the procedure, at which point the patient is likely to be sedated, intoxicated, disinhibited, and/or delirious for up to 6 hours. Another common mistake is to prescribe only short-acting opioids, a decision that does reduce accumulation and can help with procedures, but it leaves the patient in significant pain between medication dosages and can reliably induce drug-seeking behavior and pseudo-addiction. For incident pain such as that experienced by Mrs. Ewing, the combination of the two types of medication is critical. While it is reasonable to be attentive to the national problem of prescription substance abuse, such concern is generally not pertinent to severely ill cancer patients such as Mrs. Ewing.

The Psychodynamic Consultation

Milton Viederman, M.D.

THE psychodynamic consultation is designed to engage the medically ill patient through an ongoing, nuanced dialogue. Tailored to the patient, every such interview is unique. While there may be multiple goals to the consultation, it is vital that the patient feel seen and recognized. This process of feeling understood allows the patient to recognize the consultant as a therapeutic presence who can offer relief from the loneliness that often accompanies a medical crisis. How is this done? What sort of questions should the consultant ask? And, more importantly, how does the psychiatrist establish an intimate connection with a difficult, medically ill woman like Mrs. Ewing?

By reading the chart and having a discussion with the primary physicians, the psychiatrist has some knowledge of the patient's predicament before the consultation begins. In the case of Mrs. Ewing, we might wonder if she welcomes the consultation with an expectation of gain. Is she resistant? Does she see the consultation as something imposed upon her? Does she worry that her primary physician sees her as psychiatrically disturbed?

What has she been told about her illness and prognosis? Has she actively inquired about her medical condition, or is she inclined to avoid such a discussion and its serious implications? What are her particular worries? To what extent is she still affected by her delirium? The consultant's initial approach to the patient will likely be based on one of these questions.

In the case of Mrs. Ewing, we know that she is in pain, angry, and skeptical about the value of a psychiatric consultation. After initial introductions and a general inquiry into her health, the consultant might want to specifically explore her greatest immediate concern, which is likely to be the pain. While this may not be the area that most interests the psychiatrist, connection with the patient mandates that the patient's chief complaint be explored. Initial questions might focus on the pattern, intensity, and quality of the pain. While the consultant may be able to make substantive recommendations for pain medications, the initial consultation is also an opportunity to explore the patient's anxieties, concerns, and fantasies related to pain. Pain is a subjective experience. Ever since Beecher's seminal observations during World War II, we have known that the experience of pain depends significantly on its meaning to the patient and the surrounding context (Beecher 1946). For example, pain may be particularly disturbing if it is part of a terminal process that seems to be out of control or if it occurs at night, when the patient is more vulnerable to fearful fantasies. This can be explored through open-ended questions such as "When you are awake at night, what thoughts and feelings dominate your experience?" As part of a basic professional responsibility and as a sign that the chief complaint is taken seriously, the psychiatrist may conclude this phase of the interview with an offer to discuss medication options with the primary team. During this initial exploration, however, the consultant may recognize a hesitancy or hostility that would match the skepticism that had already been noted in Mrs. Ewing. The consultant may decide to acknowledge that skepticism is reasonable given the reality that many doctors had thus far been unable to provide complete pain relief. The consultant could add that it is not clear whether a psychiatrist will help but that such efforts have been helpful to other people.

Mrs. Ewing had been a woman in charge of her life, and the clinician might acknowledge that the passivity of the patient role presents special problems for assertive people like her. What elements of control could be afforded her? The consultant might suggest that she manage aspects of her daily routine such as her as-needed pain medication. Concrete suggestions are clinically helpful and indicate to the patient that she has been heard. The consultant could also say that she is a woman who has prided herself on her independence. The hospital would be a difficult place for such a person. If Mrs. Ewing recognizes this to be true, she may be asked to follow her thoughts, to go back to other times in life when independence was threatened. This would be an effort not to explain her behavior but rather to see where the thoughts lead. The product of the inquiry may lead to the formulation of a psychodynamic life narrative (Viederman 1983) that can be therapeutically useful. The life narrative is a construct that defines a current reaction or characteristic behavior and places it in the context of the patient's life, where it is shown to be a logical and inevitable product of early life experience.

The consultation would continue with an encouragement of openness and curiosity. The consultant might ask Mrs. Ewing whether she has experienced the doctors as having been frank. Had they promised more than could be delivered? Had they not adequately warned her about the possibility of a cancer recurrence? As Mrs. Ewing describes her irritation, the psychiatrist might tactfully explore any long-standing inclination toward mistrust. If such an inclination is acknowledged, the patient could again be asked to go back to her early life and reveal the memories or thoughts that come to mind. Has she experienced other important people as deceptive or hurtful? Was there a pattern of deficient nurturance? This might lead the psychiatrist to consider whether Mrs. Ewing has particular conflicts relating to Erikson's phase of trust versus mistrust (Erikson 1959).

The interviewer might ask how the patient feels about her family's hostility toward the doctors. By asking about this in a nonjudgmental way, the consultant reveals curiosity and encourages the patient to address this issue with greater thoughtfulness. The tone of this question might contrast with that of earlier physicians whose perspective and sense of time constraints might have led to a question that would serve primarily to alienate her (e.g., "Why are you so *angry*?"). To extend this line of inquiry, the consultant might address the family power structure. What is the nature of the ongoing conflict with her husband, and is this now reflected in his lack of understanding of her current situation? Is the patient alone in her suffering, with a sense that no one understands her lonely confrontation with death? What is her fantasy about being punished by God? It is common for patients to have such fantasies, but what thoughts does she have about guilty transgression? How do these relate to her angry renunciation of God?

Apparently, the patient is all too aware of her impending death. It is unclear which aspect of death especially troubles her. This may be asked directly, or by asking how she imagines her future. What was her mother's experience with cancer? Does she fear that her own illness will parallel her mother's? Does she fear intractable pain, helplessness, loss of bodily function, body image changes, dependency, loss of control, or separation from loved ones? It is important to clarify her own understanding of her primary fears, which may be quite different from the fear of death.

The consultant's ability to elucidate and crystallize these concerns will decrease isolation and loneliness, feelings that confront dying patients who have a limited support network. This exploration might lead the psychiatrist to say:

> It seems as though you have been highly successful, both in business and with your kids. Much of this success stems from your independence and willingness to work hard, and these are qualities that you are proud of. And now that you are sick, these same qualities are getting you in trouble with your doctors, who want you to behave and take your medicine. This may be fine for some people, but it doesn't work so well for someone who wants to be in charge.

We do not yet know enough about Mrs. Ewing to be certain about such a statement, but a successful psychodynamic intervention should not try to be a reductionistic summary of a long, complex life. Instead, it is an active, ongoing, imaginative construction of what she is experiencing, an effort that takes into consideration her personality and life experience and the nature of her current stress. This understanding should be communicated to her with the recognition that while it is a start, it is only an approximation. She may then help to refine and clarify her own life story so that the conversation can safely move into uncharted territory, an effort that is, in itself, often deeply therapeutic.

Working With the Family

David W. Kissane, M.D.

PALLIATIVE care has long focused on the family, both because the family has special needs and because the family can provide invaluable support to the person who is sick. While "family" consists of anyone the patient considers family, primary support for a dying patient is most commonly drawn from among the spouse, close members of the extended family, and female kin—daughters, sisters, granddaughters, and in-laws. These people bring with them patterns of coping with illness that include religious and ethnic beliefs and rituals that have been transmitted across the generations. The diverse richness of this transgenerational mix is crucial to the family's ability to respond to the strain of illness and the finitude of life. Families respond to the stress of illness not only through culturally informed supportive strategies but also with varying degrees of adaptation. The psychosocial care of Dorothy Ewing might take both of these dimensions into account, first through an initial family meeting that can identify and make use of the existing supports and then through ongoing family meetings that focus on predictable relationship patterns that may be healthy and supportive but can become, for example, hostile or sullen.

Psychiatric involvement with the Ewing family would begin when the mother becomes delirious. The sudden onset of confusion is often frightening to the patient but may be even more upsetting to family members, who worry not only about the indignity and potential for falls but also about the possibility of permanent cognitive deficits. Further, delirium is often accompanied by irritable dysphoria and demoralization in the patient, and such emotional reactions are contagious and quickly shared with worried family members. Intense feelings can quickly translate into anger, predisposing family members to complicated grief (Kato and Mann 1999), especially among family members with unresolved family conflicts.

A family meeting is often organized when an important change develops in the medical status of the chronically or terminally ill patient. Its aims are to facilitate understanding of the goals of care, promote care provision, and nurture adaptation to the emergent clinical reality. The resultant process integrates the biological with the psychosocial, optimizing a cohesive approach to care giving and support.

The meeting should include key representatives from the family, the medical team, and the psychosocial care team, though its exact composition will depend on a variety of factors that include availability, preexisting family conflicts, and cultural traditions such as a patriarchy or matriarchy that might lead to the exclusion of certain family members. Mild cognitive impairment is not an absolute contraindication to patient involvement, but delirious or agitated patients will not make a useful contribution. Otherwise, patients should generally be asked to participate.

Prior to the meeting, the medical and psychosocial teams should seek clarity about diagnosis, treatment plan, disease progression, and prognosis. Clinicians who are attached to their patients overestimate future length of life by error rates of two- to fivefold. Families tend to maintain similarly optimistic viewpoints that depend less on actual information than on hopes, fears, and expectations. While the exact life expectancy is rarely certain, some sort of consensus should be reached in this pre-meeting, even if it is only an awareness of physician disagreement. In the course of the meeting, the patient and/or family members may collude to avoid the diagnosis or prognosis. If so, the clinician should use the language of the patient and/or family and avoid an immediate confrontation, trusting that an ongoing alliance will allow adequate care provision and continued tactful negotiation regarding a shared understanding of the illness. Underlying this attitude is the acknowledged uncertainty of disease progression alongside the existential drive to continue life until death intervenes.

In regard to the structure of the meeting, it generally begins with the dispensing of medical information and gradually becomes more interactive and more focused on psychosocial concerns. Throughout, the goal is improved understanding, an appreciation of challenges and concerns, and the creation of a consensus about the care plan.

In the case of Mrs. Ewing, for example, the medical team might meet with the family during her delirium and then, once she is cognitively clear, meet with the family and the patient. Throughout these meetings, the psychiatrist should be prepared to ask questions that help explore the needs of the family. Initially, linear questions might provide basic information. As the family relaxes, more open-ended questions can help Mrs. Ewing and her relatives reflect and describe their perspectives on relational and support patterns. As these sessions unfold, the clinician can offer increasingly thorough summaries that might underscore tensions, ambivalences, and strengths within the family. As is generally the case, the therapist should retain neutrality and avoid being drawn into potentially entrenched differences of opinion or style among the family members (Kissane at al. 1998).

One or two such meetings can help some families regroup and adapt to the difficult situation in ways that are creative and resilient. These *adaptive families* can be recognized through their mutual support, intimacy, and open communication in responding to adversity. They may argue among themselves, but they can tolerate conflict and remain cohesive. Adaptive families make good use of community resources; their relational styles are supportive and conflict resolving; and they exhibit very low rates of psychosocial morbidity among their members. These families demonstrate a robust ability to successfully adapt to the most difficult of challenges (Kissane and Bloch 2002).

Other families develop predictable difficulties that can be assessed on the basis of three variables: the family's communication skills, level of cohesiveness, and ability to resolve conflict. The most dysfunctional families communicate poorly; conflict causes fractures and separations; and they struggle to provide support for a sick family member. Such families have a pattern of relating termed *hostile*. While they may appear to be in desperate need of psychotherapeutic intervention, they often reject offered help (Kissane and Bloch 2002).

A second dysfunctional pattern is marked by more muted conflict and is associated with *sullen families*. Less outwardly angry than hostile families, sullen families demonstrate poor communication skills and limited levels of cohesion. These problems lead to high rates of depression and poor coping in family members. These family members are more help-accepting than hostile families, and therapeutic interventions are more effective.

Given their levels of conflict and anger, Mrs. Ewing's family may profit from family focused grief therapy (FFGT), which is a preventive model of family-centered care that begins during the diagnosis of a terminal illness and is extended into bereavement. *Grief* refers here to the many losses caused by illness, as well as the potential loss of the sick family member. The model aims to optimize relationships within the family, promote adaptive coping, and maximize family strengths. The patient's involvement in treatment can be helpful in a variety of ways, including the deepening of the therapist/family alliance during the eventual bereavement. A recent randomized trial demonstrated that FFGT led to reduced distress and depression in family members 13 months postdeath compared with untreated controls (Kissane et al. 2006). Better effect sizes occurred in families of the *sullen* type. Depending on the needs of the family, therapy can range from 4 to 12 sessions over as many months.

FFGT treatment of the Ewing family might begin during the delirium. The psychiatrist would draw out the family's understanding of delirium and its etiology, frame a treatment strategy, and emphasize that delirium is often transient. After the delirium clears, a second meeting might be used to explore the meaning of pain and the varied approaches to its management. At this meeting, the psychiatrist might also lay out the medical plan for ongoing treatment of the patient's cancer and its related symptoms. As an alliance develops, the patient and family might be interested in discussing the meaning of the illness, which would provide an opportunity to learn about religious and cultural issues that are often ignored in the hospital. What was hard about Mrs. Ewing's mother's death? Did any benefits ensue? What approach might help Mrs. Ewing and her family explore the spiritual implications of her disease? What is their understanding of the genetic risk to the daughters? Are there any long-standing conflicts between different family members that are currently causing problems? How are different family members dealing with the illness? How is the husband coping? Throughout these sessions, the psychiatrist would try to help uncover the deepest and most long-standing values that are shared by Mrs. Ewing and her family. Such shared beliefs could enhance family cohesion during times of conflict. Any demoralization could be addressed as a group, with the invitation for them to rally in celebration of her life. The emerging affection between Dorothy and her husband could be underlined as an indication of this family's desire to support and help one another.

While it cannot be predicted in advance whether the Ewing family fits the criteria for a hostile, sullen, or adaptive family, their anger, tendency to blame others, lack of trust, and the distant marital relationship are hints that they are at risk for conflict and a poor outcome. While culture is handed down across the generations, so are patterns of dysfunctional relationships that can be the target of a focused intervention. A crisis may be painful but it can also be an opportune moment to harness family strengths and optimize the ability to cope with adversity.

The Difficult Patient

Sharon Alspector Mozian, M.D.
Philip R. Muskin, M.D.

WHILE not a diagnostic category in itself, "the difficult patient" is a frequent precipitant for psychiatric consultation in the general hospital. This heterogeneous group of patients have a central common trait: they induce strong emotional responses—or countertransference—in clinicians. Some difficult patients are calmly recognized by members of their primary medical team, but many others are identified by the psychiatric consultant through the internist's tone of voice or offhand comment. The psychiatrist must, therefore, listen to both the words and the music of the consultation. To increase the likelihood of a successful intervention, the psychiatrist should also look explicitly for variables that might make someone "difficult" to his or her treatment team. While we cannot know for sure why this particular treatment team finds Dorothy Ewing to be difficult, she does manifest a number of key variables that are commonly found among difficult patients. These include her behavior, complex family issues, her status within the hospital, and character traits.

Patient Behaviors

Patients commonly behave badly in the hospital, at least partly because the crisis of illness often leads to regressive behavior and utilization of primitive defense mechanisms (Groves and Muskin 2005; Muskin 1995). Depending on the patient, the difficult behavior can range from florid psychosis and physical aggression to extreme neediness and depression, all of which make doctors uncomfortable and can quickly create barriers to care.

How did Mrs. Ewing's behavior become difficult for the treating team? The initial psychiatric consultation was called after Mrs. Ewing refused a chest X ray and blood work. The "words" of the consult request a determination of whether depression or drug addiction was interfering with Mrs. Ewing's capacity to consent for medical procedures. The accompanying "music" informs the psychiatrist that this refusal has become a significant problem for a primary team that is now unable to carry out its treatment plan.

Why has Mrs. Ewing refused? Is her refusal due to depression or drug addiction as implied by the primary team? Is she angry at the doctors and refusing the procedures out of spite? Has she regressed to the point of using borderline defenses such as splitting and projection? It quickly becomes clear to the psychiatrist that Mrs. Ewing's initial refusals were manifestations of a delirium. The psychiatric consultant's identification of the delirium was critical, while the issue of capacity became secondary. Additionally, helping the team recognize that the patient's refusal was not intentional may help manage the team's countertransference and improve its performance.

How else has Mrs. Ewing's behavior been perceived as difficult? After the delirium resolved, she complained of severe pain, refused to leave her bed for tests, and made frequent requests for pain medication. The staff became concerned that she was becoming a drug addict. Complaining patients, especially those who demand pain medications, are viewed as needy and entitled; doctors and nurses instinctually ignore such demands, regardless of their validity (Groves 1978). This common situation in the medical hospital should prompt several questions in the psychiatrist's mind. First, are the doctors treating the patient's pain adequately? Bony pain is notoriously difficult to treat and frequently requires high doses of opioids to make the patient comfortable. Doctors fear turning their patients into drug addicts and commonly—if unintentionally—undertreat pain (Marks and Sachar 1973). This can create, as it does in Mrs. Ewing's case, a cycle of worsening interpersonal interactions. In the eyes of Mrs. Ewing and her family, the staff is mean-spirited and withholding, while in the eyes of the staff, Mrs. Ewing is a complaining drug addict with a family that threatens lawsuits. In response to these perceptions, the staff avoids giving prn pain medications and the patient refuses to cooperate with tests and procedures. The psychiatrist recognizes this situation and adjusts the pain medications, and the patient and staff are more comfortable. The psychiatrist might also seize this opportunity to talk to Mrs. Ewing's doctors and nurses. While empathizing with their anxiety about prescribing high doses of opioids, the psychiatrist can educate about the treatment of bony pain and provide reassurance that the patient will not become an addict. To do so in a nonjudgmental and uncritical way is one of the arts of psychiatric consultation.

Other questions should come to mind with a patient like Mrs. Ewing who is demanding pain medications. For example, is she attempting to medicate an anxiety disorder? If so, the anxiety can be assessed and treated. Some of Mrs. Ewing's desperation may be secondary to her fear that she will suffer the way her mother did when she died of breast cancer. If so, we would want to understand more about this experience and how it is affecting her current hospital experience. The assessment of dangerousness, as always, is crucial in this patient as well: is she attempting to hoard narcotics so that she can overdose and commit suicide?

Family Issues

The "difficult" label can stem from the patient, but Mrs. Ewing is also seen as difficult because her family is threatening litigation. Few things stir up fear in doctors like the threat of impending lawsuits. It is crucial to identify the meaning behind the family's threats. Why are they so angry? Do they believe their mother is suffering unnecessarily? Do they fear that the daughters will have breast cancer like the mother and grandmother? Do they feel the patient is being mistreated? Are their threats a reaction to their feelings of helplessness or guilt? Most actual malpractice suits stem not simply from a bad outcome but from a poor relationship between the patient and doctor. The psychiatric consultant can often be central in understanding the needs of the patient and family. Through this clarification, the treatment team can more effectively manage the difficult family and reduce untoward legal events.

Patient Status

All patients are not created equal. Depending on the clinician's own biases, low status might, for example, be conferred by homelessness or alcohol dependence. Low status is often reinforced by rendering the patient distant and anonymous through using a diagnosis as the person's primary identifier. For example, patients may become "a 65-year-old GI bleeder" or "a 50-year-old homeless alcoholic." While shorthand may improve efficiency, the psychiatric consultant can help humanize the patient by mentioning that the 65-year-old with a GI bleed is a math professor or the 50-year-old homeless alcoholic is the father of a hospital employee. In this way, almost any patient can become a special patient in a more positive way.

Special status also depends on the degree to which the patient promotes identification. For example, some of Mrs. Ewing's clinicians might be especially admiring of her durability and business acumen. While her attending physicians might be affected by the fact that she is dying at the relatively young age of 60, some younger trainees might view 60 as being quite old. Some of the doctors might identify more readily with the patient's daughters, who are likely to be their own age.

Like most other people, members of the medical staff may be affected by VIP patients. Mrs. Ewing lacks fame and wealth and may not seem unusual, but her sister is a senior administrator at the hospital. Most doctors do not actually know what administrators do, but they are aware that such people control salaries and jobs. In hospitals, then, the sister of a senior administrator becomes a VIP patient. Such a status may improve her care, but, in the case of Mrs. Ewing, her sister's perceived intrusiveness seems to have intensified the medical team's avoidance and irritation.

Mrs. Ewing showed improvement during her hospital stay, but her overall prognosis is grim. Dying patients have their own status within hospitals. This leads some staff members to show special interest and patience, while other doctors—and family members—avoid interactions with the patient. Such behavior can exacerbate the patient's feelings of loneliness, abandonment, and anger, creating a cycle of staff avoidance, patient loneliness and anger, and more staff avoidance. The psychiatric consultant can intervene by outlining for the medical team how the patient will benefit from clear, brief strategies and by helping the patient find more adaptive coping mechanisms than lashing out at her doctors and nurses.

Character Traits and Pathology

Patients with certain character traits or pathology are frequently experienced as difficult. Mrs. Ewing has been "hard-edged and mistrustful," qualities that were apparently adaptive in the business world. These same traits are problematic in the hospital, however, where doctors expect and need to be trusted. An edgy, wary patient can make doctors feel devalued, inadequate, and anxious. Further, her fear of dying may combine with the mistrust and lead to projected blame and a belief that the doctors are inflicting harm on her. At this point, the psychiatrist can recognize Mrs. Ewing's need for control and suggest to the team that they be as "transparent" as possible, providing the patient with specific details of her workup and treatment. This might include anything from the rationale for tests to the potential side effects of medications. Although these interventions may be time and labor intensive, her fatigue will prevent these discussions from stretching too long, and transparency will help develop a rapport with Mrs. Ewing and her family.

There is no formula that can be applied to resolving the problem of the difficult patient. Textbook chapters never do justice to the complexity of a particular case, nor can they replace the creativity of the psychiatric consultant. What seems to be most useful is recognizing that a difficult patient can be *difficult* for a myriad of reasons. A psychiatric consultant, through the process of listening to the consult request, recognizing familiar themes that result in the label of "difficult," interviewing the patient, and gathering information from others, can successfully demystify the difficulty (Lipowski 1967). In so doing, the consultant can help to reestablish the alliance between the treating team and the patient.

Genetic Counseling

Mary Jane Massie, M.D.

CANCER has been diagnosed in four members of the Ewing family, and it is not surprising that they want to learn more about its inheritance. The psychiatric approach to such a situation includes evaluation that leads to a diagnosis and some combination of education, support, and treatment. Before any effective intervention, however, the psychiatrist must possess an understanding of relevant cancer genetics.

Breast cancer is the most common cancer in women. In the great majority of cases, breast cancer develops without significant familial clustering. Such cases are considered *sporadic*. When constructing Dorothy Ewing's family history, the psychiatrist would focus on all cancers, but particularly cancers of the breast, ovary, prostate, and colon. Mrs. Ewing's mother was diagnosed with breast cancer at age 46, her aunt with ovarian cancer at age 49, and her uncle with prostate cancer at age 50. A *familial pattern* is likely when there is a family history of breast and ovarian cancer or two or more cases of breast cancer diagnosed before the age of 50, and so the Ewing family conforms to one criterion (cancer of the breast and ovary).

Such knowledge may well drive the Ewing family to seek genetic counseling and DNA testing. They have had several years to consider such testing, however, and have so far deferred the option. There may be many reasons for such a delay, but an important issue may be that knowledge of a genetic predisposition to cancer can be very upsetting and could be driving some of the family's current hostility. In addition to fears of developing cancer, many people worry about the possibility of employment and insurance discrimination based on genetic test results (Offit and Thom 2007). The discussion of genetic testing would therefore require a knowledgeable approach and would often be carried out by clinical geneticists or specially trained genetic counselors.

The family may be specifically worried that Mrs. Ewing is one of the 5%–10% of women with breast cancer who have *hereditary* breast cancer. A significant proportion of hereditary breast cancer can be attributed to mutations in one of two breast cancer susceptibility genes, *BRCA1* or *BRCA2* (Garber and Offit 2005; Robson and Offit 2007; Smith and Robson 2006). These mutations are passed in an autosomal dominant fashion, and so if Mrs. Ewing tests positive for either of these gene mutations, there would be a 50% chance that the mutation would be passed along to each of her children. If one of her daughters does inherit such a mutation, she would have an 80% chance of being diagnosed with breast cancer during her lifetime (Antoniou et al. 2003) in contrast to the 12.5% risk in the general population. She would also have a greatly elevated lifetime risk of ovarian cancer, ranging from 54% with the *BRCA1* mutation to 23% with *BRCA2*. These risks compare unfavorably with the 1%–2% lifetime risk of ovarian cancer in the general population. Men with these mutations carry elevated risks of breast, prostate, pancreas, and colon cancers.

During genetic counseling, the family would be informed that most people who develop breast cancer will not test positive for the currently available genetic testing. If Mrs. Ewing does have a negative test, the results will be of limited value to her daughters. If a *BRCA* mutation is found in Mrs. Ewing, however, testing can be informative. If she tests positive and her daughters test negative, then the family will have the reassuring news that the daughters did not inherit the greatly elevated cancer risk. If Mrs. Ewing tests positive and one (or more) of her daughters is also positive, then the daughter will have inherited the high risk of cancer. Such news is a major reason that some people choose not to get tested, but throughout the process and regardless of the ultimate result, the therapist should remain alert to psychological reactions that may include fear, anxiety, anger, relief, and guilt.

If the daughters are found to be at high risk, they may decide to actively minimize their chance of becoming ill. Their efforts might include enrollment in a high-risk surveillance clinic. Such clinics provide education about cancer prevention and detection while providing multiple types of support. Psychoeducation tends to begin with *primary prevention,* which might include lifestyle changes such as exercise and healthy eating and the consideration of chemoprevention with a medication like tamoxifen.

Secondary prevention strategies for high-risk women are aimed at early cancer detection and include breast examination and mammography and may include magnetic resonance imaging and ultrasound. Women at increased risk should also receive ovarian cancer screening that includes pelvic examinations, transvaginal color-Doppler sonography, and CA-125 screening. Both men and women at increased risk should also receive colon cancer screening, while men should be regularly screened for prostate cancer.

Patients in high-risk surveillance clinics would also learn about the risks and benefits of prophylactic risk-reducing surgery, in which bilateral mastectomy or salpingo-oophorectomy is performed to significantly reduce the likelihood of later cancer (Friebel et al. 2007; Rebbeck et al. 2002).

These prophylactic surgeries would not, of course, be performed before the consequences were thoughtfully considered. In some cancer centers, psychiatric consultation is an essential part of the evaluation process for the woman who considers risk-reducing surgery (Massie and Greenberg 2005). This evaluation includes a review of the woman's family and personal psychiatric history with a focus on psychiatric conditions that might impact on the decision (e.g., body dysmorphic disorder, depressive disorders, anxiety disorders, or personality disorders). It would also include exploration of the family history of all cancers and the person's perceptions and fears related to her own cancer risk.

In order to predict the woman's response to prophylactic surgery, the psychiatrist might explore her satisfaction with previous plastic surgery; her history of litigation; and her history of abuse, rape, or assault. Since these surgeries impact on reproduction and breast feeding, the evaluation should clarify her sexual, pregnancy, and breast-feeding histories, with some focus on her desire to have (more) children. If loved ones are involved, their points of view are discussed, but surgery is, of course, the woman's decision. This evaluation provides an opportunity to clarify information, discuss decisions and the decision-making process, and obtain psychological understanding and support. The evaluation would also be an opportunity to diagnose and treat psychiatric disorders and to discuss strategies to manage situation-specific anxiety. Finally, the counselor could explore ways in which the patient might feel pressured to have or not have the surgery. This latter concern is of particular importance since it has been found that the women who later express regret about having had prophylactic mastectomy are those who feel that the decision was driven by their surgeon (Payne et al. 2000).

Genetic counseling makes use of some of the most technologically sophisticated tools in medicine. It is now routinely done for diseases that begin in childhood, such as sickle cell disease and Tay-Sachs disease, to hereditary cancer syndromes, like breast cancer, that occur throughout the life cycle. The psychiatrist has an important role through counseling, advocacy, education, and research.

Spirituality

Colleen Jacobson, Ph.D.

IN the context of her serious illness, Dorothy Ewing seems to have become preoccupied with God, a concern that is central to the "existential crisis that is terminal illness" (Kearney 2000). In particular, she appears to be displacing her anger at her cancer onto God, a common reaction to a terrible diagnosis. Her search for causation and meaning may be somewhat adaptive but may also alienate her from a religion that had previously provided comfort as well as from her doctors who are trying to treat her illness.

To maximize the effectiveness of Mrs. Ewing's treatment, her clinicians should make use of the growing body of literature on the interaction between religion and health. In concert with an increasing focus on the terminally ill, for example, there is increasing evidence that certain types of religiosity and spirituality may promote adjustment to physical illness and ensuing death (Fehring et al. 1997; McClain et al. 2003; McClain-Jacobson et al. 2004). Exploration into religion and spirituality is not intended, of course, to change fundamental beliefs. Instead, it has two fundamental purposes: to help the person feel understood and to find meaning in the life that is remaining.

Such a pursuit can be facilitated by understanding some of the recent literature. Researchers typically divide religiosity into two types. *Intrinsic religiosity* relates to living life according to one's own religious beliefs, while *extrinsic religiosity* refers to the use of religion for social connectedness. *Spirituality* typically refers to feeling a connection to a greater being or to understanding life in relation to existential values. Intrinsic religiosity and spirituality overlap in their focus on a search for meaning, and higher levels of each have been associated with lower levels of depression, hopelessness, and suicidal ideation among terminally ill patients. It appears that it is this meaning-making that is most closely linked to positive psychological states (Fehring et al. 1997; McClain et al. 2003; Nelson et al. 2002). In talking to Mrs. Ewing, the clinician might want to explore the ways in which she pursues her religious faith and what she means when she says that she fears that her illness has resulted from His wrath. Such a discussion might also include ways in which her religion has been helpful in finding meaning in the world.

TABLE 5–1. PSYCHIATRIC INVOLVEMENT IN RELIGIOUS AND SPIRITUAL ISSUES

Level	Approach	Examples of techniques	Case example
1	Exclude religious issues from assessment and therapeutic stages.	Do not discuss religious or spiritual issues; if patient mentions religion, refer to pastoral care.	Ask Mrs. Ewing if she would like to discuss religion with a priest.
2	Include religious/spiritual issues within assessment phase only.	Include a series of questions about religious issues. If this assessment identifies distress, refer the patient to pastoral care.	When Mrs. Ewing worries that God is punishing her, ask about her belief system. If she still struggles, refer to priest.
3	Support and encourage exploration within therapeutic relationship.	In addition to the approach of level 2, explore how religious and spiritual beliefs affect patient's psychological state and vice versa.	Explore Mrs. Ewing's theories about God's role in her illness and that of her mother. Consider other options and whether her current beliefs are affected by depression.
4	Specifically address religious and moral dilemmas within the therapeutic relationship.	In addition to the approaches of levels 2 and 3, ask patient to explore conflicts about religion. Tactfully point out contradictions that may be hurtful. Judiciously reveal personal conflicts and resolutions about religion.	Point out that Mrs. Ewing's God is both all-loving and all-punishing. Explore alternative explanations and perhaps include examples of how you have resolved tragedy within religion.

Source.   Adapted from Josephson et al. 1999.

Coping style is also important. Health has been positively correlated with active and collaborative coping styles, while "deferred religious coping"—passively relying on God—has been negatively associated with health (Pargament et al. 1998). Additionally, belief in an afterlife has been associated with lower levels of end-of-life despair in one study of terminally ill patients (McClain-Jacobson et al. 2004). If done nonjudgmentally and tactfully, such an interview could help Mrs. Ewing regain some perspective on her religion and her relationship to God.

A basic understanding of the major religions can aid in differentiating a delusion from a religious belief. For example, one could conceptualize Mrs. Ewing's belief that her illness is a result of God's wrath as a delusion that warrants antipsychotic medication. At the same time, Mrs. Ewing's Catholicism endorses the belief in the punishment for one's sins. The mention of religion should not de-skill, however, and so the interviewer should tactfully try to understand both the patient and her belief system in order to uncover treatable psychiatric conditions. This might lead to a tactful exploration of the extent to which her fear of punishment is consistent with her religious belief and the extent to which it reflects depression, a delusion, or a transient projection of her own anger and hostility. For example, Mrs. Ewing's fear of God's punishment might quickly resolve with a reduction of pain medications or with psychological support that helps lift her out of a regressive, depressive position. Conversely, tactful questioning might reveal a lifelong belief that all good and bad events are the result of prior behaviors and misbehaviors, and she may forever believe that her cancer was the result of some prior malfeasance. While this may not be a view shared by the consultant, it would not necessarily warrant psychiatric treatment.

Table 5–1 outlines four levels of involvement available to clinicians as they approach spirituality in their patients. While the depth of interaction will vary based on the patient and the therapist, it should be underlined that the pursuit of meaning does lie within the psychotherapeutic task. For example, both meaning-centered psychotherapy and the psychodynamic life narrative can help patients find meaning during the final phase of life (Breitbart et al. 2004; Viederman 1983). Increasing evidence demonstrates that good clinical practice requires at least level 2 involvement.

Meaning-Centered Therapy

Shannon R. Poppito, Ph.D.

William Breitbart, M.D.

THE case of Dorothy Ewing is complex, but such complexity is the rule rather than the exception in psycho-oncology. The complexity is derived, in part, from the "all-too-human" players in this drama of pain and suffering—players who include not only Mrs. Ewing and her family and friends but also the doctors and nurses. These care providers appear to have a limited understanding of both the patient and their own sense of helplessness, and so they quickly label Mrs. Ewing "difficult" and a "drug abuser." Such an approach allows her physicians to feel a sense of control, but they then miss the reality that their patient is grappling with fundamental questions of human existence. In the face of such adversity, Mrs. Ewing may benefit deeply from psychotherapy that is based on Victor Frankl's writings that focus on helping people find meaning in the face of great suffering.

Existential Pain and Suffering

When we look beyond Mrs. Ewing's "severe bony pain," we will find an existential suffering that includes the physical pain as well as anguished changes in her familial relationships, psychological functioning, cognition, and spiritual life. In order to understand Mrs. Ewing, we will need to explore all of these spheres. Cancer will also have a personal, historical meaning to Mrs. Ewing. She bears the genetic legacy of a mother, aunt, and uncle who all died early of cancer, and she is likely to fear that she might pass on her genetic vulnerability to her own daughters. Moreover, she carries the emotional wounds of witnessing her own mother die an eerily familiar "wrenching, horrendous" fate of metastatic breast cancer. Without attention, any one of these concerns may seriously impact on the quality of her final days.

Mrs. Ewing's suffering is multifaceted. For example, she complains of shortness of breath that may stem from disease progression, but it could also stem from anxiety related to memories of her own mother's terrifying death, anticipation of her own demise, or worries about God. She may be suffering from death anxiety, or existential *angst,* a word that derives from the Latin *angere,* meaning "to squeeze" or "to strangle." When patients dread death, they may feel as if they are being strangled to death.

Relieving Existential Suffering

Victor Frankl championed the importance of finding meaning in suffering. In his seminal work *Man's Search for Meaning,* Frankl (1959) wrote that even when all else has been stripped away—physically, mentally, emotionally, spiritually—one may still find meaning in life. Frankl (1959) challenged,

> We must never forget that we may find meaning in life even when confronted with a hopeless situation, when facing a fate that cannot be changed. For what then matters is to bear witness to the uniquely human potential at its best, which is to transform a personal tragedy into a triumph, to turn one's predicament into a human achievement. When we are no longer able to change a situation, such as inoperable cancer, we are challenged to change ourselves. (p. 116)

Meaning-centered therapy, developed from Frankl's meaning-oriented ("logotherapeutic") framework, was particularly created for the unique existential needs and concerns of advanced end-stage cancer patients (Breitbart 2002; Breitbart et al. 2004; Greenstein and Breitbart 2000). The therapist attempts to engage dying patients by helping them find meaning through an acknowledgement of their grief and sadness while fostering a sense that life-meanings can again be found. In so doing, the therapist and patient can help convert a tragedy (cancer) into a human triumph (legacy), a core theme of Meaning-Centered Therapy.

Exploring Sources of Meaning

Unlike an open-ended exploratory therapy, meaning-based treatment features a guided exploration of distinct aspects of the patient's life. The approach takes into consideration the realities that people are not naturally prone to discussing both the best and the most difficult aspects of their lives, that a longitudinal understanding is important, and that time is limited. Such an effort can lead to the discovery of personal meaning in the midst of the most difficult set of circumstances.

We might begin our work with Mrs. Ewing by asking her to recall experiences, loves, losses, and accomplishments. Such an effort might remind her of her unique humanity, thereby bolstering her self-worth and dignity. In addition, we would help explore her personal view of history, culture, and the human condition, universal constructs to which we all belong; such a discussion can help her feel connected to humanity and reduce her existential isolation.

This exploration would gradually deepen to include a broader understanding of Mrs. Ewing's history, an understanding that can be viewed as her *living legacy.* We would subdivide this legacy into three parts (see Figure 5–1).

Sources of Meaning

❖ **Historical Sources** – *"Life as a Living Legacy"*
  • Legacy that has been given (past)
  • Legacy one lives (present)
  • Legacy one will give (future)

❖ **Attitudinal Sources** – *"Encountering Life's Limitations"*
  • Turning personal tragedy into triumph via the attitude taken toward given circumstances (e.g., physical suffering, personal adversity, one's mortality)

❖ **Creative Sources** – *"Actively Engaging in Life"*
  • Via roles, work, deeds, accomplishments
  • Re: courage, commitment, and responsibility

❖ **Experiential Sources** – *"Connecting With Life"*
  • Via relationships, beauty, nature, humor

FIGURE 5–1.   Sources of meaning.

The first involves the unalterable past and includes her inherited legacy (e.g., her genetic predisposition to cancer), her upbringing, her loves (e.g., her family), and her losses (e.g., her mother). In the second we would focus on the present and address her here-and-now relationships with her husband, three children, and close friends. Finally, we would help Mrs. Ewing develop a future legacy, which would be framed as the meanings of her life that will be passed on. The meaning-centered therapist would explore her sadness and resentment as well as things about which she is proud or happy. Such a dialogue might lead to the sense that Mrs. Ewing is especially upset by her terminal illness, since it will prevent her from seeing her grandchildren grow up. After sitting with these hopeless feelings, however, the therapist would encourage and even challenge Mrs. Ewing to consider that her attitude toward life and suffering could be a living testament of courage that can be shared with her grandchildren for years to come. Choosing one's attitude toward life in the face of suffering and death is a core value of meaning-centered work, in which it is termed an *attitudinal source of meaning.* The meaning-centered therapist helps Mrs. Ewing see that beyond physical limitations, there lies a freedom in choosing her attitude at any given moment.

Using this framework, Mrs. Ewing's therapist would continue the treatment by encouraging her to explore *creative and experiential sources* of meaning by talking about moments when she was engaged in life through being a mother, wife, and worker, as well as through recalling moments when she experienced love, beauty, and humor. Such memories are elicited using direct questions and the assumption that each of us has experienced a range of deep, gratifying experiences. Meaning-centered dialogue often leads dying patients to new perspectives on the people around them and may lead them to direct expressions of love, gratitude, and even forgiveness toward the important people in their lives. Some people resist opening up old wounds or facing the realities of serious illness, but many people are hungry for the opportunity for such a dialogue.

In sitting with Mrs. Ewing, the therapist acts not only as a guide in the pursuit of meaning but as a physical reminder that she has not been abandoned, thereby functioning as a comforting transitional presence as death approaches. Further, the work provides a model for intimacy for her family and friends. Strong emotions may well up when she talks about such issues as her own mother's early death, her business, her pain, and her difficult marriage. Like happy memories, regrets are inevitable, and they can be framed back to the patient as an example of the richness and complexity of life. In bearing witness to both the positive and negative meanings that emerge in the therapeutic process, meaning-centered therapy allows for an unfolding dialogue that offers Mrs. Ewing the space and time to bring meaningful closure to a well-lived life.

The Doctor–Patient Relationship

John W. Barnhill, M.D.

Joseph J. Fins, M.D.

THE psychiatric service can help Dorothy Ewing in a variety of ways, but from the perspectives of a psychiatrist and an internist-ethicist, we would suggest that her medical team has the primary role in reducing her suffering and that many of Mrs. Ewing's problems stem from her primary team stepping away from its responsibilities. Psychiatrists can—and should—play a vital role as consultants in complex cases and in situations where primary psychiatric issues affect the hospitalization. They are often useful in ethical dilemmas and in situations where doctor–patient communication is especially difficult.

All of these indications for a psychiatric consultation play some role in Mrs. Ewing's hospitalization, but it remains true that Mrs. Ewing's nonpsychiatrist physicians missed her delirium, overdiagnosed substance abuse and depression, undertreated her pain, and got into a squabble with both the patient and her family. These behaviors are significant, but perhaps the most serious error is the apparent absence of any medical perspective on her terminal illness. Such lapses are all too common in American hospitals and may reflect our increasingly narrow view of our role as physicians. Instead of accepting the responsibility of ministering to the suffering, physicians are increasingly ignoring the biopsychosocial needs of their patients, leading to fragmented care and to the loss of the powerfully therapeutic aspects of the doctor–patient relationship.

While we do not actually know the workings of this particular medicine team, we do know that many modern physicians see death as a medical failure (Wanzer et al. 1984). Much of medical training revolves around a similar notion of underachievement, and even though medicine is filled with uncertainty, physicians of all ages are often plagued by the concern that they might make a mistake. This can lead them to a pseudo-objectification of their roles as physicians, so that they believe that they have succeeded if they fulfill a series of more-or-less technical tasks (Danis et al. 1999; Fins and Nilson 2000). This narrow, superficial approach might lead members of the medical team to look at Mrs. Ewing's sad face and diagnose depression, glance at her medication list and diagnose substance abuse, and assess her family as "difficult" as soon as they question anything about her care.

Despite Mrs. Ewing's terminal illness, there seems to be little communication between the doctors and the patient and family. Left in an information vacuum, Mrs. Ewing and her family become increasingly frustrated and upset. How might her primary medical team have improved this difficult situation? Perhaps the most important intervention would be a discussion of her situation as well as an exploration of the values of the patient and family. Such a discussion may involve the psychiatric consultant, but internists handle most of these conversations alone.

The discussion about the treatment plan should be an exploration rather than an effort to help Mrs. Ewing decide whether or not to sign the Do Not Resuscitate (DNR) paperwork. DNR is not a care plan (Fins et al. 1999). Mrs. Ewing's prognosis may be poor, but there are always options in regard to treatment, and the internist should try to develop this particular patient's and this particular family's philosophy about treatment and about palliation. This discussion need not happen on the day of diagnosis, but the primary physician might make clear that such a discussion can begin anytime and that the discussion will be a process rather than something that requires an immediate, set-in-stone decision. Throughout this discussion, goals should drive the therapies rather than available therapies driving the goals (Fins 2006).

The primary physician should be careful about terms when talking to patients. For example, many patients may say that in cases of medical futility, they would not want "extraordinary measures." This term derives from Catholic moral teachings and, as such, is unlikely to be of great benefit to anyone who is not well versed in Catholic moral philosophy. In regard to most patients (including most Catholics), it is a term that is difficult to define. One family may refuse an IV, since it may seem extraordinary to have a needle in one's arm. Another may specifically accept one pressor but not another. Another may be unsure about a specific procedure until they know the patient's likely lifespan and quality of life with and without the procedure.

During the discussion of the situation with Mrs. Ewing, it might become clear that in the event that she loses the capacity to make her own medical decisions, she would prefer that the decisions be made by someone in her family, probably her husband. While she might prefer to make herself DNR or to create a living will, designating a durable power of attorney—or what is generally termed a *health care proxy*—offers the most flexible option, as well as the option that is most likely to reflect the patient's wishes.

Proxies have a powerful moral authority (Fins 1999). Not only does the proxy know what the patient has explicitly stated, the proxy is the person most likely to know what the patient would want under unforeseen circumstances and be trusted to use discretion in interpreting the clinical context in light of the patient's prior preferences (Fins et al. 2005). The physician's relationship with the proxy can allow for a more subtle understanding of what the patient would want and take advantage of that proxy's discretionary moral authority in order to provide a treatment that is tailored to the patient (Danis et al. 1991).

Mrs. Ewing's physicians are busy, and these discussions may seem tangential to the medical enterprise, an enterprise that is increasingly focused on length of stay, governmental regulations, and avoidance of liability. Structures of care, such as the hospitalist movement, may also create tensions. While many hospitalists fill the breach as internists with a comprehensive view of care, they operate without the benefit of a preexisting relationship with the patient.

Perhaps an even greater obstacle to Mrs. Ewing's good care is a hospital ethos in which cure is all-important, while death implies failure. While some may say that the optimal medical approach to Mrs. Ewing would be the gradual transition from curative efforts to palliative care, modern medical centers are built and maintained with a very different bias. Hospitalized patients are generally cared for by teams of doctors, each assuming responsibility for an organ system or a discrete technological intervention. Further, as noted by the historian and medical sociologist, Rosemary Stevens, the twentieth-century hospital grew up as the workshop for surgeons and acute care medicine (Stevens 1989). Such a model may be technically proficient but does not necessarily meet the needs of today's chronically and terminally ill populations.

For multiple reasons, then, physicians tend to miss the cues that would allow a smooth transition from acute curative care to palliation and hospice. Although the Hospice Medicare Benefit is 6 months, for example, the average length of stay in a hospice is less than 3 weeks (Haupt 2003; Hoyer 1998; Miller et al. 2003). At times, people have even died in the ambulance on the way to hospice.

How does this happen? Why the delay? The answers are complex and beyond the scope of this brief essay, but communication failures are often at the root of the problem. Institutional and reimbursement systems that promote fragmentation of care heighten the patient and family's sense of estrangement and abandonment. Further, many practitioners avoid frank conversations about difficult themes like death, finitude, and medical failure. It is sometimes too easy to simply call a "psych consult" (and in some settings an ethics consult)—and "turf" the case—rather than to take personal responsibility for the broader psychosocial needs of patient and family. Consultation-liaison psychiatry and ethics consultation services are there to help, but they should never replace the full engagement of the clinicians providing direct medical or surgical care.

Our message here is simple: the humanistic dimensions of patient care cannot—and should not—be delegated to consultants, whether they are from consultation-liaison psychiatry, palliative care, or ethics. While helpful, consultants cannot replace an ongoing and comprehensive doctor–patient relationship. Indeed, by not taking personal responsibility for the broader psychosocial needs of the patient and family, generalists deprive not only the patients entrusted to their care but also themselves of the great professional satisfaction of being a healer.

Overview of Hospital Psychodynamics

John W. Barnhill, M.D.

THE stress of the hospital environment provokes characteristic responses in people, and many of these responses are useful. Adaptive denial, supression, and an immediate positive transference combine with desperation to allow sick people to accept often-risky care from strangers wearing hospital uniforms. At the same time, these strangers—the health care workers—are generally willing to work long hours with people who are sad, regressed, sick, and wary. Despite the potential for problems, the system works well: most patients are satisfied by their hospital experience, and most medical people find their jobs gratifying. Nonetheless, problems do occur, leading to efforts to better understand characteristic psychological responses to being sick and to the development of psychotherapies that take into consideration typical patient and staff responses.

Most classification schemas grew out of the ego psychological literature, particularly as that school evolved from dealing with completely intrapsychic conflicts (e.g., the ego combating the id) to a model that conceptualized the ego—or self—as significantly adapting to the outside world. Post–World War II writings on ego strengths and weaknesses led to a series of books by popular writers whose work could be adapted to the medically ill. For example, Erik Erikson (1963) used ego psychology to describe how people navigate psychosocial crises. His final stage—integrity vs. despair—is especially useful to an understanding of the plight of the seriously ill, regardless of the patient's age. George Vaillant (1977) described a hierarchy of defenses ranging from the primitive (e.g., denial and projection) to the advanced (e.g., altruism, sublimation, and humor); with illness, most people regress toward the use of the more primitive defenses. Elisabeth Kübler-Ross (1973) outlined stages of dying that begin with denial and anger and culminate in acceptance of the situation. In each of these schemes, there is an implicit goal, whether it is Erikson's "integrity," Vaillant's "sublimation," or Kübler-Ross's "acceptance." These schemas make intuitive sense, and Dorothy Ewing fits these models: she projects bad feelings onto her caretakers and God, who are then seen as malevolent. She is angry. She appears to be falling apart, which conforms to one pole of Erikson's conflict between integrity and despair. She refuses crucial tests because of pain and delirium, but refusal may reflect denial of aspects of her dire medical situation. Similarly, denial probably contributed to her decision not to seek medical help in the weeks prior to hospitalization despite increasing symptoms and a recent history of breast cancer. Psychological reactions to illness can be seriously maladaptive, then, and warrant focused therapeutic strategies.

Effective hospital-based psychotherapies tend to base themselves on object relations and self psychology, psychoanalytic schools that grew out of the strengths and limitations of ego psychology. Object relations theory emphasizes the importance of relationships, the dyadic connection between infant and mother, the importance of deficit rather than conflict, and the idea that children develop in the gaze of the parent; it is through this gaze—or mirroring—that the child internalizes a self in relationship to the object. Similarly, self psychology emphasizes deficits and mirroring and, importantly, stresses the importance of disintegration anxiety.

While these theories developed out of work with people with psychosis and severe personality disorders, we can see many of the same issues in normal people who are dealing with the abnormal stress of severe medical illness. This stress leads many seriously ill people to feel like Mrs. Ewing: they are falling apart, and they manifest noncompliance, denial, and depression. Such patients have a relative inability to tolerate interpretations or confrontations, a limitation that tends to distance, frustrate, and deskill their therapists.

One type of psychotherapy involves taking a *life inventory*. By exploring important memories, people, and activities, Mrs. Ewing would be able to develop a story of her life that brings comfort and coherence. We see such a process in earlier discussions when, for example, Viederman describes the psychodynamic life narrative and Poppito and Breitbart outline meaning-centered therapy. Such therapies help Mrs. Ewing return to the life trajectory that had been derailed by the illness.

Underlying these therapeutic approaches is an unstated but important aspect of the treatment. By sitting attentively with the medically ill person and creating an empathic alliance, the therapist allows the patient to introject the consultant as well as the consultant's construct, which creates a transference gratification and leads to the feeling of being understood. In other words, Mrs. Ewing's self worth is strengthened by being seen, and her shaken values and ideals are reaffirmed through collaboration with the therapist. As Henry James (1893/2004) noted, "It is glory to have been tested, to have had our little quality and cast our little spell. The thing is to have made someone care" (p. 126). The specific intervention may be less important than devising a tool that helps Mrs. Ewing develop a sense of coherence and meaning in a world that feels like it is dissolving.

Implicit in these discussions is the importance of the bio-psycho-social-spiritual approach to the patient. The relative importance varies, but the alert clinician should be prepared to shift smoothly from one to the other, prioritizing based on the needs of the patient, family, staff, and psychiatric situation. Treatment teams and individual clinicians can get stuck, however, and focus on only one of the four aspects of patient care. Mrs. Ewing's hospitalization is marked by periods during which the medical team focuses on procedure acquisition at the expense of the patient-as-person, while, at other times, the medical team focuses on personality issues when it should be diagnosing delirium or optimizing pain control.

Such oversights are sometimes attributable to lopsided training, personal bias, and inexperience, but the underlying cause can often be a group dynamic that leads to a cognitive and emotional constriction that impairs medical and psychiatric care. In attempting to understand such tendencies, it is useful to review the group process literature that grew out of work done by such people as Wilfred Bion and Melanie Klein.

According to current theories, groups operate on two levels. On the first level, the group consciously focuses on completing a task (i.e., the *work group*). On the second, group members act as if they had made unconscious, *basic assumptions* about the purpose of the group—assumptions that may be different from what the group is consciously intending. These basic assumptions are seen as a way for the individual to deal defensively with the regressive pull of being in a group. One of Wilfred Bion's (1961) most seminal ideas was to relate these unconscious group assumptions to theories that were originally elaborated by Melanie Klein in regard to the development of infants (Klein 1948). For example, Bion's *fight/flight* assumption corresponds to Klein's *paranoid-schizoid position* in which the group either fights with or flees a perceived persecutor. In the case of Mrs. Ewing, for example, the primary medical team has responded suboptimally to this "difficult patient." As discussed by Mozian and Muskin, the team sees her as someone who behaves badly, stirs up family conflicts, and angers the medical team. By all accounts, she frustrates exactly the sort of people who very much want to be seen as helpful and good. The patient is also noted to be mistrustful and paranoid, which implies that she uses a defense in which badness is projected out into her world, so that she is likely to project badness into the nearest-available people, her doctors, nurses, and social workers. The medical team is unlikely to want to accept this projective identification of being bad, which—under the stress of hospital work—can lead them to a group process in which the badness is projected back into the patient. At the same time, the group can identify with this projection of badness and act unprofessionally by either fighting with the patient or fleeing the steady, attentive responsibility that is their usual approach to complex medical situations.

In addition to the infantile paranoid-schizoid position, Klein postulated an *infantile depressive position*. Several decades of writings on group process have led to the view that a "depressed" reaction can lead to two different outcomes. In the first, the group members act unusually weak and dependent; their demoralized attitude pulls for someone (e.g., the therapist or the leader of the group) to be seen as a powerful rescuer. A second group reaction to depressive anxieties is a hypomanic effort to repair the badness that is felt within the group. These two reactions are common within hospitals. For example, the team might become demoralized and "give up" on difficult patients like Mrs. Ewing. On the other hand, they might ignore important subtleties and hypomanically treat her well past the possibility of positive clinical effect, which is one reason for delayed shifts to a palliative focus and hospice care.

These dynamics are certainly not limited to medical teams but are found wherever groups gather, whether within a class of students, a sports team, or—as seen in group-process workshops—randomly assembled people gathered in a room for a few hours with a mission of talking about anything they want.

Such dynamics may also help us understand the ways in which families deal with the terminal illness of a loved one. In his research into terminally ill cancer patients, Kissane describes three types of families: healthy, hostile, and sullen (Kissane and Bloch 2002). *Healthy families* deal with sadness, conflicts, and disappointment in a creative and robust way. These families might correspond with Bion's "work group" in that the family has not succumbed to regressive pressures and is able to approach problems without debilitating, unconscious basic assumptions. These families may be especially gratifying for medical staff, since they not only appreciate our efforts but do well regardless of our actual interventions. Kissane's *hostile families* are contentious, lack cohesion, and are unable to resolve conflicts. They tend to reject outside help. Such families appear to have regressed under the stress of the illness and the sudden return to being a family unit; even previously healthy family members get sucked into the vortex of mistrust. Their unconscious basic assumption appears to correspond to Klein's paranoid-schizoid position. This model may best fit the Ewing family, which is noted to be fractious, paranoid, and "difficult." The third type, *sullen families,* also have impaired communication, cohesion, and ability to resolve conflict, but they appear to be less mistrustful and more depressive. These families may correspond to Klein's depressive, demoralized position. While a difficult group to work with, they may be relatively amenable to treatment because they lack hostile paranoia.

Conscious awareness of individual and group dynamics allows the clinician to sidestep regressive tendencies and remain attentive, helpful, and professional. Aside from its important role in making our jobs more pleasant, the ability to retain our skills during difficult times can help us reduce the sense of isolation and despair that is common among the seriously ill and help them develop a newfound sense of connection, achievement, and integration.

Summary Points

- Delirium is common in hospitals. Its diagnosis should lead the psychiatrist to seek its precipitant; reassure and counsel the patient, family, and staff; and recommend small amounts of antipsychotic medication for insomnia, fear, and confusion.

- Pain is common in hospitals. Psychiatrists can be especially useful when patients are being undermedicated and/or when incident pain confuses the treatment picture.

- Powerful psychological reactions to illness are common in hospitals. Psychiatric intervention can reduce the regression, hostility, and noncompliance that may contribute to psychological pain and poor medical care.

- Within the general hospital, medical and surgical teams handle most interpersonal conflicts, reactions to illness, and discussions about end-of-life issues.

- The request for a psychiatric consultation generally indicates that something unusual has developed with the patient, family, or team.

- Psychiatric work within the general hospital requires a reasonable grasp of general medicine and a specialized knowledge of common psychiatric presentations among the medically ill.
- Most psychiatric consults in a general hospital are triggered by the development of some impediment to diagnosis, treatment, or discharge.

Chapter 6

AGITATION
AND
STEPHEN FRANKEN

Part A

SOON after taking over a shift in the psychiatric emergency department (PED), a psychiatrist was startled by shouting and the shuffle of many feet. At the time of the interruption, the psychiatrist was interviewing a recent arrival to the PED, a man with schizophrenia who needed a medication refill. The psychiatrist looked out into the hall, where two policemen escorted a young man in handcuffs. Four hospital security guards waited nearby. His face contorted, the new patient screamed at the police to leave him alone.

The psychiatrist glanced at the rest of the patients in the PED. While he had not yet met any of them, the patients fit the descriptions provided by the psychiatrist from the previous shift. The pregnant manic woman had apparently awakened since sign-out and was now partially disrobed; the alcoholic, depressed, suicidal man was edgily awaiting admission; the drug-abusing teenager was bickering with his parents; and the elderly woman with dementia appeared frightened. The final patient—an unkempt young woman who was briskly pacing down the hall—had apparently been admitted to the PED while the psychiatrist was interviewing the man who needed the medication refill.

The nurse handed him an intake form: "Stephen Franken, age 32. EDP, fought with police." Aside from the information that the patient was an "EDP," or "emotionally disturbed person," the psychiatrist had no outside information.

The psychiatrist looked carefully at Mr. Franken. His clothing appeared to be new and clean, and his hair was trimmed. While somewhat disheveled, he did not appear homeless or to have been agitated for more than a few hours. The patient refused to answer questions or sit. "No reason to trust any of you," he said rapidly. "This place is just a sham way to imprison innocent people." As Mr. Franken paced up and down the hall, the uncertain and somewhat overwhelmed psychiatrist noticed that a medical student was trying to keep the manic woman from disrobing; the alcoholic man had begun to argue with a nurse; the adolescent was shouting at his parents; the elderly woman had retreated to her room and placed a blanket over her head; and the new patient was having an animated conversation with a second medical student.

The psychiatrist walked Mr. Franken to a corner of the PED and tried to calm him down. The security guards, police, nursing staff, medical students, and other patients watched as Mr. Franken engaged the psychiatrist in a dialogue about his arrest, the military-industrial complex, and conditions for an immediate release. The psychiatrist felt a sense of embarrassed chagrin that the PED had rapidly spiraled out of control but did feel confident that Mr. Franken was the person who most acutely deserved attention. After extensive negotiation, Mr. Franken received haloperidol (Haldol) 5 mg, lorazepam (Ativan) 2 mg, and benztropine (Cogentin) 1 mg. He fell asleep.

A review of Mr. Franken's old chart revealed that he had been evaluated for headaches in the emergency room 3 months earlier. His laboratory results were normal at that time, but in the ensuing three months, he had apparently lost 20 pounds.

When he awoke a few hours later, Mr. Franken appeared strikingly different. He spoke minimally and appeared fearful. While he denied seeing things, he often blinked and looked oddly at the television and into the air. Over the ensuing hours, he became feverish, diaphoretic, and coughed frequently.

Mr. Franken was diagnosed with a pneumonia and delirium and admitted to the inpatient medical service.

Summary

Stephen Franken was a 32-year-old man who was brought to the PED by the police because of agitation. The discussants in the first part of this case explore Mr. Franken's initial evaluation and management. The second half of the case follows Mr. Franken through the first week of his hospitalization.

Discussions of the Case of Stephen Franken, Part A

Managing Multiple Patients in the Emergency Department . . 215
  Peter J. Freed, M.D., and John W. Barnhill, M.D.

Evaluating an Emergency Patient. 219
  Peter J. Freed, M.D., and John W. Barnhill, M.D.

Stimulant Abuse 225
  Petros Levounis, M.D., M.A.

Part B 230

Managing Multiple Patients in the Emergency Department

Peter J. Freed, M.D.
John W. Barnhill, M.D.

THE psychiatrist in this case has lost control of the psychiatric emergency department (PED) even before the handcuffed Stephen Franken is dragged through its doors. Not having been warned by triage, the psychiatrist knows nothing of Mr. Franken; other patients are wandering freely; and no one has prepared the sedating medications and restraints that would—at the least— be part of negotiations with this patient. More worrisome, the department's level of agitation was already too high when Mr. Franken arrived. The manic, pregnant woman should have been controlled; the suicidal man should have been receiving medications for his likely alcohol withdrawal; and the adolescent's parents should have been in the waiting room if they could not keep their son at least as calm as he would be without them. Medical students have been left unsupervised, and while well intentioned, they may inflame patients and someone could get hurt. Many people are working or being evaluated in this PED, but the psychiatrist has spoken only with the quietest, least dangerous patient—the man who has presented for a medication refill—neglecting even to meet the potentially dangerous woman who has not yet been evaluated by any psychiatrist. This chaos could end in disaster.

Calm safety in the PED is the foundation upon which evaluation of individual patients must be built. To accomplish this goal, the psychiatrist must develop an ear for the acuity of the PED as a whole. Concentrating only on one patient at a time, as one would in an outpatient clinic, is not enough. The PED is, in a sense, an ecosystem, and when one or two patients get out of control, the entire group can quickly follow suit. Therefore, it is crucial to develop a sense of the maximum level of anxiety, tension, or confusion that the PED can have without its becoming chaotic. If this threshold is crossed and the PED gets "too loud," care of individuals should stop while the clinician anticipates and deals with problems affecting the PED ecosystem. An intentional stance toward safety would have led the psychiatrist to quickly deal with the agitated Mr. Franken, for example, but it would also have prompted the clinician to move beyond the customary focus on a single patient and take responsibility for the other patients who are likely to become upset by nearby turmoil and for the colleagues, staff, and trainees who are also working in the PED. At a more psychological level, the PED psychiatrist must come to terms with being an authority who is willing to administer involuntary medications and restraints and order hospitalizations. While we know little of the psychiatrist's thoughts about the situation, we could guess that the unusual responsibilities of the PED led to anxiety that led to the unfortunate decision to start off the shift with the most straightforward patient. Such an error would be less likely after the psychiatrist becomes more adept and comfortable with his or her expanded role.

Three aspects of the PED experience are particularly important to the creation of a safe, effective environment: the *sign-out*, the *meet-and-greet*, and the *triage*, all of which have to do more with the overall management of the PED than with the management of any particular patient.

Sign-Out

Safety in the PED begins during the sign-out from the previous clinician. For each patient, there should be discussion of the bottom-line reason that each patient is in the PED, the worst-case scenario, and an anticipated response to that scenario (Table 6–1).

TABLE 6–1.	EXAMPLES OF "WORST CASE SCENARIO" PREDICTION AND TREATMENT IN PSYCHIATRIC EMERGENCY DEPARTMENT (PED)	
Bottom-line patient type	Worst-case scenario	Likely worst-case response
Arrested	Legal complications	Call administrator; clarify obligation to police
Borderline personality	Acting-out behavior	Employ limit setting, 1:1; medicate
Doesn't need to be in PED	PED worsens condition	Discharge; transfer to medicine
Intoxicated	Withdrawal	Benzodiazepines; call medicine
Medically ill	Physical decompensation	Observe closely, call medicine
Pregnant	Harm to fetus	Individual room, call ob/gyn
Suicidal	Suicide attempt	Employ 1:1; medicate

Each new patient should prompt the same thought process. Prior to Mr. Franken's arrival, for example, the psychiatrist might have envisioned potential problems from the six patients who had already been admitted to the PED. While all of these patients might have been relatively calm upon admission, it should be anticipated that the manic patient might behave provocatively, that the teenager might fight with his parents, that the suicidal man might hurt himself, and that the elderly woman with dementia might become frightened. Sign-out should also focus on patients who are unknown in some way, either because their presentation is unusual, potentially dangerous, or unpredictable or because they have not yet been evaluated; these patients should generally be seen immediately after sign-out is over.

An intentional stance toward safety does not require memorization of "worst case scenarios" but would likely have led to a series of rapid responses and a calm PED by the time of Mr. Franken's arrival. That stance would also have led the psychiatrist to take one look at Mr. Franken, the police, and the history ("EDP, fought with police"), and rapidly develop a cluster of possible diagnoses and pertinent issues (e.g., intoxication, suicidality, homicidality, medical illness, and police involvement). With a more intentional stance toward safety, the psychiatrist would likely feel ready to work with Mr. Franken rather than feeling "uncertain and somewhat overwhelmed."

Organization during the sign-out helps the psychiatrist maintain a sense of control. PEDs tend to use a white board to accurately track each patient in tabular form. Sign-out is an opportunity to update the white board's summary of dispensed medications, completed notes, and planned dispositions; frequent updates of the board can be critical to a safe, efficient PED.

Sign-out is also an opportunity to meet other members of the medical, nursing, and security staffs. A good relationship with staff and trainees not only makes for a more pleasant experience but also allows the psychiatrist to work more effectively with multiple patients at the same time. Sign-out is an excellent place to think out loud and help clarify the psychiatrist and staff's thinking. In addition, trainees and staff will likely appreciate an expansion of their perspective and the opportunity to provide second opinions.

Meet-and-Greet

After sign-out, but before individual case management, the psychiatrist should tour the PED and get a personal sense of how things are going. The meet-and-greet is an opportunity to make observations and introductions, get a sense of what brought the patient to the PED, and provide an active, reassuring presence. It is not the time to get a thorough history but rather an opportunity to determine two particular things: First, does the patient match the sign-out? Cases often evolve between evaluations, and prior to changeover, the disrobing manic patient might have been asleep, and the parents might have been calming to their adolescent son. Second, does anyone appear dangerous? If so, that person is likely to require immediate attention. In addition to assisting in the evaluation, the meet-and-greet allows the psychiatrist to begin to develop an alliance with patients and potentially calming families. It can be tempting to skip this important step, but a brief meet-and-greet informs the psychiatrist's work and helps make the PED a safer place.

Triage

Triage consists of deciding which patient should be seen first. The process of triage occurs throughout the day and night and requires an ongoing evaluation of patients, communication with staff and trainees, and listening for overall chaos and dangerousness. The most urgent patient may be the most acutely agitated, but it can also be the patient who should be most quickly discharged from the PED or most rapidly admitted to the inpatient service. Work with Mr. Franken would have been significantly easier, for example, if the depressed, alcoholic man had already been admitted to psychiatry or medicine (or at least received medications for his alcohol withdrawal); if the disrobing pregnant woman had been controlled in her room; if the adolescent boy's parents had already been asked to wait outside the PED; and if the pacing, argumentative woman had at least been evaluated. The decision to see the man with schizophrenia who has presented for a medication refill might allow for a quick discharge from the PED, but that triage decision has contributed to havoc in the PED and may lead someone to get hurt.

The most obvious and exciting aspect of working in the PED is the management of an agitated patient like Mr. Franken. His successful diagnosis and treatment does demand a special set of skills and attitudes, most of which revolve around anticipating problems, managing the PED's overall acuity level, building relationships with coworkers and patients, and maintaining an organized, ongoing sense of each patient. Through such efforts, the psychiatrist can reduce the shock effect of Mr. Franken's entry into the PED ecosystem and begin an effective individual evaluation.

Evaluating an Emergency Patient

Peter J. Freed, M.D.
John W. Barnhill, M.D.

THE central goal in the psychiatric emergency department (PED) is a safe, appropriate, efficient disposition. Alliance, patient confidentiality, a definitive diagnosis, and immediate symptom relief are useful and desirable, but they are less important than safety and disposition. Disposition inevitably falls into one of three categories: discharge into either an existing or new treatment program; deferral of a decision pending a diagnostic or stabilizing intervention; or admission to an inpatient facility. Colloquially reduced to "split, sit, or admit," disposition is a focus of every evaluation in the PED.

Evaluation of safety and disposition tend to occur contemporaneously, though safety is paramount. For example, Stephen Franken has been brought to the PED by two policemen and four hospital security guards. He is agitated and handcuffed. The intake form is brief: "Stephen Franken, age 32. EDP, fought with police." This particular psychiatrist turned immediately to the "emotionally disturbed person," but it may have been more useful to have the team escort the patient to a quiet room, ensure that the other patients had been led away from the potentially dangerous new patient, and talk directly to the arresting officers, who likely had a more complete story than was on the intake form. In addition, a glance at the vital signs might have pointed the psychiatrist toward intoxication or withdrawal. In other words, before entering the room, the clinician should try to understand the context in which the patient presents.

The Initial Interview

As the psychiatrist approaches Mr. Franken, it is reasonable to ask him what led to his being brought to the PED. Many agitated patients calm quickly when allowed to tell their stories, but it is also true that emergency psychiatric patients are unknown and are prone to violence. While the interview with Mr. Franken may go smoothly, the psychiatrist should have an escape route (i.e., stand or sit near the door) and back-up (i.e., police or security guards should be nearby). If threatened, the psychiatrist should back off and work with the security guards to reestablish a sense of safety. While he may be adamant, Mr. Franken does not immediately need to present his entire story or recognize the wisdom of his arrest; he does, however, need to calm down.

When it becomes clear that Mr. Franken is out of control, a series of steps may be necessary to calm him. To maximize the likelihood of safety, the psychiatrist needs to be clear and prepared. Instead of the "lengthy negotiations" that are described in the case report, the psychiatrist should present Mr. Franken with a series of either/or choices that begin with the least restrictive option and proceed, if necessary, to the most restrictive. The first is a behavioral choice:

> Mr. Franken—you are too excited right now to be safe. I would like to offer you a choice. Either you go to your room and remain quiet, or you can take some medication to help you calm down.

If he accepts the low-conflict option, he should be thanked and a follow-up plan arranged with nursing and security. If he does not calm down, he should be offered a medication choice:

> Mr. Franken, you haven't been able to calm down by yourself. You need some medication—would you like to take it by mouth or would you like us to inject it?

Prior to presenting this series of options, a nurse should be standing by with oral and intramuscular medications, and security should be ready to restrain the patient should intramuscular medication be necessary. Mr. Franken received "5, 2, and 1": a regimen of 5 mg of haloperidol (Haldol), 2 mg of lorazepam (Ativan), and 1 mg of benztropine (Cogentin). This regimen sedated him, but if it had not, he should have been offered a restraint choice:

> Mr. Franken, you haven't been able to calm down enough to be safe. You need to be in restraints for a little while—would you like to get in them yourself, or should we place you in them?

The psychiatrist should allow very little time for agitated patients to discuss these choices—no longer than 30 seconds. Security guards should be standing by, ready to each grab a limb. Nursing or security should have prepared restraints and a bed.

The presence of adequate staff and a confident, no-nonsense approach help organize the patient and increase the likelihood of rapid compliance. Such controlling behavior is unusual within psychiatry and can elicit concerns about patient's rights. Done properly, however, forced treatments and emergency management can increase safety and be the first step to Mr. Franken's recovery.

The Diagnosis

Mr. Franken has been triaged to psychiatry, but there are many medical emergencies that can cause a behavioral disturbance. As the evaluating physician, the psychiatrist must do a physical exam and evaluate Mr. Franken's vital signs and basic labs and consider ordering additional tests. It can be a fatal error to ignore medical problems such as infections, delirium, and substance abuse, just as it can be disastrous not to examine wounds produced by self-cutting and to not consult medicine after learning of a drug overdose in a patient who "seems fine."

While Mr. Franken sleeps, the psychiatrist should try to calm and assess the other patients in the PED. While it might be tempting to respond to the stress of such an encounter by rehashing the event at length with co-workers, it is important for the other patients to see that the psychiatrist remains available and in charge.

The period of sedation can be an important time to find out more about Mr. Franken. Are there collateral sources of information? Is the patient suicidal? Might he have hidden weapons? Are there children or dependent elderly people at home, alone, waiting for his care? What is Mr. Franken's legal situation? Does he take standing medications? Have labs been drawn? Does he need special labs, such as medication levels, toxicology, or imaging? Are vital signs being taken regularly?

Pattern Recognition:
The Search for a Patient's "Type"

While psychotherapy often consists of exploring a patient's issues and conflicts and uncovering the details that make that person unique, the initial goal of the emergency psychiatric evaluation is to actively match the patient to a "diagnostic type" that allows for the efficient development of a treatment plan. In regard to Mr. Franken, we do not need to ask him any questions during his initial moments in the PED to develop a working diagnosis. Using the patient types as outlined in Table 6–2, we can surmise that he is "agitated/ impulsive" and in need of safety. Additional historical information might be useful, but its importance is outweighed by the risk of injury during the delay. In other words, it might feel satisfying to attempt an exquisite, hour-long social history on Mr. Franken, but such an effort helps no one.

TABLE 6–2.   PATIENT TYPES

Patient type	Key considerations
Agitated/Impulsive	Ensure safety and then proceed with assessment.
Anxious	Evaluate for medical causes and psychiatric comorbidities. Persons with primary anxiety and panic are rarely admitted.
Arrested	Beware of one's own assumptions about law enforcement.
	Protect staff and self (have police nearby) and the patient (do not let the police listen; document carefully).
Borderline (and other personality disorders)	Assess suicidality and outpatient support system.
Demented/Delirious	May require transfer to a medical unit. Not all behavioral problems are psychiatric.
Depressed	Assess suicidality and outpatient support system.
Frequent fliers	Review records and look for changes. Much of the history has already been taken.
Homicidal	Consult others and get a consensus. Legal and ethical issues abound.

(continued)

TABLE 6–2. PATIENT TYPES *(continued)*

Patient type	Key considerations
Intoxicated (drugs/ alcohol)	Manage medical aspects of withdrawal.
Malingering	Be skeptical of the unbelievable (especially regarding suicidality and hallucinations).
Manic/Mixed	Distinguish mania, schizophrenia, substance abuse, and personality disorders. Assess for impulsivity. Low threshold for control with medications.
Medically ill	Transfer to Medicine.
Minimizing	Remember that suicidal, psychotic, and danger- ous people will often try to talk their way out.
Narcissistic	Can be especially demeaning and demanding.
Pregnant or children/ dependent elderly at home	Ask if the patient is pregnant or has a dependent at home. If so, you are responsible for more than the one patient. Involve social services.
Psychotic	Accept that underlying etiology is often not determined in the PED, but if the symptoms are new and not transient, the patient likely warrants admission.
Suicidal	Generally admit, though assess for transience as seen in personality disorders and intoxication.
VIP	Remember that deviations from routine can worsen care.

The Second Interview and the Disposition

Mr. Franken awoke several hours later, at which point he barely spoke, was fearful, and seemed to be having visual hallucinations or misperceptions. He also became febrile, with rapid breathing and frequent coughing. Mr. Franken's lab results included a toxicology screen that was positive for cocaine and amphetamines, a positive RPR (rapid plasma reagin), a low white blood cell count, a fever, and pneumonia (Table 6–3). The evolution of his medical condition shifted him from being a psychiatric patient to being a medically ill patient who warrants an admission to a medical unit.

TABLE 6–3.   STEPHEN FRANKEN'S TEST RESULTS IN THE PSYCHIATRIC
EMERGENCY DEPARTMENT

Labs	Results
Toxicology screen	Positive for cocaine and methamphetamine
RPR	Positive
WBC	1700
T (°C)	38.1
Chest X ray	Widespread pulmonary infiltrates

Note.   RPR=rapid plasma reagin; WBC=white blood cell count; T=temperature.

Such a transfer would not, however, occur instantaneously. It would likely take several hours for Mr. Franken to wake up and for his tests to demonstrate the medical problems. What should the psychiatrist do during this time? While safety is the first concern, acquisition of additional history becomes critical during this second phase of the evaluation. The psychiatrist should, therefore, search out old medical records and tactfully ask the patient for the name and phone number of friends, family members, and physicians.

While Mr. Franken's situation is urgent, some effort should be made to maximize his privacy, both inside and outside the PED. Psychiatrists do not generally call friends and family members, but in emergency situations, it is ethically, legally, and clinically warranted for the treating clinician to make judicious inquiries without the patient's permission. That said, it is generally wise to ask for permission and to give the patient a chance to explain why particular people should not be contacted. We can make contact over objection, but it is best to try to remain allied with the patient. Breaches in confidentiality can be minimized by listening and asking questions and contributing little information to the patient's family and friends.

Throughout the initial evaluation, effort should be directed at uncovering medical and psychiatric diagnoses, substance abuse, previous treatments and complications, any history of suicidality, allergies, and social and financial supports. While focused pursuit of social history is unlikely to be useful in this mistrustful, delirious man, in other situations it can be critical to diagnosis and disposition. For example, if Mr. Franken's delirium clears but he remains impulsive or suicidal, his discharge from the PED will likely hinge on outpatient support systems.

Given his medical situation, however, Mr. Franken is admitted to an inpatient medical service. Careful, serial assessments will be particularly useful to the colleagues who will take over Mr. Franken's care. These include recordings of vital signs to help assess for withdrawal and/or intoxication as well as documentation of his evolving mental status. Quantifiable cognitive assessments might include the Mini-Mental State Examination (MMSE) or the Clock Drawing Test (CDT), either of which can help differentiate, for example, a psychosis from a delirium. Perhaps most important to Mr. Franken's care was, however, the rapid recognition that his behavioral disturbance was not psychiatric in origin, thereby leading to his safe disposition to the medical service.

Stimulant Abuse

Petros Levounis, M.D., M.A.

STEPHEN Franken is agitated and paranoid and has tested positive for cocaine and amphetamines. How do we treat his intoxication, cushion his withdrawal, and help reduce the chance of relapse? Further, how do we understand his substance use and organize our medical thinking to help him improve his life?

Intoxication

Mr. Franken presents to the psychiatric emergency department (PED) with psychomotor agitation, confusion, fever, and diaphoresis. Such symptoms can be explained by an infection-induced delirium, but the paranoia, hostility, and combativeness point toward either substance intoxication or withdrawal. The observation that the patient "frequently blinked and looked oddly at the television and into the air" is particularly suggestive of the stereotypical behaviors—like the grinding of teeth (bruxism) and staccato eye movements (tweaking)—that stimulant users experience during intoxication.

The toxicology screen indicates that Mr. Franken uses two stimulants, cocaine and crystal methamphetamine. The first, cocaine, is used widely throughout the world. The second, crystal methamphetamine, has expanded from being almost exclusively a rural drug used by heterosexual men and women to also being an urban club drug used by gay men. As he becomes more cognitively clear, he should be asked about same-sex encounters. While his recent 20-pound weight loss is consistent with the anorectic effects of sympathomimetic drugs like cocaine and methamphetamine, it could also result from an HIV infection or a medical condition such as a malignancy. Amphetamine is a metabolite of methamphetamine in a very similar way that norepinephrine is a metabolite of epinephrine. All four chemical compounds have striking structural similarities, which largely account for their related clinical properties (Figure 6–1).

Like most young people who abuse substances, Mr. Franken uses his drugs in combination. The drugs he is using are, however, from the same class, which simplifies the initial evaluation and treatment. We do not have an antidote for cocaine or amphetamine overdose like we do for heroin (naloxone) or benzodiazepines (flumazenil). Stimulant intoxication is treated symptomatically and supportively with the judicious administration of antipsychotics, benzodiazepines, and antihypertensives.

Withdrawal

We often think of crystal methamphetamine as the turbo cocaine. Just as the high from "crystal meth" is more extreme than that from cocaine, acute withdrawal leads to more intense depression, cognitive difficulties, and insomnia. The intensity of the depression can lead to suicidality, though many depressed, stimulant-abusing patients also suffer from coexisting major depression; for some patients, the cocaine and/or crystal methamphetamine are used as self-prescribed "antidepressants" which do transiently improve mood before withdrawal intensifies the despair. Cocaine withdrawal typically lasts 24–48 hours, which allows weekend users to go to work on Monday. Crystal methamphetamine is not as forgiving, however, and users often find themselves unable to go back to normal living for several days.

The treatment of stimulant withdrawal is supportive. We educate about dependence, anticipate withdrawal symptoms, and provide reassurance. Such psychoeducation and support can reduce the acute despair of stimulant withdrawal. Pharmacotherapy has not yet been shown to be effective, although there is now an interest in studying modafinil (Provigil), which can reduce the fatigue and sleepiness that tend to lead patients to self-medication with more cocaine and/or crystal methamphetamine in order to stay awake at work. Withdrawal symptoms are, however, the major deterrent to stimulant use. Reducing these symptoms could lead patients to the belief that they own a "get out of jail card," thereby increasing the abuse of these substances.

Methamphetamine

Amphetamine

Epinephrine

Norepinephrine

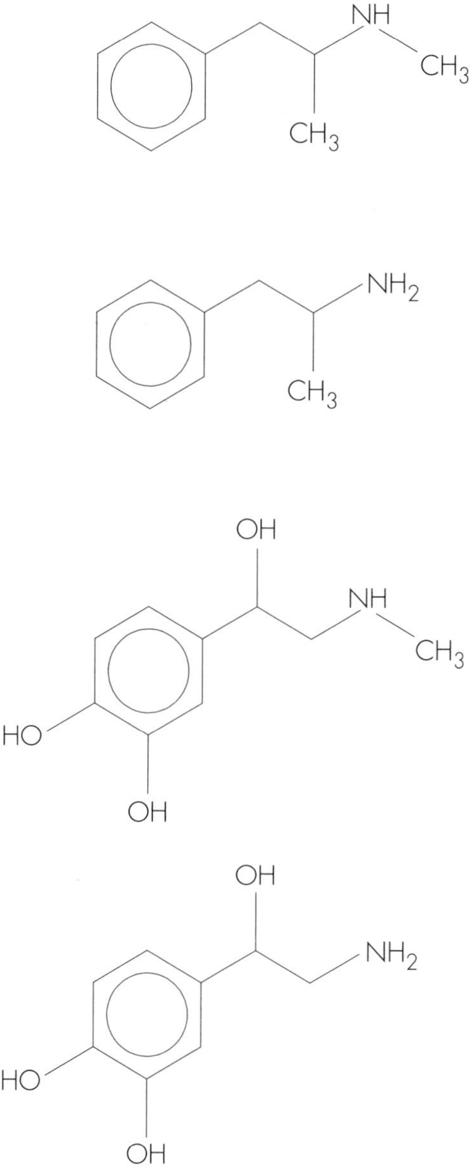

FIGURE 6–1. Structures of sympathomimetic drugs.

Relapse Prevention

Mr. Franken's drug use likely meets the criteria for *cocaine and amphetamine dependence.* While Mr. Franken's precise history, and therefore diagnosis, remain uncertain, we do know that his use of cocaine and methamphetamine is a problem and can have grave medical and psychosocial consequences. For example, crystal methamphetamine is particularly implicated in unsafe sex practices among men who have sex with men. Further, amphetamines damage the serotonin and dopamine systems, increasing the risk of depression, anxiety, and cognitive impairment. While the neurotoxic effects of alcohol and drugs have often been overestimated, amphetamines have been clearly shown to harm the brain, and at least some damage may be permanent. In order to halt the progression of illness, possibly reverse brain injury, and restore psychosocial function, then, Mr. Franken needs treatment of his substance abuse. As therapeutic efforts to prevent relapse are most likely to be effective during crises, they can be started even while the patient is in acute intoxication or withdrawal.

The classic treatment model, consistent with the traditions of Alcoholics Anonymous (AA), aims at complete abstinence. This model is supported by a neurobiological understanding that once the dopaminergic pleasure-reward pathways of the brain have been hijacked by the drug(s) of abuse, the patient is vulnerable to relapse, possibly for a lifetime. Similar programs have been started that focus on cocaine and on crystal methamphetamine, but they all tend to focus on the use of the twelve steps, self-help groups, individual sponsors, and an effort to stay completely clean and sober.

Twelve-step programs contrast with the *harm reduction model,* in which the clinician helps the patient reduce and control the use of substances in order to avoid his or her most dangerous consequences. Also called *moderation management,* harm reduction recognizes that many patients may not want, or may not be able to achieve, abstinence but can still benefit from counseling and treatment. In general, the more severe the abuse pattern, the more likely that abstinence is necessary.

The debate between proponents of these two approaches may have been resolved by the introduction and wide acceptance of *motivational interviewing,* a therapeutic technique that is based on the stages of change: precontemplation, contemplation, preparation, action, maintenance, and sometimes relapse. Motivational interviewing bypasses the question of abstinence versus harm reduction by narrowing treatment to three tasks: 1) understand the patient and make sure that she or he feels understood; 2) identify the stage of change, which may even be no desire to change at all (equivalent to precontemplation); and 3) help the patient move forward to the next stage (Miller and Rollnick 2002). This therapeutic technique capitalizes on the reality that all people are ambivalent about their abuse of drugs. The interviewer makes use of this ambivalence by allying with the part of the person that does want to quit. Not only does motivational interviewing help the patient take a more mature ownership of the problem, it helps reduce the tendency of the clinician to feel frustrated or moralistic. It can be used for any type of substance abuse and dependence.

Many relapse-prevention programs base treatments on cognitive-behavioral principles. Positive drug screens might lead, for example, to a reduction in privilege level, with the expectation that such a "punishment" will reduce relapse. *Contingency management* uses behavioral principles to reinforce positive behaviors rather than try to extinguish negative behaviors. For example, a program might reward negative toxicology screens with gift certificates for movie theaters and restaurants. This positive reinforcement seems to work well in a population whose drug use has inevitably impaired the brain regions that control risk and reward.

Pharmacologically, the treatment of stimulant dependence is at the experimental stage. In contrast to other substance abuse treatments, there are no FDA-approved medications to help prevent stimulant relapse (Table 6–4).

TABLE 6–4. FDA-APPROVED MEDICATIONS FOR SUBSTANCE DEPENDENCE

Nicotine	Alcohol	Opioids	Stimulants
Bupropion (Zyban)	Acamprosate (Campral)	Buprenorphine (Suboxone, Subutex)	None
Nicotine replacement	Disulfiram (Antabuse)	Methadone (Dolophine)	
Varenicline (Chantix)	Naltrexone (ReVia, Vivitrol)	Naltrexone (ReVia)	

Mr. Franken is at high risk for co-occurring psychiatric disorders, and these should be carefully explored as he returns to his baseline. Treatment of comorbid conditions reduces the likelihood of relapse, but he would still warrant treatment aimed at his substance abuse. Once the addiction has been engraved in the mesolimbic pleasure-reward pathways of the brain, it develops a life of its own and requires it own attention and treatment.

As Mr. Franken recovers from his acute episode of agitation and confusion, a treatment plan should be developed. To do this, the clinician should tactfully explore the possibilities of such interventions as twelve-step programs, psychotherapy, and medications. Mr. Franken's ultimate prognosis depends on his level of motivation, but it also depends on our ability to treat comorbid conditions, create an alliance, and foster the motivation to quit, a desire that exists in everyone whose life has been damaged by substances of abuse.

Part B

DURING the first 4 days of his medical hospitalization, Mr. Franken demonstrated fluctuating levels of attention, fear, paranoia, agitation, and insomnia. The medical team asked a consultation-liaison psychiatrist for help with medication management. The psychiatrist suggested a low dose of an antipsychotic medication to help with the delirium. Mr. Franken admitted to using crystal methamphetamine and cocaine but denied other drugs and alcohol. He denied being homosexual but seemed to agree when asked if he had sex with men. During a period of lucidity, the patient agreed to an HIV antibody test that was requested because of the neuropsychiatric symptoms that had developed in the context of drug use and high-risk sexual behavior.

By the sixth hospital day, Mr. Franken appeared consistently calm, cooperative, lucid, and apologetic. With some hesitancy, he described using cocaine and crystal methamphetamine as part of his nocturnal sexual pursuit of anonymous men. He was sickened at the possibility that he might be gay and ashamed that his sexual fantasies concerned faceless men and never women. When asked why he was so upset by homosexual fantasies, he joked that he had a "strong case of internalized homophobia." He said that he had never had a boyfriend but had occasionally dated women. Sexual relations with women were stressful but manageable with the help of an erectile dysfunction drug and fantasies about men. He estimated that he had anonymous sex with men every 2–3 weeks. He usually used some sort of drug to "overcome inhibitions about sex." These encounters had begun while he was in college.

On day six, Mr. Franken's internist told him that he had AIDS. After consultation with the hospital Infectious Diseases HIV/AIDS Program, Mr. Franken was educated about antiretroviral and other treatments for HIV/AIDS, about the importance of adherence to medications, and about the vital importance of ongoing attention to safe sexual practices. After this discussion, he was appropriately sad and worried about the diagnosis, but felt he had a plan of medical treatment and was more optimistic about his future. He said that this diagnosis was a wake-up call and that he needed to address his behavior, his lack of intimate relationships, and his perceptions of himself. He asked about starting an exploratory psychotherapy and said that he felt particularly comfortable talking to the consulting psychiatrist. The psychiatrist wondered whether Mr. Franken would be a suitable patient for therapy.

Personal History

Mr. Franken had been raised in a series of foster homes after the death of his mother when he was 4 years old. He had never known his father. He graduated from a local college with a degree in accounting, and while he had never sought a high-flying Wall Street career, he had become financially and professionally successful. He said he loved being around people but spent most of his time alone.

Personal Psychiatric History

The patient described chronic feelings of loneliness. He reported feeling panicky when he got "too close" to people but denied other prominent anxiety symptoms.

After using crystal methamphetamine or cocaine, Mr. Franken said he tended to feel "a little paranoid" for a few days but denied that this affected his work or relationships. When he was not coming down from drugs, he denied paranoia.

Family Psychiatric History

None known.

Medical History

Recent weight loss, night sweats, and coughing.

Mental Status Exam, Part B

The patient was alert, calm, and cooperative. He made good eye contact and did not have abnormal movements. His speech was goal directed and of normal rate and rhythm. He described feeling exhausted but not depressed. His affect was appropriate and included smiles. He denied all suicidality and homicidality. He was cognitively intact (MMSE 29/30; CDT 4/4). His insight and judgment were intact at the time of the interview but impaired by history.

Summary

After Mr. Franken was admitted to a medical unit, his cognition cleared, and he was diagnosed with AIDS. The following discussions focus on his hospitalization, psychological development, interpersonal relationships, and treatment options.

Discussions of the Case of Stephen Franken, Part B

Consultation-Liaison Psychiatry 233
  John W. Barnhill, M.D.

Informed Consent 235
  Charles P. Stowell, M.D.

HIV and AIDS 239
  Stephen J. Ferrando, M.D.

Internalized Homophobia 243
  Richard C. Friedman, M.D.

Sexuality and Sexual Dysfunction 246
  Robert Kertzner, M.D.

Jekyll and Hyde 249
  Hilary J. Beattie, Ph.D.

Psychotherapy Selection 251
  Carolyn J. Douglas, M.D.

Overview of Connection 254
  Francine Cournos, M.D.

Summary Points 256

Consultation-Liaison Psychiatry

John W. Barnhill, M.D.

WHILE half of the patients in a general hospital have a psychiatric diagnosis, most of these problems are transient or mild and handled by the primary medical and surgical teams. Not infrequently, however, such patients profit from a psychiatric consultation. Such an intervention demands a cluster of skills and attitudes that are unusual for a psychiatrist, and the consultant who tries to make use of a traditional psychiatric approach will frustrate the primary team and do a disservice to the patient.

Stephen Franken was admitted to a medical inpatient service with a delirium that seemed to stem from some combination of stimulant intoxication and HIV infection. At the time of admission, the internist asked for suggestions regarding medications and management of disruptive behavior. The medical team was also communicating something else: "We would like to take care of his medical problems, so would you please take charge of his psychiatric and behavioral problems?" Mr. Franken's delirium cleared after the fourth day, at which point the team would likely have a second request: "Please make sure that psychiatric issues don't delay his discharge." These two needs are generally silent but are often crucial to the success of the consultation.

The consultation-liaison (C-L) psychiatrist is working within a hospital system, then, that mandates quick decisions and suggestions. In as little as a session or two, the C-L psychiatrist should plan the patient's discharge. For example, how long should Mr. Franken continue the antipsychotic medication that may have helped resolve his delirium? How best to address his substance abuse? Motivational interviewing might help clarify the possibilities, but what level of treatment should be encouraged? Possibilities include an inpatient rehab, individual therapy, and twelve-step programs. But can a man with a resolving delirium and a new-onset HIV infection make an educated decision? What should be done about the chronic social isolation that has likely been driven by his shame over his homosexuality and by his experience in foster homes? What treatments should be considered for chronic anxiety and depression that may—or may not—have predated the substance abuse? There are only modest hard data upon which to base such decisions, and hardly any evidence that is specific to Mr. Franken, yet the primary medical team would generally like a treatment plan on the day of the consultation. The subspecialty within psychiatry that may be closest to medicine is also a specialty that relies heavily on clinical experience and unsubstantiated personal convictions.

Given the enormous possible scope of Mr. Franken's problems, how does the C-L psychiatrist function? The first step is to clarify the consultation question with the medical team. About half of their questions will turn out to be inaccurate. For example, many people who are supposedly "depressed" turn out to be delirious and many people who are supposedly "anxious" turn out to be in alcohol withdrawal. Nevertheless, the consultation question is important. In addition to helping organize the consultation, direct communication can reveal the team's underlying concerns. In regard to Mr. Franken, the initial consultation goals are to confirm Mr. Franken's delirium, suggest medications, help control his fear and agitation, and contribute to the search for an underlying diagnosis. Given his confusion, initial goals did *not* include substance abuse counseling, rehab placement, or psychotherapy referral. Premature focus on secondary goals serves primarily to sidetrack and dilute the effectiveness of the consult.

After clarifying the goals, the C-L psychiatrist should carefully review Mr. Franken's chart, paying particular attention to his labs, list of medications, nurse's notes, and doctor's notes. The consultation is often marked by a complex medical situation, a thick (and frequently unavailable) chart, and a lack of privacy. Nevertheless, attention to this patient's chart will likely reveal such words as "confusion" and "agitation" as well as the presence of cocaine and crystal methamphetamine on the toxicology screen. Such information points toward a delirium diagnosis that will likely be confirmed within moments of observing the patient's cognitive disorganization, inattention, and fearfulness. The history of crystal methamphetamine use in an urban area should have alerted the medical team and the psychiatrist to the possibility of unsafe sex with other men, but at the time of the first contact, the patient has not revealed much history. While the hospital-based psychiatrist may spend an unusual amount of time studying external reality, the interview remains central, and it is from the interview that the consultant first adds significantly to Mr. Franken's care. While delirious, Mr. Franken understood the warmth and patience behind the consultant's words and was able to reveal his high-risk sexual behavior.

The delirium diagnosis, the history of high-risk behavior, and the medication recommendations are useful only when clearly communicated to the primary team. Such information should be related in two ways: first, via phone or in person, and second, in a chart note. Such notes are written primarily for the medical team, not for other psychiatrists, and they should be brief and focused. They may also eventually be read by the patient, the patient's family, the hospital administration, and malpractice attorneys. Notes should be informative and accurate, but they should not feature "chart wars" or indiscrete information. Thorough discussion of psychosocial issues is rarely pertinent. For example, Mr. Franken's personal history might indicate that he has a history of substance abuse and unsafe sexual practices that put him at risk for HIV. Such a note might include whether or not he used drugs intravenously, but it need not include embarrassing and unhelpful information about the patient's personal life.

As Mr. Franken's delirium resolved, the consultation became less neuropsychiatric and more focused on loneliness, his life in foster homes, and his difficulty accepting his homosexuality. Little of this need be reported in the chart or to the primary team, a group that would be most interested in an effective, efficient discharge plan.

Informed Consent

Charles P. Stowell, M.D.

THE term *informed consent* refers to a situation in which someone agrees to an action based on an understanding and appreciation of pertinent facts and implications. It is a core ethical and legal principle in modern medicine. During 6 days of delirium, however, Stephen Franken received numerous interventions that ranged from involuntary—and potentially toxic—medications to a variety of medical tests, including one for HIV. How should informed consent be applied in the many situations in which the patient has limited capacity? In regard to Mr. Franken, did his medical team break laws or violate ethical standards? What exceptions are made to these standards? How might the concept of informed consent have been used differently if Mr. Franken had been hospitalized in another country?

Two ethical principles underlie informed consent. The first is *autonomy,* in which the physician tries to maximize the degree to which the patient is an active and knowledgeable participant in medical decisions. The second principle is that of *beneficence,* in which the physician tries to maximize the good that is done to the patient without regard to personal gain. Beneficence might include providing information that allows an autonomous decision, but there are also times in which these core ethical principles conflict, such as during Mr. Franken's delirium, when medical delay in the interest of autonomy might lead to significant harm to the patient.

There are legal standards for informed consent throughout the world. These standards have evolved significantly during the last century and are marked by differences between states and between countries. The doctrine of informed consent in the United States grew out of a series of important 20th-century court cases. In *Schloendorff v. Society of New York Hospital* (1914), Judge Benjamin Cardozo determined that a surgeon had committed battery against a woman by performing a surgical procedure to which she had not consented, a procedure that led to gangrene and the amputation of several fingers. While the hospital argued that it was doing what was best for the patient and acted without financial gain or an intention to hurt the patient (i.e., with beneficence), Cardozo ruled in favor of one's "right to determine what shall be done with his own body." The provision of information was added to the notion of informed consent in the case of *Salgo v. Stanford University* (1957), when a physician was found negligent for failing to explain to his patient the potential risks of an angiographic procedure that resulted in the patient's permanent paralysis. The ethical principles that underlie medical research are spelled out in the 10 points of the Nuremberg Code, a document that emerged from the postwar trials of Nazi doctors who performed human experimentation. Later incorporated into such guidelines as the Declaration of Helsinki, the Nuremberg Code underlined the right of self-determination and informed consent and is the basis for international laws regarding the doctor–patient relationship.

At present, informed consent is composed of five elements: 1) disclosure, 2) capacity, 3) understanding, 4) voluntariness, and 5) consent. There is ambiguity inherent in each of these, and standards vary between states and between countries. For example, in England, adequate disclosure is based on risks that are *ordinarily* provided (i.e., "sufficient consent"), while laws in the United States emphasize a broader standard for disclosure so that the patient must be informed of significant risks as well as risks that would be of particular importance to that patient (i.e.,"informed consent"). Nevertheless, while there are variations, there seems to be general consensus that informed consent requires disclosure of 1) the nature of the patient's condition; 2) the nature of the proposed intervention, including possible risks and benefits; and 3) alternatives to the intervention, along with their associated risks and benefits. The most widely accepted standard used to determine how much information regarding the risks, benefits, and alternatives of the proposed treatment should be disclosed is the *reasonable person standard,* by which the physician discloses the information that a reasonable person would want to know in order to make an informed decision.

The second and third principles—*capacity* and *understanding*—are generally assessed by the primary physician without explicit testing. In cases of uncertainty, which are relatively common, a psychiatrist or ethicist may be consulted to determine the patient's capacity; if the patient is found to be incapacitated, a proxy can provide informed consent. *Voluntariness* is another principle that appears clear-cut in theory but that is often ambiguous in practice. While undue influence and coercion are forbidden, there are certainly times in which families and doctors try to convince or coerce patients to accept medical interventions. Such behavior can be ethically and legally wrong, but it is often acceptable in the interest of beneficence, especially when the coercion is an effort to help the patient make the decision that he or she would make if voluntariness were not being acutely constricted by circumstances (e.g., pain, fear, or psychological regression).

These rules do not seem to help us with Mr. Franken, since he is clearly unable to provide informed consent during his first days of hospitalization, and there are no known relatives to provide consent. For such situations, there are exceptions to the rules. For example, in urgent situations, physicians are allowed to treat without consent. This exception applies to the unconscious gunshot victim who needs surgery and to the out-of-control psychiatric patient, like Mr. Franken, who needs sedating medication in the emergency room. Assuming the medical team failed in its efforts to locate family and friends while the patient was incapacitated, the team can ethically and legally act in ways that are clearly in his best interest, particularly in making such low-risk/high-gain interventions as routine blood work, a chest X ray, urine drug screen, antipsychotic medication, and antibiotics. If he had required higher-risk interventions, the team would likely have needed to involve an independent authority. In some hospitals and jurisdictions, that authority rests in "patient services," a hospital-funded group of professionals who are expected to act independently. For example, they can act as the patient's proxy in regard to informed consent and treatment planning. In other jurisdictions and hospitals, intervention decisions are not made internally but require a judge's decision. In cases of uncertainty and exceptional risk, it is often wise to arrange a meeting of involved members of the team, patient services, and the hospital's ethics committee to ensure that the patients' rights are being upheld.

A second exception to informed consent occurs when a patient waives the right to make medical decisions, preferring to let the decision be made by family or the physician. Often invoked by patients (and families) from outside of the United States, this exception may be reasonable, but the physician should tactfully ensure that the patient independently agrees with the request and is not being coerced by family members. A third exception occurs when the physician invokes "therapeutic privilege" to withhold information about a diagnosis or treatment from a patient who the physician believes is psychologically vulnerable. For example, if members of the medical team believe that Mr. Franken might become suicidal with the news of an HIV infection, the primary physician might decide to delay the release of the information until Mr. Franken either felt more stable or was in a protected setting. The use of therapeutic privilege is rare in the United States but common in many other countries, where news such as cancer or terminal illness is frequently withheld from patients in the interest of their mental health.

Regardless of whether or not he was delirious, no one would have asked Mr. Franken to sign a consent form for routine blood draws. Considered a fourth exception to informed consent rules, "implied" or "presumed" consent has inspired a variety of defenses. Perhaps the most widely accepted justification refers to a notion of proportionality: the greater the risk incurred by the intervention, the greater the need for a formal disclosure and consent process. By this principle, for a routine blood draw, it would suffice for the clinician to inform Mr. Franken that he would like to draw blood and for Mr. Franken to hold out his arm to signify consent. For more risk-laden interventions like surgical procedures, a formal, written consent is required.

The case report indicates that—alone among his interventions—Mr. Franken's HIV test required his capacity to provide informed consent. The special status of HIV testing in the United States reflects unusual aspects of the history of the disease, particularly its initially grim prognosis and the stigma of being seen as dying, gay, and/or substance abusing. HIV/AIDS is no longer an inevitable death sentence, however, and stigma has generally lessened. Critics of the current privacy laws argue that they are anachronistic barriers to diagnosis and treatment. In particular, they refer to the estimated 250,000 Americans who do not know that they are infected with the virus and to the 40,000 new cases of HIV infection that occur annually in the United States. Proponents of new laws argue that updated testing requirements would allow wider-scale testing, promote earlier diagnosis and initiation of treatment, decrease the incidence of opportunistic infections associated with HIV/AIDS, and reduce the rate of transmission by those who are unaware that they are infected. Some opponents argue that significant stigma still exists and that routine testing threatens patient privacy and may drive people away from needed medical care. Others argue over who would pay the additional expense. Nevertheless, the Centers for Disease Control and Prevention (CDC) announced a change in its testing guidelines in 2006: specific consent would be replaced by the right to opt out of HIV testing.

Not yet widely implemented, the CDC guidelines are likely to pave the way for more flexible informed consent rules. As such, HIV testing is an example of how the principle of informed consent is complex and evolving, not only in the United States but also worldwide. While "getting a consent" may sometimes feel like a burden to a busy medical team, the underlying ethical and legal issues are integral to modern medicine.

HIV and AIDS

Stephen J. Ferrando, M.D.

SINCE the beginning of the AIDS epidemic, it has been recognized that there are complex relationships among psychiatric illness, substance abuse, and the viral infection. Both psychiatric illness and substance abuse increase the risk for acquiring HIV, and both may complicate its diagnosis and treatment. Further, HIV and its treatments may produce neuropsychiatric symptoms. For these reasons, Stephen Franken's situation provides an excellent basis for a discussion of diagnostic and therapeutic issues regarding HIV, substance abuse, and neuropsychiatry.

While HIV remains epidemic in much of the world, the use of combination antiretroviral therapy has reduced morbidity and mortality to such an extent that HIV is now generally viewed in developed countries as a chronic illness that may not be curable but is definitely treatable. This has led to an underestimation of the ongoing impact of HIV in countries like the United States, particularly among several relatively disenfranchised subgroups of the population. Persons of color are disproportionately represented among the newly infected. High-risk sexual behavior remains prevalent among young gay men, for example, while substance abuse leads to HIV infections through contaminated injection equipment and through the association of drugs—especially psychostimulants—with sexual risk behavior. As a consequence, HIV remains endemic in the United States, with the rate of new HIV infections remaining steady at approximately 40,000 per year (Centers for Disease Control and Prevention 2001a, 2001b).

Mr. Franken presented with confusion and agitation, methamphetamine and cocaine abuse, fever, and a low white blood cell count. HIV infection should have been considered even before the medical team uncovered his history of having had sex with men. Many hospital-based physicians and trainees, however, have become progressively less familiar with the neuropsychiatric complications of HIV/AIDS as its management has become increasingly based in specialty outpatient clinics. An understanding of the varieties of disease presentation is critical if the psychiatrist is to accurately diagnose this treatable but potentially lethal infection.

No one knows the current rates of undiagnosed HIV infection in the general hospital. Blinded HIV seroprevalence studies that were done over a decade ago indicate HIV seroprevalence rates ranging from 0.1% to 14%, with up to 10% of cases going undiagnosed at discharge (St. Louis et al. 1990). With reduced awareness of HIV-related complications, it is likely that cases of HIV continue to go undiagnosed and untreated.

Fortunately, an astute medical and psychiatric staff identified the likelihood of HIV infection in Mr. Franken. In addition to making the diagnosis, however, the treating team needs to consider a broad range of neuropsychiatric conditions that are commonly associated with HIV and AIDS (Table 6–5).

TABLE 6–5.   DIFFERENTIAL DIAGNOSIS OF HIV-ASSOCIATED
NEUROPSYCHIATRIC DISTURBANCES

Delirium (from multiple possible etiologies, often superimposed on underlying HIV-associated neurocognitive disorder)

Primary or comorbid psychiatric disorder (e.g., bipolar disorder, depression)

Primary or comorbid neurodegenerative disorder (e.g., Alzheimer's disease, vascular dementia)

Systemic illness (i.e., pneumonia, sepsis)

Central nervous system opportunistic illnesses and cancers (e.g., cytomegalovirus or herpes simplex encephalitis, progressive multifocal leukoencephalopathy)

Substance intoxication and/or withdrawal

Neuropsychiatric complications of hepatitis C and its treatments

Neuropsychiatric side effects of HIV medications

Metabolic complications of HIV medications (e.g., diabetes, cerebrovascular, and cardiovascular disease)

Drug interactions

Endocrinological abnormalities (e.g., hypogonadism, adrenal insufficiency)

Given Mr. Franken's fever, lowered white blood cell count, abnormal chest X ray, and a positive urine toxicology screen for amphetamines and cocaine, it is likely that the delirium was precipitated by the psychostimulants and an infection that might be as straightforward as a pneumonia or urinary tract infection. In addition, patients with central nervous system (CNS) opportunistic illnesses and cancers can present with a wide range of cognitive and neuropsychiatric symptoms, most often in the context of delirium. The medical workup should search for the major CNS opportunistic illnesses and cancers: toxoplasmosis, cryptococcus, herpes simplex, cytomegalovirus, progressive multifocal leukoencephalopathy, and lymphoma.

One of two HIV-related neuropsychiatric disorders might have contributed to Mr. Franken's initial presentation: HIV-associated minor cognitive motor disorder (MCMD) and HIV-associated dementia (HAD). Both disorders involve cognitive and behavioral symptoms associated with functional impairment (mild in MCMD, moderate to severe in HAD) and have been found to predict shorter survival (Wilkie et al. 1998). The associated cognitive symptoms are characteristic of other subcortical–frontal disorders and include impairment in psychomotor processing speed, executive function, and verbal memory. Behavioral symptoms range from apathy and depression to mania and psychosis. While Mr. Franken has cleared from his delirium and appears cognitively intact, neuropsychological testing should be considered because of the frequency of sometimes-subtle cognitive problems in HIV.

Mr. Franken has multiple current concerns, including his social isolation, his homosexuality, and his reaction to the HIV infection, each of which is likely to cause distress that can be significantly improved with psychotherapy. Perhaps the most pressing issue is, however, the successful initiation of antiviral medication. Known specifically as highly active antiretroviral therapy (HAART), these regimens attack the virus at various stages of replication and have been shown to be effective in preventing and treating CNS complications of HIV. HAART has greatly reduced HIV-associated morbidity and mortality and has converted HIV/AIDS into a largely chronic illness among people who are adherent to their medication regimens, and so it becomes urgent that Mr. Franken receive the support and education that can optimize his treatment.

HIV does replicate independently in the brain and body, and antiretroviral medications have variable degrees of CNS penetration, and so there had been concern that antiviral medications could extend life without protecting against dementia (Ferrando and Tiamson-Kassab 2006). While antiviral medications with the highest degree of CNS penetrance may lead to the greatest cognitive improvement (Letendre et al. 2004; Marra et al. 2003), the overall risk of dementia has dropped in half during the HAART era (Sacktor et al. 2001). Heterogeneous HAART regimens have been shown to reduce cerebrospinal fluid viral load to undetectable levels (Gisslen et al. 1997), to reverse white matter lesions on magnetic resonance imaging (Filippi et al. 1998), to reverse brain metabolic abnormalities detected by proton magnetic resonance spectroscopy (Chang et al. 1999), and to improve neuropsychological test performance (Ferrando et al. 2003; Tozzi et al. 1999). Despite these hopeful findings, however, functionally significant cognitive and behavioral disturbances, without frank dementia, may persist in up to 22% of HAART-treated patients (Ferrando et al. 1998), impeding adherence to treatment (Hinkin et al. 2004) and ability to work (van Gorp et al. 2007).

Not only do HAART medications *not* fully protect against neuropsychiatric conditions, in some instances they may have neuropsychiatric side effects. The most widespread clinical concern has been generated by reports of sudden-onset depression and suicidal ideation after treatment with interferon α2 and/or efavirenz. Reported effects are protean and include depression, suicidal ideation, vivid nightmares, anxiety, insomnia, psychosis, cognitive dysfunction, and antisocial behavior. The antiviral medications may also inhibit or induce the metabolism of psychotropic medications and illicit drugs (including methamphetamine) through interaction with the P450 enzyme system, particularly the P450 3A4 and 2D6 isoenzymes.

Mr. Franken's HIV infection puts him at risk for endocrinological derangements that may produce neuropsychiatric symptoms. These include deficiencies of thyroid hormone, testosterone, adrenal glucocorticoids, and adrenal androgens, particularly dehydroepiandrosterone (DHEA). All are associated with fatigue, low mood, low libido, and loss of lean body mass, and all of these symptoms may be ameliorated by correction of the deficiency state.

Mr. Franken's substance abuse puts him at high risk for infection with hepatitis C, a virus that is transmitted primarily through transfusions and the sharing of needles (e.g., illicit substance abuse, tattoos). While less likely to directly cause an agitated confusion than is HIV, hepatitis C is frequently characterized by multiple neuropsychiatric complaints such as fatigue, depression, anxiety/agitation, and cognitive dysfunction (Crone and Gabriel 2003). Compared with patients with HIV alone, patients with comorbid HIV and hepatitis C are more likely to have dementia (Ryan et al. 2004), and patients with end-stage liver disease and cirrhosis do experience superimposed delirium ("hepatic encephalopathy"). If Mr. Franken does have hepatitis C, treatment with combination pegylated interferon α2a or α2b and ribavirin treatment for hepatitis C can cause dysphoria, suicidal ideation, anxiety, sleep disturbance, fatigue, mania, psychosis, confusion, and cognitive dysfunction.

Fortunately for Mr. Franken, his HIV infection was properly diagnosed. His delirium cleared. He appears to be addressing the challenges of establishing HIV care and the multiple psychological issues related to his sexuality and his infection. This initial evaluation period may be a good time to explore his prior concerns about HIV, particularly if he felt infection to be a death sentence, a punishment for prior behavior, or out of his control. Such preconceptions may lead to distress, avoidance, ongoing high-risk behavior, and poor adherence to treatment. The clinician should also assess for depression, anxiety, and suicidality, since multiple studies have found that 60%–70% of patients with HIV infection have one or more primary psychiatric disorders prior to an AIDS diagnosis. Interestingly, while anxiety runs high prior to HIV testing, anxiety tends to dissipate after testing, regardless of the test results, especially when psychological support and medical care are made available to those who are diagnosed HIV positive. Moving forward, Mr. Franken should be monitored for substance abuse relapse, for denial about his illness with associated nonadherence and high-risk sexual behavior, and for a variety of psychiatric disorders such as major depression, anxiety, and HIV-associated neurocognitive disorders. Nevertheless, the diagnosis of HIV may serve not just to save his life through the initiation of antiretroviral medications but also to stimulate him to take a more active approach toward promoting his health and to address long-standing, partially recognized fears and anxieties that relate to infection, intimacy, and homosexuality.

Internalized Homophobia

Richard C. Friedman, M.D.

CLINICAL issues involving sexual orientation are best conceptualized from a developmental perspective. Stephen Franken's homosexual and heterosexual impulses are obviously a source of conflict at present, but his problems probably began long before adolescence. Particularly suggestive is his childhood history of having been raised in multiple foster homes or institutions, an experience that is frequently traumatic and suggests the possibility of a number of major psychopathological consequences.

First is possible impairment in the capacity to form meaningful attachments. There is no evidence from the available history that Mr. Franken has ever had an enduring intimate relationship. This man's sexual relational style may, therefore, be part of a general impairment in all of his interpersonal relationships. While he has requested psychotherapy, all types of psychotherapy depend on the patient's capacity to form a working relationship with the therapist. A further elaboration of the quality of his relationships during the course of his life would help assess his capacity for participating in a psychotherapeutic process.

A second issue concerns his personality structure and function. It is possible that his childhood experiences were traumatic enough (interacting with unknown genetic factors) to influence the formation of some type of personality disorder. If this were so, the abnormal mental *states* that characterize his present illness would be experienced and expressed in the context of more enduring pathological personality *traits*. If present, these would have influenced and been influenced by his sexual experiences and activities.

Mr. Franken's childhood dislocations may have also influenced the occurrence of gender identity and/or sexual disorders. It would be helpful to learn more about his childhood gender role behavior, since gender role behavior that is atypical—such as preferring girls' to boys' clothing, or playing exclusively with girls—may trigger abuse from other boys. This abuse may include bullying, physical attacks, or ostracism, and if present, these painful interactions would have contributed to a fragile sense of masculine self-esteem.

Mr. Franken indicates that his homosexual activity is motivated by homoerotic fantasies/desire, whereas the reasons for his heterosexual activity are unclear. We know that he can perform heterosexually with the assistance of an erectile dysfunction drug and homosexual fantasy. If he is not motivated by erotic fantasies, why does he engage in heterosexual activity? Another question concerns his capacity to form erotic relationships. Why has all his sex with men been with anonymous strangers rather than with someone with whom he has formed a meaningful relationship?

At this point let me define some basic concepts. The term *sexual fantasy* refers to conscious experienced imagery associated with psychophysiological manifestations of sexual excitement/arousal. The onset of erotic fantasy usually occurs during childhood. By the time of puberty almost all boys masturbate, and their masturbatory imagery has usually been in place for some time. Once a boy's erotic programming is in place—as exclusively heterosexual, bisexual, or exclusively homosexual—it usually remains fixed for life. There are exceptions, however, and some men appear capable of a greater degree of erotic object plasticity than are most (Friedman 1988, 2006; Friedman and Downey 1994, 2002; Laumann et al. 1994).

The sense of identity as gay or heterosexual occurs much later in development, during adolescence or young adulthood. Mr. Franken has repeated sexual encounters with anonymous men but is "sickened" by the thought that he might "be gay." Being gay refers to a person's sense of identity and, if advertised to others, his social role. A person's sense of identity as gay or heterosexual may be congruent or incongruent with his erotic fantasies and/or erotic activity. The reasons for the incongruity in Stephen Franken's case remain to be established.

Mr. Franken jokes that he has a case of "internalized homophobia." The term *homophobia* was coined in the late 1960s to connote an irrational aversion to homosexual people (Weinberg 1972). So-called homophobia is often learned and based on false assumptions about nonheterosexual people. It may also be associated with cognitive and emotional styles that are more paranoid than phobic (Herek 1996). The term *internalized homophobia* was introduced into the clinical literature in the early 1980s to connote the psychopathological effects among homosexual individuals of internalizations during childhood of antihomosexual authority figures (Malyon 1982).

Let's return to Stephen Franken's history with these basic concepts in mind.

The *onset* of his sexual fantasies during childhood almost certainly was associated with self-condemnation. By late childhood, therefore, he had probably experienced painful conflict between homoerotic programming and prohibitions of conscience. He wanted to have sex with males but felt guilty and ashamed.

Self-condemnation in response to homosexual fantasies/desires is commonly caused by antihomosexual religious convictions and by internalizations of homophobic and/or heterosexist caretakers. With respect to the former, it is necessary to ascertain the history of Mr. Franken's religious value system. Sometimes an adult may consider himself to be secular, but nonetheless antihomosexual religious beliefs assimilated during childhood may still retain their behavioral effects. Of course, other authority figures may be internalized in addition to religious ones. Sometimes such caretakers might not actually directly condemn homosexuality, but rather may be "heterosexist." That is, they may privilege heterosexual family forms as being the only "normal" way to live. In order to adequately assess Stephen Franken's conflicts, it is necessary to explore the development of his moral belief system about sexual matters.

One aspect of his history might be particularly helpful in attempting to learn more about Mr. Franken's conscience. Here I am referring to his ideas about "safe sex," both historically and at present. How did he feel about high-risk sexual activities during the course of his life? Did he believe that he deserved to become HIV positive? Was he so guilty about homosexual desires that he actually sought to contract HIV? At this point, what are his ideas about managing his HIV positive status with respect to sexual activities with others?

Additional interviews will help clarify the meaning of homosexuality and heterosexuality to this patient and may help clarify his ability to tolerate the intimacy of psychotherapy. As Mr. Franken is better understood, treatment planning can be placed into an appropriately complex perspective.

Sexuality and Sexual Dysfunction

Robert Kertzner, M.D.

WHILE perhaps not as urgent as his delirium or HIV infection, Stephen Franken's sexual issues warrant specific therapeutic focus because they contribute to his unhappiness, social isolation, and substance abuse. In addition to exploring sexual dysfunction and conflicts about homosexuality, Mr. Franken's psychiatrist should also aim to understand his overall sexual well-being in the larger context of his physical health, psychological and interpersonal functioning, and culture.

The psychiatrist might begin by exploring Mr. Franken's behavior, fantasy life, and sexual identity. Mr. Franken has sex with men and women, fantasizes exclusively about men, and does not consider himself to be gay. Self-identification that is discrepant with sexual behavior or desire may be indicative of psychological conflicts (as with Mr. Franken), but the psychiatrist should not presume this to be universally true. Many adolescents, young adults, and women have same-gender partners but do not identify as gay or lesbian, without an implication of psychological conflict.

In addition to his difficulties accepting homosexual feelings, Mr. Franken describes problems in sexual function. Details are important, and so the history should include when the problems began and whether the problems vary based on the partner's gender, the situation, or the degree of intimacy. It appears the Mr. Franken uses an erectile dysfunction medication in order to have sex with women. Since he apparently only fantasizes about men and is unable to get an erection with women, the implication is that he has a homosexual orientation about which he is conflicted. That would not, however, be the end of the history. We do not know the details of his fantasies, nor do we understand why he has sex with women when he is sexually uninterested. What is—and has been—pleasurable about heterosexual relations? Do relations with women make Mr. Franken less anxious about same-sex attractions? Does he find it easier to experience emotional intimacy with a woman than with a man, as some bisexual men report? Is he ashamed of homosexual behavior? Why does he want people to view him as heterosexual? The exploration of his sexual life with women would most likely develop in concert with discussion of a variety of other issues, including the ways in which his experience with intimacy and sexuality were influenced by having been raised in foster care.

It would be equally important to explore his relationships with men. If his fantasies are exclusively homosexual, why does he need to take stimulants in order to have sex with men? Perhaps he feels physical discomfort during receptive anal intercourse that requires his use of cocaine to facilitate penetration. Perhaps sex has become entangled with "bad" behavior, leading him to associate sexual activity with anonymous partners and illicit substances. Or perhaps stimulants allow him to overcome inhibitions about having sex with men. Until these are discussed, the therapist will be unable to fully understand Mr. Franken's sexual desires and behaviors.

Diagnostic assessment should include a broad psychosocial and sexual developmental history that provides a psychological context for understanding current sexual problems. This history includes a characterization of the patient's sexual drive (subjective experience of seeking sex), motivation (aspirations for having a sexual experience), and conflicts (wishes vs. fears, impulses vs. values) (Levine et al. 2003). In this way, an evaluation of sexual health becomes intertwined with such concerns as attachment, self-esteem, intimacy, and love. It is likely that Mr. Franken has not previously spoken about his sexual life and so may not have a very clear understanding of his own motivations, desires, and inhibitions. A thorough interview that considers developmental and psychosocial factors would help Mr. Franken with an understanding of his sexuality by developing a tentative narrative of what had previously been a bewildering set of impulses and behaviors. In this respect, a thorough assessment can be therapeutic as well as inform the formulation of diagnoses and treatment planning.

The psychiatrist should also consider whether Mr. Franken's erectile dysfunction is related to psychiatric or biomedical conditions for which specific interventions are indicated. Mood, anxiety, psychotic, and personality disorders (particularly those marked by impulsivity or compulsivity) are associated with sexual dysfunction. Furthermore, a wide variety of psychotropic medications are associated with sexual side effects. For example, Mr. Franken may have been taking a selective serotonin reuptake inhibitor (SSRI) antidepressant that diminished his libido. While none of these is mentioned in his history, it is also clear that Mr. Franken is not the most transparent of historians. Many nonpsychiatric medical conditions can also impact upon sexuality. Vascular, neurologic, and endocrine disorders are well known to cause sexual dysfunction, as are a variety of other systemic illnesses and medications. HIV can cause sexual dysfunction through a decrease in testosterone and/or other hormones, peripheral neuropathy, and medication treatments such as protease inhibitors (Collazos et al. 2002). Regardless of coexisting illnesses, duration of HIV infection is independently associated with sexual dysfunction (Asboe et al. 2007).

Treatment should reflect this biopsychosocial evaluation. Substance abuse treatment is a priority and would provide a structure in which Mr. Franken could discuss his problematic association of drug use with sexual desire, arousal, and behavior. Individual psychotherapy could help Mr. Franken accept his sexuality and explore ways to realize sexual desires that enhance sexual well-being and psychological health. Although less clearly indicated, possible modalities for treating his sexual problems include behaviorally based sex therapy, group therapy, and psychoeducational interventions.

Mr. Franken might also benefit from medication treatment for depressed mood or anxiety, in which case the psychiatrist would carefully consider and discuss the potential sexual side effects of psychotropic medications. Mr. Franken might prefer medications less likely to affect libido or orgasm such as bupropion (Wellbutrin). The best-established pharmacologic treatments for erectile dysfunction are the phosphodiesterase-5 inhibitors such as sildenafil (Viagra), tadalafil (Cialis), and vardenafil (Levitra) (Taylor 2006). These medications generally work well for many causes of erectile dysfunction, including the use of SSRIs. Low testosterone levels are frequently found among the elderly and people with HIV infection and often respond to exogenous testosterone.

While a nonjudgmental approach is essential to all aspects of psychiatric care, it is particularly important in regard to sexuality. Many patients experience shame or guilt about aspects of their sexuality; some may be concerned that a psychiatrist holds stigmatizing views of their sexuality. The psychological burden of a disowned sexuality or impaired sexual functioning undermines mental health; conversely, the enfranchisement of sexuality in a patient's life and enhancement of sexual function are core elements of well-being. Psychiatrists are in a unique position to assist these aims by virtue of understanding the link between sexuality and mental health. For Mr. Franken, efforts to promote sexual well-being may be as important to his quality of life as any other psychiatric intervention.

Jekyll and Hyde

Hilary J. Beattie, Ph.D.

The names of Jekyll and Hyde are often used metaphorically, by clinicians and laypeople alike, to refer to cases of "split personality"—that is, to describe someone whose conventional exterior conceals a life of secret iniquity, or who is subject to abrupt and baffling personality changes in which the two selves are so extremely different as to appear unrelated. But relatively few are familiar these days with the famous "double" story, *Strange Case of Dr. Jekyll and Mr. Hyde,* published in 1886 by the Scottish author Robert Louis Stevenson (1850–1894), which made such an impression worldwide that it rapidly became part of popular folklore and "common sense" psychology.

Before outlining the ways in which the story may illuminate the case of Stephen Franken, a brief synopsis is in order. Stevenson's tale, as the title implies, is presented as a gradually unfolding case study in abnormal psychology. We first meet the youthful but repulsive-seeming Edward Hyde on his nocturnal roamings, as he commits an act of casual, wanton aggression (trampling a little girl) and then sneers defiantly at the citizens who apprehend him. Later, he compounds his crime by brutally murdering a distinguished older man who had "accosted" him in a dark, deserted street. It emerges that Hyde has a close but mysterious connection with a respectable, middle-aged, celibate physician, Dr. Henry Jekyll. Suspense and terror mount as Jekyll's friend and lawyer, Utterson, vows to track down Hyde, whom he suspects of blackmailing the doctor over some secret sin. Only at the end do we learn (through a posthumous, confessional statement) that Jekyll had developed a drug that enabled him to assume at will the split-off persona of Hyde and thereby secretly pursue the shameful and evil pleasures that were incompatible with his social position and scientific ambitions. As the evil self grew stronger, the change became involuntary and ever harder to reverse, and when the original supply of the salt used to make the drug ran out, Jekyll found himself forever trapped (fatally infected, as it were) in the loathsome being of Hyde, with no recourse but discovery or death.

There are some uncanny parallels with the case of Stephen Franken (whose name also alludes to another nineteenth-century classic about scien-

tific experimentation resulting in an out-of-control alter ego, Mary Shelley's
Frankenstein). The patient makes his first, Hyde-like appearance late at night,
as an "emotionally disturbed person," fighting with the police as he is
brought to the hospital. He too is angry, hostile, suspicious to the point of
paranoia, and uncooperative. Later, in the light of day, he appears strikingly
different; though still intermittently confused and agitated, he becomes more
lucid, apologetic, and socially conforming. It emerges that Mr. Franken is a
fairly successful professional (like the respectable Dr Jekyll) who suffers from
chronic loneliness and isolation. He is unable to form a satisfying personal
and sexual relationship with a woman and is so concerned with controlling
social appearances that his sexual desire for men (still less the idea of being
"homosexual") is completely incompatible with his self-image. Like Dr.
Jekyll, in order to release and indulge his unacceptable, "hidden" Hyde, Mr.
Franken has to resort to the use of addictive, mind-altering drugs. These
make possible both his reckless, angry, nocturnal pursuit of what he considers illicit and shameful sexual encounters, and his resulting, permanent, HIV
infection (just as the Jekyll to Hyde change becomes impossible to reverse).
Mr. Franken's final exposure and self-confrontation do not result in suicide,
as in the case of Jekyll/Hyde, but we are left with questions as to the extent of
the physical and emotional damage he has inflicted on himself and how
much of it is reparable. Can he, unlike Jekyll, use therapy to integrate the re-
pudiated aspects of himself into a more realistic self-image, or will he pursue
his self-destructive course?

Strange Case of Dr. Jekyll and Mr. Hyde has given rise to endless discussion
since its first publication, and has often been interpreted in terms of illicit sexual desire, especially for men. The story actually had deep roots in the author's
own life, Scottish Calvinist upbringing, and youthful dissipations, and originally came to him in the form of a terrifying nightmare (Beattie 2001). Part of
Stevenson's genius in constructing the tale lay in a careful refusal to specify the
exact nature of Dr Jekyll's "moral turpitude" and disgraceful pleasures, leaving
generations of readers to project on to it their own worst imaginings. Since all
the major characters are men (celibate, professional, emotionally isolated like
Jekyll himself), it has been easy to give it a homosexual interpretation, reinforced by the fact that in 1885 homosexuality had been criminalized in English law (in the so-called Blackmailers' Charter). Certainly, the absence of
women throws into relief the darker implications of sadism and perversion in
male sexuality (one may recall that Krafft-Ebing's *Psychopathia Sexualis* was
also published in 1886). But many other interpretations are possible. The
story ultimately has its origins in the Romantic "double" genre of the early
nineteenth century, popularized by such writers as E.T.A. Hoffmann, Poe, and
Dostoevsky, which reflected a growing secular interest in psychology and the
darker side of human nature. By the end of the century it also tapped into

widespread fears of social Darwinian regression to primitive instincts, criminal degeneracy, urban violence, and social unrest. *Jekyll and Hyde* can be read as a comment on contemporary theories of abnormal psychology, such as hysteria and multiple personality, found in the work of Charcot and others. (Stevenson was said to have been "deeply impressed" by a paper he read in a French scientific journal on "sub-consciousness.") The story likewise foreshadows Freudian notions of the repetition compulsion and the return of the repressed, as well as object relations theories of internalized objects and egos (Beattie 1998). Stevenson himself later stressed that Jekyll's real sin had nothing to do with sexuality per se, but with cruelty, selfishness, cowardice, and, above all, hypocrisy, which deform and distort human nature (this last point being particularly apt in the case of Stephen Franken).

In short, *Strange Case of Dr. Jekyll and Mr. Hyde,* the classic narrative of self-alienation, can illuminate many diverse cases. It still retains its ability to disturb and shock, and well repays close reading in one of the excellent modern editions available.

Psychotherapy Selection

Carolyn J. Douglas, M.D.

IN this era of highly educated consumers, Stephen Franken's specific request for "exploratory psychotherapy" is not especially unusual. Patients may well come to us having investigated psychodynamic psychotherapy (both exploratory and supportive approaches), cognitive, behavioral, interpersonal, dialectic, and existential therapies, 12-step programs and other self-help groups, biofeedback, relaxation training, motivational interviewing, eye movement desensitization (EMDR), and Gestalt therapy, to name just a few—not to mention all of the biologically based interventions, including psychotropic drugs, alternative medications, herbal remedies, light therapy, and vagal nerve stimulation. It is beyond the scope of this discussion to describe the differing characteristics of and indications for all of these treatment modalities. However, I would be curious about the specificity of this patient's request and would want to ask him how and why he came to ask for this particular form of treatment, what he knows about it, and how he hopes it will help him.

The psychiatrist in the story asks whether Mr. Franken is suitable for individual exploratory therapy, but it may be more useful to ask whether such treatment is optimal for a young man with his particular history and constellation of strengths, vulnerabilities, problems, current internal stressors, and present life circumstances. I would consider not only the principal type of psychotherapy to be used but also whether psychotherapy should be offered in conjunction (or sequentially) with any other psychological treatments (e.g. psychotropic medication, substance abuse treatment, or a support group for patients newly diagnosed with HIV); where the treatment should take place (inpatient drug rehabilitation facility, intensive outpatient program, or private office); how frequently to meet; whether it should be offered in an individual or group format; how long the treatment is likely to last (brief or time-unlimited); and finally, who should provide it. The patient seems to have attached himself quickly to the consultation-liaison psychiatrist, but if it is not feasible, practical, or in the patient's best interest for the psychiatrist to take him on personally, to whom should he be referred? Since he will be taking medication when he leaves the hospital, at least provisionally, he would presumably need to see a psychiatrist. But would it be desirable for the treating therapist to have special expertise in treating conflicts about sexual orientation, substance abuse, or psychiatric problems in the medically ill, specifically in patients with HIV/AIDS? Should the therapist be male or female? Does it matter if the therapist is gay or straight? In short, what are this particular man's needs, short and long range, at this particular time in his life, with his particular array of problems, assets, and resources? What he is likely to tolerate, what is he motivated to pursue, and what is he apt to benefit from the most?

The treatment decision should take into consideration the possibility that the delirium and/or the HIV infection could lead to persistent cognitive problems that could interfere with his ability to participate in an exploratory psychotherapy. It would also be important not to ignore his history of substance abuse. Assuming inpatient drug treatment was not the treatment of choice, outpatient treatment could be pursued in parallel with our work. Mr. Franken may choose, of course, to reject my advice. Some therapists might make abstinence from alcohol and drugs a condition for taking this man on as a patient, but I think it is unrealistic to require people to simply stop doing what brought them to treatment in the first place. In Mr. Franken's case, his drug use is clearly bound up with and fueled by considerable uncertainty and conflict about his sexual orientation, and these issues will take time to sort out in psychotherapy. If he chooses not to pursue targeted substance abuse treatment, I would at least discuss with him possible negative consequences of his continuing to use drugs, including its impact on the work he hopes to do with me. As the patient–therapist alliance develops and as the treatment unfolds, the substance abuse could be re-explored.

Before recommending a specific psychotherapy, I would try to assess the severity of his psychopathology, and specifically how much "support" (or modifications in the usual techniques of exploratory psychotherapy) may become necessary. From Freud's era through the 1960s, the prevailing belief about patients' "suitability" for psychodynamic psychotherapy was that "healthier" people with sufficiently intact "ego functioning" (including reality testing, impulse control, object relations, and psychic defense mechanisms) should generally be prescribed the more intensive, uncovering modes of therapy—variously referred to as exploratory, psychoanalytically oriented, expressive, insight-oriented, interpretive, or transference-based therapy—with the aim of exploring feelings, needs, motivations, and repetitive conflicts, along with some of the childhood origins of these conflicts. Such exploration would bring about personality change and growth. "Sicker" patients with chronically "fragile" egos—or people whose generally good ego functioning had been temporarily overwhelmed in the face of an acute crisis—were thought to require a more supportive approach, with greater emphasis placed on relieving painful feelings, building self-esteem, instilling hope, supporting deficient psychological functions, and improving coping skills and overall functioning (Dewald 1971; Perry et al. 1983).

Like most people, however, Mr. Franken presents with a mix of personality strengths and vulnerabilities and defies neat pigeonholing as either "healthy" or "sick," "suitable" or "unsuitable" for uncovering work. He seems to have a number of possible "ego weaknesses" in the areas of identity cohesion, self-esteem, object relations (difficulty forming stable and lasting relationships), and impulse control (use of drugs to manage painful emotional experiences), and has also been recently diagnosed with a serious, life-threatening illness. All of these are well-recognized indications for adopting a more "supportive" approach.

At the same time, he seems to have long-standing conflicts around attachment, dependency, intimacy, and sexual orientation, with possible long-term precursors that would seem to call for a more uncovering psychodynamic mode of treatment. Further, he has numerous personality strengths that would augur well for such an approach (including motivation, a capacity for introspection, evidence of some positive emotional connection to the evaluating psychiatrist, and a demonstrated capacity for work despite long-standing internal conflicts).

Rather than deciding between supportive and exploratory therapy, Schlesinger (1969) has suggested that a prescription for psychotherapy should be explicit about what needs to be supported, and when, and why, and what needs expression and why. Mr. Franken may need an uncovering psychodynamic treatment, for example, but, given his long-standing need to maintain emotional distance, I would at least initially focus on outside relationships rather than the transference relationship. Further, at least at the beginning of treatment, he may also need help with problem solving, a referral to a self-help group, instruction on relaxation techniques, and direct encouragement of realistic optimism and healthy behaviors. Such supportive interventions do not necessarily detract from Mr. Franken's self-understanding, as often suggested in the literature. Instead, such supportive interventions enhance the "holding function" of psychotherapy, which can allow investigative work to proceed at a reasonable pace and a comfortable depth (De Jonghe et al. 1994; Modell 1976; Pine 1986; Winnicott 1965).

Finally, I would anticipate that the therapy will need to be open-ended rather than time-limited. Mr. Franken is very much alone in the world. People who have suffered significant early losses tend to have considerable anxiety about attachment, dependency, and separation. Despite the apparent ease with which Mr. Franken seemed to engage with the consultation-liaison psychiatrist, I would anticipate there will be strong resistances against dependency in the therapy. Once achieved, a genuinely engaged relationship with the therapist may be hard—if not contraindicated—for Mr. Franken to give up. It is not difficult to imagine that for some time to come, perhaps quite a long time, the therapist may be the only person Mr. Franken allows himself to need.

Overview of Connection

Francine Cournos, M.D.

LIKE many psychiatric patients, Mr. Franken has multiple problems and diagnoses. Nonetheless, working with him successfully requires a unified and integrated understanding of his situation. One way to achieve this is to create a longitudinal story of Mr. Franken's life, a set of hypotheses that will be continuously tested as we learn more about him.

Using our limited information, we might construct the initial narrative as follows: Mr. Franken was born to parents who were themselves isolated—a father who maintained no connection with him, and a mother who was not sufficiently close to family or friends to ensure that someone would step forward to take in her young son when she died unexpectedly. Through a process sometimes referred to as the *transgenerational transmission of trauma*, which may have genetic as well as experiential and psychological roots, young Stephen was left to grow up with multiple caretakers, none of whom kept him for long. His 4 years with his mother, although perhaps barely remembered, may have contributed to his strengths, including the discipline and drive he would need to become a successful professional, a goal that many foster children never achieve.

Because children can grow and heal only in the context of relationships, the lack of a suitable substitute for his deceased mother interfered with Mr. Franken achieving an integrated and stable sense of himself as a good and worthy person who could love and be loved. Sometimes aspects of childhood trauma and loss can be worked through at a later stage of development in the context of creating an adult family, although achieving this often requires considerable psychotherapy. This path is more difficult for gay men, who must confront a lack of formal social structures and acceptance of gay relationships, creating yet another hurdle for Mr. Franken in re-establishing himself in a family of his own. And so, Mr. Franken found himself on an ambivalent search for intimacy with men and women.

It is also likely that Mr. Franken emerged from foster care with one or more psychiatric illnesses, which is the case for the majority of children in foster care. Mental illness and substance abuse increase the risk for HIV infection. This association, combined with his history of unsafe sex with men, made becoming HIV positive almost inevitable. Substance use and undiagnosed HIV infection put Mr. Franken at significant risk for delirium, which brings us to his arrival in an agitated state in the emergency department.

Creating an integrated hypothetical picture of Mr. Franken helps ground the clinician, but it does not alter the complexity of Mr. Franken's treatment, nor the likelihood that this treatment will be fragmented. Each of our discussants offers a thoughtful analysis of how to proceed with various aspects of diagnosis and management, but few clinicians possess the full range of such expertise, however, and few treatment systems can offer the full range of suggested services. We need not be unduly discouraged. No single psychiatrist needs to memorize every possible cause of delirium, for example, as long as the medical/psychiatric team searches for causes, assesses risk, and maintains safety. As Mr. Franken's delirium clears, the clinician is faced with a series of issues: his substance abuse, his risky sexual behavior, his strategies for coping with AIDS, and the pervasive impact that early trauma and loss have had on his current ability to accept his sexuality and to overcome his state of social isolation. The risk of treatment fragmentation is significant but reduced by the fact that there has been greater emphasis on providing integrated care for HIV/AIDS than for many other medical disorders.

Had Mr. Franken presented with this medical picture at the beginning of the HIV epidemic, his life span would have been severely limited. Today, HIV has become a chronic and manageable illness, although antiretroviral treatment is best initiated before the CD4 count drops below 200 or when the patient first becomes symptomatic. Given the advanced state of his immunosuppression, and the association of substance use with poor adherence to antiretroviral treatment for HIV, Mr. Franken's life depends on his ability to accept and strictly adhere to his AIDS treatment regimen without allowing substance use to interfere with his doing so. How can this be achieved?

From a psychological perspective, the repeated image in our discussants' remarks is of Mr. Franken as a man who is alone in the world. Such a profound sense of aloneness can rob a person of the meaning and purpose that is essential to self-preservation. Mr. Franken is at a critical juncture. On the one hand, he has discovered that he is seriously ill with an incurable infection. On the other, he is finally getting the care and attention that he has needed for some time. The fact that Mr. Franken is seeking a relationship-focused treatment is a very positive development. In fact, it may be critical, for if Mr. Franken is to save himself, it may only be possible in the context of the therapist's conviction that Mr. Franken is worthy of the investment.

Summary Points

- Managing psychiatric patients in the emergency room requires an unusually active stance and a focus on safety, disposition, and the group as a whole.

- Abrupt changes in behavior should prompt a search for substance abuse and neuropsychiatric illness.

- Twelve-step programs and motivational interviewing are effective at least partly because they take into consideration typical reactions in the therapist and typical behaviors and attitudes in the person who abuses substances.

- Managing psychiatric patients in the general hospital requires an unusually active stance and a focus on the medical team's needs as well as those of the patient.

- Early deprivation affects the ability to develop adult relationships.

- Early experience as a stigmatized other affects the ability to develop adult relationships.

- A psychotherapy recommendation requires an assessment of distress, cognition, motivation, interpersonal relationships, ego strengths and weaknesses, and treatment availability.

Chapter 7

ADOLESCENT BEREAVEMENT AND AMELIA GUTIERREZ

THE headmaster of a local private school referred Amelia Gutierrez, a 16-year-old bilingual tenth-grader, to an outpatient psychiatrist after she began to scratch her wrists and tell classmates she wanted to die. According to the headmaster, Amelia's grades and attendance had declined since the death of her mother 1 year earlier, and he wondered whether Amelia would be better off in a school that was less socially and academically stressful. The headmaster added that the school would pay for psychotherapy to help ease her transition to a neighborhood public school but did want the psychiatrist's opinion about the wisdom of expulsion.

The psychiatrist called the father in order to obtain further history. According to him, Amelia had not adjusted to his wife's death from breast cancer. Formerly an attentive and lively student and daughter, she had become increasingly morose, tearful, and hostile.

After talking by phone with the headmaster and father, the psychiatrist met with Amelia. She broke into tears almost immediately, saying that she knew that she was a horrible daughter and student and that she deserved to get kicked out of school. She felt especially guilty since her mother had pushed so hard for the scholarship but that nothing seemed especially important anymore. She described intense loneliness. Not only did she miss her mother, but she missed the two elderly neighbors who had watched over her throughout her childhood. All of the local families had moved as part of an urban renewal project, and while she knew that her current apartment was nicer, she missed the old neighborhood. She had a few friends at school but spent most of her evenings reading novels and avoiding homework. Little interested her. She slept 10–12 hours per night, often sleeping past noon on weekends. She admitted to missing school frequently, explaining that she just didn't want to go.

Amelia viewed her deceased mother as the center of the family. Her mother had been the primary breadwinner, homemaker, and disciplinarian, checking Amelia's homework for thoroughness and her room for cleanliness. Since her mother was diagnosed, her father had seemed distracted and overwhelmed and been unable to pick up the slack. She viewed her father as "a nice guy but kind of a loser." Amelia denied feeling angry at anyone but did say that she had no patience for her father, teachers, younger brother, and classmates. She also had no patience for herself and said that she worried that the stress of raising children had somehow contributed to her mother's death.

Personal History

The patient was born in the Dominican Republic and immigrated to the United States at age 3 years. She attended local public schools until, during eighth grade, she was recruited by an elite private school after she had won an essay contest. She believed that her writing talents stemmed from a daily diary she had begun on her tenth birthday. Her diary, she said, was her best friend. She used it to confide her secret thoughts and feelings and also to practice her skills as a writer. In it she wrote poems and fragments of stories.

Amelia had a 9-year-old brother who was "a pest." Her mother had been an executive secretary, and her father was a part-time handyman in a large apartment building. The family had attended mass weekly until her mother became too ill, at which point the priest and her mother's friends began to visit the home. After Amelia's mother died, the visits tapered off, and no one had visited in over 6 months.

When asked if she was or had been been sexually involved with anyone, Amelia asked if the sessions were confidential. When this was affirmed, Amelia said she had begun to date a 21-year-old college student who lived in the neighborhood. They tended to meet in his apartment on Saturdays and that getting together with him was the only time she felt alive. They drank alcohol and smoked marijuana each week, but she "didn't have a problem with it." He was also Dominican, and she liked speaking Spanish with him, since hardly anyone spoke Spanish in the neighborhood or at her school.

Personal Psychiatric History

Amelia said she began to cut herself 2 years earlier in an effort "to feel real, not numb." These episodes were often triggered by worries about her mother, who had been ill for several years prior to her death. Amelia was embarrassed that anyone had found out about the cutting. While she did sometimes wish she were dead so that she could see her mother again, she denied ever having had active suicidal intention or a plan. She did not know why she had told some of her friends that she wanted to die. She denied ever having made a suicide attempt, adding that the cutting was never intended to be seriously damaging. She denied alcohol and substance abuse beyond the marijuana and alcohol mentioned above. She denied eating problems.

Family Psychiatric History

None known.

Medical History

None.

Mental Status Exam

The patient was a casually dressed adolescent girl whose makeup and posture suggested someone a few years older than her stated age. She spoke rapidly with a slight Spanish accent. There were no abnormal movements, and her gait was normal. She said she was sad, and she appeared glum. Her frequent tears and occasional smiles were appropriate to content. Her thoughts were goal directed. She denied wanting to kill herself, but she did say that she sometimes felt so hopeless that she wished she were dead. No psychotic symptoms were elicited. The patient was cognitively intact. Her insight and judgment were considered fair.

Summary

Amelia Gutierrez was a 16-year-old girl who became depressed in the context of her mother's death, a move to a new neighborhood, and the possibility of school expulsion. The following discussions explore ways in which ethical, cultural, and developmental issues impact her evaluation and treatment.

Discussions of the Case of Amelia Gutierrez

An Ethical Dilemma. 261
Paul S. Appelbaum, M.D.

Adolescent Bereavement 264
Cynthia R. Pfeffer, M.D.

Suicide. 267
J. John Mann, M.D.

Interview of the Adolescent. .269
Ayame Takahashi, M.D.

Psychological Impact of Dislocation 273
Mindy Thompson Fullilove, M.D.

The Dominican Patient 276
Ian Canino, M.D.

Virginia Woolf: On Being Ill 280
Katherine Dalsimer, Ph.D.

Neurobiology of Attachment .283
H. Jonathan Polan, M.D.

Pharmacology of Adolescent Depression 286
P. Anne McBride, M.D.

Interpersonal Psychotherapy .289
Laura Mufson, Ph.D.

Psychodynamics of Depression. 292
Fredric N. Busch, M.D.

Overview of Adolescent Bereavement. 296
Theodore Shapiro, M.D.

Summary Points 298

An Ethical Dilemma

Paul S. Appelbaum, M.D.

Aᴍᴇʟɪᴀ Gutierrez is a depressed student with suicidal ideation who has come to the attention of authorities at a private high school. After making an appropriate referral for psychiatric evaluation, the headmaster ponders his next step. Perhaps the school itself is part of the problem? Maybe Amelia would be better off in a less-demanding environment? Indeed, given that she is speaking openly to her classmates about her thoughts of death, perhaps it would be less disturbing to all concerned if she simply went somewhere else.

Unfortunately, this is not an uncommon scenario, though it is one that usually plays out at the college level rather than in high school. Sometimes for good reasons, but often for less charitable ones, academic administrators may require students who manifest suicidal ideation to leave campus immediately; they may preclude their return for a semester or even an academic year—and then only allow them to resume their studies after assurances that their disorder has remitted. Indeed, some schools classify suicidality as a violation of their disciplinary codes and remove students on that basis. Since psychiatrists are often involved in these cases, it is worth thinking seriously about the complex ethical/clinical matrix in which they arise (Appelbaum 2006).

Why do schools expel suicidal students? In some cases, administrators may genuinely believe that the school environment is overly stressful and that it would be in the student's best interests not to have to cope with high-level academic demands. And sometimes they are concerned about the impact of one student's mental state on other students, especially in dormitory settings, where roommates may find themselves caring for a distraught friend rather than attending classes or doing assignments. However, these are not the only motivating factors. Recent court cases have suggested that college officials who know of students' suicidal ideation and fail to act appropriately may be held liable if students later harm themselves (*Schieszler v. Ferrum College 2002*; *Shin v. Massachusetts Institute of Technology 2005*). Although courts have generally been protective of schools and colleges (Lake and Tribbensee 2002), getting a suicidal student out of school and off campus may seem like a reasonable risk management strategy (Capriccioso 2006). Moreover, there are other risks for educational institutions besides legal ones. The adverse publicity stemming from a student committing suicide—especially if it occurs on campus—can tarnish a school's reputation, diminish its competitiveness for top applicants, and thus increase the school's incentives to suspend or expel suicidal students.

Although the justifications offered publicly for expelling suicidal students, as with Amelia, usually relate to the student's interests, there are many reasons to believe that suicidal students may not benefit from changing schools. Often already isolated as a result of their depression, expelled students may be cut off from their remaining social networks, rendering their depression still harder to treat. Being in school, especially a prestigious institution, may enhance a student's self-esteem. At a difficult time in his or her life, academic performance may be the only area of accomplishment left to the student. For students away at college, sending them home may mean moving them from the relative sanctuary of the campus to the locus of their difficulties in a dysfunctional or hostile family environment. Remaining in school may also be freighted with great personal significance for students. Were Amelia to be expelled, one suspects that Amelia would feel even more as though she had let down her deceased mother, who fought so hard to get her daughter into this private school. Thus, administrators' assertions notwithstanding, it will often not be in students' interests to be forced out of school.

Are there ethical principles that we can recruit here to help analyze the situation? Schools and colleges confronted with suicidal students may be tempted to act in their own interests, which may not be the same as the student's interests. But why should we expect them to act otherwise? One might respond that schools are different from other entities with which we have purely commercial relationships, where payment is exchanged for a discrete product or service. Unlike our dealings with the cobbler, from whom we expect nothing more than to competently affix a new pair of heels, we entrust our children to schools and colleges in the expectation that these institutions will help to shape them as people. That means something beyond just teaching them mathematics or French. It implies a fiduciary obligation to act in ways that will promote students' development, even if it might be easier or safer for the school to ignore their needs. To be sure, there are limits to this expectation—one would not expect a teacher or headmaster to become involved in a student's personal life. But when an academic institution expels a student because it may benefit the school, even if it harms the student, such action violates our expectations of the fiduciary responsibilities of the school.

Psychiatrists can play a positive role in these cases. Whether they are working for a school or college health service, or are seeing the student elsewhere, it is likely that school officials will turn to them for advice. Obviously, a treating psychiatrist cannot discuss a patient's case without the patient's consent. But students will often give consent—more or less freely—because they want to do what they can to remain in school. And nontreating psychiatrists who consult with the school administration are free to make recommendations without these concerns. Perhaps the key point to communicate to educational administrators is the need for an individualized assessment of the student's situation. Blanket policies, such as those that require suspension of suicidal students, make no sense and may cause more harm than good (Pavela 2006). In addition, they may violate federal and state law, including the Americans With Disabilities Act and Section 504 of the Rehabilitation Act (Appelbaum 2006).

Some students are truly burdened by excessive academic pressure that would be relieved by taking time off or by transferring to a less-demanding setting. Others may find the social pressure or interpersonal relationships at school to be problematic. For these students, leave or transfer may be indicated. Indeed, to the extent that a student's academic work is being impaired by symptoms of a psychiatric disorder such as depression, allowing the student some time away to have effective treatment may enable a successful return to school at a later date.

For many students, though, leaving or changing schools will be exactly the wrong answer. Forcing a depressed student to adapt to a new academic and social environment all but ensures failure. Expulsion may be a humiliating experience that reinforces the student's sense of hopeless depression. Take away the structure of high school or college life, and many depressed students may find little reason to get out of bed in the morning, or may turn instead to increased drug and alcohol use. Time off from school is no panacea. Students who fall behind their age cohort are at increased risk of subsequently dropping out of school, and they experience higher rates of suicide as well. These are the probabilities that need to be weighed in the case of suicidal students.

How can we apply these principles to Amelia? Given her depressed and socially withdrawn state, forcing her to a new school at this point will only make things harder for her. Her sole remaining social outlet would likely be the older college student with whom she is already using alcohol and drugs, and apparently engaging in sexual activity—behaviors that are likely to be good neither for her depression nor for the course of her life. Leaving the private school will also mean disappointing the dreams of her mother, exacerbating the guilt she already feels about her mother's death. It is difficult to identify any way in which being expelled from this private high school would be in Amelia's interests.

Instead, the school's headmaster should be encouraged to view Amelia as having a treatable, time-limited disorder that may require some temporary accommodation. This should be a familiar situation to administrators who have to deal with students who contract mononucleosis or other disorders that may impair their school performance. The headmaster should be assured that once she receives adequate therapy, she is likely to return to her prior functional status. It may also be helpful to talk with the headmaster about the different levels of suicidal ideation and behavior, encouraging him to distinguish between superficial scratches that may represent a plea for help and more serious attempts at suicide. A psychiatrist who supports the headmaster and teachers in allowing Amelia to continue in school while therapeutic interventions take place will have made an important contribution to this young woman's life.

Adolescent Bereavement

Cynthia R. Pfeffer, M.D.

AMELIA Gutierrez is grieving the death of her mother. This reaction is not simply emotional but physical, cognitive, and behavioral, and it leads to crises that are social, religious, and philosophical. In order to reduce the acute suffering and the likelihood of enduring complications, it is useful to understand such terms as grief, bereavement, depression, and mourning and also explore some of the interventions that can help grieving teenagers.

While *grief* is a reaction to loss, *bereavement* is a more enduring state or condition. Both are normal human reactions but can also become abnormal. In the acute setting, uncomplicated—or normal—bereavement can look like major depression, with the presence of symptoms such as sadness, diminished interest and pleasure, physical complaints (e.g., problems with sleep, appetite, energy), and a variety of behavioral problems that reflect the developmental age of the child. While some children and adults will need professional help after the loss of a loved one, most rebound within weeks or months without psychiatric intervention, especially when there is a supportive psychosocial network. These supports stem from family and friends, but because the reaction to death is such a central human experience, cultures and religions have developed behaviors and rituals that help people *mourn* such losses.

Amelia faced this major loss, however, without the benefit of her most intimate support—her mother—or the ongoing support of her old neighbors, community, and church. Her private school may be abandoning her, and her father is suffering the loss of his wife. Amelia's symptoms have become both intense and persistent, and she would now be considered to have *complicated bereavement*. She is sad and has a constellation of intrusive thoughts and feelings about her mother that interfere with her life. These include anger, guilt, longing for reunion, intrusive memories, and worries about her life without her mother. These reactions are not, however, the primary reasons that she was referred to a psychiatrist. Most notable to her school and father are suicidality and misbehaviors that may be signs of newly developing psychiatric disturbances. This 16-year-old girl has begun to drink alcohol and smoke marijuana, cut her arms, and tell her friends that she wants to die. Such suicidality may reflect an intense desire to rejoin her mother, and may not lead to an actual attempt to kill herself, but it is worrisome and requires further exploration.

Developmental age influences coping style. Puberty is often accompanied by cognitive and emotional sophistication, for example, and some grieving teenagers respond to loss by becoming "over-achievers." Puberty also opens up opportunities for problematic behaviors. Turning her back on peers, school, and family, Amelia is experiencing a lonely sadness that appears to be ameliorated only by a connection with an older boyfriend who is introducing her to a world of sex and substance abuse; while temporarily reassuring, such behavior may lead to school failure, estrangement from friends, and pregnancy. Amelia's reaction contrasts with that of her younger brother, whose grief is likely to be expressed as sadness, irritability, and an uncertainty about the meaning of death. He might also become more needy, fearing abandonment by important adults. No wonder she sees him as "a pest." If he had been a few years younger, we would expect him to exhibit mood instability with periods of crying, insomnia, restlessness, and withdrawal from others, but he would lack the cognitive maturity to appreciate the finality of his loss. Regardless of the details, it is likely that her younger brother is also suffering from the absence of an empathic adult and an intact community; the psychiatrist might want to tactfully explore whether he, too, is suffering a complicated bereavement.

Amelia has been seriously impacted by her mother's physical decline and death, and so it would be important to evaluate her for *traumatic grief,* a serious type of complicated bereavement that is similar to posttraumatic stress disorder (PTSD). Related research is complicated by the reality that while parental deaths can be categorized, the children's experiences vary significantly. A parental suicide rarely occurs out of the blue, for example, and so the effect on the child is not just the death but the presuicide parental psychopathology that might have led to neglect and abuse. In situations such as Amelia's, terminal illness can lead to widely varying exposures to emotional and physical pain and to a strangely frightening hospital environment. Traumatic grief is marked not just by depression but by a cluster of PTSD symptoms: reexperiencing of traumatic events, avoidance of reminders of the deceased, and physiological hyperrarousal. Suicidality is common. It is not clear whether Amelia has any of these symptoms.

Exploration of such symptoms might increase the likelihood of successful treatment of bereavement-induced physiologic changes. A 2-year study of bereaved children whose parents died in the September 11 terrorist attacks demonstrated persistent hyperarousal of the hypothalamic-pituitary-adrenal (HPA) axis, manifested by elevated salivary cortisol levels and an abnormal dexamethasone suppression test (Pfeffer et al. 2007). This finding is important not just because it underlines the physiological effects of complicated bereavement, but because chronic HPA axis hyperactivity can lead to such health problems as cognitive impairment, reduced bone density, and insulin resistance. It can also lead to efforts to self-soothe with such substances as alcohol and marijuana.

Uncomplicated bereavement is generally treated by the family, community, and important institutions. These interventions include ongoing adult availability, mourning rituals, the support of the surviving parent by other adults, and an array of signs that life remains safe and enduring. Depending on developmental level, grieving children and adolescents are typically encouraged to think about positive aspects of their own lives and develop new supportive relationships. They are encouraged to talk about the deceased parent, including their inevitably ambivalent feelings about a parent who loved them and then abandoned them. Such reflections are often aided by mourning rituals such as funerals, memorial services, and wakes, in which adults discuss their own feelings of sadness, regret, and gratitude toward the deceased. These rituals help integrate the reality of the loss with memories of the deceased while laying the groundwork for a life without the parent.

The line between a normal and abnormal reaction to death is uncertain, and there is ambiguity as to when professionals are needed to help with the grieving process. In the initial stages of grief, it would be considered normal for Amelia to have all the symptoms of a major depression and, at times, to describe dissociation, shock, and the experience of having seen or heard her dead mother. While DSM-IV-TR (American Psychiatric Association 2000) defines bereavement as lasting less than 2 months, this is an artificial dead-line, since for many people, some symptoms of grief can persist a lifetime. Nevertheless, there are situations in which bereavement becomes patholog-ical and interferes not only with the pursuit of a gratifying life but with en-gaging people and the world in ways that can help lift the bereaved person out of his or her bereavement.

Psychotherapy and pharmacotherapy have both been shown to help com-plicated bereavement. The goals of these treatments are to reduce trauma-related symptoms and to facilitate normal grief. Exploratory psychotherapy would be an opportunity for Amelia to talk about her feelings without the usual concern that she might be upsetting her father or friends. This might be done individually or in groups of people who have suffered losses. Cog-nitive-behavioral therapy (CBT) might focus on stress management, im-proved coping skills, problem solving, and affect regulation. CBT could also focus on some of her behaviors that are self-defeating and that distance her from friends and family. Her depressive and anxiety symptoms might re-spond to an antidepressant medication, and her alcohol and marijuana use might be addressed by an intervention such as motivational interviewing.

Loss is a core part of the human condition and has long been central to psychiatric and psychoanalytic theory. Most of this interest has been focused on adult recollections of early separation and trauma, particularly in regard to how such experiences contribute to later mental illness. It has become in-creasingly clear, however, that early intervention may not only prevent later psychopathology but also help grieving children and adolescents return to a normal developmental trajectory and a happier life.

Suicide

J. John Mann, M.D.

AMELIA Gutierrez describes a history that illustrates the relationship be-tween the development of mood disorders and suicidal ideation. From the description of the case, she has not made a suicide attempt, but we cannot know whether she falls into the category of individuals who experience a mood disorder but are relatively resilient to making a suicide attempt. It appears that she had been an excellent student until the death of her mother, at which point her grades and attendance began to decline. In relation to that decline, she describes tearfulness, poor self-esteem, low mood, loss of interest or anhedonia, difficulty concentrating, difficulty completing her homework, oversleeping, missing school, and having occasional thoughts that life is not worth living. The patient meets, therefore, the criteria for a major depressive episode. These observations are supplemented by the father's description that she was formerly an attentive and lively student and daughter and now has become morose, tearful, and hostile. There is an identification with her mother that may magnify the impact of the loss.

Ms. Gutierrez's risk for suicide depends on these mood symptoms as well as on a variety of other factors. For example, she describes occasional feelings in which she wishes she were dead but denies a specific plan for suicide. While there is no history of an actual suicide attempt, the patient does describe self-mutilation over the prior 2 years. There is some association between suicide attempts and self-mutilation, but that association is not as strong as an association between an actual past suicide attempt and the risk of future suicide attempts. The uncertain association is likely related to the clinical reality that while some cuts are intended to cause serious harm or death, other cutting serves a nonlethal, self-soothing function.

While suicidal behavior most often occurs within the context of psychiatric disorder, particularly depressive disorders, suicide and certain types of suicide attempt appear to have distinct neurobiological correlates. Individuals who make nonfatal suicide attempts or die by suicide have altered serotonergic function, evidenced by lower cerebrospinal fluid (CSF) levels of 5-hydroxyindoleacetic acid (5-HIAA), a serotonin metabolite, and by alterations in the serotonin transporter and serotonin 5-HT_{1A} and 5-HT_{2A} receptor binding (Mann 2003). These alterations appear to differ from those attributable to mood disorder (Arango et al. 1995; Mann et al. 2000). The serotonergic system influences impulse control and is related to aggression and mood regulation. These abnormalities in the serotonergic system may contribute to the risk of suicidal behavior through a loss of inhibition and greater pessimism that cause an individual to be more likely to act on suicidal thoughts. There is also evidence of dysfunction in the stress response system of the hypothalamic-pituitary-adrenal axis (HPA) in suicide (Mann et al. 2006). Thus stressful life events such as a loss of a parent or the episode of depression itself may elicit an abnormal stress response that increases the risk of a suicidal act in an individual with the underlying biological diathesis for suicidal behavior.

The biological characteristics of nonfatal suicidal behavior are less clearcut. The biological variations are largely attributable to the fact that a suicide attempt can range from a high-lethality attempt survived only by chance to a low-lethality attempt that may be better characterized as a gesture or cry for help. The former have been found to be more akin to completed suicide with respect to indices of serotonin function; these include low CSF levels of 5-HIAA (Mann and Arango 1999); HPA dexamethasone resistance (Coryell 1990); and more platelet and brain 5-HT_{2A} binding but blunted signal transduction (Malone et al. 2007; Pandey et al. 1999). People who make low-lethality attempts are more similar to people who do not attempt suicide than to people who do.

There is no biological "test" available to confidently determine the suicide risk of an individual patient. Given that Amelia is in her first episode of a major depression, it is too early to tell whether she has a predisposition (or diathesis) toward suicidal behavior. She lacks a known family history of psychiatric illness or suicidal behavior, and she does not have a history of aggressive-impulsive personality traits, any of which would increase her overall suicide risk. While these are reassuring historical facts, only time will tell whether this patient has a diathesis for suicidal behavior, and the reality is that two-thirds of the adolescents who commit suicide do so on their first attempt. Given these uncertainties, careful clinical monitoring will obviously be important to assess the emergence of serious suicide risk in this young woman.

Interview of the Adolescent

Ayame Takahashi, M.D.

THE diagnostic interview of the adolescent is heavily influenced by the patient's shifting developmental level. The interviewer must also attend to parents, who have a legal and financial authority. Finally, the therapist should be prepared for powerful transference and countertransference experiences as the patient and clinician explore this especially intense period of human maturation.

Within moments of meeting Amelia Gutierrez, each of the above issues is likely to present itself. As with an adult, it is often useful to ask Amelia why she came to the office. This question might lead her to talk about her mother's death, her school, her family, and her own situation, but it might also allow her to express the degree to which she is interested in therapy. During these opening minutes, it is more important to help develop an alliance than to elicit information, and so the therapist should be attentive to Amelia's hesitations and evasions.

It would not be surprising if Amelia proves to be a "difficult interview." While teenagers tend to become increasingly verbal with age, they also become increasingly wary. The concern may be that the therapist will reveal secrets, but it can also be a more diffuse apprehension about the therapist's motivation. For example, Amelia might be curious about the extent to which the therapist is an agent of either the father or the school, given that she may view therapy as something being decided—and performed—by adults. Her concern would be particularly reasonable, since the therapist has already spoken with both the father and headmaster. Further, the therapist may be getting paid by the school to help extract a troublesome student.

Amelia's interviewer must, therefore, interact spontaneously with an alert, cautious girl who has recently had her mother die, her father become "a loser," and her school headmaster consider expulsion. To prevent a new parental figure—the therapist—from quickly becoming a similar disappointment, it is useful for the clinician to be direct about what is known and not known. For example, the therapist can explain that the contacts with the father and the headmaster helped lay some overall groundwork but that the real work would be done by the two people in the room. The therapist can often tell the late adolescent that their work will be entirely confidential except when there is a risk of danger or when they agree that the therapist should talk with the father. This promise of confidentiality depends to some extent on the patient, the family, and the clinical situation, however, and brings with it some risks. Some of Amelia's issues involve her father and little brother, and it might be overly restrictive for the therapy not to include them. Further, many parents want updates and involvement, and if they are dissatisfied or uncomfortable, they may refuse to bring in the patient or pay the bill. It is also difficult for all involved people to agree on the definition of dangerousness. At the time of this first interview, for example, this 16-year-old girl is cutting herself, claiming suicidality, smoking marijuana, drinking alcohol, and having sex with an older boyfriend. While the cutting and suicidality seem to have precipitated the consultation, the other behaviors are actually illegal, and it becomes difficult to clearly know which of these, if any, should necessarily be relayed to the father. It would not be unreasonable to explain the twin goals of safety and honesty to Amelia and have her help in deciding which of these risky behaviors need to be discussed openly with her father, which behaviors can remain confidential but need to be worked on in therapy, and which are not immediate problems. Honesty is an important paradigm in working with parents as well, and Amelia's father should be told that the sessions are generally confidential. This is not simply true but also reduces the chance that an uncovered secret would undermine the relationship between the parent and therapist.

In addition to honesty, neutrality is critical. Neutrality is not the same as acting wooden or unfeeling, and adolescents will generally not react well to therapists who are unempathic and unfriendly. Instead, neutrality helps the therapist from too readily agreeing with one side of the patient's point of view. If the therapist agrees that the patient's father is "a loser," for example, Amelia may then find it difficult to discuss parental idealizations.

Instead of becoming an agreeable friend, the clinician should try to tactfully learn Amelia's perspectives on her mother's death, her family, her school, her friendships, her boyfriend, and herself. The interviews should aim to feel like conversations, with the usual tangents and uncertainties. Much of the evaluation will consist of issues and feelings that are difficult or embarrassing, but the clinician should also make some attempt at uncovering strengths and passions. In the case of Amelia, for example, it might be useful to ask about her interest in writing. Not only does this help the therapist understand the three-dimensional teenager, but it strengthens the therapeutic alliance and encourages the patient to show all sides of herself.

As is the case with adults, adolescents tend not to enjoy interrogations. If Amelia seems wary of discussing her own feelings about such risky behaviors as sex and drug use, it can be useful to ask her about the behavior of her friends. Her attitudes toward other people's behaviors can reveal beliefs that underlie her own behavior. For example, Amelia has admitted to marijuana and alcohol use but said that she "doesn't have a problem with it." This might lead to questions about how she'd know if someone had a problem. How often would they smoke and drink? How would they behave? This line of conversation can lead to a discussion of over-the-counter drugs, herbal supplements, and any other substances that can affect mood and behavior. Adolescents should also be explicitly asked about substances that can be used for weight loss and about symptoms of anorexia and bulimia.

Similarly, it is important to ask specifically about sexual behavior. Some adolescents will discuss their behavior straightforwardly, while others will appear shocked at the idea of discussing sex with an adult. If so, it is useful to not only appear nonjudgmental but to specifically say that such questions are routine and part of all evaluations. It is also important to understand normative behavior. While it is illegal for a 16-year-old like Amelia to have sex with a 21-year-old man in most parts of the United States, sexual activity is likely to be the norm for many of her peers, with oral sex having become especially commonplace. In discussing sexuality with Amelia, it would be useful not only to hear what she does and the degree to which she protects herself from disease and pregnancy but also to understand how she feels about it.

Amelia's cutting is the third important piece of risky behavior that deserves exploration during an initial evaluation. It is important not to assume that cutting reflects suicidal intent. Try to understand her mindset. How often does she cut? What does she use to cut? What are the triggers? Does anything else help when she feels that way? Cutting is often a means to feeling something instead of feeling dead or numb. It can also be a way to gain relief from such intense emotions as rage and sadness. The potential dangerousness of these cuts is not necessarily proportionate to the stated suicidality, so you may want to see some of the cuts, which can range from superficial scratches to deep wounds. The therapist's nonjudgmental curiosity into such behavior can be a deeply moving interaction for a girl who feels misunderstood and abandoned by the important adults in her life. Such a discussion can also segue into the possibility of earlier sexual abuse and to actual desires to be dead.

Not only is Amelia's behavior worrisome, but she may have subconscious desires to attach to adults through "getting under their skin." An average expectable paternalistic response might lead Amelia to angrily fleeing treatment, while a minimal response might lead her to believing that the therapist doesn't care. Amelia's interviewer should also be prepared to re-feel some personal feelings of adolescence as well as some feelings of being a parent; self-monitoring is the key to avoidance of a countertransferential enactment in which issues from the therapist's life interfere with the treatment.

Finally, it is important to remember that Amelia is depressed. Her mother has died. Her father and brother are presumably preoccupied with their own sorrows. She has been geographically dislocated from her old neighbors. She may be kicked out of her school. Amelia may be behaving in dangerous ways, but she is doing the best that she can to keep her head above water. At this point, she doesn't need another friend or another parent or another lecture. She also doesn't need a therapist who will focus only on the misbehaviors that obscure her strengths but may also serve to cover up her psychological pain. Instead, Amelia needs a clinician who can tolerate the ambiguities of adolescence and work to understand her lonely sadness.

Psychological Impact of Dislocation

Mindy Thompson Fullilove, M.D.

IT is easy to overlook the brief allusion to "urban renewal" in the gripping story of a suicidal 16-year-old girl. After all, how can loss of neighborhood compare with other losses in the child's life, such as the death of her mother? In this discussion, I will propose that, contrary to general assumptions, the loss of neighborhood is a significant contributor to the illness that has brought Amelia Gutierrez into treatment.

George Engel, one of the founders of consultation-liaison psychiatry, wrote a seminal article in which he examined a parallel issue: the possible contribution of the hospital unit to distress in a cardiac patient (Engel 1980). By carefully tracing the multiple systems within which the patient was embedded, he was able to show that issues extending far beyond the man's body had deleterious effects on his cardiac system. Indeed, Engel pointed out, we all live in an array of systems that have complex and important relationships with one another. In his paper, he noted that "environment" is an important larger system affecting the individual. My research team has found that *place*—the individual's near environment—influences, and is influenced by, individual mental activity (Fullilove 1999). We define place using an archaic definition from Webster's Dictionary which states that place is the material contents of a three-dimensional object. Assume that we can define the three-dimensional object as a neighborhood. We are then interested in the neighborhood's contents and internal workings as well as the personal meaning of loss of place.

People have a sense of place. They construct an internal image of their three-dimensional environment that includes not just its physical contents but its internal workings and associated social and personal meanings as well. People have a sense of any place they encounter, but they develop deep and complex relationships with places within which they live, work, or play—relationships that are a mix of knowledge, identification, dependence, and appropriation. These are not trivial operations. The ability to move safely and surely in space enables the individual to find shelter, nourishment, water, and companionship. Forced displacement fractures bonds, and this may lead to relational disruption that can, in turn, result in disorientation, nostalgia, and alienation (Fullilove 1996).

Equally important, a network of relationships is also broken. These embedding bonds are an essential secondary system of homeostasis without which the individual suffers a loss of social strictures on behavior, social reinforcement for conformity to group norms, and companionship for processing of grief and loss, among other features of collective social life (Bowlby 1973).

Forced Displacement Due to Urban Renewal

Urban renewal programs are sponsored by governments working in conjunction with private developers (Fullilove 2004). The goal of such programs is to permit conversion of urban habitat from one use to another. In general, such conversions are interesting to the real estate industry because the construction of new buildings is often more profitable than maintenance of old buildings. Substantial in size, such projects destroy a cluster of buildings or even whole neighborhoods to prepare for the new construction. In so doing, they clear-cut the land in the same manner as industrial forestry or strip mining. Neighborhood families and businesses are forced out and randomly scattered.

Social networks are shredded in this process. Friends and even family members can lose contact with one another. Social and cultural organizations fall apart. People lose political power and cultural knowledge. The social systems that organized prosocial behavior, including the socialization of the young, are destroyed. Such systems are not easily replaced. The creation of new relationships tends to be slow and is often difficult. When displaced people are inserted into an existing social system, it might seem that integration would naturally follow, but displaced newcomers tend to be slow to form connections. This can be understood as a form of *hysteresis,* a term from physics that describes the lag in reaction in a system that has been altered in some way. For example, a study of residents displaced from a neighborhood in Washington, D.C., found not only that former residents felt a deep sense of loss 1 year later, but also that 25% had not made a single friend after being forced from their old neighborhood (Fogelson 2001).

Understanding Forced Displacement in Amelia's Life

An understanding of dislocation and place may shed light on Amelia's sense of isolation and may be an important underlying contributor to her suicidal ideation and self-destructive behavior. What Amelia has lost, according to our theory, is more than an apartment: she has lost the whole neighborhood system of which she was a part. That system included supportive neighbors, an attentive and normalizing church community, and a cluster of informal contacts with people like the newspaper seller or candy-store owner. With the loss of this interpersonal fabric, she has very little to remind her of who she is or who she wants to be. In the old world, she would not have been allowed to sleep in and not do her homework. She would have gone to school. And she would not have been left alone on Saturday afternoons so that she could smoke, drink, and have sex with an older boy. In her new world, she has been cast adrift, and the relationship with the boyfriend feels like all she has.

The impact of the neighborhood losses is magnified by the loss of connections with her parents. Not only has her mother died, but her father has become emotionally distant, perhaps grieving his own losses. Amelia's sense of isolation may be further intensified by the fact that this is the second forced displacement in her life, the first being her family's immigration when she was 3 years old. We don't know anything about what that first removal meant for her, but we know that it was a massive shift in the family's life-world. Such reorganizations of family life always leave traces, the central attribute of systems with hysteresis.

While clearly problematic for Amelia and her family, urban renewal is generally billed as "progress," and the people who are displaced are seen as "whiners." The psychological cost of the dislocation is minimized for many reasons, including the desire of the developers to maximize profit and limit liability, but the societal minimization leads people like Amelia to having no language for their distress. Cut off from an ability to communicate her distress and cut off from her old neighborhood, Amelia's cutting of herself takes on a particularly poignant symbolic meaning.

How to Ground Amelia

Our practice focuses on neighborhood groups rather than individuals, and we work to give these groups the opportunity to express their feelings regarding the loss of home and neighborhood. Their words unleash a critically important flow of emotions (Robins et al. 1999). The pain and sorrow, once articulated, can be managed in a variety of ways. One of the ways in which we work with neighborhood groups is to walk together, examining the lost landscape in order to make sense of it. These walks typically involve both people who lost their homes and others who were outside the story. The insider/outsider dynamic opens up storytelling on both sides. Through this process, the ache of the unspoken loss is tempered, and healing can begin.

In an individual therapy with Amelia, a visit to the old neighborhood should be considered. Generally, people are curious about the new buildings and tend to have a psychological connection to areas that extend past the core site of destruction. These trips are spooky for people because they can and cannot imagine the way things used to look. Despite this dissonance, visits open up a storehouse of thoughts, images, and ideas, and permit the working-through process to commence.

As the loss is brought into focus, the therapy can begin to tackle the formation of new relationships. There is a lag—the hysteresis—in developing connections, but therapy can serve as a catalyst for meeting people. We find that the lingering bitterness after upheaval can interfere with connections to new places, in this case church and school. The therapy must address this alienation. For Amelia, the need for a new church is great, as is acceptance at her school.

As a final note, the therapist must urgently work against expulsion from school. This would be a third forced displacement, and perhaps the fatal one. The school must commit itself to being part of a hopeful world for Amelia. In this regard, schools are often very interested in issues of space. A history project about Amelia's neighbors' memories of home might be fun and instructive for her classmates and would help Amelia make something positive of her pain.

The Dominican Patient

Ian Canino, M.D.

THE biopychosocial model is a familiar paradigm within medicine, but whereas biological and psychological issues are widely studied, sociological and cultural issues tend to be relatively ignored. In the case of Amelia Gutierrez, an understanding of her Dominican culture is important to both an understanding of the girl and to the development of an effective treatment. At the same time that she belongs to a Dominican subgroup, however, cultural norms are also significantly affected by her gender, social class, and age (Lewis-Fernandez and Kleinman 1995). Further, an adolescent's cultural identity is based not only on ethnicity but also on national origin, religious background, language, and current sociocultural experiences (Canino and Gonzalez 2003; Phinney and Rotheram 1986).

From the case, we know that Amelia is 16 years old and is grieving the death of her mother. In addition, her father is overwhelmed, she is using marijuana and alcohol and is having school difficulties, and she has an older Latino boyfriend. Each of these facts is influenced by her Dominican culture. Like two-thirds of the Dominicans in the United States, Amelia lives in the New York City area. As is common among Dominicans, her father is underemployed, has a relatively low income, and—related to his recent immigration—probably has poor language skills (Vazquez 2001). As with many Dominican families, however, school is important, and both educational attainment and growth in human capital have gradually increased (Hernandez and Rivera-Batiz 2003).

In common with people from their sister Caribbean countries of Puerto Rico and Cuba, Dominicans descended from American Indian, African, and Spanish ancestors. In contrast to the personal independence that is often encouraged in American families from other ethnic backgrounds, Dominicans rely on extended families and kin networks. They tend to respect the elderly without question, maintain clear-cut gender roles, expect obedience and good manners from their children, and support the concept of virginity before marriage (Vazquez 2005). In general, their religious beliefs are a combination of Catholicism and mystical African traditions; some may practice spiritualism and folk healing in conjunction with their Catholic beliefs (Vazquez 2001).

It is likely that all of these factors add stress to Amelia's father, who lacks a mother, grandparents, and a social network for his children. Raised in a culture with defined gender roles, it can be assumed that he never expected to be the primary caretaker for his children and that he would likely lack some of the skills that make a home function efficiently. Further, he may expect that his children will be obedient, religious, and sexually inactive, but his children are spending most of their time in a culture whose values are quite discordant to his. No wonder his daughter considers him "a loser."

Amelia's evaluation and therapy will likely be similar to work with other adolescents. In addition to such general issues as suicidality, depression, and the structure of treatment, the culturally aware clinician should explore several additional topics. These include *religion, the family,* and *development.*

Religion

It might be useful to explore Amelia's views on her Catholicism. Is she religious? Does she feel guilty about having sex? Has her relationship with God changed since the death of her mother? It is also important to ask about other spiritual beliefs that may support ideas of reunification and/or communication with spirits of the dead, particularly her mother. Such beliefs can be reassuring, scary, or a reflection of suicidality. These may, in turn, hinder or facilitate the process of bereavement. Even if Amelia discounts the influence of Catholicism and spirituality, the question will communicate to her that the therapist recognizes that such issues are important within the Dominican subculture and is willing to take seriously whatever issues are important to her.

The Family

Mrs. Gutierrez's illness likely meant that Amelia, as eldest daughter, would have taken on her mother's gender-specific roles. In addition, she would likely be seen within the family as more adult and maternal, adding to her stress. Immigration removed her extended family, and relocation separated her from neighbors and the clergy. This loss of a social and familial network means that she is handling her increased responsibility without adequate support. Therapy would help Amelia explore her own changing status within the family, as well as such feelings as pride, resentment, and worry.

Development

Developmental issues need to be considered, especially in regard to how culture interacts with maturation. As a first-generation Dominican adolescent, Amelia is bilingual. Not only does she have to deal with the differences between Spanish and English, she is struggling with the competing values and expectations of her two cultures. As a bilingual child she probably had to serve as a language broker between the English-speaking public agencies and her Spanish-speaking parents. This may have prepared her for her current parentified role, but, taken on too early, such a role can feel overwhelming and scary. While she lives within a Dominican family that presumably values interdependence, cooperativeness, and clearly defined family and gender roles, she is living in an American society that treasures individuality, independence, and a different set of gender and family roles. This tension is heightened by her age and developmental stage, particularly in regards to her own need to mature and become more adult while also needing to feel protected and part of a stable home. While her father is likely to cringe at signs of her Americanization, her classmates may be befuddled by some of the Dominican values that remain important to her. A culturally astute, non-judgmental therapist may be the only person to whom Amelia can openly explore her conflicted feelings.

This tension is exacerbated by her strong identification and attachment to her Dominican mother, the current emotional unavailability of her father, and her likely connection with friends from school. Her relationship with an older boyfriend may be substituting for the absence of her distressed father and the eroded extended adult network. The sexual aspects of the relationship with her boyfriend likely conflict with her cultural and religious values, especially in regard to the importance of premarital virginity. This can partially explain her initial hesitancy to discuss this relationship with the interviewer.

Summary

Cultural awareness helps clinicians understand their patients. Cultural differences influence definitions of mental health and illness and lead to variability in expressions of distress, which can, in turn, influence the duration and number of symptoms required for impairment and treatment response (Mezzich et al. 1996). Sociocultural patterns may also influence health seeking behavior and health literacy as well as the content, meaning, and intensity of symptoms (Rubio-Stipec et al. 2008). Cultural beliefs influence case definition, disability criteria, interviewer response, and the reporting of child behavior (Hacket and Hacket 1999). Finally, on an individual level, recognition of cultural complexities helps clinicians build a stronger therapeutic alliance with patients who might feel outside of a system that often includes few members of their subculture.

Virginia Woolf: On Being Ill

Katherine Dalsimer, Ph.D.

FOR all that has been written about Virginia Woolf, the most vivid portrait of her remains the one she wrote herself, in her diaries and letters over the course of a lifetime. They document not only the extremes of feeling that ravaged her at times but also, quietly and movingly, her capacity to savor the ordinary rhythms of life—her contentment in the quiet weeks in the country with her husband, Leonard Woolf, the pleasures of London, the frequent visits of friends, long afternoon walks after mornings of writing. Her diaries and letters preserve, too, the rhythms of her inner life—the ebb and flow of thoughts, fantasies, feelings and memories, the shifts of light and dark. She describes symptoms that now would be diagnosed as bipolar disorder; she experienced mood swings from severe depression to manic excitement and episodes of psychosis. Today there are effective treatments for the illness that haunted Woolf from the age of 13; in her own lifetime, however, psychiatry had little to offer her. The inevitable prescription, rest in bed with no reading and no writing, deprived her, she felt, of the only effective therapy she knew—the practice of her art.

Virginia Woolf was born in 1882 into a large and very accomplished family—born, as she wrote, "not of rich parents, but of well-to-do parents, born into a very communicative, literate, letter-writing, articulate late 19th century world" (Woolf 1985). Her father was an eminent Victorian man of letters, Sir Leslie Stephen; her mother, Julia Duckworth Stephen, was celebrated for her beauty by the artists and poets of their circle. Both parents had previously been married, and both had been widowed with children. Together, they had four children—Thoby, whose friends from Cambridge would become the nucleus of the "Bloomsbury group"; then Vanessa, who would become the painter Vanessa Bell; Virginia; and Adrian, who would become a psychoanalyst. When they were young the Stephen children collaborated on a weekly newspaper, *The Hyde Park Gate News,* filled with news from a child's eye perspective—the visits of cousins, a toy sailboat lost, the adoption of a puppy (Dalsimer 2001). This high-spirited chronicle of family life ceased abruptly when Virginia was 13 years old and her mother died.

Like the young Virginia Woolf, Amelia Gutierrez experienced the death of her mother during adolescence. And like Woolf, too, she found comfort in reading and writing—specifically through writing in her diary. For Amelia, keeping a diary also fostered the development of her gift for writing and led to her recruitment by a school that offered the sort of intellectual opportunities prized by her mother. For many adolescents the keeping of a diary can be of crucial importance, particularly in the face of loss. The most famous adolescent diary of our time, *The Diary of Anne Frank,* was begun in the face of catastrophic loss (Dalsimer 1986). In her diary Anne conjured into being an imaginary confidante she called "Kitty," whom she used to "comfort and console" her. But a diary can serve a number of different purposes. Virginia Woolf used the diary she began when she was 15, and still reeling from the death of her mother, as a factual day-by-day chronicle of her activities: it was her effort to hold on to ordinary reality, when she felt her grasp of that reality slipping. Amelia Gutierrez, in the shadow of impending loss, perhaps tried to contain in her diary her sense of sadness and rage, helplessness and guilt—feelings that, after her mother's death, she expressed through her symptoms.

The death of Virginia Woolf's mother, of rheumatic fever after an 8-week illness, was shattering. Soon afterward, Virginia had her first severe depression and psychotic episode. She was thought still to be recovering when there was another death in the family, that of her 25-year-old half-sister Stella. Virginia was now 15. Other deaths would follow: when she was 22, the death of her father; when she was 24, the death of her brother Thoby. Vulnerable as she was—"skinless" was her word—she looked back on these as "sledge-hammer blows." In the period after her mother's death, she heard for the first time what she would later call "those horrible voices." She would hear them for the last time in the weeks before her death, in 1941: "It is just as it was the first time," she wrote in a note to her sister. "I have fought against it, but I can't any longer." Putting stones in her pockets, she walked into the River Ouse, committing suicide at the age of 59.

When illness prevented her from beginning work on the novel she envisaged—it would be her great autobiographical novel *To the Lighthouse*—Woolf recorded in her diary "a whole nervous breakdown in miniature": "Oh its beginning its coming—the horror—physically like a painful wave swelling about the heart—tossing me up. I'm unhappy unhappy! Down—God, I wish I were dead...I've only a few more years to live I hope. I can't face this horror any more...Does everyone go through this? Why have I so little control?" (*Diary* 3:110–111).

Her diary documents a period of weeks when she was paralyzed by depression, withdrawn from human contact, unable to write, unable even to speak, when the horror and terror of her experience made her long for death.

And yet after emerging from this state, she looked back on it as something valuable: "These 9 weeks give one a plunge into deep waters…There is an edge to it which I feel of great importance…One goes down into the well & nothing protects one from the assault of truth" (*Diary* 3:112).

In a letter to a friend, she reflected on the protracted psychotic episode that began when she was 30, following both the completion of her first novel and her marriage: "And then my brains went up in a shower of fireworks. As an experience, madness is terrific I can assure you, and not to be sniffed at; and in its lava I still find most of the things I write about. It shoots out of one everything shaped, final, not in mere driblets, as sanity does" (*Letters* 4:180). Earlier she had mused in her diary, "I believe these illnesses are in my case— how shall I express it?—partly mystical. Something happens in my mind. It refuses to go on registering impressions. It shuts itself up. It becomes chrysalis…Then suddenly something springs" (*Diary* 3:287). Similarly when she was writing *The Waves*: "These curious intervals in life—I've had many—are the most fruitful artistically—one becomes fertilised—think of my madness at Hogarth [House, in Richmond]—& all the little illnesses" (*Diary* 3:254). Yet she could also declare, "Give me no illnesses for a year, 2 years, and I would write 3 novels straight off" (*Letters* 3:232).

She railed against the inactivity that was enforced when she was ill: "Here I am chained to my rock: forced to do nothing: doomed to let every worry, spite, irritation & obsession scratch & claw & come again. This is to say that I may not walk, & must not work…No one in the whole of Sussex is as miserable as I am; or so conscious of an infinite capacity of enjoyment hoarded in me, could I use it" (*Diary* 2:132–133).

For Woolf, writing was an "extraordinary exhilaration," "a divine kind of relief," and "the greatest rapture known to me." And there were also times when writing was simply hard work, something she made herself do. She knew that it was necessary that she keep writing in order to keep depression at bay. It was for this reason, no doubt, that she began to imagine each of her books just as she finished the one before, so that there would never be a gap in which she was not writing: "I pitched into my great lake of melancholy. Lord how deep it is! What a born melancholic I am! The only way I keep afloat is by working…Directly I stop working I feel that I am sinking down, down. And as usual, I feel that if I sink further I shall reach the truth" (*Diary* 3:235).

To sink under water: it is a metaphor that recurs, with shifting valence, throughout Woolf's writing. It is the metaphor she uses to describe her method of working: "I let myself down, like a diver, very cautiously into the last sentence I wrote yesterday. Then perhaps after 20 minutes or it may be more, I shall see a light in the depths of the sea, and stealthily approach—for one's sentences are only an approximation, a net one flings over some sea pearl which may vanish; if one brings it up it won't be anything like what it was when I saw it, under the sea" (*Letters* 4:223). To sink underwater was Woolf's metaphor for succumbing to depression—and for reaching the truth. We read such passages with a chill sense of foreboding, knowing that ultimately, to sink under water was the way she would seek her death.

At times Virginia Woolf railed against her illness, feeling frustrated and impeded by it, and at other times she felt it was essential to her. In diaries and letters she returned to the question repeatedly without coming to a resolution: was her illness a terrible obstacle to her art—or the necessary condition for it?

Neurobiology of Attachment

H. Jonathan Polan, M.D.

AMELIA GUTIERREZ is mourning the loss of her mother. She has also lost—or is in the process of possibly losing—her school and classmates; her old apartment with its nearby church, priests, and maternal neighbors; her previously intimate connections to her father and brother; and the language and values of her homeland. She may even have lost her will to live. The possibility that all of these losses contribute to her depression fits with Freud's assertion that mourning can stem not only from the loss of a loved one but also from the loss a substituted abstraction such as the motherland or an ideal (Freud 1917[1915]). Grief following loss can present in many ways (Lindemann 1944) and can affect people who range from infants reared in foundling homes (Spitz 1945) to elderly widowers (Parkes 1969). The pain of lost attachment has been studied, but it has also been the focus of some of mankind's greatest fiction, poetry, drama, and art. By any measure, attachment is important to humans.

The prototypic human attachment is between the infant and mother. Not only does the baby obtain food, warmth, and protection from its parent, their dynamic behavioral interactions influence all later attachments, including the infant's eventual mating and parenting. The infant's bond to its mother—also called *filial attachment*—became the focus of scientific study in the mid-twentieth century with clinical observations that institutionalized infants demonstrated apathy and slowing of physical growth, despite adequate nutrition and a clean, safe environment (Spitz 1945). This tragic syndrome, known as *anaclitic depression,* is of particular interest to researchers since it develops in people who have not yet developed the sophisticated mental structures that are often implicated in depression and, therefore, suggests that grief and depression may be fundamental biological reactions.

These observations led to the first animal models of filial attachment. These studies have implications for humans because many of the basic attachment behaviors that are seen in people have direct analogs in other mammals. Harlow found, for example, that anxious infant monkeys sought "contact comfort" rather than their source of milk, thereby demonstrating that attachment is a motivational system that develops independently from the physiological need for nutrition (Harlow and Zimmerman 1959). Hofer (1975) showed that infant rats responded to acute maternal separation with a variety of responses, including calling, activation, and sleep dysregulation, thereby suggesting the ubiquity of attachment-like phenomena in mammals. Hofer (1996) also demonstrated that the elements of what the mother provides, such as warmth, nutrition, or tactile stimulation, regulate the infant's separation responses in distinct ways.

More recently, it was shown that newborn rats approach and orient to specific thermal, tactile, and olfactory properties of the mother while their world is still sightless and soundless. Further, these maternally directed orienting behaviors were found to develop before separation responses (Polan et al. 2002), and are the behavioral building blocks of the infant's filial attachment. These physiologic interactions form the basis of the infant's attachment to the mother and may be phylogenetically the oldest manifestations of attachment relationships; they appear to be evolutionarily preserved, even in primates and humans, because they shape the infant's fundamental relationship to its environment.

Studies on mother–pup behaviors in rats indicate that early interactions shape response patterns for life. Licking and grooming of the pups are mainstays of the mother's care during the first 2 weeks of life, performed during nursing and in bursts upon returns to the nest. As with most behaviors, these behaviors are normally distributed in a population on a more or less bell-shaped curve. Those mothers who lick and groom their pups very frequently have offspring who are resilient to stress when they become adults, as manifested by reduced fear behavior and glucocorticoid (stress hormone) production, compared with the adult offspring of mothers who licked and groomed them relatively infrequently (Cameron et al. 2005). These stress-sensitive adults are also more susceptible to depression, as determined by tests that model depression in animals. The stimulation provided by maternal licking initiates a cascade of physiologic events in the pup's central nervous system that alters the course of brain development. In particular, high licking upregulates the production of glucocorticoid receptors by neurons of the hippocampus. This higher level of receptors downregulates the stress response by dampening the central signals that stimulate stress-induced glucocorticoid release. Dysregulation of the stress system has been found in children who were deprived of maternal care while being reared in orphanages or neglected or maltreated in homes and can persist into adulthood (Carpenter et al. 2007). Furthermore children who were neglected or maltreated are more vulnerable to acute stress and stress-induced depression when they become adolescents (Harkness et al. 2006) and are at significantly increased risk of depression as young adults (Widom et al. 2007). Such variations in maternal care may induce alterations in brain development in young children that are similar to those in developing rats. Working out the mechanisms of these changes in the animal models will help us understand the analogous processes in humans.

Molecular genetic analysis is now being used to study the pathways that affect the development of attachment relationships. One method is through genetic engineering, which alters specific genes that are believed to provide critical instructions for the assembly, maintenance, and environmental response of a particular behavior.

In one study of mice, our collaborators deleted, or "knocked out," the gene for glutaminase type 1 (GLS1), which is the enzyme responsible for most of the brain's main excitatory neurotransmitter, glutamate (Masson et al. 2006). The newborns that lacked both copies of the gene—called "knockouts"—died in the first day or two of life and were found to lack milk in their stomachs. Their heterozygote siblings—those with one copy of the GLS1 gene—survived and, to casual inspection, appeared to be no different from their normal, or "wild type," siblings.

The knockouts' failure to obtain milk was not due to behavioral debilitation. They were as active as their heterozygote and wild type litter mates but did not orient to their mother in such a way that allowed belly-to-belly contact. Without such an orientation, the pup was unable to locate a nipple and nurse. This suggests that they either failed to recognize the mother or could not organize an appropriate response to her. The heterozygotes, which had a partial deficiency of glutamate neurotransmission, were midway between the knockouts and the wild types in the organization and efficiency of their maternally directed behaviors. Thus, glutamate appears to be an important regulator of the earliest attachment behaviors.

Although animal models can never explain the intricacies and subtleties of the human infant's interactions with his or her mother, they do provide an important window into the basic mechanisms of attachment and loss. The neural processes that we learn about from animals are the base from which people develop the complexity of psychological processes that allows for the creation of some of our greatest works of art and for the intense feelings of loss following the death of a loved one. While it does not replace psychology, the biology of attachment helps inform our understanding and may lead to more focused and effective treatments for depressions, such as Amelia Gutierrez's, that are brought on by loss.

Pharmacology of Adolescent Depression

P. Anne McBride, M.D.

AMELIA Gutierrez is reeling from a number of traumatic events that have left her sad, lonely, angry, and lacking in confidence. Once "attentive and lively," she is now sad and withdrawn, showing none of her former enthusiasm for school, hobbies, and friends. She sleeps excessively but has little energy. She can concentrate only on reading novels. Guilt ridden, Amelia believes she contributed to her mother's death. She views herself as essentially worthless, a "horrible daughter and student" who deserves to be expelled from school. She is hopeless and endorses passive suicidal ideation. Her symptoms are intense and persistent. She has a major depression.

Having arrived at this diagnosis, the clinician should review the range of potential treatment interventions with Amelia and her father. These options will include medications and psychotherapy, though recent evidence indicates that the best outcome stems from the use of both of these interventions rather than one or the other (March et al. 2004).

Underlying the pharmacologic discussion is the reality that only one medication—fluoxetine—has been approved by the U.S. Food and Drug Administration (FDA) for pediatric depression. This approval stems from two large studies that demonstrated that fluoxetine (Prozac) was more effective than placebo among children and adolescents with major depression (Emslie et al. 1997, 2002). Another large study demonstrated the modest superiority of sertraline (Zoloft) over placebo (Wagner et al. 2003), though findings from other studies have been equivocal or negative. The literature supports the impression that tricyclic antidepressants, particularly those with predominantly noradrenergic effects, are generally ineffective in depressed pediatric patients. Research on psychopharmacology for children and adolescents has generally been plagued, however, by a limited number of studies as well as methodological problems such as small numbers of subjects, a high placebo response rate, and the inclusion of multiple study sites with relatively few subjects per site. In other words, currently available antidepressant medications may be less effective for children and adolescents than they are for adults, but confirmatory data are lacking.

In addition to the information about the effectiveness of antidepressant medication, Amelia or her father may be concerned that medication could increase suicidality, a subject that has received significant news coverage. It appears that antidepressant medications do slightly increase the risk of suicidal ideation (Hammad et al. 2006), particularly during the initial weeks of treatment (Jick et al. 2004). Such a statistical approach should be balanced by the very small number of completed suicides in this age group and the significant impairment and suffering of untreated depression. Suicide rates of adolescents have fallen, for example, in regions of the United States where antidepressant medications have become more commonly prescribed (Olfson et al. 2003). While the use of antidepressant medications may initially raise serotonin levels that lead to the occasional, transient suicidality, a bigger problem may be not using these medications. This concern has been substantiated by two postmortem studies that conclude that most children who kill themselves are found to lack detectable amounts of antidepressant medication in their blood (Hammad et al. 2006; Leon et al. 2006).

Prior to writing a prescription, the psychiatrist should discuss potential side effects, particularly psychomotor activation and induction of mania. Since the risk of noncompliance is high, it is important to emphasize that improvement would not be expected for a few weeks and may take a couple of months. In addition, Amelia and her father might need to set up a system to ensure that she remembers to take the medication daily.

The choice of initial medication for Amelia is straightforward, since fluoxetine is the only antidepressant medication that has received FDA approval for children and adolescents. Typically, the fluoxetine would be started at a low dosage (generally 5–10 mg/day), with gradual increases.

Pharmacologic management necessitates relatively frequent visits in order to monitor side effects and suicidality, encourage compliance, and provide both support and psychoeducation. Many teenagers become noncompliant because they want to feel "normal" or do it on their own. Similarly, adolescents may not want to share their feelings with an adult, particularly feelings that may lead to an increase of medication or—if they mention risky behavior or suicidality—a decrease in their personal freedom. During medication monitoring visits, Amelia's physician not only can work toward the development of trust but also can help the youngster to view depression as a treatable medical condition rather than an indication of weak character or "being crazy." Sessions provide an opportunity to review behavior that could interfere with treatment response, such as poor sleep hygiene or the use of alcohol and drugs. An ongoing relationship also reduces the risk that every small change in mood or behavior leads to an unnecessary medication adjustment. If psychotherapy is provided by a second professional, it is crucial for the psychiatrist and therapist to keep in close contact. According to FDA research guidelines that are now widely used in clinical practice, Amelia should be seen weekly during the first month of antidepressant treatment and twice during the second month. Subsequently, no more than 3 months should elapse between follow-up visits.

Standard pharmacologic intervention with fluoxetine indicates that Amelia has an approximately 60% chance of moderate improvement and a 40% chance of remission during the first 2–3 months of treatment. Thus, there is a significant possibility that she will not respond sufficiently and will therefore require a reevaluation of her medications and psychotherapy. In the absence of adequate data among depressed children and adolescents, expert psychopharmacologists developed the Texas Children's Medication Algorithm Project (Hugher et al. 1999).

In accord with the recommendations of the Texas consensus panel, most pediatric psychopharmacologists would place Amelia on an alternative selective serotonin reuptake inhibitor (SSRI) if she did not show at least moderate benefit from fluoxetine. Sertraline is probably the best alternative given that it is FDA approved for the treatment of pediatric obsessive-compulsive disorder and was found to be superior to placebo in one published double-blind, placebo-controlled trial among depressed youth (Wagner et al. 2003). If Amelia shows a partial but insufficient response to an SSRI, the physician might want to augment with lithium, bupropion (Wellbutrin), thyroid hormone, or buspirone (Buspar). If treatment with two consecutive SSRIs yields a minimal response, the SSRI should be replaced with an antidepressant from a different category, which might be bupropion, venlafaxine (Effexor), mirtazapine (Remeron), or a tricyclic antidepressant. One may try adding one of these latter compounds to fluoxetine or another SSRI. A monoamine oxidase inhibitor (MAOI) could be considered in cases of truly treatment-refractory depression, but the risk of dietary or illicit drug-induced toxic reactions is a particular concern in adolescents.

Psychopharmacology among adolescents is complicated by the paucity of evidence, the immaturity of the nervous system, and the frequency of noncompliance. Nonetheless, it is clear that antidepressant medications can be judiciously combined with psychological and social supports to help reduce the suffering and morbidity that are associated with depression in this age group.

Interpersonal Psychotherapy

Laura Mufson, Ph.D.

AMELIA Gutierrez has become depressed in the context of grief over her mother's death and transitions to a new school and neighborhood. She is, therefore, a potentially good candidate for interpersonal psychotherapy (IPT), a treatment that makes use of the link between interpersonal issues and the onset or maintenance of depressive symptoms. In fact, grief and role transitions are two of the interpersonal areas that can become the focus of IPT (the others are role disputes and interpersonal deficits). While originally developed for adults (Weissman et al. 2000), it has been adapted as a 12-week treatment for depressed adolescents, IPT-A (Mufson et al. 2004a, 2004b). Both versions of IPT work by helping the patient improve interpersonal effectiveness and relationship satisfaction.

Amelia's *grief* stems from her mother's death and the impact of that death upon herself and her family. In regard to *role transitions,* Amelia has had to adjust to leaving a public school in her neighborhood with other Latino adolescents for a private school with a very different group of adolescents. By moving to a new neighborhood, she lost her relationship with the two women who functioned like supportive grandparents. Her profound loss of attachment figures and social support appears closely linked to her depression. The dearth of people to whom she can talk about her feelings has left her unable to cope with these strong emotions, and when upset, she has turned to scratching her wrists and having thoughts of wanting to die. Her father, grappling with his own loss, has been unable to step in to serve as a support to Amelia; even previously helpful members of her church are no longer reaching out to the family with support.

Assuming Amelia agreed to IPT, the therapist would begin by confirming for Amelia that she has a depression. In addition, the therapist would emphasize that depression is a real illness that sometimes develops when people lose someone they love and then have to take on new roles. Amelia would also be counseled that she should maintain a "limited sick role," which means that she should maintain normal activities as much as possible; skipping school might, for example, make her feel temporarily better but would quickly make her feel worse. Safety is a major concern in working with depressed adolescents, and it is important to clarify the intensity and nature of her suicidal thoughts and feelings. The therapist might contract with Amelia for safety, but it may be more useful to create a safety plan for her to follow if she begins to feel dangerously suicidal. These initial tasks can be done directly with Amelia, but her father should also be involved for at least a brief meeting.

The therapist would then conduct a *closeness circle,* which would allow the therapist and Amelia to identify the important people in Amelia's life and assess how close she is to each one. Given her recent losses and transitions, it is likely that Amelia's closeness circle reveals a paucity of important people. The therapist would discuss with Amelia the people she does turn to for support. They would then conduct an *interpersonal inventory,* reviewing which of her most important relationships are currently stressful. They would explore the nature of the difficulties, the possibilities for increasing support from the remaining people in her life, and ways that she could develop supportive and healthy relationships. Finally, the therapist and Amelia would formulate the problem area(s) for the remaining sessions.

These main initial tasks—confirming the diagnosis, explaining the limited sick role, conducting a family meeting, and developing a closeness circle, an interpersonal inventory, and a problem area—are integral to IPT for depressed adolescents and tend to take about four sessions.

Once the therapist and Amelia agree on the identified focus for treatment, the therapist begins the work of the middle phase, which typically spans sessions 5 through 9 but continues throughout the treatment. Amelia's IPT-A therapist might first focus on the grief problem area by carefully reviewing Amelia's mother's illness and eventual death and their impact on Amelia's feelings and relationships. The therapist would try to explicitly link Amelia's depressive symptoms to interpersonal events and also try to identify Amelia's strengths and her interpersonal skills that need strengthening. The goal of the middle phase would be to help Amelia improve her ability to express herself and get support so that she does not feel the need to engage in self-injurious behavior. Role playing is one way in which the therapist might teach Amelia how to better connect with people. While this might include bringing the father in for coaching, the majority of the therapy sessions would be individual ones with Amelia. After role playing a targeted interaction, the therapist might assign her "work at home" that might include engaging her father in an activity or conversation. Throughout the treatment, the therapist would continue to monitor Amelia's depressive symptoms, specifically linking mood changes to interpersonal events.

While discussing the impact of her mother's death, the IPT-A therapist would also link her depression to *role transitions* that might include any of the following: the move to a new apartment and the loss of supports; the move to a new school and the loss of her old friends; the experience of seeing her father stressed, sad, and unavailable; the experience of having new responsibilities as the eldest female at home; and the experience of dating and becoming sexually involved. The IPT-A therapist might choose to focus on any of these role transitions as a way to help Amelia learn ways to

- Communicate feelings more directly and effectively
- Problem-solve through the use of decision analysis
- Become more adept at getting support and making herself heard

These strategies also might be applied to her relationship with her boyfriend, with whom she has been smoking marijuana, drinking alcohol, and engaging in sex—all of which seem to be atypical behaviors for her. She might learn to express herself more clearly and refuse to do things that make her uncomfortable. Therapy might lead her to conclude that it would be better to find a relationship with someone more her peer and with more similar expectations for a relationship.

As the depressive symptoms resolved, the final few sessions would focus on assessing Amelia's progress in treatment and need for any further treatment. Amelia and the therapist would review her warning symptoms of depression so she could identify future relapses or recurrences earlier and get help sooner. They would review the specific strategies that were the focus of her sessions, discuss her accomplishments and successes, and brainstorm the use of these strategies in future situations. Finally, they would discuss her feelings about ending treatment. The therapist might suggest continuing in a maintenance phase of treatment (if Amelia had recovered) to decrease the risk of relapse. They might meet once a month for 6 months to support her use of the new strategies and monitor her symptom improvement. Although maintenance IPT-A has not been formally studied in clinical trials, it is a reasonable suggestion in light of the adult literature (Frank et al. 1990), the recommended practice parameters for treating child and adolescent depression (American Academy of Child and Adolescent Psychiatry 1998), and accepted clinical practice.

IPT-A has been proven efficacious for depressed adolescents treated in both university hospital-based clinics (Mufson et al. 1999; Rosselló and Bernal

1999) and school-based mental health clinics (Mufson et al. 2004b). It has not yet been systematically studied with depressed adolescents who engage in self-injurious behavior like Amelia. Clinically, IPT-A has been used with such adolescents with the belief that the self-harm behavior will dissipate as the adolescent learns more effective communication strategies and her relationships improve. Given that antidepressant medication is not always the preferred initial treatment nor always effective for adolescents, it is important to have other treatment options to offer. Finally, since it focuses on increasing independence and negotiating interdependence, IPT-A is relevant and appealing to teens.

Psychodynamics of Depression

Fredric N. Busch, M.D.

PSYCHODYNAMIC treatments of depression have not been studied with the same rigor as have medications and cognitive-behavioral therapy (CBT), and so evidence-based recommendations are premature. Nevertheless, psychodynamic models of depression and its treatment have a long history within psychoanalysis (Abraham 1911; Bibring 1953; Freud 1917[1915]; Jacobson 1971; Rado 1928). Further, clinical experience and some systematic studies suggest that psychodynamic treatment can effectively relieve mild to moderate depressive disorders and may be a useful adjunct in the treatment of moderate to severe depressions that are also being addressed with medications or CBT (Busch et al. 2004). In addition, psychodynamic psychotherapy may be particularly effective in addressing psychological vulnerabilities that can lead to persistence or recurrence of depression.

Amelia Gutierrez's brief case history suggests psychodynamic factors may have contributed to her depression and may prove pivotal in her treatment. A psychodynamic approach can also stimulate further lines of inquiry that may not only assist in her treatment but help this young woman feel better understood.

Ms. Gutierrez's depression occurs in the context of the death of her mother, the loss of supportive neighbors, and the threatened loss of her school. Psychoanalytic theorists have posited that loss, and the meaning of that loss, are significant in the etiology of depression. Freud (1917[1915]), for example, in his highly influential paper "Mourning and Melancholia," suggested that the individual identifies with the lost person in order to cope with the pain of separation. Ambivalent feelings toward the lost person, including anger, then become directed toward the self, leading to guilt and self-criticism. As will be described below, the interactions among feelings of sadness, anger, and guilt are central to depressive dynamics.

People vary in their sensitivity to such losses. Although Ms. Gutierrez has suffered clear-cut external trauma, some depressions seem to result less from external hurt than from narcissistic vulnerability, which is a sensitivity to perceived or actual separations or rejections (Rado 1928). Individuals with narcissistic vulnerability will tend to experience more events as rejections or losses and react to them with a drop in self-esteem, depressive affects, and rage.

After the death of her mother, we would anticipate Ms. Gutierrez would experience reactions of sadness and deprivation. In addition, she would likely be angry, perhaps unconsciously, at her mother for abandoning her. Depressed patients often have conflicts about such anger, which can feel intolerable or unacceptable. This anger can trigger self-criticism and guilt, which may be more conscious than the original sadness. The anger can also be displaced onto people who feel more acceptable than her deceased mother. While Ms. Gutierrez denies anger, she does admit that she gets impatient with "her father, teachers, younger brother, and classmates." Further, her headmaster describes her as "hostile." Her difficulty acknowledging the evident anger suggests the possibility that the anger and disappointment that she felt when her mother died has been denied, made subconscious, and then directed at the important people in her life.

While often directed outward, Ms. Gutierrez's anger is also directed inward in the form of self-criticism and guilty accusations. She has "no patience for herself" and describes herself as a "horrible daughter and student." She feels guilty about not working harder at school and believes she deserves punishment for her laziness. She even fears that she contributed to her mother's death. These self-criticisms are evidence of a punitive conscience, or superego. People who are vulnerable to depression are likely to have a particularly harsh or rigid superego in which self-observation is imbued with intolerant self-criticism for a variety of feelings, including anger, sexuality, and envy. This self-criticism leads to a lowering of self-esteem and an expectation of punishment. According to analytic theory, these reactions may reflect a turning of anger against the self, which can exacerbate depression.

While psychological defenses unconsciously protect the individual from painful feelings, they can also worsen depression by preventing direct resolution of feelings and conflicts. Ms. Gutierrez's thoughts and behaviors are typical of defense mechanisms found in depressed patients (see Busch et al. 2004). For instance, Amelia's anger may be unconsciously denied and then projected into other people, who are then experienced by her as negative or critical, leaving her feeling wronged and alone (Abraham 1911). Her inability to complete tasks and her declining academic performance may reflect the poor energy and motivation that are frequently found in depression, but these failures might also reflect an indirect expression of anger, or a sign of *passive aggression.* Such behavior tends to arouse ire in others and may have contributed to the threat of expulsion. While Amelia sounds very pleasant, that same quality may reflect *reaction formation,* a defense in which she is overly nice to the same people who anger her. Reaction formation, however, prevents her from being aware of her anger and expressing it in an effective manner toward others. Thus, her unconscious rage may increase, triggering further frustration and depression, or sometimes erupting in aggressive or provocative behavior. While these defenses can be adaptive, they may confirm her belief that she deserves criticism, deepen her sense of isolation, and undermine her ability to directly communicate her feelings and needs.

Related to the strictness of the superego, depression is often accompanied by *idealizations* and *devaluations* of self and others. Idealization of others is fueled by the fantasy that the idealized other will relieve low self-esteem. Self idealizations represent an effort to compensate for feelings of inadequacy. At the same time that they idealize, depressed patients may devalue others to prop up their own self view and to protect themselves from feelings of rejection. However, devaluation leaves little room for others to be experienced as caring and responsive. Idealizations are often fragile and likely to lead to further feelings of disappointment and depression. In regard to Ms. Gutierrez, we have hints that she may idealize the boyfriend and devalue her father and herself. The therapist should be alert for indications of these perceptions, as they could heighten Ms. Gutierrez's experiences of disappointment and loss when the idealized boyfriend disappoints her.

Conflicts involving the dynamics of depression lead to vicious cycles that intensify depressive affects (Busch et al. 2004). For instance, Ms. Gutierrez likely had had some propensity toward depression before her mother became ill, perhaps through some combination of genetic loading, low self-esteem, and narcissistic vulnerability. Ms. Gutierrez likely experiences feelings of loss and rejection in response to her mother's death. While she would probably not consciously understand the link, Ms. Gutierrez's feelings of rejection and loss would lead to anger at her mother. Hostile feelings toward her mother would be consciously unacceptable, so she would then direct her anger inward and wind up feeling guilty and self-critical. At this point, the feelings come full circle: the guilt and self-criticism intensify her narcissistic vulnerability and low self esteem, creating a vicious cycle of depression (see Figure 7–1).

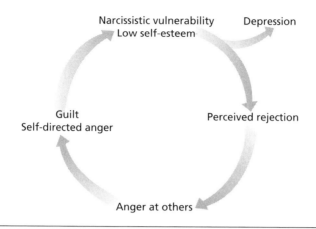

FIGURE 7–1. Vicious cycles in depression: narcissistic vulnerability/anger.
Source. Reprinted with permisson from Busch et al. 2004.

In a second vicious cycle, not clearly demonstrated by Ms. Gutierrez, low self-esteem leads to a propensity to idealize self and others to ease these feelings (see Figure 7–2). This idealization triggers disappointment, which leads to a devaluation of self and others, with a further lowering of self-esteem. The self-devaluation triggers a further pressure to idealize.

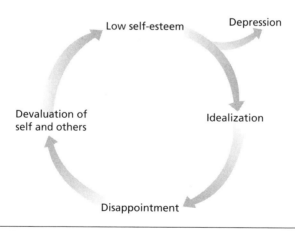

FIGURE 7–2. Vicious cycles in depression: low self-esteem and idealization/devaluation.
Source. Reprinted with permisson from Busch et al. 2004.

In regard to her self-cutting, a psychodynamic clinician would consider the meanings of Ms. Gutierrez's behavior in addition to assessing suicide risk. Such self-destructive acts could represent another form of anger being turned against the self, a means of punishment for her angry feelings, or punishment to relieve her guilt for being a "horrible" daughter. Self-cutting can also represent an expression of anger toward others, a means of seeking help and attention, and a technique to self-soothe.

Ms. Gutierrez's suicidal feelings certainly deserve exploration. She does describe the common fantasy of reunion with her mother through suicide. Such a fantasy does not necessarily mean that she would try to kill herself, but it does indicate that her threats and thoughts should be taken seriously.

A psychodynamically oriented therapist would make use of this understanding of Ms. Gutierrez to help her explore not only her sadness and disappointment but also her anger and guilt. Goals would include helping her work through these feelings and become more tolerant of them. Increased tolerance of angry feelings would help the patient express them more directly and effectively, rather than through a variety of suboptimal defenses. Guilty reactions would be explored with the goal of easing the patient's intense and unfair self-criticisms, including concerns about having damaged her mother. The therapist's nonjudgmental, humane, and inquiring stance would be crucial in helping this young woman identify and accept painful feelings and move on with her life.

Overview of Adolescent Bereavement

Theodore Shapiro, M.D.

WHILE modern psychiatric generalists focus on diagnostic categories and pharmacology as well as on brain imaging and genetics, child and adolescent psychiatrists consider all of these from a developmental perspective. Such an advantage is especially useful when considering the case of Amelia Gutierrez, whose difficulties threaten to derail her successful progression from adolescence into adulthood.

Maturation is a concept that combines the species-specific unfolding of genetic potential within the physical environment and surrounding culture. This interplay leads to predictable achievements that vary based on genetics, diet, and child-rearing practices and include walking at about 12 months, speech and language competencies at about 3 years, and puberty at about 9–16 years. Adolescence is defined as the period between puberty and adulthood, although from a developmental/biological point of view, such a middle ground does not exist: one is either pre-procreative or procreative. Adolescence is, then, a cultural invention that Eric Erikson called a "moratorium" (Erikson 1950). In it, childhood dependency is gradually shed while the body and mind mature. Many of Amelia's problems stem from this adolescent dilemma: decked out in her newly acquired secondary sexual characteristics, this 16-year-old girl was confronted with her mother's illness and death just as she was struggling with her own autonomy and dependence. Pertinent life cycle issues are as important to an understanding of Amelia as symptom clustering and specific diagnoses.

The history indicates that Amelia had been close to her family, particularly her mother. After the mother's death, Amelia seemed to have backed away from her family and school friends and become depressed and suicidal. She has also begun to date a 21-year-old man, with whom she is smoking marijuana and drinking alcohol. Such behavior is worrisome, but understanding the behavior should be informed by the concept of developmental psychopathology.

The normally developing adolescent becomes increasingly independent through a variety of means that are variably acceptable to adults. One of the ways that adolescents develop is through peers who introduce the values and mores of the surrounding society. Adolescent independence is most visible in the ways in which the teenager connects with an outside subgroup or lover, a theme elaborated, for example, in Philip Roth's novel *Letting Go*. Similarly, the film *Breaking Away* focuses on the gradual alienation of an adolescent while he is being accepted by the subculture of the girl he pursues. These popular themes underscore the conflicted dependency of adolescence. They also hint at the transient identifications that grow out of crushes and idealization—and that may be sexualized—but that may serve different psychological purposes than does adult sexuality.

The understanding of likely developmental hurdles, needs, and fantasies informs the exploration of a patient like Amelia. We might anticipate that her independence would be fueled by her growing attention to community norms that include the dating patterns and language of the dominant culture. Individual imagination and fantasy color maturation, including the intrapsychic conditions that enhance sexual arousal. These conscious and unconscious fantasies must also mature in order to promote an adult level of sexual maturity and readiness. Amelia's sexual relationship can, therefore, be assumed to have personal, psychodynamic meaning. In tactfully discussing her relationship, the clinician might anticipate that her Spanish-speaking boyfriend might have become a new receptacle for the love that she had for her Spanish-speaking mother. In this way, Amelia may be using sexuality as a way to fulfill dependency needs rather than as a means to deepen mature intimacy.

Similarly, death and immortality have their own unique meanings within both the culture and the individual psyche. Not only do we follow religious rituals, we create our own versions of the post-death story. These fantasies may be magically tinged with hope for reunion and continuing protection, especially if the deceased is one's mother. Given her developmentally normal urge toward independence with resultant ambivalence toward her mother, it becomes likely that her depressive symptoms stem at least partially from anger at her mother's abandonment that is then turned towards herself. Her suicidality might stem from guilt that would arise from anger at her mother as well as a conscious or unconscious fantasy that she can reunite with her mother through death.

Developmental and psychodynamic possibilities need to be confirmed, of course, through ongoing exploration with the patient. In addition, the adolescent psychiatrist must attend to demographics and evidence-based symptom clusters. For example, while boys are far more vulnerable to psychiatric illness as children, depression besieges our teenage girls. In addition to the possibility that she is developing a major depression or pathological mourning, Amelia is developing a personality style that may lead to heightened emotionality that would be consistent with a budding personality disorder marked by suicidality, mood lability, and identity diffusion.

Amelia Gutierrez's more immediate diagnosis will depend on her symptoms, which include grief, suicidality, cutting, and declining school performance. Her treatment should also include an exploration into the meaning of her losses, her behavior, and her inner experience. Perhaps most importantly, however, any intervention must consider her developmental stage with an understanding that the central goal of treatment is the successful transition into adulthood.

Summary Points

- Psychiatric work involves ethical conflicts, cultural norms, and sociological disruptions, as well as descriptive diagnosis and pathophysiology.

- Normal adolescent development includes increasing independence while holding onto dependency.

- Some independent behaviors can derail normal adolescent development.

- Antidepressant medications have been tentatively implicated in suicidal thoughts among depressed adolescents, but not suicide.

- Antidepressant medications have been tentatively implicated in reducing the rates of suicide among depressed adolescents.

- Loss can lead to depression, and treatment that focuses on loss can reduce depression.

- Depression can be perpetuated by cycles of thought, feeling, and behavior, and conscious recognition of those cycles can reduce depressive symptoms.

Chapter 8

ANXIETY
AND
SOPHIA HASTINGS

Part A

SOPHIA Hastings, a single, 28-year-old seventh-grade teacher, was referred by her primary care physician for psychiatric evaluation. She had initially seen her internist because of recurrent shortness of breath, sweats, a choking sensation, and a feeling of always being on edge. A thorough medical workup found no physical cause for these complaints, and the internist suggested that she might have an anxiety disorder.

Ms. Hastings had first experienced these symptoms as a freshman in college in anticipation of a fraternity party, but they had gradually become more frequent and intense, until they began to occur multiple times during the course of a week. The sensations generally occurred in social settings, particularly in the teacher's lounge when "everyone else seemed to be enjoying themselves."

While describing her situation to the psychiatrist, Ms. Hastings was obviously uncomfortable. She explained that most social settings made her anxious but that she could "get by." She indicated that the current coed school at which she taught was difficult for her; she had felt more comfortable during her four years teaching at an all-girls school, where almost all of the teachers were women. She said she wanted to socialize but had rarely gone to parties or dated. She denied ever having had a boyfriend but described a dozen "one-night stands" while "really drunk." These were "stupid and humiliating," she said, but "no big deal." She denied sexual attraction to women. The presence of romantically appropriate men tended to elicit anxiety and the cluster of physical symptoms described above, although she insisted these feelings occurred at other times, as well.

In order to treat this discomfort, the patient described drinking an "airplane bottle" of vodka a few times during the school day. To treat early and mid-insomnia, she tended to have several "stiff drinks" every night. She said that she felt tremulous and anxious if she skipped her morning alcohol but said she did not know if that meant she was "in withdrawal or just my usual anxious self." Over the past year, she had begun to worry about whether she was an alcoholic. To test this, she had twice stopped all alcohol for a week; the abrupt discontinuation led to no medical complications, but she had been barely able to leave her apartment. She denied ever having had blackouts and seizures. She denied legal difficulties related to the drinking but said that before moving to New York City, she would occasionally "drive drunk." She denied abusing other substances.

At the conclusion of the interview, Ms. Hastings asked about possible treatments that might help her relax and have a better life. She also asked if she was an alcoholic, and, if so, whether she needed alcohol treatment.

Personal History

Ms. Hastings was born and raised in a nearby city. She never knew her father and was raised by a substance-abusing mother who had multiple boyfriends during her childhood. While her mother and her boyfriends were "colorful," Ms. Hastings describes herself as having been a "straight arrow," with excellent grades and perfect school attendance. She denied significant difficulties during her childhood and adolescence, adding that she was busy with studying and "bailing out" her mother who was "always getting in trouble." While she admitted to few early memories, she denied physical and sexual abuse. She attended a prestigious women's college on scholarship and then taught at a girl's school in her hometown. After 4 years, she impulsively quit that job and moved, declaring that it was time to get on with her life. She talked to her mother almost every evening, and their discussions focused primarily on the mother's struggles with men and Alcoholics Anonymous (AA).

Personal Psychiatric History

Ms. Hastings saw a school psychologist at age 15 after her mother found her diary in which "I hate me" was repeated many times. She went to several sessions before deciding she "didn't need it."

As described earlier, she used alcohol to control her anxiety. She estimated that she drank one or two liters of vodka per week.

Family Psychiatric History

The patient's mother was addicted to multiple substances, including alcohol, heroin, and cocaine, with multiple failed rehabs. Her biologic father had also been dependent on substances and had been incarcerated at least twice for robbery.

Medical History

None.

Mental Status Exam

The patient was well-groomed, cooperative, and engaging. She appeared shy and younger than her stated age. She tended to avert her eyes when discussing personal issues. Her speech was soft and fluent, and her thoughts were goal directed. She demonstrated no abnormal movements. She described her mood as "edgy and anxious." Her affect was tense and generally constricted. She denied depression, suicidality, and psychosis. She was cognitively intact. Her insight appeared good, though her judgment appears to have been impaired sporadically by alcohol.

Summary

Sophia Hastings was a 28-year-old woman who was referred to an outpatient psychiatrist for evaluation of anxiety symptoms. The discussions in Part A focus on Ms. Hastings' anxiety and alcohol abuse and review multiple treatment modalities. The second half of the case focuses on Ms. Hastings after 1 year of treatment.

Discussions of the Case of
Sophia Hastings, Part A

Anxiety Disorders 302
  Laszlo A. Papp, M.D.

Alcohol Abuse 305
  Bruce Phariss, M.D., and Jennifer Cooper Stelwagon, M.D.

Neurobiology of Alcohol 310
  Daniel Herrera, M.D., Ph.D.

Pharmacology of Anxiety 313
Smit S. Sinha, M.D., and Franklin Schneier, M.D.

Cognitive-Behavioral Therapy 315
Susan Evans, Ph.D.

Panic-Focused Psychodynamic Psychotherapy 319
Fredric N. Busch, M.D.

Part B 322

Anxiety Disorders

Laszlo A. Papp, M.D.

NORMAL anxiety can enhance preparation, concentration, and performance, while excessive anxiety may interfere with functioning but tends to be brief and self-limiting. *Anxiety disorders* are characterized by persistent and disabling anxiety. Most people are able to distinguish between these three types of anxiety and seek treatment only when overwhelmed by the psychological sensation of anxiety or by one of its many somatic expressions. Physical complaints are a central part of the anxiety disorders, and many people seek initial consultations with general practitioners or specialists in cardiology, pulmonology, or gastroenterology. Negative medical evaluations are often followed by inadequate treatments, and people with anxiety disorders frequently turn to street drugs and alcohol.

Sophia Hastings reports that her symptoms began as she entered college, are worsened in social situations, and have increased in intensity over the years. She has multiple somatic complaints and originally sought help from her internist. She self-medicates with alcohol. Her history is typical of a patient with an anxiety disorder.

Which diagnosis best fits Ms. Hastings? While a venerable DSM tradition, establishing one central diagnosis may not be particularly relevant to her treatment. Most treatments target symptoms that cut across Axis I and Axis II categories.

That Ms. Hastings' symptoms mostly occur in social situations suggests the DSM-IV diagnosis of *social anxiety disorder* (SAD), the condition also known as *social phobia*. Her desire for social interaction rules out a number of diagnoses also characterized by social avoidance, such as schizoid personality disorder and autism. As is typical, her symptoms, initially limited to a few specific situations (termed *specific SAD*), became widespread, leading to the more severe diagnosis of *generalized SAD*. Generalized SAD tends to run in families and to be treatment resistant. It is often comorbid with depression, other anxiety disorders, eating disorders, and substance abuse. Extensive avoidance could lead to social isolation, restricted functioning, hopelessness, and suicidality.

Ms. Hastings may also meet DSM criteria for *avoidant personality disorder*. Some argue that avoidant personality disorder is a severe form of SAD. Indeed, SAD-focused therapies seem effective for avoidant personality disorder, supporting the potential advantages of a dimensional diagnostic approach in which the symptoms of social anxiety are seen on a continuum from episodes of mild performance anxiety to severe, lifelong pathology.

The dimensional view easily accommodates the clinical reality that most anxiety disorders feature similar symptoms, comorbidities, and complications. With few exceptions, they respond to the same medications. For instance, panic attacks used to be thought of as a pathognomonic feature of panic disorder. The clinical reality is that the panic symptoms reported by Ms. Hastings are very similar to those experienced in most anxiety disorders.

Ms. Hastings appears to be abusing alcohol. In most cases of comorbidity, the SAD precedes the substance abuse. In Ms. Hastings' case, the family history of alcoholism suggests the possibility of a different sequence. She may have begun to use alcohol and then experienced anxiety during periods of withdrawal. Regardless of the initiating pattern, it is likely that the anxiety disorder and the alcohol abuse are connected in a crippling cycle. The alcohol/anxiety interaction is a good example of how multiple diagnoses are most effectively treated when addressed concurrently. For example, prolonged abstinence from drugs and alcohol is no longer the precondition for initiating treatments for anxiety and mood disorders. Educating Ms. Hastings about the interaction between alcohol use and anxiety will have to be a treatment priority.

Ms. Hastings has, therefore, a number of possible diagnoses, including SAD, avoidant personality disorder, and alcohol abuse. Although she denies it, she probably suffers from depression as well.

In addition to symptom assessment, it is important to better understand the development of Ms. Hastings' anxiety. Not only was her substance-abusing father absent and imprisoned at least twice, she was raised by a polysubstance-abusing mother in an environment in which adults were constantly needing her to "bail them out." She might have genetically inherited a tendency toward unpleasant feeling states and/or a tendency toward substance abuse. Further, her chaotic and unsupportive home environment may have overwhelmed her, and it would also have increased the likelihood of more explicit trauma, perhaps even sexual abuse by one of her mother's multiple boyfriends. Any of these factors would help explain her anxiety and alcohol abuse. Further exploration of her history might also lead to a diagnosis of posttraumatic stress disorder (PTSD).

The role of early trauma in the development of psychiatric disorders is controversial. By the 1980s, many biologically oriented psychiatrists had rejected the traditional psychoanalytic notion that most psychiatric disorders originate from early trauma. The currently prevailing, more balanced, and increasingly evidence-based view is that for a subset of psychiatric patients, major life events and traumas in early childhood play a significant role in anxiety and mood disorders. Rather than predicting a specific illness, early trauma seems to confer general vulnerability to a spectrum of disorders. The specific disorder stems from a confluence of factors, such as genetics, upbringing, experience, medical illness, substance use, and sociocultural influences. Just as no particular early trauma leads to a specific psychiatric disorder, no disorder stems from a particular experience.

Ms. Hastings' diagnosis will not be complete until her formative experiences, early relationship patterns, and family dynamics are explored. These explorations can facilitate the therapeutic alliance, help make sense of her symptoms, and prepare the therapist for potential problems. For example, a patient who describes intimacy-induced panic may well become anxious in any sort of exploratory psychotherapy. Revealing and addressing previously hidden handicaps, real or perceived, such as a physical deformity or speech impediment, could be particularly therapeutic for patients with social anxiety. In the case of Ms. Hastings, we might want to tactfully explore her rationale for writing, "I hate me" in her diary, her feelings about being perfect, and her experience living in such a chaotic household. The evaluation of Ms. Hastings' level of insight and her ability to withstand the intimacy of therapy will help determine treatment selection.

Despite the many strikes against her, Ms. Hastings has many strengths. She overcame difficult early experiences, excelled in school, and found a meaningful career. She appears motivated and may have the resources and health insurance to pursue treatment. It is likely that the course of her therapy will be complicated by the same mistrust of parental figures that may have contributed to the initial anxiety, but it can be predicted that she will benefit from some combination of medications, substance abuse treatment, cognitive-behavioral therapy, and exploratory psychotherapy.

Alcohol Abuse

Bruce Phariss, M.D.
Jennifer Cooper Stelwagon, M.D.

THE successful treatment of alcohol abuse begins with the development of an accurate diagnosis and treatment plan. The patient's motivation to change and the therapeutic alliance are also crucial, and both are adversely affected by the chronic abuse of alcohol. These characteristic psychological sequelae to chronic alcohol abuse have led to the development of specific interview techniques that are useful not only for patients but for clinicians who might have a tendency to move away from their usual position of tactful, helpful curiosity when working with people who abuse substances.

Sophia Hastings' evaluation should begin with her story of anxiety and alcohol. At some point during the first session, however, it is mandatory to assess her risk of serious withdrawal phenomena, since untreated alcohol withdrawal can be fatal secondary to a seizure or delirium tremens (DTs). Ms. Hastings does complain of tremor and anxiety when she stops drinking. These complaints—along with such symptoms as sweats and nausea—are consistent with mild alcohol withdrawal. Her two trial weeks of abstinence are somewhat reassuring but do not necessarily mean that discontinuation will be safe. She may have developed more of a dependence since her trial weeks, for example, or she may not be providing an accurate history. If she is able to tolerate an outpatient detoxification, the psychiatrist will need to carefully monitor symptoms. If the symptoms are either dangerous or intense enough that relapse is likely, she may require a benzodiazepine taper. The taper can be done as an outpatient if the withdrawal is not severe and the patient is reliable, has a strong support system, and has no history of benzodiazepine abuse or dependence. When withdrawal symptoms are mild, an alternative approach would be to avoid the dependency and abuse risks of the benzodiazepines and instead focus on psychosocial interventions and use low doses of an antipsychotic medication (e.g., quetiapine [Seroquel]) to alleviate episodic anxiety. In the following discussion, we will assume that she has mild withdrawal symptoms and does not require an inpatient detox.

A second important diagnostic issue is the interaction between her alcohol abuse and other psychiatric disorders. She says that she drinks alcohol in order to ease her anxiety and insomnia, but it is important to assess whether she has indeed been "self-medicating" or whether the alcohol use actually predated her anxiety. She has a strong family history of alcohol and substance abuse, and she—like many people—might prefer to see herself as an anxious person rather than an alcoholic. It is useful to hypothesize that she may be able to discontinue the alcohol if the anxiety disorder is successfully treated, but alcohol abuse often takes on a life of its own and, regardless of how it began, requires a focused treatment that is different from a typical psychiatric treatment.

Laboratory tests can help confirm the extent of alcohol abuse. For example, mild elevations in mean corpuscular volume and liver function tests would support the diagnosis and help direct treatment. Many people abuse multiple substances, and a toxicology screen would help identify people who do not readily admit polysubstance abuse. The evaluation for anxiety will be covered elsewhere, but thyroid abnormalities should certainly be checked, since they are an especially common cause of anxiety and mood disorders. Finally, a thorough physical exam can help identify the many medical illnesses that tend to accompany chronic alcohol abuse.

In addition to making a diagnosis, assessing the need for detoxification, and ordering lab tests, the clinician at the first session has an opportunity to assess Ms. Hastings' level of insight and motivation for change. According to the case report, she sounds unsure as to whether she is an alcoholic despite the fact that she drinks throughout the day, needs alcohol to sleep, and has recurrently put herself into danger while intoxicated (e.g., driving and sexual situations). In order to engage Ms. Hastings in the treatment process, it is useful to review the stages of change in recovering from alcoholism (see Table 8–1).

TABLE 8–1.   THE SIX STAGES OF CHANGE IN ALCOHOL ABUSE

Stage	Definition
1. Precontemplation	Not aware of a need for change
2. Contemplation	Uncertain about change
3. Preparation	Making a commitment to an action, plan, or program
4. Action	Practicing the plan for 3–6 months
5. Maintenance	Consolidating behavior into a lifestyle
6. Relapse	Redefining as a learning experience; reevaluating the treatment plan

Source.   Adapted from DiClemente 2003.

During the first session, Ms. Hastings spontaneously wonders whether she abuses alcohol, so she has already moved from the precontemplation to the contemplation stage. A primary therapeutic task is to help Ms. Hastings move through the rest of the stages of change. Although any good, active psychotherapy should help, *motivational interviewing* is an excellent complementary model to help patients move through the stages of change (Miller and Rollnick 2002). Motivational interviewing is a directive, client-centered counseling style for eliciting behavior change by helping clients resolve ambivalence. How is that done? Miller and Rollnick (2002) emphasize that in addition to technique, the spirit of the method is important and can be characterized as follows:

1. Motivation to change is elicited from the client and not imposed externally.
2. It is the patient's job, not the therapist's, to resolve the ambivalence.
3. Direct persuasion is not an effective way to resolve ambivalence.
4. The interviewing style is quiet and eliciting.
5. The therapist is directive in helping the patient to examine and resolve ambivalence.
6. Readiness to change is not a patient trait, but a fluctuating product of interpersonal interaction.
7. The therapeutic relationship is more like a partnership than like an expert/recipient relationship.

In addition to these general characteristics, motivational interviewing outlines specific behaviors that the therapist can use when discussing alcohol and substance abuse. These include seeking to understand the patient's frame of reference via reflective listening; expressing acceptance and affirmation; eliciting and selectively reinforcing the patient's own self-motivational statements; monitoring the patient's degree of readiness to change and not jumping ahead of the patient; and affirming the patient's freedom of choice and self direction. Implicit in motivational interviewing is the view that the therapist should act as a guide rather than a moral policeman, a view that is sometimes forgotten when working with people whose behaviors are generally condemned by the society at large.

The therapist does, however, have a responsibility to impart useful information, and psychoeducation would be an important part of Ms. Hastings' treatment. For example, we would explore the interaction between alcohol and anxiety by explaining that alcohol calms her temporarily but leads to mild alcohol withdrawal and rebound anxiety. We would also explain that the first step to treating her anxiety is to stop drinking. If the anxiety persists, the underlying psychiatric comorbidity can be accurately diagnosed and treated in an alcohol-free setting. In order for Ms. Hastings to stop drinking, however, we would need to immediately address the intense anxiety and panic.

There are several medications that could help Ms. Hastings' anxiety. Benzodiazepines treat anxiety in a similar fashion to alcohol, but they also create a cross-tolerance to alcohol and can lead to alcohol craving. Further, the combination of alcohol and benzodiazepines can be lethal. We tend to use benzodiazepines only after other options have been exhausted and a recovery network is well established. Some addiction experts completely avoid benzodiazepine use with former alcohol abusers. Others might use benzodiazepines during the initial phase of alcohol abstinence, either to treat withdrawal symptoms or to reduce anxiety before other treatments have begun to work.

Instead of benzodiazepines, selective serotonin reuptake inhibitor (SSRI) antidepressants are the mainstay of pharmacologic management of comorbid anxiety and depressive disorders in alcohol abusers. In regard to Ms. Hastings, the antidepressant could be started immediately with the explanation that she would see full benefit several weeks after she stops drinking. We would also consider using a sedating atypical antipsychotic medication, such as quetiapine. A low dose could be used as needed for anxiety during the day, with a somewhat larger dose at bedtime if Ms. Hastings is having trouble sleeping.

The decision to start an SSRI immediately is controversial. An alternative approach is to evaluate the anxiety after a period of abstinence. Since Ms. Hastings' anxiety appears to have predated her alcohol abuse, it will likely persist after she quits drinking, and so we would choose to begin the SSRI prior to abstinence. In a case with less clear chronology, waiting up to a month before beginning the SSRI might be prudent.

Many alcohol-abusing patients are reluctant to enter a treatment that insists that they never drink again. Instead, we request abstinence for 90 days, a period of time that often seems manageable and would, in the case of Ms. Hastings, allow her the longest period of sobriety since she was a teenager. Ms. Hastings might disregard our request and try to cut down her drinking. Although this might work briefly, she is likely to quickly relapse. Relapses are common enough in substance abuse treatments that they are one of the stages of changes that are outlined earlier. As long as the therapeutic relationship is intact, such "failures" can be used as learning experiences to effectively tailor the treatment through ongoing education and efforts to resolve the inevitable ambivalence. Ninety days of abstinence are likely to lead her to the recognition that ongoing abstinence is preferable; relapses will remain a threat, however, as referred to in the AA maxim "One Day at a Time."

There are three ways in which this therapeutic plan can be enacted: 1) individual psychotherapy; 2) referral to a twelve-step program in addition to individual psychotherapy; and 3) referral to an outpatient substance abuse treatment expert or treatment facility to parallel the individual treatment.

Twelve-step programs such as Alcoholics Anonymous are a cornerstone of most treatments. AA is an organization run by its members, and many alcoholics are able to maintain abstinence by attending regular meetings and following "the twelve steps." These steps can be summarized as "trust God, clean house, and help others." The emphasis on God and a "spiritual awakening" is one of the reasons that many people resist AA. Much of this resistance stems from a resistance to stopping alcohol, however, and many nonreligious people have found AA to be very useful. In addition, AA provides a ready-made group of people who are motivated to maintain sobriety in both themselves and other members, and this safety net can be invaluable (Khantzian and Mack 1994). AA meetings are held throughout the world and have dramatically different attitudes and demographics. We generally suggest that patients attend at least five different AA meetings before settling into a "home group" or dropping out. Once a comfortable group is uncovered, we suggest that the patient ask other members to suggest groups that have a similar feel.

Resistance to AA may indicate a wish to continue drinking, but Ms. Hastings' social anxiety could keep her from groups unless accompanied by a friend or relative. Other patients fear that if they go to AA and do not stop drinking that they are hopeless. In order to address such resistances and provide more personal therapy, we would probably suggest that Ms. Hastings begin with, for example, an individual treatment at one to three times per week or an outpatient treatment program where professionals lead small groups. Any combination might work, and we use relapses and dropouts to help guide future treatments.

Ms. Hastings probably does not need any of the three medications that are currently used for alcohol abuse and dependence. All can be used in conjunction with AA and/or psychotherapy but are not generally used with someone like Ms. Hastings, who does not appear to have alcohol dependence and has never before been treated. Naltrexone (Revia) has been shown to reduce craving in alcoholic persons and might be tried if she should relapse. Naltrexone is an opioid receptor antagonist that appears to modulate the dopaminergic mesolimbic pathway that ethanol is believed to activate. Acamprosate (Campral) is also used to reduce craving, though its efficacy and mechanism of action are uncertain. Disulfiram (Antabuse) causes severe "hangover" in people who drink alcohol by blocking an enzyme (acetaldehyde dehydrogenase) that is crucial to alcohol's metabolism; accumulated acetaldehyde (an alcohol metabolite) leads to a severe "hangover" that can last for hours.

Treatment of Ms. Hastings' anxiety will likely prove impossible until she eliminates her alcohol use. A variety of techniques can help, but her attendance and effort are crucial. Underlying her participation is the therapeutic relationship, which, in turn, is based on the clinician's attitude of respectful curiosity. This therapeutic attitude is not simply "being nice" but rather a re-flection of the clinician's having developed an understanding of alcohol that allows the clinician to overcome the preconceptions that stymie many such treatments.

Neurobiology of Alcohol

Daniel Herrera, M.D., Ph.D.

ALCOHOL is a simple molecule that has profound effects throughout the body. Through its impact on the cytochrome P450 system, alcohol not only induces its own tolerance but increases the metabolism—and reduces the effectiveness—of multiple other drugs. Alcohol also increases the mu-tagenicity of tobacco, thereby contributing to many cancers. Implicated in myriad nutritional deficiencies, organ abnormalities, and endocrinopathies, alcohol would appear to be a poor choice for human ingestion. Like many people, however, Sophia Hastings appears to use alcohol to reduce anxiety and decrease her behavioral inhibition. She and her therapist worry whether she is dependent on alcohol and worry about the possibility of withdrawal and delirium tremens. They are considering medication to reduce her alco-hol craving, and there is uncertainty over whether complete abstinence is preferable or necessary. Advances in neurobiology can inform their evalua-tion and treatment plan.

Four decades ago, it was thought that ethanol reduced neuronal activity by altering the fluidity of the cell membrane (Tan and Weaver 1997). In re-cent years, focus has shifted to alcohol's specific effects on subcellular activ-ity, with an emphasis on its effects on important neurotransmitters, certain brain regions, and neurogenesis.

Neurotransmitter Systems

The two most-implicated neurotransmitter receptors—NMDA (*N*-methyl-D-aspartate) and GABA$_A$—are important receptors for the brain's two most widespread neurotransmitters: glutamate and GABA (gamma-aminobutyric acid), respectively. Glutamate is an excitatory transmitter, whereas GABA is inhibitory.

Alcohol is a very potent antagonist of the NMDA receptor and a potent agonist of the $GABA_A$ receptor (Davis and Wu 2001). Both of these pharmacological actions translate into acute inhibition of neuronal activity, which would lead to diminished anxiety. Sophia Hastings reports this effect but also reports a need for increasing amounts of alcohol and exacerbation of anxiety when she is briefly abstinent. What is the mechanism for these effects?

In order to maintain normal neuronal excitation during chronic exposure to alcohol, the implicated transmitter systems undergo compensatory changes. For example, the chronic antagonism of the NMDA receptor leads to upregulation of the receptor (Narahashi et al. 2001), which leads to increased sensitivity of the brain to a lack of alcohol. In other words, when Ms. Hastings does not expose her brain to alcohol, her glutamatergic system becomes unusually active, leading to increased excitation and increased anxiety. Sudden withdrawal in someone with long-standing heavy alcohol exposure can lead the glutamatergic system to such a high state of activity that a seizure ensues. Similarly, alcohol's agonist effect on GABA leads to a downregulation of the $GABA_A$ receptor. Withdrawal following chronic use of alcohol leads to underactivity of the GABAergic system or a reduction in the inhibitory neurotransmitter, or to anxiety.

These compensatory changes in NMDA and $GABA_A$ can persist for several months (Kumar et al. 2003) and lead to a need for increasing amounts of alcohol to induce the same effect (i.e., tolerance) and side effects when the alcohol is stopped (i.e., withdrawal). These effects combine to make alcohol an acutely attractive and chronically devastating drug of abuse. These neurobiological findings enrich the dialogue about treatment. The common guideline of starting treatment with 3 months of abstinence (similar to the suggestion within AA for "90 meetings in 90 days") conforms to the finding that transmitter systems may take several months to normalize following chronic use. Similarly, the drug acamprosate may diminish alcohol craving by partially antagonizing NMDA receptors and enhancing the balance of the glutamate/GABA actions (Rammes et al. 2001).

Neurobiologic research is shedding increasing light on the details of these compensatory changes. For example, upregulation of the NMDA receptor may be mediated by an increase in glutamic acid release from presynaptic terminals or by sensitivity changes at the level of the NMDA receptor. The inhibition of NMDA response with chronic alcohol use appears to be secondary to alterations in the subunit composition of the NMDA receptor that is secondary to changes in subunit messenger ribonucleic acid (mRNA) expression; the newly formed receptors are either more sensitive to NMDA or less sensitive to ethanol (Narahashi et al. 2001). NMDA receptors have been shown to be necessary in certain learning and memory processes, which may explain the short-term memory problems that are pervasive in people with alcohol dependence.

Chronic exposure to alcohol leads to $GABA_A$ receptor adaptation through multiple mechanisms: gene expression, posttranslational modification, subcellular localization, synaptic localization, regulation by other receptor interactions, intracellular signaling, and neurosteroid responses to ethanol (Kumar et al. 2004). Other $GABA_A$ receptor modulators include benzodiazepines, barbiturates, and neuroactive steroids. The cross-tolerance between benzodiazepines and alcohol is likely the result of these molecular effects.

Direct Brain Effects

Alcohol damages specific neuronal populations such as the cerebellum, certain thalamic nuclei, and the hippocampus. The damage is especially severe following the ingestion of large amounts of alcohol in a short period of time. Such binge drinking can damage more neurons than steady drinking of even larger amounts of alcohol.

Alcohol seems to directly damage neurons through oxidative stress. Alcohol ingestion in large amounts generates *reactive oxygen species* (ROS), which damage DNA and key enzymes and may trigger apoptotic cell death. Recently, we have shown that alcohol can directly impair *neurogenesis* (Herrera et al. 2003). Neurogenesis is the process through which new neurons proliferate and differentiate. This process takes place throughout the life cycle, including in humans, most specifically in the dentate gyrus of the hippocampus. ROS produced by alcohol diminishes neurogenesis. Interestingly, neurogenesis is heavily implicated in the effectiveness of antidepressant medications (Santarelli et al. 2003), and it is likely that both depression and alcoholism have an adverse impact on neurogenesis. For these reasons, neurogenesis may be fundamental to the recovery from both disorders.

Although further research is needed, the biological basis for ethanol's effects on the brain is increasingly understood. In the case of Ms. Hastings, such research helps to explain alcohol's anti-anxiety effects, its overlap with the benzodiazepines, the effects of intoxication and withdrawal, and a variety of issues that relate to treatment, including the usefulness of abstinence. The complexity of the different mechanisms that mediate alcohol's effects is still an obstacle to effective treatments for alcoholism. Alcoholism occurs in individuals who have their own genetics, life histories, psychologies, and social context, and any evaluation must take this complexity into consideration. Nevertheless, advances in neurobiology have increasingly explained the clinical and therapeutic aspects of alcohol use and should prove increasingly helpful in more precisely targeting the treatments of the future.

Pharmacology of Anxiety

Smit S. Sinha, M.D.
Franklin Schneier, M.D.

IN approaching the issue of whether Sophia Hastings might benefit from pharmacotherapy, the clinician needs to consider whether she has a diagnosis or symptom cluster for which there is evidence for a specific intervention. In other words, judicious pharmacotherapy does not mean wholesale use of the pharmacopeia or the use of medications just because they are available. It is also helpful for the clinician to conceptualize anti-anxiety medications as an aid to the patient's own active efforts at recovery. These efforts should include either informal or professionally directed efforts at graduated self-exposure to feared situations and the practice of cognitive or relaxation strategies to manage anxiety symptoms. Treatment goals will vary with the individual patient, but it should be recognized that while the majority of persons with anxiety disorders will attain clinically meaningful improvement, complete remission is relatively uncommon.

While Ms. Hastings' specific diagnosis is uncertain, the intensity and duration of her symptoms indicates that she has an anxiety disorder. Social anxiety probably fits her best, though she also has significant panic attacks and some symptoms that are consistent with PTSD. As in many "real world" cases, her symptoms transcend a single diagnostic category. Such diagnostic uncertainty is not surprising given the substantial overlap that exists among the anxiety disorders with respect to both neurobiological underpinnings and pharmacological response profiles. Indeed, serotonin, norepinephrine, and neural network models of fear have been implicated to varying degrees in all the pathological anxiety conditions listed in the DSM-IV.

An initial approach to the pharmacotherapy of Ms. Hastings would be to target her social anxiety with panic attacks as the primary condition while being carefully mindful of her ongoing alcohol abuse. Currently, the most widely recognized first-line medication treatments for social anxiety disorder are the selective serotonin reuptake inhibitors (SSRIs). While SSRIs are more commonly linked to treatment of depression, there is abundant evidence linking serotonin to anxiety. For example, SSRIs have been shown to have clear anxiolytic effects resulting in increased social interaction among patients with social anxiety. Low levels of serotonin have also been found in subordinate primates who behave in ways that are akin to social fear in humans.

Given that Ms. Hastings has no medication history, a trial of one of the SSRIs is warranted. Equally effective for the generalized subtype of social anxiety disorder would be one of the serotonin-norepinephrine reuptake inhibitors (SNRIs), but she is also experiencing panic attacks, for which SSRIs are more effective. Panic patients tend to be sensitive to activation side effects such as jitteriness, however, and so the SSRI should be introduced at a very low dose and increased cautiously. A potential regimen for Ms. Hastings would be to start paroxetine (Paxil) at 10 mg/day, and the dosage would then be gradually increased to a maximum of 50 mg/day. If the medication is effective in reducing social anxiety and panic, Ms. Hastings should be encouraged to maintain it for at least 6–12 months. Not only do some patients expand their gains with extended treatment, earlier discontinuation increases the risk of relapse of both social anxiety and panic.

Ms. Hastings appears to use alcohol because of its powerful anti-anxiety effects. Her psychiatrist may decide to use one of the benzodiazepines to reduce her anxiety, especially during the weeks before the SSRI is likely to be effective. All of the benzodiazepines act through the GABAergic system to exert widespread inhibitory influence over several neurotransmitter systems implicated in the pathogenesis of diverse anxiety states. When used appropriately and under supervision, these medications are safe alternatives or adjuncts to typical antidepressant medications, and can be particularly useful for patients unable to tolerate antidepressant side effects. Benzodiazepines are highly effective for decreasing social anxiety and have marked anti-panic effects. Given their risk of physiological and psychological dependence, however, they are not considered first-line treatments for the anxiety disorders. In patients with social anxiety disorder or panic disorder who have no risk factors for substance abuse, a benzodiazepine such as clonazepam (Klonopin) can be initiated at a dosage of 0.25 mg bid, and the dosage can be increased every few days as tolerated by 0.5 mg per day to a target total daily dose of 2–4 mg. Such a suggestion is complicated with Ms. Hastings, who abuses alcohol and has a strong family history of abuse and dependence. Assuming she is not physiologically dependent on alcohol, clonazepam may be used to limit her anxiety and mild withdrawal symptoms, but the dosage should be tapered after the SSRI is introduced. The taper should be slow, on the order of a 0.25-mg reduction each week. Such a pace should allow the clinician to determine whether her symptoms can be managed by the SSRI and psychosocial interventions. It would not be unusual for episodes of panic to persist despite the resolution of much of her social anxiety. In that case, it might be prudent to prescribe an as-needed benzodiazepine that works quickly, such as 1 mg of lorazepam (Ativan). Because of the risk of ongoing abuse and dependence in a patient like Ms. Hastings, any benzodiazepine prescription mandates close monitoring and psychoeducation.

Although Ms. Hastings' personal and family histories do reduce the pharmacologic options, there are a variety of options if the initial SSRI is unsuccessful or only partially successful. The SSRI could be switched to an SNRI such as venlafaxine (Effexor), which is an effective first-line agent for social anxiety and an effective second-line anti-panic agent. If consecutive 8- to 12-week trials are inadequately effective, different classes of medications should be considered.. The anticonvulsants gabapentin (Neurontin) and pregabalin (Lyrica) have each shown efficacy for social anxiety disorder. Tricyclic antidepressants such as imipramine, though largely ineffective for social anxiety, are remarkably effective anti-panic drugs that could be considered if Ms. Hastings' social anxiety improves but the panic persists. Monoamine oxidase inhibitors (MAOIs) are also effective for social anxiety, but they carry the risk of hypertensive crisis if patients fail to follow a strict low-tyramine diet that excludes certain alcoholic beverages and aged foods. MAOIs could only be considered for Ms. Hastings after a prolonged period of sobriety.

Cognitive-Behavioral Therapy

Susan Evans, Ph.D.

WHILE Sophia Hastings' alcohol abuse should be addressed immediately, cognitive-behavioral therapy (CBT) can teach skills and strategies that would help her more effectively manage her anxiety. CBT is based on the tenet that emotional and behavioral responses are shaped by patterns of thought and, more specific to Ms. Hastings, that anxiety is precipitated by the appraisal of a stimulus as dangerous.

Psychoeducation is the first, critical step in the treatment of anxiety disorders. It is essential that Ms. Hastings understand that her thoughts affect her emotions, her bodily reactions, and her avoidance behavior. Patients often feel better by simply understanding the pattern of their symptoms, and so the initial phase of treatment would focus on identifying patterns that are specific for Ms. Hastings. The initial phase of CBT also makes use of *relaxation skills*. These include progressive relaxation, diaphragmatic breathing, and guided imagery. All of these can be taught and practiced in sessions. For example, guided imagery might involve Ms. Hastings envisioning herself calm and confident in the teacher's lounge.

As Ms. Hastings begins to understand her anxiety and some ways to deal with it, treatment would continue to clarify the automatic thoughts that contribute to the anxiety or embarrassment. Ms. Hastings might think, "People will see I'm nervous," followed by, "And if they see I'm nervous, they'll think there's something wrong with me." Further, she is likely to doubt that she has adequate resources to handle the perceived threat. These thoughts and expectations put her body's alarm system on alert so that her "fight-flight response" releases adrenalin, which contributes to a cascade of reactions that are emotional (e.g., anxiety), physiologic (e.g., palpitations, sweating, tension), and behavioral (e.g., avoidance, use of safety behaviors). A clear understanding of the cycle of the thoughts, feelings, and behaviors that lead to the cycle of anxiety is critical for the creation of a treatment that depends on *cognitive restructuring* and *behavioral desensitization*. Central to CBT is an accurate assessment of this cycle. In the first couple of sessions, the therapist would get a detailed accounting of the frequency and nature of Ms. Hastings anxiety attacks. When she enters the teacher's lounge, what does she physically experience? What goes through her mind at that moment? The immediate goal is to link her emotional, physiologic, and behavioral response to these automatic thoughts.

Consider a hypothetical dialogue:

Therapist: What were you feeling when you went into the teacher's lounge yesterday?

Ms. H: I felt really nervous and scared.

T: Were you having any physical sensations?

Ms. H: I felt my heart was racing, bounding out of my chest. I felt like I was gasping for air; my throat was all clogged up. It was horrible.

T: What do you think was going through your mind in that moment?

Ms. H: I don't know, I just felt scared.

T: Take a minute and ask yourself what you were thinking when you went into the teacher's lounge.

Ms. H: Initially, that everyone seemed to be enjoying themselves.

T: And then what did you think?

Ms. H: It's hard to remember but I may have thought that I didn't belong. I got so nervous that I started to think I might faint or something and make a complete fool of myself.

In the case of Ms. Hastings, a panic sequence might be conceptualized as in Figure 8–1.

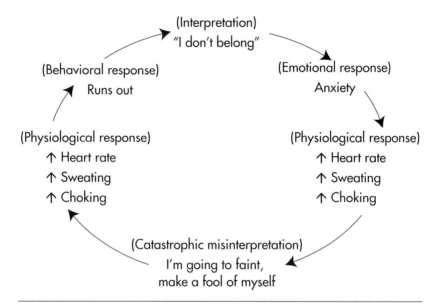

FIGURE 8–1.   Panic cycle.

Stimulus: Walks into the teacher's lounge and automatically thinks, "I don't belong here."

As the panic sequence becomes clear, the therapist would help Ms. Hastings examine the accuracy of her interpretations and assumptions. The *Dysfunctional Thought Record* (DTR) could help patients capture automatic thoughts, critically examine them, and restructure the thinking more realistically. Figure 8–2 is an example of a DTR that might have been completed by Ms. Hastings a few weeks into her treatment.

Situation	Automatic thought	Emotion	Adaptive response	Outcome
Walk into teacher's lounge	I don't belong	Anxious	I teach here, so I belong here as much as anyone else.	Anxious
		100%	It makes me nervous to talk to people I don't know, but I can try to meet one person—ask them how they like the school, what grade they're teaching	60%
				Spoke to another teacher

FIGURE 8–2.   Example of a Dysfunctional Thought Record that might have been completed by Ms. Hastings a few weeks into her treatment.

The therapist would help Ms. Hastings better understand the automatic thoughts through a series of questions. "What's the evidence this thought is true?" "Is there another way of looking at this?" "What would I tell a friend who had this thought?" Laid out clearly, these thought patterns will likely appear dysfunctional to the patient and lead to cognitive restructuring. As she recognizes that catastrophic distortions contribute to panic, she will learn techniques to think her way through situations by asking herself, "What's the worst that can happen?" "What's the best case scenario?" and "What's the most likely outcome?"

Role-playing is a useful example of *social skills training* in which adaptive responses are reinforced, rehearsed, and modeled. For example, the therapist might play the role of Ms. Hastings and start a conversation with a hypothetical co-teacher. The two could then shift roles so that Ms. Hastings could practice and prepare for actually entering the faculty lounge.

After this initial phase of therapy, Ms. Hastings would use these core CBT principles and skills in the real world through exposure exercises and behavioral experiments. The first step would be to grade a set of social situations from least to the most anxiety provoking. Ms. Hastings' *graded hierarchy* might appear as shown in Figure 8–3.

Percent anxiety	Situation
10	Asking for help in a department store
40	Calling up a friend from college
70	Starting up a conversation in teacher's lounge
100	Going out on a blind date without self-medicating

FIGURE 8–3. Example of how Ms. Hastings' graded hierarchy might appear.

Ms. Hastings and her therapist would focus first on the least anxiety-producing exposure—asking for help in department store—and then apply the skills that had been learned, including cognitive rehearsal, social skills training, and relaxation techniques. Success with low-anxiety stimuli reinforces confidence and affords the opportunity of practicing the techniques. She is likely to greet her familiar, disabling anxiety with the thought "I can do this."

Ms. Hastings could receive a course of CBT while taking medications and receiving other forms of psychotherapy, including exploratory psychotherapy and treatment for substance abuse. CBT is generally acceptable to patients, as indicated by attrition rates that are significantly lower than found in medication studies for panic (Butler et al. 2006; Haby et al. 2006). Toward the end of treatment—which typically lasts approximately 20 sessions—Ms. Hastings and her therapist would outline a treatment plan to help her make use of the cognitive and behavioral skills that she learned in treatment. Monthly booster sessions are often useful to review progress and address relapses, while a more exploratory therapy may help her deal with issues that continue to bother her.

Panic-Focused Psychodynamic Psychotherapy

Fredric N. Busch, M.D.

PSYCHOANALYSTS have generally approached the various anxiety disorders with nonspecific exploratory and interpretive techniques. Psychodynamic models have led to more focused treatments of anxiety and panic and even to manuals of dynamic therapy (Milrod et al. 1997; Wiborg and Dahl 1996) with demonstrated efficacy (Milrod et al. 2007). One psychodynamic model integrated neurophysiological vulnerabilities, findings from psychological research, and clinical experience (Busch et al. 1991; Shear et al. 1993). According to this model, individuals susceptible to developing panic disorder have a fear of unfamiliar situations based on neurophysiological vulnerabilities or traumatic developmental experiences. This fear causes them to feel dependent on parents or caretakers to provide a sense of safety, leading them to being especially vulnerable to emotional or physical separations or disruptions.

Psychodynamic models of social anxiety, to the extent they have been developed, overlap with this formulation for panic disorder, with internal fears of rejection and abandonment informing the experience of social situations (Busch and Milrod 2004).

Psychodynamic therapy would likely be quite helpful to Sophia Hastings, who appears to be fearfully dependent. Her illness began, or at least intensified, when she separated from her mother. Her childhood background, while described as "colorful," was chaotic. It is likely she would have been unable to depend on adults for safety and would have chronic fears of abandonment. It is also likely that she would have felt episodic anger at her mother and other caretakers for their substance abuse and likely unpredictable, unsafe behavior. Such powerful, painful feelings would have threatened the child's relationship with all-important caretakers, since expressions of need and/or anger could lead to abandonment.

People tend to use characteristic mechanisms to keep such unpleasant feelings out of their consciousness. According to psychoanalytic theory, these memories and conflicts remain present in the unconscious, however, and create anxiety when situations or internal experiences threaten to bring them into consciousness. In regard to Ms. Hastings, it is likely that she uses clusters of defenses that are typically found in people with anxiety and panic. For example, she describes few childhood memories, which is consistent with *repression,* a defense mechanism in which painful memories or frightening fantasies are kept out of consciousness. A related defense mechanism in panic disorder is *denial,* in which patients deny the presence of angry or dependent feelings and fantasies, which remain unconscious (Busch et al. 1995).

Fearful dependency and a perceived inability to independently manage situations lead to an ongoing, humiliating narcissistic injury. This intolerable internal state is projected onto the parent, who is then seen as unreliable. The child may also become angry at the parents' perceived or actual critical or rejecting behavior. Anger and angry fantasies trigger additional problems: not only might anger drive the needed parent away, but hostile, angry feelings toward a beloved parent also lead to guilt. These emotional states can cycle into one another, intensifying anxiety and inducing panic.

Difficulty expressing anger can lead to another defense mechanism that is typically found in panic patients, *reaction formation,* in which a feeling or associated behavior that is felt to be threatening is converted into its opposite. The presence of this defense mechanism is indicated by her description of her mother and boyfriends as "colorful," her recurrent efforts to "bail them out," and her ongoing, nightly phone calls with her mother. She makes all of these helpful efforts without the resentment that would be seen in the average-expectable person.

In addition to denial, repression, and reaction formation, Ms. Hastings may make use of *undoing,* a defense mechanism in which a threatening feeling is "taken back" as a way to make amends. For example, Ms. Hastings might say, "I hate my mother, but I really love her." Another defense is *somatization,* in which patients become preoccupied with something being wrong with their bodies, displaced from fears about feelings or fantasies. These defense mechanisms, however, are not entirely effective. By denying anger and anxiety, people are unable to successfully address their frustrations or fears. Further, defenses can lead to an intensification of unpleasant feelings, since they can lead people to helping and/or depending upon people at whom they are unconsciously angry.

Given this psychodynamic understanding, Ms. Hastings' therapy would focus on exploring her fears related to separation and anger, with particular focus on her defense mechanisms. For instance, Ms. Hastings might say that she is annoyed that she has to call her mother every night but undo that feeling of anger by adding, "but at least she's going to AA." The therapist could point out that the anger appears to have triggered some discomfort, a comment that might lead Ms. Hastings to discuss her chaotic early life as well as her feelings about her absent father and the presence of her mother's drug-abusing boyfriends. Exploration of her feelings regarding loss, separation, and safety might help her identify feelings of resentment and might also lead to the recognition that dependency and resentment do not necessarily disrupt relationships. If Ms. Hastings continued to deny anger at her mother, the therapist might point out that someone in her position would likely be angry at her mother but suggest that it might be difficult to experience anger given her fears about the safety of her attachment. Implicit in this theory is that the unconscious defenses that she developed in order to survive are now causing more harm than good.

In identifying the psychodynamic origins of panic, the therapist and patient would explore the nature of specific panic symptoms as well as the circumstances, feelings, and stressors surrounding panic onset. Ms. Hastings says her panic and anxiety began during college, implying issues related to separation. In addition, the panic seems to intensify around men, indicating the possibility of anger and separation fears related to sexuality and the absence of a consistent father figure. The therapist would likely theorize that Ms. Hastings' chaotic childhood put her at risk for verbal, physical, and/or sexual abuse, and would use this tentative formulation in the tactful exploration of Ms. Hastings' relationships with her mother, her mother's boyfriends, and men to whom she had become attached.

As the therapy develops, it is likely that Ms. Hastings would experience increasing trust in the therapist and the process of treatment. This sense of trust might allow her to explore previously uncharted parts of her life, which can be exhilarating but can also intensify her anxiety. While the overall trend might be increasing feelings of calm, periods of discomfort should be expected. Rather than reflecting relapse or therapeutic stalemate, such anxious moments can be important clues and opportunities. These moments offer opportunities to explore, for example, transference, in which feelings about the therapist reflect earlier experience. Ms. Hastings might become, for example, fearful of the therapy or therapist, which might reflect her earlier concerns related to her home situation. Similarly, she might become anxious about angry feelings toward the therapist. The effectiveness of the treatment will depend at least partly on her experiencing the anger and anxiety without losing the connection to the therapist.

Psychodynamic manuals have been developed that attempt to more precisely capture the nature of the therapeutic experience and to provide a blueprint that allows for replicable research into treatment of specific disorders. One such manual led to a randomized controlled trial that focused on the likelihood of relapse in panic disorder. When 3 months of weekly psychodynamic therapy were added to the antidepressant clomipramine, the risk of panic relapse at 18 months was reduced from 91% to 9% (Wiborg and Dahl 1996). A second manualized approach is *panic-focused psychodynamic psychotherapy* (PFPP) (Milrod et al. 1997), which was explicitly based on the psychodynamic model outlined above. PFPP has shown a high rate of remission in panic in an open trial (Milrod et al. 2000, 2001) and was found in a randomized controlled trial to be superior to a less active treatment, applied relaxation therapy (Milrod et al. 2007).

Regardless of whether or not the treatment takes into account one of the above manuals, a therapist who explores Ms. Hastings' conflicts and fears with tactful, nonjudgmental, empathic curiosity can help her become more comfortable with previously unpalatable feelings and fantasies. These explorations can lead Ms. Hastings to reduced symptoms of anxiety and panic through a lifting of repression and denial, greater honesty with herself, and an increasing tolerance of unpleasant feelings, thoughts, and memories.

Part B

AT the conclusion of a two-session evaluation, the consulting psychiatrist diagnosed Sophia Hastings with alcohol abuse and social anxiety disorder. It was not clear whether she might also have an avoidant personality disorder on Axis II. The patient had no known medical problems. Initial lab work revealed several values just outside the normal range, including a low magnesium level, elevation of her red blood cell mean corpuscular volume, and an elevated aspartate aminotransferase—values that were consistent with alcohol abuse. There were no other abnormalities, and the thyroid panel was normal. She had no known medical illnesses. Her primary psychosocial stressor was her isolation, and she was seen to be functioning with mild to moderate impairment. The psychiatrist assessed her risk of suicide to be low.

The most pressing initial issue was the possibility of alcohol withdrawal. Given her lack of serious withdrawal phenomena in the past and her recent history of having twice been able to abruptly stop all alcohol for 1 week, the psychiatrist decided that it would probably not be physiologically necessary to do a detoxification. At the same time, the psychiatrist was attentive to the possibility that she could still have significant withdrawal problems.

The initial treatment plan was marked by a series of negotiations. Sophia and the psychiatrist agreed on goals, and the patient appeared genuinely motivated to eliminate alcohol use, reduce her anxiety, and increase her ability to socialize and date. She was willing to learn techniques to reduce anxiety (e.g., breathing, muscle relaxation, and visualization) and appeared interested in learning how anxiety can cause physiologic changes and panic. Ms. Hastings agreed to attend weekly psychotherapy sessions to meet these goals. While she said she wanted to stop drinking, she was unwilling to go to AA meetings, explaining that groups made her anxious. She was also unwilling to discontinue her alcohol without adjunctive "anxiety pills," but she did agree to start sertraline (Zoloft), which would aim to reduce her anxiety after several weeks. Clonazepam (Klonopin) was begun at a dosage of 0.25 mg twice daily, but Ms. Hastings rapidly increased this dose to 1 mg twice or three times daily. She did not, however, drink alcohol after the first evaluation session, and her therapist decided that this dose was an acceptable starting point for a gradual taper.

The therapist's own reactions were quite positive toward the patient. Eager to please and cheerful, the patient praised the therapist's efforts, and unlike most people who abuse alcohol, she became abstinent on day one. The therapist silently hypothesized that Ms. Hastings' immediate discontinuation of alcohol was akin to her perfect school attendance and that such compliance might be somehow linked to her chaotic childhood and anxiety. The therapist also noticed that Sophia was quite attractive and endearing, qualities that would complicate her twin desires of becoming intimate with men and avoiding the anxiety that is precipitated by intimacy with men.

During the initial sessions, the psychiatrist discussed the cycles that appeared to contribute to Sophia's anxiety. Most obviously, the alcohol reduced her anxiety enough so that she could engage socially, but escalating dosages led to recurrent mild withdrawals with exacerbations of her anxiety and tremulousness. This cycle of intoxication would not address underlying psychological or physiologic issues that contributed to the anxiety, would reduce the likelihood that she would learn techniques to manage anxiety, and appeared to have led to impulsive sexual behavior that was likely to have made her feel worse about herself. Clarification of this cycle led to efforts to reduce anxiety through breathing exercises, visualization, and muscle relaxation exercises.

A second anxiety cycle was elaborated between the patient and therapist over the first few sessions. In that cycle, it appeared that Sophia would enter a potentially stressful situation like the teacher's lounge and have an automatic thought that would induce the sensation of anxiety, which would lead, in turn, to a physiologic response, a catastrophic misinterpretation of those physical sensations, an exacerbation of those sensations, and a need to flee the situation. Not only did this series of events conform to a classic CBT paradigm that allowed for a series of therapeutic interventions, but clarification of the cycle helped reduce her sense that the panic was inexplicable and completely out of her control.

Several months into therapy, many of the initial goals had been met through the focus on alcohol abuse and CBT strategies for anxiety. The sertraline was gradually increased to 150 mg in the morning (higher doses led to an exacerbation of anxiety); the clonazepam was tapered and discontinued; and as-needed quetiapine (Seroquel) was begun at low doses for episodic insomnia and exacerbations of anxiety. The use of relaxation techniques and the development of a graded hierarchy and a series of efforts at exposure therapy led to a significant diminution of her anxiety while teaching and while at home. She remained unable to date men, however, and her out-of-school activities remained minimal. At this point, Sophia said she was satisfied with having eliminated the constant feelings of panicky anxiety and the alcohol abuse. She asked whether it would be okay to stop treatment.

During these months, the therapist had tried to develop a more complete understanding of the development of Sophia's anxiety. This effort had been significantly stymied by the patient's apparently minimal interest in her childhood and her general reluctance to explore issues that were not directly related to practical interventions. The therapist felt certain that there would be more to her story than simply a recollection that the mother and her series of boyfriends were "colorful," but Sophia insisted that there was nothing more to report. The therapist wondered about the extent to which the patient was repressing and denying important experiences from her childhood. The therapist also noticed that Sophia never seemed overtly angry. Instead, she would describe a scenario in which she had been taken advantage of, pause, and blithely move on to another story. As these stories were told regularly, the therapist began to feel protective of the patient, angry for her, and frustrated that the patient would then deny any strong feelings about the situation. When the therapist would occasionally make a mistake, such as lateness or a delayed telephone call, it seemed notable that the patient would be effusively gracious and nonblaming. The therapist had recurrently linked Sophia's experiences with feelings and reactions that seemed likely, such as anger, but the patient appeared uninterested.

The therapist wondered about Sophia's use of denial, repression, and reaction formation, hypothesizing that these defenses were linked to her anxiety and that they had been ingrained since childhood. The therapist went on to silently hypothesize that Sophia had needed to defend against childhood feelings of anger and dependency that had been too intense for her at the time. It seemed likely that Sophia's childhood experiences had been significantly more traumatic than she had been admitting (or remembering), and it seemed to the therapist that her request to stop the treatment was a way to discontinue a painful process, keep the therapist safely away, and reassure herself that authority figures were unhelpful (an unhappy belief, but one that would fit with a repetition compulsion in which people repeat traumatic events in order to unconsciously deal with them).

To the request to discontinue treatment, the therapist said that they had a choice. They could stop. They could reduce sessions from once per week to monthly and continue to focus on CBT and relaxation exercises. They could continue once per week and try to focus more intensely on social anxiety. The therapist recommended, however, that they increase sessions to twice weekly and try to treat more of the underlying issues that were contributing to the anxiety. The therapist offered this recommendation with some hesitation. Such a suggestion might be an abuse of Sophia's tendency to do what was expected of her, and the therapist did not want to be overly intrusive or controlling. Further, it was not clear whether Sophia would be able to tolerate the intense feelings that would be aroused by a more exploratory therapy. At the same time, a less intensive treatment seemed likely to lead this young woman to being forever shackled by her fears.

Sophia agreed to both the increase in sessions and shift in focus, and they began a more open-ended, exploratory therapy. This change was met with a phase of wariness, but Sophia gradually became more able to discuss situations of loneliness and anxiety that were related to both her current life and childhood. During these descriptions, she would frequently appear distracted and scared, though all feelings were generally denied, even after being pointed out by the therapist. Most of her tumultuous childhood memories were fuzzy, as if Sophia, herself, had "been on the acid trip." She said she had decided to be a teacher because school had always seemed clean and predictable. She could describe most current experiences with clarity and dispassion unless they related to chaotic scenes or men who made advances to her. She expressed minimal curiosity into transference phenomena, even when they seemed obvious to the therapist. The therapist's own feelings included protectiveness, an irritation over the patient's lack of curiosity, and a desire to encourage Sophia into seeking out a sexual, intimate relationship. At other times, the therapist felt distanced and numb. Each of these responses felt unusually intense and induced a sense of chagrin and hesitation and some consideration as to whether or not the patient was suited for an exploratory therapy. This feeling of uncertainty would sometimes lead the therapist to discuss medications or a CBT technique such as a breathing exercise, a tendency that she assumed was both reasonable (these interventions were continued throughout the treatment) and a reflection of countertransference (a lack of confidence in her psychotherapy technique in the face of a distancing patient).

After a year of treatment, the patient announced that she had gone on two dates with one of her fellow teachers. A third date was planned for the evening of that session. The therapist was not surprised by this after-the-fact announcement, since Sophia had a tendency to report her experiences rather then discuss her plans, a tendency that the therapist assumed reflected her fears of closeness. Choosing to support the patient's efforts, the therapist shifted to a discussion of strategies on how Sophia could calm her anxiety as well as some discussion of Sophia's thoughts and feelings about the dates and the young man. For the first time in her treatment, the patient canceled the next two sessions.

When Sophia came for her session the following week, she said that she had canceled because she wasn't feeling good, but when the therapist asked about the date with the fellow teacher, Sophia paused and became pale. In a hushed voice, she said, "When we started to fool around, I just panicked. I had to escape even though it was in the middle of the night, and he was upset and everything." She had been miserable ever since, saying she couldn't "get away from the feeling." She had missed therapy sessions because it was "just too much." Interspersed within long stretches of silence, she said she couldn't sleep and was having bad dreams. She said her stomach hurt all the time and that she kept seeing one specific image, that of the lamp on the desk that was in her room while she was growing up. She whispered the word *he* several times but did not finish her sentence. Hunched in her chair, appearing miserable, Sophia sat quietly with her eyes closed.

While Sophia had long denied any sort of childhood trauma, this episode convinced the psychiatrist that the patient had been sexually abused. As that became clear to the therapist, the patient quietly said that she needed to quit therapy. The therapist made several comments that were intended to be supportive, but Sophia gradually doubled further over in her chair and quietly trembled. She whispered, "He can hear us," and then lapsed back into silence. Fifteen minutes before the session was to end, the patient got up to leave. The therapist felt an unusual surge of desperation and protectiveness. As the patient walked by, the therapist gently touched her arm and asked her to stay. Sophia appeared distracted and terrified, began choking and gagging, and slid to the ground.

The therapist felt inclined to reach down and help Sophia back to her chair but stopped, quickly recognizing that the collapse was induced by the touch on the arm and the request to stay when she felt that she needed to leave. Feeling powerless and guilty, the therapist paused and quietly apologized for not having been adequately protective. While Ms. Hastings sat cross legged on the floor with her head in her hands, the therapist explained that they would work this out together, that they had gotten to an important point in the treatment, that Sophia had been dealing with this by herself for a long time, and that they would try to make this effort as safe as possible. After 10 minutes, Sophia went back to her chair and appeared to gradually become more alert and was able to leave the office under her own volition.

Summary

Sophia Hastings' initial complaint of anxiety led to treatment of her alcohol abuse, as well as pharmacotherapy, CBT, and psychodynamic psychotherapy. As her symptoms improved over the course of a year, she was able to begin dating for the first time. A crisis developed when sexual involvement reactivated memories of childhood abuse. In the following discussions, the discussants explore the after effects of child sexual abuse as well as some of the countertransference difficulties that typically arise when working with this population of patients.

Discussions of the Case of
Sophia Hastings, Part B

After Effects of Sexual Abuse 328
    Daniel S. Schechter, M.D., and Erica Willheim, Ph.D.

Overview of Countertransference. .332
    John W. Barnhill, M.D.

Summary Points 336

After Effects of Sexual Abuse

Daniel S. Schechter, M.D.
Erica Willheim, Ph.D.

AFTER a year of treatment, Sophia Hastings panics in the context of sexual involvement with a fellow teacher and then appears to reexperience childhood sexual trauma during the ensuing therapy session. While the possibility of a traumatic childhood was considered throughout her treatment, Ms. Hastings consistently denied abuse. How might the childhood sexual abuse have been identified earlier, and how should this history affect the diagnosis and treatment?

In patients presenting with a wide array of symptoms but no report of early sexual abuse, the assessment of sexual trauma rests upon the clinician's understanding of traumatic sequelae and careful attention to the available material. Since symptoms such as depression, substance abuse, anxiety, panic attacks, phobias, eating disorders, and self-harming behaviors are not specific to trauma alone, their comorbid presentation frequently leads clinicians to make a number of discrete diagnoses that may overlook a triggering traumatic experience or set of experiences, and/or a related primary diagnosis of posttraumatic stress disorder (PTSD) (van der Kolk et al. 2005).

Linking symptoms to adverse experiences can organize seemingly disparate and randomly acquired comorbid conditions into a coherent constellation of trauma-associated psychobiological reactions and meaningful psychological symptoms. This process of clarification requires a patient and open-minded approach that confronts posttraumatic avoidance but avoids "leading the witness" during the clinical interview.

A diagnosis of PTSD, as found in DSM-IV-TR (American Psychiatric Association 2000), requires at least one precipitating event wherein the patient experiences or witnesses a life-threatening event that creates overwhelming feelings of fear and helplessness, and then a temporal link between the event(s) and the symptoms. The diagnosis of PTSD includes symptoms across three categories: increased arousal, avoidance and numbing, and reexperiencing. When trauma occurs in an interpersonal context and repeatedly over time, it may result in complex PTSD (Herman 1992). The sequelae of complex PTSD include such additional symptoms as chronic somatization, substance abuse, dissociative phenomena, traumatic reenactment (which often includes self-harm or harm by others), feelings of self-hatred and disgust, and impaired interpersonal relationships (traumatic bonding).

Ms. Hastings is initially referred to treatment because she is experiencing anxiety and an array of somatic symptoms that have no apparent physiological basis. While nonspecific to a history of trauma, these somatic symptoms are commonly found posttraumatically. Breuer and Freud (1895) emphasized shortness of breath and choking sensations as "hysterical" symptoms commonly associated with sexual abuse or overstimulation within their "seduction theory." The patient's description of "always being on edge" can be construed as generalized anxiety, but Ms. Hastings may be describing her experience of chronic posttraumatic hyperarousal. Additionally, the circumstances of Ms. Hastings' early history—her substance-abusing mother and the presence of "multiple boyfriends"—should immediately alert the clinician to a high-risk environment with the potential for early childhood abuse. We know that children who live with a chronically substance-abusing caregiver are at relatively high risk for maltreatment (abuse and/or neglect) and/or family violence exposure (Anda et al. 2002). Research also suggests that sexually abused girls frequently have disturbed relationships with their mothers that can complicate subsequent caregiving relationships (Schechter et al. 2002).

While certainly not definitive, posttraumatic avoidance is suggested by Ms. Hastings' graduation from a women's college, employment at an all-girls school, and lack of dating. Such avoidance would reduce exposure to external cues that cause conscious or unconscious recollection of the overwhelming affects that occurred during the original trauma. When we then hear that the presence of "romantically appropriate" men increases anxiety and somatic symptoms, that the onset of symptoms occurred in anticipation of a fraternity party, and that discomfort is experienced in the coed teacher's lounge where social interaction is unstructured, we are reminded that avoiding interactions with men is a common posttraumatic response to abuse by a male perpetrator. "Appropriate" men—with their potential for intimate involvement—become traumatic reminders of the original abuse experience and therefore must be avoided. As we see in the case of Ms. Hastings, symptoms of anxiety break through when avoidance is not possible.

Ms. Hastings' history of a "dozen one-night stands" is evocative. Freud's original notion of "remembering, repeating, and working through" trauma (Freud 1914) encourages us to question whether the patient was drawn to repeat (reexperience) the original sexual trauma in order to master the experienced helplessness. Alcohol would have numbed her from the associated affects of shame, rage, anxiety, and excitement. Further, the fact that Ms. Hastings had never had a sexual encounter while sober is perhaps one of the strongest indicators of early sexual abuse. The comorbidity of substance abuse and PTSD in patients with histories of childhood sexual abuse has been well documented and frequently overlaps with severe borderline spectrum personality disorders (Zanarini et al. 1998, 2006). Although substance abuse by both of Ms. Hastings' parents certainly indicates a genetic vulnerability to addiction, the presence of PTSD alone is a powerful risk factor for substance abuse. Benzodiazepines, cocaine, and alcohol are often used to numb or self-medicate PTSD symptoms. The disinhibition resulting from intoxication typically leads the patient into risky or dangerous situations in which she may be retraumatized as we see with Ms. Hastings' one-night stands and driving drunk. The ensuing PTSD from the secondary traumatization then fuels continued substance abuse. Ms. Hastings' abuse of alcohol is complex, then, and while most practitioners would agree the substance abuse should be addressed early in therapy, an exclusive focus on substance abuse or even on anxiety typically ends in relapse for such patients. Treatment strategies for substance abusers with a history of sexual abuse have been developed that emphasize the treatment of the underlying trauma in order for the patient to successfully maintain sobriety (Najavits 2002). In addition, selective serotonin reuptake inhibitors (SSRIs) can help alcoholic patients with comorbid anxiety, depression, and PTSD symptoms.

Further clues to the early origins of Ms. Hastings' symptom picture are found in the story that she saw a school psychologist at age 15 after it was discovered that she had written "I hate me" in her diary. Feelings of self-hatred, disgust, loathing, and blame are commonly held by traumatized individuals, and particularly by sexually abused children. The rage felt at the perpetrator, and often at the caregiver who failed to keep them safe, is turned inward upon the self in order to preserve the illusion of good protective caregivers (Fairbairn 1952). Ms. Hastings' discontinuation of that earlier treatment and her initial "obvious discomfort" in the current psychiatrist's office point to the avoidance of a therapeutic relationship that would involve the confrontation of traumatic memories and associated affects.

Ms. Hastings recalls little of her childhood, which is consistent with traumatic amnesia for early sexual abuse. Williams (1994) documented that 38% of women with emergency room admissions for childhood sexual abuse had amnesia for the event 17 years later. The appearance of being "distracted" and "scared" when trying to recall childhood memories further suggests to the clinician that dissociative processes are at work. The question is also raised as to whether Ms. Hastings does in fact remember certain events but avoids and withdraws in order to not become flooded by negative affect.

At the 1-year mark, the content of the final session elucidates and confirms the clinician's hypothesis of early sexual abuse. Ms. Hastings goes on a third date with a fellow teacher and panics when there is sexual involvement.

Likely her first sexual encounter experienced while sober, the experience apparently triggered painful, traumatic memories. She subsequently misses two sessions, signaling her avoidance of both the intolerable trauma-related affect that therapy would certainly have elicited and the unknown response of the therapist. When she does return to therapy, she recounts a dramatic increase in PTSD symptoms, with insomnia (hyperarousal), nightmares (reexperiencing), and somatization. Most telling is her recollection of the lamp on the desk in her childhood room. Experiences of derealization are common during the event of sexual abuse. In one frequent scenario, the child dissociatively fixates on one object in the room. Such dissociative experiences often remain as long-held screen memories for the traumatic event. Person and Klar (1994) have written that "trauma must be told" and if not in words, then through reenactment. When Ms. Hastings whispers, "He," she experiences overwhelming anxiety. She repeatedly fails to finish the sentence, expresses her need to stop treatment, and attempts to flee from the session. She appears "distracted, terrified, ill" as her defenses fail, and she is flooded by traumatic memory. Ms. Hastings maintains only a fragile hold on reality and collapses when the psychiatrist touches her arm with an intention of keeping her in the room. She is reliving the trauma, complete with the physiological sensations of choking and gagging and the perceptual belief that "he can hear us." This may well be a form of "flashback," which would be a reexperiencing symptom that is pathognomonic of PTSD. The seeming loss of time-and-space continuity is also consistent with dissociative phenomena, which are commonly associated with chronic, complex PTSD. Such dissociative phenomena may protect the psyche against the actuality or memory of overwhelming, life-threatening experience at the expense of an integrated autobiographical memory. When her usual psychological defenses fail and the trauma is fully reexperienced, Ms. Hastings loses consciousness.

By the time of the crisis, Ms. Hastings has received a series of treatments that have helped with her alcohol abuse, social anxiety, and panic. Even though Ms. Hastings consistently denied abuse, her earlier treatments appear to have been successful, perhaps because each of those clinicians considered the possibility of abuse and were sensitive to her need to proceed at a pace that she controlled. Since fear and helplessness activate the symptomatology for which she is seeking help, early work would ideally have explored how she feels in the consultation room, how she feels in her own body in the here-and-now, how to identify initial sensations of anxiety, and how to use relaxation, breathing, and muscle relaxation techniques to increase affect regulation. In short, patients like Ms. Hastings must be helped to establish a sense of safety within the therapeutic relationship and within herself—namely, the capacity to internally manage negative affect in order that she not flee from treatment when traumatic material finally emerges.

Overview of Countertransference

John W. Barnhill, M.D.

SOPHIA Hastings' diagnosis and treatment evolve during her year in therapy, and while she winds up on the floor, stricken into what appears to be a dissociative re-creation of childhood sexual abuse, she appears to have improved significantly and seems to be on the way to further gains. One way to understand the complexity of this case is through an exploration of the therapist's own reactions to Ms. Hastings. Also known as countertransference, the therapist's internal response influences the initial diagnosis and treatment plan, heavily informs many of the moment-to-moment interactions between the two people in the room, and can provide invaluable insight into the patient's inner experience. Countertransference can also lead the therapist into errors, enactments, and a neglect of the person who has come for treatment.

Immediate countertransference reactions depend on the gender, theoretical background, and professional experiences of the therapist, as well as on the fit between the clinician and patient and the therapist's own personality and acute personal issues. For example, within moments of entering the consulting room for the first time, Ms. Hastings might elicit a variety of reactions. One therapist might dismiss her as a substance-abusing woman prone to denial and avoidance. Another therapist might find himself physically attracted to her, while a third might find herself competitive. Does the clinician "need" the patient, perhaps for financial or training purposes? Is the therapist feeling acutely bereft so that the treatment of Ms. Hastings might fill a hole that has been created by death, divorce, or separation from a child, lover, or friend?

These feelings can influence the treatment in a number of ways. For example, a therapist who feels a powerful need to work with Ms. Hastings might avoid the topic of substance abuse and/or prescribe increasing doses of clonazepam. A clinician who feels irritated by—or attracted to—Ms. Hastings might insist on immediate alcohol abstinence without adjunctive medication for her anxiety. Such a decision might be reasonable, but it might also lead the patient to discomfort, mistrust, and a premature termination that leads, in turn, to self-righteous surprise in the clinician. Knowing that Ms. Hastings shies away from sexualized situations, the therapist may avoid personal information and intimate connection. Or, if annoyed, provoked, or intrigued, the therapist might become intrusive in a way that resembles the behavior of the men who Ms. Hastings encountered as a child. Countertransference can, therefore, distort the therapeutic alliance, the creation of an accurate diagnosis, and an optimal treatment plan.

The therapist writes, "Sophia was quite attractive and endearing." We do not know either the gender or sexual orientation of the therapist, but we are being told not only that the patient is likable and potentially sexually appealing but also that the therapist has shifted from calling her "Ms. Hastings" to the more familiar and intimate, "Sophia." These are relatively meager revelations, however, and we gain immediate access to few initial feelings toward the patient. These feelings are important not just because they might influence the therapist's interventions but because they provide the therapist with some understanding of how others might respond to the patient as she goes through her life; such an understanding is reflected in the therapist's comment that being attractive and appealing might "complicate her twin desires of becoming intimate with men and avoiding the anxiety that is precipitated by intimacy with men."

A patient like Ms. Hastings is an excellent introduction to the topic of object relations, a psychoanalytic school of thought that focuses on the idea that we exist only in relationships with one another. Shaped by experience, strong feelings, and childhood fantasy, early relationships leave us with enduring psychological schema called "object relations" which consist of mental representations of the self in interaction with others. Our object relations forever shape our experience of others and influence how we interact with them. To some extent, emotional health can be defined by the degree of flexibility and realism with which we interact with others so that we recognize them as "whole objects" (or complete, complex individuals with good and bad qualities) rather than "part objects" who are idealized, devalued, or otherwise distorted.

The impact of child sexual abuse on psychological development varies on the basis of a variety of factors, including the age, personality, and resilience of the child; the degree of coercion and violence; the chronicity of the abuse; and the availability of additional support systems. Such variables determine the later effect of the trauma as well as the development of object relationships. For example, a characteristic object relations dyad that might follow early sexual abuse would be the enduring experience of oneself as the abused, helpless child in the hands of a mean, scary abuser. This dyad (helpless child/

scary abuser) is often defended against with avoidance and emotional/cognitive blunting as appears to be the case with Ms. Hastings. The dyad becomes more prominent at certain times, like during psychotherapy, and can lead the patient to feeling frightened and the therapist—through projection and projective identification—to feeling and even acting like an abuser.

A second prominent dyad might include the experience of oneself as abused and helpless in the hands of a rescuer. The second dyad (child/rescuer) may be more quickly enacted and may be one reason that Ms. Hastings presents herself as endearing and likable to a therapist who is presumably primed to be a helper. The child/rescuer dyad may allow the therapy to proceed, but the creation of some sort of difficult, frightening transference/countertransference constellation would almost certainly develop in an intensive treatment with someone who was significantly abused in childhood. Recognition of this transference paradigm requires internal monitoring on the part of the clinician. As the treatment develops, for example, the therapist might perceive an internal, uncharacteristic sensation of anger or sexual intrigue. This unusual sensation might be the first clue as to the patient's history of abuse, especially when combined with the patient's childhood history of parental neglect and her panicky avoidance of sexual partners.

In order to survive early sexual abuse, children tend to physically and emotionally tune out—or dissociate—and focus instead on something like a lamp. Dissociation leads traumatic memories to remain outside of consciousness or to be recalled as images or physical sensations. While the patient may have avoided discussing the abuse because it felt dangerous or shameful, it is at least as likely that she lacked words to describe somatic memories (e.g., gagging, nausea, pelvic pain) or memories that are recalled as distant snapshots from someone else's roll of film. As Ms. Hastings' therapy continues, her psychiatrist reports unusually intense feelings of distance, numbness, and uncertainty. Such wordless confusion can be critical to a successful treatment. Sitting with those unusually intense and uncertain reactions can help the therapist develop greater empathy for the patient's internal world. Further, the effort of putting words to Ms. Hastings' inchoate inner experiences can lead her to more manageable memories, thoughts, and feelings.

Awareness of the importance of countertransference can also reduce the likelihood that the therapist will try to flee from these feelings through a focus on medications or behavioral goals or a shift to other, more palatable topics for discussion. At the same time, however, topic shifts can be helpful. For instance, work with Ms. Hastings should never become a singular pursuit of some sort of historical truth. Safety, prevention of suicidality, medications, and cognitive-behavioral techniques will likely be part of Ms. Hastings' treatment for the foreseeable future.

The therapist may recognize the likelihood of sexual abuse months or years before the patient is prepared to openly discuss events from her childhood. In such cases, it is important to pay attention to the tendency to pressure the fearful patient into premature disclosure. Errors in this regard can lead the patient into feeling—once again—that she is being forced into an overwhelming, unprepared-for situation. Threats made by the abuser may carry clout for decades, partly because the abuser often played a dominant role in the family. Even more insidious are the patient's own likely childhood fantasies. One common, deep-seated belief stems from the young child's hard-wired view of parents as being all-important to survival, and, as such, beings who behave in reasonable ways. In the minds of young children, abuse is a punishment for the child's badness. Even adults who "know" that they are no longer threatened by their childhood abuser tend to be haunted by unconscious fears, somatic pains, traumatic memories, overwhelming guilt, and a sense of themselves as terrible.

As her therapy progresses, Ms. Hastings does begin to feel safer and more able to take on new risks and opportunities. Before the abuse is explicitly discussed, however, she describes her new sexual relationship as "too much" and describes nightmares, abdominal (pelvic?) pain, and the image of the lamp. She whispers the word, "He"; says she needs to quit treatment; and begins to walk out of the room. How might therapists respond to this desire to terminate? One clinician might feel relief that a difficult treatment could end. Another therapist might feel angry. Ms. Hastings' therapist describes feeling "an unusual sense of desperation and protectiveness," and reached out to stop the patient's exit from the room. A well-meaning countertransference reaction, it led to what appears to be an intensification of a dissociative episode, marked by "choking and gagging" and the patient's sliding to the ground. The therapist's initial reaction was intrusive and appears to have led to a re-creation of childhood trauma, but the next intervention—to apologize and talk quietly and without a sense of coercion—may have laid the groundwork for a deepening of the alliance and the safe exploration of the traumas that have crippled Ms. Hastings.

Such episodes may also lead to therapeutic transgressions (Gabbard 2003). For example, Ms. Hastings might express the desperate wish to feel physically safe with the therapist, a wish that can lead the vulnerable patient and therapist into a sexual relationship. Such a boundary violation may feel natural and even therapeutic to both the psychiatrist and patient, but such an enactment re-creates the experience of abuse for the patient and creates a set of legal, professional, ethical, and personal problems for the therapist. While such transgressions are written about most frequently in the psychoanalytic literature, Ms. Hastings' unconscious pull for a re-creation of her childhood sexual abuse is just as likely to occur in treatments and situations that do not explicitly focus on psychodynamics and are perhaps even more likely to be enacted by therapists who are not fully aware of the power of transference and countertransference.

Instead of re-creating the violation, treatment provides the opportunity to put the feelings, wishes, fears, and memories into words, and it is only through making sense of the unutterable that Ms. Hastings can move beyond her daily unconscious terror, digest the trauma, and convert a horrendous, ongoing bodily experience into a memory. Her collapse in the therapist's office may be the concluding moment of the case report, but, if handled with tactful restraint and an ongoing offer of safety, the moment can help Ms. Hastings move into the next chapter of her life.

Ms. Hastings is, then, a challenge to even the most experienced, best-trained, and talented of clinicians. The work requires knowledge of substance abuse treatments, anti-anxiety medications, cognitive-behavioral tools, and psychodynamics. Interventions require tact, timing, durable curiosity, and patience. Perhaps just as importantly, Ms. Hastings' treatment demands that each of us know ourselves, since it is through our own reactions that we can more fully appreciate her perspective, more effectively uncover her childhood abuse, and more carefully prevent intense transferential feeling from derailing not only Ms. Hastings' life but our own careers.

Summary Points

- Untreated substance abuse will likely sabotage all other treatments.
- Untreated anxiety will likely sabotage substance abuse treatments.
- Alcohol abuse causes a host of neurobiological changes that may take months to normalize upon abstinence.
- Anxiety disorders tend to overlap with one another.
- Antidepressant medications work at least as well for anxiety as they do for depression.
- Cognitive-behavioral therapy is effective for anxiety, as is panic-focused psychodynamic psychotherapy.
- A diagnosis of posttraumatic stress disorder can organize seemingly disparate and confusing symptoms.
- Work with victims of child sexual abuse leads to characteristic countertransference reactions that can both help and stymie the treatment.

Chapter 9

HYPOMANIA AND JENNIFER INGRAM

JENNIFER Ingram was a 32-year-old woman who referred herself to a psychiatrist to evaluate possible attention-deficit disorder. She had been working for the past 10 years as an investment banker at a series of Wall Street firms. She complained that although she was highly successful at work and had done well in school, her attention and concentration were suboptimal.

Ms. Ingram said she was tired of having to compensate for her inattention and would like to consider medication that would help improve her focus. She described a long-standing ability to work extended periods of time with limited amounts of sleep, maintain relationships with dozens of friends, and engage in a striking number of activities at the same time. She denied using drugs but admitted to being an "adrenaline junkie," saying that her need for passion led her into impulsive sexual affairs, spending sprees, job changes, and daredevil physical adventures. In retrospect, none of these behaviors had caused her lasting harm and most were good memories.

Her performance was apparently top notch, but Ms. Ingram worried that her inattention led to inefficiency. She would like to accomplish even more by not getting distracted by personal issues during the work day. When asked, she said that her "personal issues" could be divided into mood, love, and music.

The patient said that while she was generally cheerful and optimistic, she tended to get morbidly depressed when she was "just standing still." She described her depressed mood as being "like poison, deadening, phlegmatic, hateful." These down, irritable periods lasted no longer than a week and were responsive to exercise, work, and the pursuit of pleasure. She also theorized that these "black moods" occurred just prior to her menstrual periods, but the connection was not completely clear.

Her sleep was "good and bad." When in a down period, she would sleep fitfully for 6 or 7 hours and feel edgy and tired all day. When in her more typical up periods, she could get by on 5 hours of sleep and feel enthusiastic and refreshed.

In regard to love, Ms. Ingram had been involved with Sarah for 3 years. She said that being a lesbian had never been a major problem. She had not come out at work because "Wall Street isn't the place to make social change." She denied feeling ostracized by her co-workers. Indeed, she experienced pleasure at being tougher and more hard working than most of them. Prior to their deaths in a car accident when the patient was 21, her parents had accepted her lifestyle, and the patient described many straight and gay friends. Ms. Ingram's feelings for her girlfriend, Sarah, had evolved during their 3-year relationship. At the beginning, the patient felt "euphorically excited" and believed that she had met her match. The patient said that while the relationship was getting somewhat boring, the two of them were discussing having a child.

Work was intellectually exciting but "sometimes deadening, like being a cog in the machine." She frequently had thoughts of quitting her job and returning to her first love, music. If it was too late to become a top-notch classical pianist, perhaps she should get more involved in a quartet or the business aspects of a creative organization. Music was one of the main ways in which she related to Sarah, a well-regarded jazz musician.

She had two theories about her intensity. The first was that she had been heavily motivated by having an older brother, Larry, with mild-to-moderate autism. She said she felt lucky to have been born normal and felt driven to "push everything to the limit." She said she had been deeply impressed by the attention and love her parents focused on her brother. While she knew that people saw her as a "mistress of the universe," she believed her own parents were far more heroic because they had sacrificed their careers and personal lives to care for him. She denied ever resenting this brother or the attention he received: "Of course not. He needed the attention, while I could always get as much as I needed."

Her second theory related to her younger sister, Karen, who, she said, had manic depression. She wondered whether she might have inherited a "bipolar gene."

At the end of the evaluation, the patient said that she had some questions. Did she have ADHD? Was she manic-depressive? Did she need medications? How much did her family affect her? Should she quit her job? Should she break up with her girlfriend or go ahead and have a child?

Should she get into psychotherapy? The psychiatrist deferred answering these questions but did schedule a second session.

Personal History

Ms. Ingram was the second of three children born to middle-class parents. She was raised in the suburbs of a large city. She maintained good grades in school despite a very busy extracurricular and social schedule, but she always believed that her grades would have been better if she could have focused better. She attended a college with an attached music school in hopes of becoming a concert pianist. She was a junior in college when her parents died in an automobile accident. At that time, deciding that she needed to make enough money to support both herself and her older brother, she switched her career plan to business.

Since her graduation from college, she had lived in four cities and had five different jobs. Each move had led to increasing responsibilities and income. Her brother lived in a halfway house 2 hours away. She supported him and visited monthly. Her sister lived far away, but they saw each other on holidays.

Personal Psychiatric History

Patient denied previous psychiatric treatment and all substance abuse. She had diagnosed herself with attention-deficit disorder but had never received any treatment for it. Sarah was her fourth girlfriend. Each of the previous relationships had faded when the patient "became bored and then infatuated with someone new." She had not been single since she was 17 years old.

Family Psychiatric History

The patient's brother had Asperger's syndrome and lived in a group home. Her 28-year-old sister had developed a manic episode in her early twenties during a period of sleeplessness in the context of exams. While her sister's pressured speech, racing thoughts, and euphoria were obvious in retrospect, that episode had not been diagnosed or treated, but it did lead to an unplanned several-month trip to Europe and a year off from school. She returned to her baseline on her own and graduated from law school. She had functioned well as a Legal Aid attorney until she became suicidally depressed in the year prior to this consultation. She was hospitalized, and after obtaining the history of mania, her inpatient psychiatrists diagnosed bipolar disorder. Psychotherapy, lithium, and sertraline were begun, and the depression remitted. Six months after she recovered, the sertraline was discontinued, though the therapy and lithium were continued. She appeared to be functioning well.

Medical History

Not contributory.

Mental Status Exam

The patient was alert and cooperative. She wore a business suit and conservative make up; she appeared her stated age. She made good eye contact. She spoke clearly and rapidly. She was goal directed. Her mood shifted based on the topic. While she often felt and appeared cheerful, she tended to feel and appear depressed when discussing her girlfriend and her job. She denied suicidality and psychosis. She was cognitively intact. Her insight and judgment were fair.

Summary

Jennifer Ingram was a 32-year-old woman who presented for evaluation of attention deficit. In the course of their one session, she also expressed concerns about her mood, relationships, and professional goals. In the following discussions, the discussants explore these concerns and consider treatment options.

Discussions of the Case of
Jennifer Ingram

Attention Deficit 341
   James L. Rebeta, Ph.D.

Bipolar Disorder 345
   Marina Benaur, M.D.

Bipolar Spectrum Disorder 348
   Sibel Klimstra, M.D., and Robert C. Young, M.D.

Premenstrual Dysphoria 352
   Margaret Altemus, M.D.

Sleep 354
Michael Terman, Ph.D.

Autism's Effect on the Family .357
Margaret E. Hertzig, M.D.

Creativity and Mental Illness 360
William Frosch, M.D.

Being Lesbian 362
Susan C. Vaughan, M.D.

Love 366
Ethel S. Person, M.D.

Psychodynamic Psychotherapy 369
Deborah L. Cabaniss, M.D.

Overview of Hypomania 373
Cathryn A. Galanter, M.D.

Summary Points 378

Attention Deficit

James L. Rebeta, Ph.D.

JENNIFER Ingram seeks psychiatric consultation for possible "attention deficit disorder," complaining that, despite noteworthy academic achievement and professional success, she is tired of having to compensate for suboptimal attention and concentration. "Personal issues" distract her throughout the workday and lead to inefficiency. By history, she notes that she achieved good grades in school and maintained a hectic extra-curricular and social schedule, but might have done better with greater focus. More recently, she reports having lived in four different cities and having held five different jobs during the

9 years since college graduation, but concedes that each change entailed enhanced job responsibilities and income. She also describes a 3-year lesbian relationship that is actually her fourth since age 17 years, with the others having ended after a period of "boredom" and then "infatuation" with someone else. Having diagnosed herself with "attention-deficit disorder," she wishes to consider medication to improve her focus and functioning.

To an extent, this 32-year-old woman's diagnosis depends upon when one asks the question. Historically, attention-deficit/hyperactivity disorder (ADHD) has been associated with children and adolescents, consistent with 18th-century philosopher John Locke's comment on students who "try as they might…cannot keep their minds from straying" (cited in Doyle 2006, p. 2). The etiology of the disorder has been controversial. For example, in 1902, English pediatrician George Still attributed childhood overactivity and inattentiveness to a lack of "moral control," connecting impulsivity with character (Barkley 2006). Soon afterward, however, characteristic symptoms of ADHD were found in children who had been victims of a 1917–18 encephalitis epidemic, indicating a possible neurological etiology. By 1937, clinicians had found that central nervous system (CNS) stimulants facilitated improved academic and social behavior (Doyle 2006). The more recent diagnostic nomenclature has evolved to capture the changing conceptualization of the syndrome, with the underlying focus shifting from brain damage ("minimal brain damage syndrome," "minimal cerebral dysfunction") to overt behavior ("hyperkinetic reaction of childhood"). By the 1970s and 1980s, research was emphasizing neurologic underpinnings, and ADHD was conceptualized as a heterogeneous disorder with predominant inattention or hyperactivity, or both.

Etiological theories for the disorder abound. Among them, Barkley's work points to a key deficit in response inhibition that interferes with all areas of executive functions (Barkley 2000), while Tannock posits three core areas of executive function deficit including working memory, visual-spatial orientation, and arousal state (discussed in Paule et al. 2000). However, in light of the heterogeneity of symptom presentation among those diagnosed with this disorder, it is not surprising that, as yet, no experimental data provide support for a single core deficit (Rowland et al. 2002). More recent research has provided preliminary evidence of a genetic underpinning, acting through neurological configuration and activation patterns (Fan et al. 2003; Fossella et al. 2002).

The diagnosis of adult ADHD is especially fraught with difficulty. Murphy and Gordon (2006) identified four elements that are key to the diagnosis:

- Childhood symptoms of ADHD
- Current functional impairment in more than one setting as a result of ADHD symptoms

- A lack of other explanations
- A lack of comorbid disorders

Each of these criteria is problematic. Childhood symptoms depend heavily on historical data and recall, both of which are often inaccurate. Further, 25% of adults recall having six or more ADHD symptoms "often" or "very often" during childhood (Murphy and Gordon 2006). Second, assessing functional impairment of adults is difficult, as occupational and relational demands markedly vary, and children are much more likely than adults to be independently observed and rated by such people as parents and teachers. Third, many psychiatric disorders whose symptoms and presentations can mimic ADHD symptoms emerge during late adolescence and early adulthood, including bipolar spectrum disorders, personality disorders, and some depressive and anxiety disorders. Furthermore, adults are more likely to have medical conditions, trauma, and prolonged stress, all of which can lead to decreased attention and focus as well as functional impairment. Finally, mood disorders, antisocial personality disorder, substance abuse, and anxiety disorders have all been found to co-occur in adults with ADHD (Biederman et al. 1993). The clinician then faces a series of diagnostic questions: Are attentional and behavioral difficulties adequately severe to warrant a diagnosis? Did these symptoms actually begin in childhood? If so, are they the result of ADHD or symptomatic of a different disorder? Further, to what extent did childhood problems with attention and behavioral control lead to later difficulties, regardless of whether the ADHD symptoms have persisted into adulthood?

Gender issues increase the difficulty of evaluating Ms. Ingram's early symptoms. She was not diagnosed as a child, but this may reflect the fact that she does not report having had hyperactivity. Excess activity is more visible and disruptive and is more common in boys, which can lead to an underdiagnosis of attentional problems in girls. Further, primary care physicians, who often see and assess children with attentional disorders, are nearly three times as likely to diagnose a male child with ADHD than a female child, regardless of symptom presentation (Wasserman et al. 1999). Although Ms. Ingram believes that her grades in school would have been better with improved focus, she reports excellent academic functioning. While there is no evidence that her symptoms caused impairment before age 7, as DSM-IV-TR (American Psychiatric Association 2000) currently requires, some challenge this criterion as being too restrictive, noting that symptoms continue to emerge throughout childhood and that the age of onset is later in girls (Taylor and Keltner 2002).

To meet current DSM-IV-TR criteria for ADHD, Ms. Ingram should endorse at least six symptoms of inattention or six symptoms of hyperactivity. She describes distractability, but this is often in response to her own thoughts and moods. She complains of difficulty with sustained attention, job changes, and episodic boredom with girlfriends, but these do not appear to be outside the norm. We do not know if she has difficulties with organization, listening to others, misplacing items, attention to detail, and forgetfulness that are typical of people with attention deficit. Regarding hyperactivity–impulsivity, Ms. Ingram's self-report and history suggest that she often feels restless and "on the go," but while her speech is apparently rapid, there is no report of excessive fidgeting or talking. More detailed questioning might elucidate more symptoms, but at this point, while she has some features of the disorder, Ms. Ingram does not appear to have ADHD.

Instead of ADHD, Ms. Ingram's inattention and impulsivity may be better explained by bipolar spectrum symptoms that include a decreased need for sleep, shopping sprees, sexual affairs, and engaging in thrill-seeking activities. In addition, she reports transient depressed mood, lasting no more than a week, but representing a significant downturn from her normally cheerful demeanor. These mood disturbances may be the primary reason for her attentional difficulties and decreased focus and concentration. Unless a more focused evaluation results in an ADHD diagnosis, stabilization of mood would appear to be a primary treatment goal, as would a therapeutic focus on intimacy and career issues.

If attentional difficulties remain troublesome after these other issues have significantly resolved, Ms. Ingram might benefit from treatment focusing on ADHD. The mainstay of treatment is central nervous system stimulants such as amphetamine (Adderal) and methylphenidate (Ritalin), though these medications are better studied in children than in adults. More recent research appears to refute previous concerns that stimulant use might increase the risk of later substance (Barkley et al. 2003), while a different study indicates that stimulant medications *reduce* the risk (Wilens et al. 2003). Atomoxetine (Strattera) is the only nonstimulant medication that carries a U.S. Food and Drug Administration (FDA) indication for ADHD, though other nonstimulant medications, including bupropion (Wellbutrin), tricyclic antidepressants, monoamine oxidase inhibitor (MAOI) antidepressants, and modafinil (Provigil), have also been found to be mildly to moderately helpful in remittance of ADHD symptoms.

Though limited data exist for adults, it appears that adjunctive psychotherapy and cognitive-behavioral therapy (CBT) can be useful, especially when ADHD is comorbid with anxiety and disruptive behavior disorders (Jensen et al. 2001). Adults with ADHD often create their own compensatory strategies that include reducing external distractions; making use of scheduling calendars and visual prompts for upcoming events; and relying upon significant others for organization, a strategy that may be effective but which can lead to interpersonal difficulties.

While perhaps not relevant to Ms. Ingram, an intervention for ADHD should include psychoeducation. This might include discussion of the symptoms, course, treatment options, and effects of ADHD on the patient's life and can include referral to useful Web sites such as www.chadd.org and www.addresources.org. Such information is especially helpful for a disorder like ADHD where the diagnostic criteria are in flux and the cardinal symptoms—problems with attention and activity—lie on a spectrum that is difficult to define and can be part of multiple psychiatric disorders.

Bipolar Disorder

Marina Benaur, M.D.

JENNIFER Ingram's attentional issues precipitated her appointment with the psychiatrist, but the possibility of bipolar disorder may have been a more long-standing concern. Not only does Jennifer have some manic and depressive symptoms, but she has witnessed the illness's impact on her sister, Karen, and worries that she might have inherited the illness. One difficulty in answering her diagnostic question relates to the fact that human behavior and psychiatric symptoms tend to lie on a continuum, and Jennifer's symptoms may or may not extend into being abnormal. A second difficulty lies in the fact that the field of psychiatry has not yet created definitive sets of symptom clusters for what presumably are multiple bipolar syndromes. There are some patients, however, who present with symptoms and history that have been clearly recognized and categorized since antiquity. Such is the case with Karen, who appears to have a clear-cut case of bipolar disorder. An exploration of Karen's symptoms and history can demonstrate how she is typical and inform our efforts to help Jennifer with her mood symptoms.

Karen Ingram's history includes an initial manic episode that appears to have been precipitated by school-induced sleep deprivation and included such symptoms as pressured speech, racing thoughts, euphoria, and uncharacteristically taking a year off from school in order to travel in Europe. As is common, she was not diagnosed at that time but was seen to be an impetuous young person. Her symptoms stabilized on their own within 6 months, and she was able to finish law school. Several years later, she became depressed and suicidal and required psychiatric hospitalization. The bipolar diagnosis was made and treatment begun. Such a story has been recognized since manic depression was first described by ancient Greek writers who noted the link between melancholy and mania.

While described extensively during the ensuing 2000 years, it was Emil Kraepelin in the nineteenth century who systematically and definitively separated the categories of recurrent mood disorders and *dementia praecox* (or schizophrenia). He identified key distinguishing features that include an episodic course, strong family history, and a relatively benign prognosis. Kraepelin described a rich spectrum of presentations, only partially captured by the current DSM-IV-TR categories of bipolar I disorder, bipolar II disorder, bipolar disorder not otherwise specified (NOS), and cyclothymic disorder. Despite an ongoing debate about the existence of a bipolar spectrum that blurs diagnostic boundaries, there is consensus that bipolar I disorder is a distinct and valid diagnostic entity.

Bipolar I disorder affects about 1% of the population worldwide, though broader bipolar spectrum may be as prevalent as 3%–9%. The diagnosis of bipolar I disorder is based on the presence of mania (i.e., it does not require a history of depression). As alluded to in the description of Karen's initial presentation, mania is characterized by euphoria, heightened sensitivity to environmental stimuli, increase in activity, grandiosity, excess energy, and decreased need for sleep. Mania can also present as a mixed state, defined as a period in which increased activity, sleep disturbance, and agitation are dominated by a dysphoric, often irritable, mood. As seems to have been true for Karen, initial manic episodes often go unrecognized because family members rationalize extreme and disruptive behavior as a reaction to some stressor or life change. Stressful life events often do precipitate mood disorders, but it is also true that manic and depressive episodes often lead to interpersonal difficulties that can exacerbate stressful situations. Subsequent episodes tend to develop with fewer clear precipitants, and the later stages of untreated illness tend to be characterized by progressively worsening mood instability. This pattern has led researchers to hypothesize that mood episodes sensitize neural networks leading to kindling phenomena and increasing vulnerability for recurrence. Early recognition and treatment are, therefore, essential and may significantly improve the course of illness. In the case of someone like Karen, who has two known mood episodes, her long-term health may depend on whether she can maintain her treatment regimen and avoid recurrences.

Perhaps the most obvious way for Karen to avoid a relapse would be for her to maintain good sleep hygiene. Her first manic episode developed in the setting of sleep deprivation during final exams, and it is well documented that reduced sleep duration predicts emergence of hypomanic and manic symptoms. For these reasons, Karen should avoid work that would require her to shift her sleeping schedule or go all night without sleep. Not only is sleep implicated in the emergence of mood changes, the quality of sleep is affected by the mood disorders. For example, depression is associated with reduction of slow wave sleep and disruptions of both sleep continuity and rapid eye movement (REM) sleep. While less well studied, sleep disturbances during mania include problems with sleep continuity and REM disinhibition.

Sleep problems do not seem to be simply epiphenomena of bipolar illness. Instead, ongoing neurobiologic research indicates that circadian rhythms may be intrinsic to the illness. For example, the 24-hour circadian rhythm cycle in the human brain is controlled by a pacemaker region in the suprachiasmatic nucleus (SCN) in the hypothalamus. The pacemaker region is controlled by so-called clock genes. Several of these genes—including *CLOCK* and *G3K3B*—have been extensively studied in patients with bipolar illness. A single-nucleotide polymorphism of *CLOCK* has been associated with higher recurrence rates of mania as well as greater insomnia. In mice, *CLOCK* mutations were associated with manic-like behavior that normalized after lithium treatment. Not only is *G3K3B* a major target of lithium, but mice that have been genetically altered to overexpress *G3K3B* demonstrate manic-like behavior that includes hyperactivity and increased startle response. Such findings offer clues as to the neurobiologic basis for the cyclical nature of bipolar illness, seasonal affective disorder, and other mood disorders.

Perhaps the most important aspect of Karen's treatment was getting the right diagnosis. Without an exploration into her history during her psychiatric hospitalization, it is likely that she would have been diagnosed with a unipolar depression and prescribed an antidepressant medication, which might have induced a manic episode. Bipolar depression is unusually difficult to treat; medication treatments for bipolar depression tend to aim to optimize mood stabilization and then to add antidepressant medication if necessary. Lithium remains the best studied and most effective treatment for bipolar mania, bipolar depression, and prevention of bipolar episodes. Lithium has also been the only medication clearly shown to reduce the risk of suicide in bipolar patients, which is quite important given that 25%–50% of bipolar patients attempt suicide in their lifetime and 6%–15% end their life by suicide. Although effective, lithium is not ideal. It has a narrow therapeutic index, meaning that even mildly elevated levels of the drug can lead to severe toxicity. Overdose can lead to dangerous neurologic, kidney, and cardiac problems, and prolonged use commonly affects the thyroid and kidney.

In addition, lithium routinely causes tremor, acne, cognitive slowing, and weight gain. Alternatives for mood stabilization in bipolar patients are valproic acid, carbamazepine, lamotrigine, and some atypical antipsychotic medications, but all have their own significant side effects.

Diagnostic evaluation of both Karen and Jennifer Ingram should consider comorbidities and other causes for mood symptoms. Anxiety, psychosis, and eating disorders are relatively common, for example, and as many as half of people with bipolar illness also abuse substances. If either sister had a history of using cocaine or amphetamines in order to elevate mood, lose weight, or stay awake, for example, it is possible that their psychiatric issues relate more strongly to the stimulant abuse than to a primary bipolar disorder. In that case, a shift of the treatment focus to substance abuse might improve long-term outcome and avoid unnecessary medications.

Karen Ingram's bipolar disorder holds several keys to Jennifer Ingram's diagnosis and treatment. Most obviously, a clear-cut bipolar diagnosis puts a sibling at a 10% risk for also having the disorder, and given Jennifer's current symptoms of hypomania, her risk is probably higher than 10%. Since mood disorders are associated with kindling phenomena, prevention is important, and Jennifer should consider a less stressful career or at least consider getting more sleep. Finally, having a grasp of bipolar I disorder provides the infrastructure necessary to consider whether or not Jennifer's condition fulfills criteria for a relatively subtle bipolar spectrum disorder.

Bipolar Spectrum Disorder

Sibel Klimstra, M.D.

Robert C. Young, M.D.

WHILE Karen Ingram's bipolar disorder is diagnostically straightforward, Jennifer Ingram presents with symptoms that may reflect mild mania and depression but may also be consistent with attention deficit disorder, premenstrual dysphoric disorder, substance abuse, and personality disorders. Her symptoms are also found in people who lack any psychiatric diagnosis, and some of her "symptoms" may be better characterized as personality characteristics that are more enviable than problematic. Such diagnostic uncertainty is common in the realm of outpatient psychiatry, where many patients do not fit neatly into established categories. While certainty may be elusive, the search for Ms. Ingram's diagnosis is important for several reasons, particularly in regard to discussing prognosis and planning treatment.

If Jennifer does have a major mood disorder, it appears to exist on a bipolar spectrum. She has manic-like symptoms that include high productivity and activity, little need for sleep, distractibility, sexual impulsivity, spending sprees, and "daredevil" activity. On mental status examination, she has rapid speech and mood lability. Depressive features include past episodes of poor sleep, low energy, and depressed mood. Collateral history from friends and family might be helpful in assessing symptom intensity, chronology, functionality, and a history of violence, but at this point, neither her manic nor her depressive symptoms appear to have caused significant distress or functional disturbance. If Jennifer does have a bipolar disorder, it appears to be quite different from Karen's single episode of behavior that was uncharacteristic for her.

There has been an ongoing effort to identify symptom clusters that might effectively differentiate between subtypes of bipolar disorder. Fundamental to the subtypes is assessment of dysfunction. Karen has manic and depressive symptoms that caused dysfunction, and she has what is considered a *bipolar I disorder*. The bipolar I diagnosis depends on frank mania, not depression, so Karen could have been diagnosed as bipolar I even prior to her hospitalization with major depression. Jennifer's mood symptoms have not led to significant impairment and so are consistent with *hypomania*. If her depressions had been more severe and lasted longer than 1 week, Jennifer would be said to have *bipolar II disorder*, a diagnosis characterized by major depressions and periods of hypomania. As it stands, however, Jennifer's depressions do not appear to reach a threshold for major depression, and so she is likely to have *cyclothymia*, which is defined by a 2-year period of numerous hypomanic and depressive symptoms that are subthreshold for a major depressive episode. Additional types have been proposed. For example, if Jennifer were chronically hypomanic without significant depressions, she might be considered to possess a "hyperthymic" temperament. Other proposed subtypes include hypomania or mania precipitated by antidepressant medication; unipolar mania without depression; depression with a family history of bipolar illness; and substance use–associated hypomania or depression.

In order to systematically investigate diagnostic possibilities, it might be useful to ask her to keep a mood diary that would include associated neurovegetative symptoms. Self-report symptom scales such as the Internal State Scale and the Self-Report Manic Inventory are useful and cost-effective (Cooke et al. 1996). Brief clinician-administered instruments for manic state severity (e.g., the Young Mania Rating Scale [Young et al. 1978]) may be used for tracking change with treatment. Ms. Ingram reports concentration and attention difficulties that can occur in both manic and depressed states and that can be assessed with the Mini-Mental State Exam. Continuous performance tests are also widely used to assess attention (Marvel 2004).

Bipolar illness can be confused with attention-deficit/hyperactivity disorder (ADHD). While ADHD lacks the pressured euphoria of mania, overlapping symptoms include impaired attention, distractibility, impulsivity, disorganized behavior, and increased motor movements and speech. To complicate matters, bipolar disorder and ADHD may occur in the same patient (Nierenberg et al. 2005), and ADHD symptoms in children may herald future development of bipolar disorder (Ross 2006). Distinguishing between these diagnoses is important, partly because pharmacologic errors are likely to be not only ineffective but harmful. For example, mood-stabilizing medications can worsen cognition, with this effect being particularly problematic for people with ADHD. More acutely worrisome is the possibility that the standard treatment for ADHD—stimulants such as amphetamine—can induce mania and psychosis. A manic response to stimulants may reflect an undiagnosed bipolar illness, a medication side effect, or a previously undetected comorbidity of ADHD and bipolar illness, but it is a potentially catastrophic outcome. In the case of Ms. Ingram, a bipolar spectrum illness appears more likely than ADHD. She complains of attention deficit, but she has apparently done well at school and has functioned at a very high level in a field that demands an ability to concentrate for prolonged periods of time. In addition, she has a strong family history for bipolar disorder.

Ms. Ingram's depressed mood appears to peak just prior to her menstrual periods. While premenstrual dysphoric disorder should be considered in the differential diagnosis, the clinician should keep in mind that there is evidence for premenstrual exacerbation of underlying mood disorders, including bipolar disorder (Miller and Miller 2001). Patients with a bipolar-spectrum illness can also manifest behaviors associated with some personality disorders (see Chapter 3, "Mood Instability and Amy Cahill").

In the face of uncertainty, a bipolar disorder diagnosis should receive priority in the differential diagnosis. Bipolar disorder is relatively well characterized, there is solid evidence to guide treatment, and it has a relatively favorable short-term prognosis. Further, a missed diagnosis can lead to adverse outcomes such as completed suicide and long-term sequelae of recurrent episodes, including possible cognitive decline.

Manic and depressive symptoms are also found in a wide variety of medical or neurologic disorders, though these commonly present with unusual symptoms or bipolar syndromes with later ages at onset. Initial evaluation of bipolar symptoms should always include a thorough medical workup, particularly when the symptoms or age at onset are unusual. Such a workup should also investigate the possibility of substance abuse. Patients like Jennifer Ingram often try to control their own symptoms through the use of a variety of medications and substances of abuse. In addition to a careful history, it is generally wise to check a toxicology screen.

Jennifer Ingram has denied suicidality, but safety issues are critical in the management of people with significant affective symptoms. While she does not appear to warrant a bipolar I diagnosis at present, she is certainly at risk for mania and/or a major depression, and the lifetime prevalence of completed suicide in patients with bipolar disorder is 10%–15% (Baldessarini 2003). It is, therefore, critical to tactfully explore Ms. Ingram's active or passive suicidal ideation, her history of suicidal thinking and attempts, and family history.

While pharmacology may be a cornerstone of the treatment of most people with bipolar disorder, Ms. Ingram is not an immediate candidate for mood stabilizing medications since she appears not to meet criteria for a bipolar I or II diagnosis. There are signs that she has difficulties with organization of her time and with relationships, perhaps related to cyclothymia or a hyperthymic temperament; if so, she might be considered for social rhythm therapy and interpersonal psychotherapy (IPT) that have been specifically designed for people with bipolar illness (Frank 2005). If Ms. Ingram's symptoms do warrant medication, education about the disorder and its treatment might be pivotal in her adherence to treatment, as might a sturdy therapeutic alliance. Regardless of her diagnosis, however, much of the effectiveness of her treatment will lie in an empathic understanding of her life story (McHugh and Slavney 1998). In other words, clarification of the diagnosis and optimization of the treatment plan will require more than an elaboration of Ms. Ingram's symptoms and an expertise in pharmacology. She will need to be carefully heard so that information that might be otherwise inaccessible can be obtained and evidence-based medicine can be informed by knowledge of the individual patient.

Premenstrual Dysphoria

Margaret Altemus, M.D.

AMONG a variety of other concerns, Jennifer Ingram reports that her
mood symptoms appear to worsen prior to her menstrual cycle, raising the
possibility that she has premenstrual syndrome (PMS) or premenstrual dysphoric disorder (PMDD). Particularly consistent with PMS and PMDD are
her complaints that her depressive periods last only a week and are marked
by depression, irritability, impaired concentration, and sleep changes. Such
complaints do not necessarily indicate one of these two diagnoses, however,
since self-reports are frequently inaccurate and other psychiatric disorders
may be present throughout the cycle but exacerbated premenstrually. In addition, most women experience mild, isolated premenstrual symptoms that
can include physical symptoms (breast tenderness, bloating/weight gain,
headache, swelling of hands or feet, muscle aches), as well as a variety of affective symptoms. Most women do not perceive these symptoms as distressing or debilitating, however, and both PMDD and PMS require evidence of
functional impairment. PMDD is a DSM-IV diagnosis that has more restrictive criteria than PMS and therefore is less common (see Table 9–1).

TABLE 9–1.   PREMENSTRUAL DYSPHORIC DISORDER (DSM-IV-TR)

Requires at least one mood symptom and four of eleven other symptoms.

Cannot represent a premenstrual worsening of another psychiatric
disorder.

Duration of symptoms: 1–14 days (average 6 days).

Symptoms must be relieved during the two weeks following menses.

Symptoms often remit at onset of menses but can persist for a few days.

Source.   American Psychiatric Association 2000.

    In contrast to PMDD, PMS is a non-DSM diagnosis that is used more
commonly in nonpsychiatric settings. According to ICD-10 (World Health
Organization 1992), PMS requires only one physical or emotional symptom

that recurs during the 4 premenstrual days of several consecutive menstrual cycles, and resolves within 4 days of menses. The 12-month prevalence rates are 3%–8% for PMDD and 20%–40% for PMS (Freeman 2003; Wittchen et al. 2002).

An accurate history is central to determining whether Ms. Ingram's condition meets these criteria. Research into PMDD has revealed that the ability to recall the timing and severity of mood symptoms is limited. Prospective ratings are therefore crucial, preferably including daily diaries for at least two complete cycles. PMDD clinical trials use such diaries, and a screening failure rate of 70% is common. A number of instruments can be used for these self-assessments (Endicott et al. 2006; Freeman et al. 1996; Mortola et al. 1990). Since the diagnoses also require functional impairment, it would be important to assess whether or not Ms. Ingram's symptoms affect her relationships or work and whether she uses illicit substances to treat her symptoms. Like many patients, Ms. Ingram would prefer that the diagnosis be made during the initial evaluation, and she would likely be frustrated by the requirement of keeping a daily mood diary for two or three months. While it is sometimes possible to mail a rating form to the patient prior to the first consultation, thereby getting an early start on the prospective rating, it is useful to remember that a failure to be rigorous about the diagnosis will likely lead to unnecessary overtreatment. Another potential pitfall of premature diagnosis could be mistreatment of a missed diagnosis, particularly bipolar disorder, a personality disorder, or ADHD.

Although PMDD is often thought of as a time-limited, recurrent depression, the symptom profile of the two disorders is somewhat distinct. Irritability, anger, and mood lability are the cardinal mood symptoms of PMDD, rather than depressed mood, worthlessness, or guilt. Women with PMDD do have increased rates of other affective disorders but appear to have low rates of comorbid Axis II personality disorders (Freeman et al. 1995; Pearlstein et al. 1990).

The pathophysiology that produces PMDD symptoms remains to be clarified. No abnormalities have been detected in circulating hormone levels, suggesting that women with PMDD have an abnormal reactivity to normal hormone fluctuations across the menstrual cycle. This hypothesis is supported by experimental studies using hormone challenges (Eriksson et al. 2005; Schmidt et al. 1998) and by observations that women with premenstrual mood disorders seem to have a greater incidence of adverse mood reactions to oral contraceptives. Because many women have symptoms that begin in the early or mid-luteal phase—before progesterone or estrogen levels start to fall—luteal hormone actions, rather than hormone withdrawal, are more likely to promote symptoms in women with PMDD. While an integrated theory of causation has not yet been elaborated, abnormalities have been found in hypothalamic-pituitary-adrenal axis regulation, luteal-phase cortical excitability, frontal lobe activation from negative stimuli, and the regulation of serotonin and GABA (gamma-aminobutyric acid).

If Ms. Ingram is found to have PMDD, her symptoms may be well treated by serotonin reuptake inhibitors (SRIs), which were the first FDA-approved treatments for PMDD. Not only can they be taken daily, there is preliminary evidence that these medications are effective when taken only on symptomatic days of the cycle (Freeman et al. 2005). Yaz-24, a new oral contraceptive with a novel progestin, drospirenone, has also been shown to be an effective treatment and was recently approved by the FDA for this indication. Other possible treatments include calcium supplementation, continuous dosing of oral contraceptives, and exercise. Psychotherapies may help both mood and behavior but have not been extensively studied in PMDD.

There are several reasons to carefully evaluate premenstrual mood symptoms in Ms. Ingram. Even though premenstrual symptoms are time-limited, the functional impairment associated with PMDD is as severe as in major depression (Halbreich et al. 2003) and might contribute significantly to her difficulties with her girlfriend and work. It would also be important to clarify whether or not she has a bipolar disorder, since the primary treatment for PMDD—antidepressant medication—might induce a manic episode. A thorough evaluation might be difficult because of Ms. Ingram's apparent impatience, but an accurate diagnosis would be well worth the effort.

Sleep

Michael Terman, Ph.D.

UNDOUBTEDLY, a clinical chronobiologist is not going to be among the first to see Jennifer Ingram. Nevertheless, insights from the vantage point of sleep could rapidly refocus the exploration of her symptoms in ways that transcend the usual Axis I diagnostic categories and point to treatments that might replace or be adjunctive to medication and psychotherapy.

Ms. Ingram reports a bipolar pattern with relatively brief periods of black mood that are sometimes premenstrual. She avoids standing still "because" this brings on the mood switch. She claims to manage well on short sleep but to sleep fitfully with more time in bed when depressed. She has probably not used sleep medications while depressed, although the question may not have been asked. Every specialist tends to focus on particular aspects of a patient, and the chronobiologist would specifically explore Ms. Ingram's sleep by eliciting answers to the following questions:

1. Is the change in sleep pattern symptomatic of the mood state, or does it trigger the switches toward either mania or depression? At what times of day does the patient fall asleep and wake up? Is her sleep pattern consistent or variable? When she reports "fitful" sleep, does she mean difficulty falling asleep (early insomnia) or staying asleep (middle insomnia)? Does she waken too early (late insomnia) or does she take more than thirty minutes to become alert in the morning (sleep inertia)?
2. Is the association of depressed mood with the menstrual cycle predominant or random?
3. When the patient is depressed, is daytime mood and energy consistent? Is depression worse in the morning (positive diurnal variation) or in the evening (negative diurnal variation)? Does she routinely slump in the afternoon or early evening but recover before bedtime?
4. Assuming the patient sleeps with her partner, how do their sleep schedules interrelate? Does her partner's sleep pattern affect hers?
5. Is the bedroom lighting environment conducive to restorative sleep?

Focused attention on sleep can help to resolve both the mood disturbance and attention deficit. However, not all the required information can be reliably extracted by interviewing; longitudinal prospective measures—that continue throughout treatment and guide the treatment regimen—are often necessary.

Sleep Pattern and Quality

Self-reports about sleep are notoriously inaccurate and are often exaggerated. For this reason, we have revamped the sleep items on the structured interview for the Hamilton Depression Scale (Williams and Terman 2003). If the patient can assume the responsibility, a daily log of sleep times and mood and energy ratings can provide a powerful key to psychiatric problem solving. The exercise becomes habit and takes only 2 minutes a day upon awakening. In regard to Ms. Ingram, we would look for displaced or drifting circadian rhythm phase (not to be confused with psychogenic insomnia), evidence of poor sleep hygiene, and sleep cycle adjustment under treatment.

Not every patient can maintain this record, particularly those with attention deficits. An objective alternative is *actigraphy,* in which the patient wears a wristwatch-like device that provides downloadable data to discriminate sleep from waking episodes and even to quantify sleep efficiency. While this technology has been a mainstay of sleep and depression studies, it merits adoption for clinical assessment and monitoring. In regard to Ms. Ingram, sleep polysomnography at a sleep disorders center is likely to be uninformative.

Light Therapy

The possibility of light therapy may appear to come out of the blue, since light therapy has historically been reserved for patients with seasonal affective disorder. But there are good reasons to think it might help Ms. Ingram, particularly if we uncover a pattern in which she has difficulty awakening after a night in which she experiences prolonged agitated sleep that leads briefly to deep slumber. In such cases, morning light therapy can serve both to ease awakening and coalesce the disturbed sleep.

There have also been successful clinical trials of light therapy for several psychiatric diagnoses that may specifically relate to Ms. Ingram. For example, light therapy has been studied during the late luteal phase of premenstrual dysphoric disorder (Lam et al. 1999). There have also been successful trials of light therapy for nonseasonal bipolar depression (Benedetti et al. 2005; Sit et al. 2007), as well as a cautious trial for rapid cycling disorder (Leibenluft et al. 1995). Especially if the patient shows a displaced sleep pattern during depressive exacerbations, light therapy might quickly improve the mood symptoms. Finally, light therapy has improved cognition in patients with ADHD irrespective of depression status (Rybak et al. 2006). As is the case with antidepressant medications, however, light therapy could induce a manic or hypomanic episode in patients with an underlying bipolar diathesis, and so an adjunctive mood stabilizer should be considered in a patient like Ms. Ingram (Terman and Terman 2005).

Dark therapy—which consists of one or more long nights of bed rest in conjunction with medication—has been used in the treatment of mania (Barbini et al. 2005; Wirz-Justice et al. 1999).

Pending further clinical information, I might suggest a relatively novel lighting intervention for Ms. Ingram: dusk-to-dawn simulation in the bedroom (Terman 1997). The patient falls asleep at the desired hour in the presence of a naturalistic dusk fade and awakens at the end of the gradual dawn signal. The time between dusk and dawn is adjusted individually. For example, we might set up a 6-hour dusk-to-dawn simulation for Ms. Ingram, who describes 5-hour sleeps while hypomanic and agitated 7-hour sleeps while depressed. The dusk transition appears acutely hypnotic, even for patients who would otherwise fall asleep much later, while the dawn signal synchronizes circadian rhythms to the external day–night cycle.

We are beginning to see a sea change in the application of light therapy and sleep–wake manipulation. Once used almost exclusively for seasonal affective disorder, these techniques are increasingly being used as adjuncts to medication for patients with a variety of mood, sleep, and attentional problems, regardless of seasonal pattern (Wirz-Justice et al. 2005). With additional clinical information, one of these therapies may be critical to Ms. Ingram's clinical improvement.

Autism's Effect on the Family

Margaret E. Hertzig, M.D.

JENNIFER Ingram speculates that she has been "heavily motivated" throughout her life by having an older brother with "mild-to-moderate autism." She wonders if his autism—or Asperger's disorder—might have contributed to her intensity and success. She does not believe that he had a negative impact on the family but instead speaks admiringly of her parents' hard work and self-sacrifice. She dispassionately describes switching her career plan from music to business following her parents' deaths—a path apparently chosen so that she could support herself and her brother, who now lives in a group home some two hours distant. This highly articulate and successful businesswoman then wonders if her brother's problems might have affected her. How might the psychiatrist address this question? What is Asperger's disorder, and what is its history? How does Asperger's disorder relate to autism and pervasive developmental delay? More specifically, how might Larry Ingram's problems have affected his sister?

Pervasive developmental disorder (PDD) is the umbrella term that includes patterns of delay and deviance in the development of social, communicative, and cognitive skills. The concept entered the psychiatric literature in 1943, when Leo Kanner described 11 young children who displayed a disturbance in social relatedness, failure to use language for communicative purposes, and "an insistence on sameness," currently characterized as restriction of interests. Autism was initially thought to be the earliest form of schizophrenia. Although schizophrenia may emerge in autistic individuals, it does so no more frequently than in the general population. The etiology of autism has long been controversial. Initially Kanner spoke of an inborn disturbance of affective contact but later suggested that the cause was faulty parenting. In much the same way that "schizophrenogenic mothers" were said to cause schizophrenia, "refrigerator mothers" were thought to induce autism. Such viewpoints were wrongheaded and hurtful to a generation of already-stressed parents. Today, PDD—like schizophrenia—is viewed as a neuropsychiatric disorder that does not result from early maladaptive environments. The PDDs have their onset in the first years of life, disrupt developmental processes, and are usually associated with mental retardation. Autism remains the prototypic PDD.

At basically the same time that Kanner was describing autistic children, Hans Asperger, an Austrian pediatrician, described four children between the ages of 6 and 11 who had marked difficulty integrating into social groups. Unlike Kanner's group of children, Asperger's patients had seemingly adequate cognitive and verbal skills while also manifesting many of the symptoms seen in more functional people with PDD. Apparently neither Kanner nor Asperger was aware of the other's observations at the time, and Asperger's work remained relatively unknown in the United States and Britain until Lorna Wing introduced the term Asperger's syndrome in 1981. Since then, Asperger's disorder has come to be applied to individuals with PDD who are of normal or near normal intelligence and whose communicative abilities are relatively well preserved early in life. In this way, the concept of PDD has broadened to include people who would not have initially met criteria for autism but would instead have been seen as odd or socially inappropriate.

Regardless of the specific name that is used to describe their conditions, affected persons may display a wide range of symptom expression, both *across* individuals and *within* the same individual at different times. Impairments in social interaction may range from withdrawal and eye avoidance to social inappropriateness. Older, verbal people with PDD may stare, for example, with an intensity that makes other people uncomfortable. They may also be unable to respond to indirect clues so that they do not recognize that "It's getting late" means "It's time to leave." They may approach relative strangers with intimate questions such as "How much money do you make?" or "Why are you so fat?" While many autistic persons remain mute or practically mute for most of their lives, others demonstrate an odd speech development. They may progress from speech patterns characterized by irrelevancies and context-inappropriate echolalia to context-appropriate echolalia to speech that, while serviceable for communication of immediate needs and wishes, is marked by pragmatic deficiencies that make conversation impossible. These people may speak with great fluency but are unable to take turns and engage in the give-and-take that distinguishes a conversation from a lecture. In addition, their speech is often characterized by an unusually constant rate, an unvarying and mechanical rhythm, and a flat tone and prosody. Their childhood play tends to be repetitive and unimaginative, and they tend to remain concrete and literal as they age. Typical repetitive motor stereotypies include hand flapping and toe walking, which tend to diminish somewhat with age. Children with PDD become upset by changes in routines, during transition times in school, or with any environmental changes, though these also tend to improve with age. Efforts toward repetition and sameness seem to underlie such early PDD behaviors as lining up toys, which may then give way to the amassing of arcane information, whether it be the names and physical characteristics of dinosaurs or the scores of all the World Series games ever played.

During adolescence, a small number of autistic individuals make marked developmental gains, while another subgroup deteriorates behaviorally. Some develop seizure disorders in adolescence. The movie *Rainman* provides a very accurate picture of the behavioral characteristics of an older, cognitively able, autistic person. The star, Dustin Hoffman, worked closely with a young autistic adult in preparation for the role. It seems possible that Larry Ingram has a similar set of behavioral characteristics as part of his high-level autistic disorder.

While Larry Ingram was born before the term *Asperger's disorder* was coined, his sister was still raised in a household in which her parents were stressed and her older brother manifested unusual behavior, idiosyncratic interests, and odd ways of relating. Of course these experiences affected her. The question is how? Siblings of individuals with a disability have long been considered to be vulnerable to adjustment difficulties, and autism seems especially likely to place family members at risk for psychological difficulties (Glasberg 2000). Nevertheless, despite their apparent face validity, the empirical evidence for these conclusions is thin. Research is fraught with methodological difficulties, and comparisons between studies are difficult because of such important variables as severity of disability, the ages and birth orders of the studied siblings, and additional stressors (e.g., the death of parents and the bipolar illness of a sister).

The results of more recent studies that have tried to systematically address these issues are more tempered. For example, one study found that although brothers and sisters of children with high-functioning autism had more behavior problems between the ages of 6 and 11 than did siblings of nondisordered children, their difficulties were not clinically significant and tended to resolve by adolescence (Verte et al. 2003). Moreover, in adolescence, sisters of high-functioning autistic children achieved higher scores on measures of self-concept and social skills than those attained by other sibling groups. In addition, raising a handicapped child can be a source of joy and happiness, increased sense of purpose, expanded personal and social networks, family unity and closeness, and increased tolerance and strength (Stainton and Besser 1998). These findings suggest that the therapist should not assume that the experience of growing up in a household with a sibling with an autistic spectrum disorder is necessarily negative. Instead, it would be important for the clinician to help Ms. Ingram clarify the nuances of her subjective experience, as well as the defensive maneuvers and adaptive strategies she has employed to cope with the periods of distress and disappointment that are an inevitable accompaniment to adulthood.

Creativity and Mental Illness

William Frosch, M.D.

JENNIFER Ingram is an investment banker, but during college, she had apparently had the potential to become a "top-notch classical pianist." Both of these occupations involve a capacity for hard, concentrated physical and intellectual work, and Ms. Ingram clearly has impressive ego strengths. At the same time, she describes multiple symptoms of hypomania and likely warrants a cyclothymia diagnosis. Such a case exemplifies the long-standing concern that creative talent and mental illness are linked.

Talent's extreme development, genius, has always attracted attention. We are puzzled by its inexplicable nature. It is often seen as "abnormal," not only in its meaning of "not usual" but also as representing pathology or as associated with disease. Aristotle linked genius to the melancholic temperament, probably implying a personality type rather than an illness. During the nineteenth and early twentieth centuries, many thought genius was part of a degenerative spectrum and related to psychosis. In the 1950s, both Lionel Trilling and Phyllis Greenacre denied that neurosis is necessary to creativity. We all have conflicts, they argued, but some people are able either to use the conflicts creatively or to work with them in productive ways. Recent retrospective studies have, however, linked affective illness, alcoholism, and suicide to creativity in visual artists and writers (Jamison 1989; Schildkraut et al. 1994). Jamison (1993) lists a lengthy roster of poets with major affective illness and/or suicidal ideation, including Blake, Byron, Coleridge, Shelley, and Samuel Johnson. American poets with affective illness include such luminaries as T.S. Eliot, Robert Lowell, Sylvia Plath, Edgar Allen Poe, and Anne Sexton. Retrospective diagnoses and anecdotally based summaries are, however, notoriously inaccurate and are incapable of definitively linking creative talent and mental illness.

Andreasen (1987) has probably been the first to study the relationship of creativity and psychopathology by using a systematically described, prospective sample, more or less matched control subjects, structured interviews, and previously agreed-upon diagnostic criteria. Her results demonstrate a remarkable prevalence of affective illness in writers in contrast to the controls, and in the first-degree relatives of the writers compared with the relatives of the controls. A similar study of musicians has not been done. My own retrospective study of composers came to the Scottish verdict of "not proven." While Robert Schumann was almost certainly manic-depressive, and Hugo Wolf at least seriously cyclothymic, it was not clear that the overall prevalence was significantly different from that of a "normal" population.

How do these findings relate to Ms. Ingram? Most specifically, they help not at all. Psychiatric evaluation and diagnosis should be applied to the individual and not to a demographic group, especially when the data are so uncertain. At the same time, the interrelationship between her mood, music, and talent can inform our understanding of Ms. Ingram, her psychological tendencies, and the possibilities for the future.

Hypomanic energy might have allowed her to work, for example, with the sort of passion that affords success in both classical music and business. After an 11-year hiatus, however, it would be virtually impossible for her to return to competitive piano. While she focused on business, conservatories turned out hundreds of talented young pianists who are hungry for careers in music (and in music management). It would be important for the clinician to pursue this dream of hers. Does she realize that it is fantasy to think that she could be a successful classical musician? If so, is the fantasy a reflection of unrealistic optimism secondary to hypomania? Does she want to return to the golden age of college before her parents' untimely deaths? Is she trying to cement her failing relationship with Sarah, a successful musician in her own right? Is she bored by banking and desirous of excitement? Does the interest in music stem from some other fantasy? Has she developed the skill set that would make her valuable in music management? Is she the very rare person who might be able to return to performance, perhaps at the level of a serious amateur? Perhaps she is one of those people who feel they absolutely must pursue their creative talent despite the long odds of success.

Ms. Ingram's aspirations will play a role in the treatment decision. Ms. Ingram's ability to practice her music and to work as an investment banker may have been fueled by hypomania's effects on energy, mood, and sleep. She may not be willing to give up those symptoms and may not even consider them symptoms but rather positive attributes of herself. Further, she may be willing to risk a frank manic episode in the interest of being creative and productive (regardless of whether it is in business or music). If we do try to affect her mood symptoms with medication, the negotiations will need to include the fact that both mood stabilizers and antidepressants may cause tremor and cognitive dysfunction, neither of which may be immediately palatable to her. Situations of diagnostic uncertainty, like Ms. Ingram's, underscore the importance of psychiatric judgment: when faced with helping to decide treatment options, do we explore, address the conflicts, or leave well enough alone?

Being Lesbian

Susan C. Vaughan, M.D.

LEARNING that Jennifer Ingram is lesbian during the course of the initial interview should cause an evaluating psychiatrist to wonder about a number of issues related to her sexuality. Although these questions may not be explored in an initial interview, an ability to think in a developmental context about a patient's sexuality is an important part of reaching an overall understanding of the patient. After reviewing a number of common developmental themes in lesbian patients, I address Ms. Ingram's specific history.

Though culture is rapidly changing, gay and lesbian patients tend to have a number of common developmental experiences, most of which are the result of societal homophobia and heterosexism. Many lesbians describe feeling a diffuse sense of aloneness and difference from peers in early life. Some clinicians speculate that this is the result of inadequate mirroring by parents who cannot or do not consider the possibility that their child is gay, creating a mismatch between parental fantasies and expectations and the child's inner world. For some lesbians, gender atypicality or "tomboyism" accounts for part of the early sense of difference; many describe their mothers' discomfort with their athleticism and encouragement of more feminine pursuits. The sense of perceived difference is not neutral, but linked to a sense that one is wrong or bad and that whatever is different should be kept hidden. In the past, playground epithets such as "lezzie" were often the first way lesbian children came to understand who they were, confirming their sense of difference and badness. One common developmental response is active, conscious suppression of aspects of the self during childhood and adolescence (e.g., concealing crushes on teachers, pretending to like certain boys), which often gives rise to a sense of secrecy and inauthenticity, as well as to conflicts about what parts of the self show on the surface. On the one hand, being "found out" would mean being known and seen, but on the other it would mean risking rejection and alienation.

To make matters more complicated, lesbian children are frequently put in situations that are sexually or sensually overstimulating. Same-sex physical interactions and nudity within families, in bathrooms and locker rooms, and at slumber parties are organized around heterosexist assumptions, grouping same-gender children and adolescents together based on the idea that only opposite-gender children are attracted to one another. For example, mothers who would never walk naked around their adolescent sons unwittingly overstimulate their lesbian daughters by doing so, and parents who would never allow boy/girl slumber parties have lesbian daughters who regularly sleep in the same bed with close female friends to whom they are often very attracted. Many lesbians respond to this overstimulation with shame, guilt, and suppression and denial of their excitement. Excitement itself becomes the enemy, threatening to expose their lesbianism to others and creating an internal struggle that can affect their later adult sexuality. The usual, intense female ties of adolescence also provide opportunities for a lesbian's budding sexuality to be simultaneously stimulated and constrained. The period of intense female involvement and friendship of early to mid-adolescence often comes crashing to an end as a lesbian's friends really do become increasingly involved in opposite-sex relationships. For many, the shift in the attentions of adored female friends precipitates substantial periods of depression and anxiety.

Being lesbian often means that women dated boys during high school and actively studied being "normal." Dating or having sex with boys is often a confusing experience for lesbian women, who can often function adequately and even enjoy heterosexual sex. Yet at some point, often in late adolescence or young adulthood, the desire to date her actual object of desire and the burden of continually hiding a fundamental aspect of the self cause lesbians to elect to tell others of their sexuality. Coming out always carries with it the risk of rejection and abandonment, and though it may be neutral news, it is rarely good news to others, especially to parents. Coming out is often a time of great inner (and often outer) turmoil as well as a relief. It sets the stage for further psychological development through what Erikson (1959) called "identity vs. identity confusion" into the phase of "intimacy versus iso-lation." Coming out is an unending process, revisited when one is changing jobs, moving to a new neighborhood, taking children for their first day at school, and so forth. Though it usually becomes easier as internalized homo-phobia resolves, it can also be a chronic, low-level stressor.

The consequences of hiding, secrecy, and suppression of desire in early life can have lasting effects on a lesbian's view of herself and her comfort in inti-mate relationships. In addition to the problems with intimacy all people expe-rience, a lesbian may internalize a societal view that she is bad or wrong for her desires, making it difficult to allow herself to be fully known by others. Lack of societal recognition of lesbian relationships often puts additional so-cial and financial stress on them. Decisions about having children are made in the face of societal discrimination; lesbians may worry that their own lifestyle may lead their children to be teased or even hated. Nevertheless, if all goes well, as lesbian patients enter midlife, their developmental concerns—di-verted for a time by issues of coming out and consolidating a lesbian iden-tity—tend to rejoin those of heterosexual counterparts: career advancement, balancing family and work, taking care of aging parents, and so forth.

Although not all of the developmental perspectives outlined above are relevant with all lesbian patients, and despite the fact that culture is chang-ing rapidly, putting a patient's history in its sociocultural context can be im-portant in helping a psychiatrist understand which aspects of the patient's history she may be minimizing or denying as well as raising areas for explo-ration that may prove fruitful.

In Ms. Ingram's case, we learn that she is 32 years old and grew up in the suburbs of a large city. Thus, she was born in the mid-1970s, only 5 years after the Stonewall riots that launched the gay rights movement and long before there were gay or lesbian characters on television or in movies. The late 1970s brought Anita Bryant's evangelical protests against gays, whom Bryant called "fruits," in response to the passage of one of the nation's first anti-discrimination laws. By the time Ms. Ingram was 10 in the mid-1980s, movies and plays with homosexual and transsexual themes, such as *Tootsie* (1982), *Victor/Victoria* (1982), and *La Cage aux Folles* (1978), were beginning to appear in popular cul-ture. By the mid-1990s, when the 21-year-old Ms. Ingram came out to her par-ents, she would still have been several years ahead of Ellen DeGeneres.

This history suggests that many of the themes outlined above may well apply to Ms. Ingram, but we have little information about her sexuality after the initial interview: Being a lesbian has "never been a major problem." She is not out at work because "Wall Street isn't the place to make social change." She does not feel ostracized by her coworkers. Prior to their deaths, her par-ents had accepted her lifestyle. She described many straight and gay friends. She has been involved with Sarah, her fourth girlfriend, for 3 years, and her feelings have evolved from "euphorically excited" that she had met her match to beginning to be somewhat bored with the relationship. Her past relationships had each faded when Ms. Ingram "became bored then infatuated with someone new," and she has not been single since age 17. The interviewer noted she appeared depressed when discussing her relationship with Sarah. The patient herself wondered whether the interviewer felt she should "break up with her girlfriend or go ahead and have a child."

Learning the impact of the common themes discussed earlier on Ms. Ingram's development would depend upon having far more information than was obtained in the initial meeting. Did Ms. Ingram experience a sense of difference in early life, and did it feel like a bad or undesirable difference? This issue might be especially loaded in her case since she probably felt driven to be "normal" given her brother's autism. How and when did she first recognize that she was lesbian, and did she have any opinions about gay people or know any gay people at that point? Was she a tomboy, and if so, how did each parent respond to this? Is she aware of actively, consciously hiding and keeping her sexuality a secret? Does she have feelings of inauthenticity based upon hiding or falsely presenting herself as heterosexual? Does she recall knowing about and hiding a crush on a friend or teacher? Did she have a best friend in adolescence and was there any sexual exploration? What was her relationship with her first girlfriend like; how did it come about and evolve? Did she ever date or have sex with men, and if so, how did she feel about it? How and why did she decide to tell her parents she was gay, what were their reactions in detail, and how did their relationship change as a result? Did she ever introduce them to a girlfriend? Did she or they tell extended family and family friends about her sexuality? Do any coworkers actually know she is lesbian? What does she herself make of her pattern of becoming infatuated with and then losing interest in women she is dating? How did the issue of having a child with Sarah come up and what do the two have in mind about it, especially given Ms. Ingram's current feelings about the relationship itself? The story of Ms. Ingram's sexuality—as well as the affect that accompanies the story—is likely to be found in details that are notably lacking in the initial interview.

In addition to the fact that these are probing and somewhat difficult questions, the interview suggests that denial, repression, and isolation of affect are Ms. Ingram's predominant defenses. For instance, she denies any resentment of her brother despite the fact that she had to change from music (her first love) to business to support him after her parents' deaths and despite the fact that he received much more of her parents' attention growing up. She speaks little about the details of her parents' deaths or her reactions and feelings to losing them; she focuses instead on what she did—pursue a business degree—rather than what she felt. In addition, she appears to use action and hypomanic defenses (probably fueled by a biological propensity for a cyclical mood disorder) to cover internal conflict. For instance, she tends to get morbidly depressed when "just standing still." Action (e.g., affairs, spending sprees, overworking, daredevil leisure pursuits) can serve as a way to fend off an awareness of inner conflict and difficult feelings such as anger, sadness, and loneliness or emptiness that can come more into awareness when such action ceases or slows down. In other words, Ms. Ingram may prefer to move at 100 miles per hour because she does not want to give herself time to think about and feel the things she would think about and feel at a slower speed, which might include conflicts about her sexuality or current relationship. This theory is supported by the fact that she appears depressed when discussing her girlfriend during the interview, describes herself as becoming bored in the relationship, and asks the interviewer whether she should break up with her girlfriend or go ahead and have a baby, two polar opposites about which she appears not to have allowed herself to think about fully. Forging ahead into motherhood can serve to quell major concerns about her relationship, at least temporarily, but at the high cost of Ms. Ingram never coming to understand what she really feels and wants.

Ms. Ingram's questions about her relationship, having a child, whether or not she should quit her job and return to music, and how much her brother and sister affected her suggest a nascent and perhaps growing awareness that she is unsure about her choices but interested in what has shaped who she is and how she came to be that way. If her self-referral was indeed prompted in part by a growing interest in and awareness of these issues in addition to concerns about ADHD, psychodynamic psychotherapy might be a good setting in which to explore these issues in more detail. An important piece of this work would undoubtedly be the understanding of the meanings of Ms. Ingram's developmental experiences surrounding her sexuality.

Love

Ethel S. Person, M.D.

IN her first session with a psychiatrist, Jennifer Ingram lays out her uncertainties: does she have depression or attention-deficit disorder; should she continue her career as an investment banker or pursue music; and should she break up with her girlfriend or have a child with her? These questions conform to her view that her problems can be distilled into "mood, music, and love." How can a focus on love help us understand and help this particular patient?

We do not know much about Ms. Ingram's relationship history. Sarah is her fourth girlfriend. She broke up with each previous girlfriend ostensibly because she had begun to be "bored and then infatuated with someone else." She has not been single since she was 17 years old. In regard to her relationship with Sarah, we do not know the extent to which each person is committed to the relationship, the meaning of considering a child, or problems aside from boredom. We also do not know the extent to which her personal history affects her current relationship. Her parents seem to have been preoccupied with caring for her autistic brother throughout her childhood, and then they were killed while she was in college. Her sister developed bipolar illness with ensuing periods of chaos and suicidality. These experiences may have contributed to her pursuit of independence as well as her desire for the psychiatrist to tell her what to do. Such information is not available from a single interview but would be central to our understanding of Ms. Ingram.

Ms. Ingram has long acknowledged her lesbianism, and she claims that it has never presented a problem for her, despite the fact that she is often silent about it. She had not come out at work because "Wall Street isn't the place to make social change." She denies feeling ostracized by her coworkers, but she experiences "pleasure at being tougher and more hard working than almost all of them." She makes a point of emphasizing that she has both straight and gay friends.

While she describes herself as assertive, her presentation to the psychiatrist is marked by uncertainty. While she felt "euphorically excited" when she first met Sarah and believed that she had "met her match," she now finds herself bored. Nevertheless, they are discussing having a child. At the same time that she seems to love her work, she describes it as deadening ("like being a cog in the machine"). This has led her to thinking about quitting her job and returning to music as a career. Such ambivalence is striking in someone who is seen as a "mistress of the universe."

It would certainly be important to explore Ms. Ingram's understanding of *why* the relationship has become boring and whether the discussion of having a child was a way of trying to cement the relationship. It would be useful to discuss her feelings about having children, her own childhood, her autistic brother and bipolar sister, and her own parents. It would be useful to explore many more details about her relationship with Sarah. For example, she describes "impulsive sexual affairs" but only four girlfriends in 15 years. Such information seems to indicate that she has had multiple affairs that did not break up her primary relationships, but that topic has probably not yet been broached in the evaluation. Has she maintained more than one relationship at a time? And if so, why?

The initial session has opened up many avenues for further inquiry, but perhaps most remarkable is that this strong, assertive woman wants the psychiatrist—a virtual stranger—to tell her what to do. In that first session with the psychiatrist, she asks if she has attention-deficit disorder, whether or not she needs medications, how much her brother affected her, whether she should quit her job, whether she should break up with her girlfriend, whether she should have a child, and whether she should get into psychotherapy. The psychiatrist, correctly, I believe, deferred answering these questions. But what is revealed in that interchange is, in part, a need for direction. Rather than exploring the issues, she is asking for answers from a psychiatrist who barely knows her. Such an attitude hints at significant conflicts over dependency.

Ms. Ingram may not even be aware of these strong dependency issues. She notes that she had not been single since she was 17 years old, which displays a kind of dependency, particularly if she is being literal in saying that she went from one girlfriend to another without any breaks in between. While Ms. Ingram is seemingly assertive, her insecurity is revealed through her desire for the psychiatrist to make all of the important decisions in her life, and it is further substantiated by her decision to not reveal her sexual orientation to co-workers. There are enough gays and lesbians on Wall Street who are "out" and are doing just fine. The problem rests in the way *Ms. Ingram herself* feels about homosexuality.

In addition to these insecurity and dependency issues, Ms. Ingram reports depressed moods that she regards as "poison, deadening, phlegmatic, hateful." Though she believes that these black moods occur prior to her menstrual period, the connection is unclear. How might these black moods relate to her relationships, ambivalence, and uncertainty? My guess is that she has a pattern in which she becomes excited about a girlfriend, job, or activity, but that this initial euphoria fades, leaving her bored and depressed. This can lead to a pattern in which she counteracts a low-level, ongoing depression with an infatuation (related to a girlfriend, job, or hobby). Such a pattern may well explain her urge to leave Sarah and her job and pursue having a child, meeting a lover, and switching careers.

The neediness, insecurity, and depression may all interact. Just as she desires that a psychiatrist direct her life, she may feel deeply dependent on her girlfriends. She may call herself a "mistress of the universe," but she does not seem to perceive herself that way. Further, she is depressed and undecided about all of the important issues in her life, suggesting some failure in her own self-identity.

When the psychiatrist is deciding on a treatment plan, however, it is more important to recognize that Ms. Ingram has said almost nothing about how her own psychological makeup might be contributing to her problems. While seemingly curious about her life, she has not been able to link her moods with her behavior and appears to have few feelings about her autistic brother, ill sister, deceased parents, and sexual orientation, all of which are likely to induce at least some ambivalence. For her, love/infatuation provides the hypomania that works as a "medication" to treat the underlying depression and neediness while allowing her the option of barely noticing the difficulties. While she is described in the case report as having fair insight and judgment, I would suggest that her judgment and insight may be less than "fair." She seems to view dramatic change as being the key to lifting her spirits, but while precipitous action might uplift her for a moment, this pattern appears to be crumbling, and she is finding herself distracted and sad. She does not appear to need medications or a quick tactical suggestion from the therapist. Instead, a more extended consultation might help uncover her capacity for a course of psychodynamic psychotherapy that might be especially beneficial in helping her gain the sort of insight that allows for conviction, confidence, and a more sturdy sense of happiness.

Psychodynamic Psychotherapy

Deborah L. Cabaniss, M.D.

PSYCHODYNAMIC psychotherapy is based on Freud's idea that conflicts, traumatic memories, and painful affects—even if they are out of awareness—can affect our moods and behavior. Given this, psychodynamic psychotherapy seeks to help people relieve their distress and cope more adaptively with their world by making them more aware of the contents of their unconscious minds.

The route from a person's conscious experience to their unconscious mind is uncharted. Perhaps someday we will have a scan or other test to guide us there—but for now we rely on many of the same techniques that Freud developed at the turn of the 20th century—all of which are based on talking and listening. Through free association, interpretation of dreams and fantasies, discussion of the patient's life, and exploration of the patient's relationship to and feelings about the therapist, patient and therapist crawl like blind moles toward material that has been hidden from the patient's awareness. Thus, to engage in a psychodynamic psychotherapy, the patient has to come, talk, and listen.

When I listen to a case like that of Jennifer Ingram, I am thinking many things at once, but three things that are at the front of my mind are the following:

1. What is the patient's multi-axial diagnosis (including level of personality organization)?
2. What types of treatment seem most appropriate for the patient?
3. What does the patient seem to be looking for from treatment?

These questions are linked but different. Any psychiatrist, from psychopharmacologist to psychoanalyst, must make a careful diagnosis during the evaluation phase, and determine what treatments are best suited to treat the patient's problems. The psychiatrist can then discuss the different types of treatment with the patient and together they can construct a treatment plan. The psychiatrist may favor one type of treatment over another and can convey this to the patient, but if the patient is either unwilling or unable to engage in that treatment, it will not be of use to the patient.

Given this, let's turn to the case of Jennifer Ingram. Ms. Ingram presented to see whether she had attention deficit disorder. She described symptoms suggestive of Axis I pathology—difficulty concentrating, decreased need for sleep, impulsivity in several areas of her life over many years, periods of depression that may be tied to her menstrual cycle, and cycles of disappointment in her love relations. Her family history is significant for her sister's bipolar illness. Proper diagnosis may require subsequent interviews and even neuropsychological testing—however, it seems reasonable to make an early hypothesis that she may have a bipolar disorder and/or a longstanding attention deficit disorder. We also know that she has had severe traumas in her life, including the death of her parents when she was 21 and being raised with an autistic brother. Finally, we know that she has many strengths (sometimes called ego strengths), including persistence, success in her career, musical talent, and the capacity for friendship and love relations. How do we best treat a patient for this and is there a role for psychodynamic psychotherapy?

Although we may recommend some type of psychopharmacological therapy for Ms. Ingram's symptoms of hypomania, depression, and attention problems, this does not mean that psychodynamic psychotherapy might not play an important role in Ms. Ingram's treatment. Ms. Ingram has lived her whole life with her symptoms, and thus her character has developed around them. We can only imagine how her sense of self, her relationships with others, and her strategies for learning and working evolved around her affective and attentional difficulties. Furthermore, we can hypothesize that she might be unaware of the extent to which her coping mechanisms (sometimes called defense mechanisms) are affecting her current adult functioning. For example, could her characterological "intensity" have developed to compensate for her attentional problems? Could her boredom in relationships parallel her moment-to-moment need to switch from activity to activity? In addition, we can speculate as to whether there are unconscious affects that may be leading to difficulties for Ms. Ingram. For example, she denied being hurt in any way by her impulsivity and did not mention any difficulties caused by her parents' death, her need to switch careers to care for her brother, her sister's bipolar disorder, or her homosexuality. Might she be repressing affects or memories that are nevertheless impacting her adult life? Further, could unconscious conflicts be contributing to her difficulties? She has been bothered by her symptoms for many years—why does she present now? Could she be conflicted about becoming a parent in light of her parents' deaths, her brother's autism, and her sister's bipolar illness? Might she want a child of her own but resent having to take care of her brother for all these years?

The answer to all of the above questions is "Who knows?"—without more information from the patient, they are purely speculative. I ask them because they represent the types of problems that, if present, can be very well addressed by psychodynamic psychotherapy. Yet this brings us back to our earlier question—what does the patient want from the treatment and would she be willing and/or able to engage in a psychodynamic psychotherapy?

The best clues as to what Ms. Ingram wants from treatment are found in her final questions. She wants to know if she has ADHD and whether she should take medication. But she wants help with other aspects of her life as well. She is interested in her relationships with her brother and sister and wants advice about her relationship with her girlfriend and about her job. She wants to know the doctor's recommendations about psychotherapy. She wonders about the extent to which her past affects her. This suggests that she is interested in more than just help with her attentional problems. As we discussed earlier, we can only do psychodynamic psychotherapy if the patient comes and talks, and listens. The patient is most likely to do this if she is interested in her inner life and if she thinks that discussion of her inner life will help with her current problems. The therapist must gauge both the patient's level of interest in her inner world and her thoughts about whether discussion of this will help her symptoms. This is best done by listening carefully to what the patient says to help engage her in thinking about her unconscious. For example, I would ask Ms. Ingram about her feelings about having lost her parents at such a young age—if she says that it was no problem, I could suggest that that seems surprising and see if she has any thoughts about that. She has already mentioned that she had a "theory" that her intensity was related to having a brother with autism—I might ask her to talk more about her theory and explore other aspects of her history that might have "motivated" her to develop in one way or another. She presents the conundrum of becoming bored with her girlfriend while talking about having a child with her—I could present this as a conflict and ask the patient her thoughts. If these sorts of questions, presented in as empathic and collaborative a way as possible, interest and engage the patient, I could then describe to the patient that it is likely that these sorts of issues, which may be out of awareness, may be affecting her behavior and leading to some distress and that psychodynamic psychotherapy would be a good treatment to address this.

Ms. Ingram has both ego strengths (mentioned earlier) and ego weaknesses (impulsivity, attentional difficulties), so part of the evaluation would focus on the degree to which she requires ego supportive therapy and the degree to which she requires and can tolerate a more exploratory psychotherapy. My guess is that Ms. Ingram's treatment would evolve over time, which is typical for the course of a psychodynamic psychotherapy. Patients present in crisis, and after early work helps with any presenting symptoms, many patients soon realize that their distress or dissatisfaction is about more than the presenting symptoms.

In this case, Ms. Ingram presents with attentional difficulties, but it is clear that the difficulties she is having with her love relationships and her work are repetitive and probably represent longstanding characterological difficulties. We should anticipate that an ongoing working relationship might be complicated by her tendency to make impulsive changes, but her intelligence and eagerness to understand herself would likely enable her to explore previously uncharted areas of her life, such as sexuality, her family, and love relationships. Early psychodynamic psychotherapy would probably be more ego supportive, helping her to shore up some of her more problematic defensive patterns, such as her impulsivity. As these initial issues resolve, it seems likely that Ms. Ingram would be able to move into a more exploratory psychotherapy or even a psychoanalysis to deal with unconscious conflicts and repressed affects with occasional forays into ego supportive work as the situation required. Adjunctive treatment with medication might improve her ability to tolerate the stress of psychotherapy. Working together, Ms. Ingram and her therapist could make an enormous difference, not only in addressing her Axis I pathology, but also in shifting Ms. Ingram toward more adaptive coping strategies and improving her satisfaction in her capacity to work and love.

Overview of Hypomania

Cathryn A. Galanter, M.D.

JENNIFER Ingram is a smart, assertive woman who has a number of concerns about her life. She wants to know if her problems fit diagnostic categories and whether they are treatable. Implicit in her questions are issues related to "normalcy" and our own expectations for our lives. Her concerns highlight some of the limitations of our diagnostic system, particularly in regard to symptom clusters that are subsyndromal or that exist on a continuum with normal human experience. The discussions highlight the many ways in which symptoms can be effectively elicited, including the clinical interview, diaries, and rating scales, but they also underline the reality that some diagnoses can only be made after the patient has become able to access feelings and experiences that had previously been defended against. The complexities of diagnosis and treatment can be organized around Ms. Ingram's initial concerns.

Attention-Deficit Disorder

The abilities to attend and concentrate lie on a continuum, and there will inevitably be an indeterminate gray zone between normalcy and the clear-cut syndrome. Further, internal and external expectations vary dramatically so that some people might complain of ADHD if they are unable to read intently for 10 hours, while others may not notice that they are unable to finish a magazine article. Ms. Ingram describes attentional difficulties, but she has functioned well at school and work. It is unlikely that someone with severe untreated ADHD would be able to function successfully in her job as an investment banker. At the same time, it is possible to compensate for mild ADHD through extra effort and/or selection of career, so that she may have worked her way into a job that features frequent attentional shifts (e.g., phone calls, e-mail, and brief meetings) and someone to organize details (e.g., a secretary, partner or spouse).

Additional information would be necessary to determine if Ms. Ingram has ADHD. In addition to the patient being asked, further history is probably best acquired through parents—since adult ADHD requires the presence of childhood symptoms. As this is not possible in Ms. Ingram's case, her girlfriend may be a useful source of information. Diagnoses are only as good as their underlying validity, however, and several authors have questioned the merits of diagnosing adults using a diagnostic framework that was developed and validated in children. Alternative models have been developed for adults. These models have focused on such important issues as the need for a retrospective diagnosis of childhood ADHD (Wender 1995) and modification of criteria so that they are developmentally appropriate for adults (McGough and Barkley 2004; Murphy and Barkley 1996).

With the currently available information, it appears that Ms. Ingram would probably not meet the criteria for ADHD. While she may have diminished attention, she has not yet reported any of the other symptoms that are necessary for the diagnosis, such as difficulties with organization and sustained attention. Since adults with ADHD tend to have impairments at work and difficulty in maintaining relationships, it would be useful to further explore the circumstances surrounding her job changes, relationship break-ups, and moves. Finally, her ADHD symptoms appear to fluctuate, and so it would be crucial to look for a mood disorder that may be the actual cause of her attentional complaints.

Mood Disorder

As is the case with her attentional problems, Ms. Ingram's mood symptoms do not clearly fit a DSM diagnosis. The patient describes depression, insomnia, fatigue, and preoccupation with personal issues, but these depressive symptoms appear to be sporadic and of less than one week's duration. She also describes symptoms that are found in mania such as a reduced need for sleep, unusual amounts of energy (with "dozens" of friends and an ability to engage in many activities), and risk taking (impulsive sexual affairs, spending sprees, job changes, and daredevil physical adventures). She denies any negative impact of the manic-sounding symptoms, and even the symptoms appear—at the worst—to be on a spectrum in which they may be a normal variant of human experience. A careful interview can often resolve ambiguity. In addition, both ADHD and bipolar disorder can be assessed with verified rating scales (Beck et al. 1961; Young et al. 1978). Collateral information might also be useful, as through an interview with Ms. Ingram's girlfriend. Additionally, having a first-degree relative with bipolar disorder increases her risk of having bipolar disorder. Her diagnosis should, however, be based on her own history and mental status exam, and not only on family history.

Ms. Ingram's disordered sleep is an example of a symptom that needs further elaboration, since sleep can be both a marker for psychiatric illness and a trigger for worsening mood states. Poor sleep might lead to worsening mood and concentration, for example, while getting less sleep in preparation for a deadline might fuel hypomania at the same time that hypomania might lead to decreased sleep and increased productivity. Monitoring sleep in conjunction with a mood diary might help clarify a mood or sleep disorder and can inform the possibility of therapeutically manipulating sleep to improve mood.

There is also the possibility that this patient's mood symptoms are simply not captured by the current classification system. Multiple investigators have tried to identify diagnostic clusters that fit the wide variety of clinical presentation, though their proposed categories are not yet well tested (Akiskal and Pinto 1999; Angst et al. 2003).

Some of the same uncertainties are found when the effort is made to link Ms. Ingram's depression to her menstrual cycles. Like ADHD and bipolar disorder, premenstrual dysphoric disorder (PMDD) and premenstrual syndrome (PMS) are characterized by symptoms that lie along a continuum of human experience. As with other mood disorders, dysfunction is an important criteria, but there are likely to be different individual thresholds for "dysfunction." To compound the diagnostic complexity, retrospective review of the timing and intensity of mood symptoms is notoriously imperfect. A mood diary may be useful to relate mood symptoms to the menstrual cycle as well as to clarify symptoms. It is also possible that Ms. Ingram has more than one disorder. Not only does DSM allow—and, when appropriate, demand—multiple diagnoses, the co-occurrence of certain disorders is not uncommon. For example, the National Comorbidity Study demonstrated that 21.2% of adults with bipolar disorder have ADHD and 19.4% of adults with ADHD have bipolar disorder (Kessler et al. 2006).

Rating scales and the initial clinical interview may not, however, adequately make the diagnosis. As many of the discussants pointed out, Ms. Ingram tends to protect herself from unpleasant feelings with defenses like suppression and minimization. Such a personality style may serve her well in many ways, but it is likely to make her an imperfect historian. An accurate diagnosis may not be possible until after she has become more comfortable with the therapist, and with herself.

Her Family

Ms. Ingram grew up with an autistic older brother, Larry, and also has a sister with bipolar disorder. She denies ever feeling resentful, claims that the experience demonstrated her parents' heroism, and believes that her brother's illness helped motivate her. Similarly, she does not appear to harbor strong feelings about her sister's bipolar disorder. As pointed out by Dr. Hertzig earlier in this chapter (see "Autism's Effect on the Family"), many people have very positive experiences growing up with developmentally disabled siblings. Nevertheless, Ms. Ingram may be minimizing inevitable difficulties. Would it really be possible for her to grow up without some degree of jealousy or irritation toward a brother who absorbed his parents' time? How might feelings of abandonment and loss contribute to her intense efforts to maintain "dozens of friends" and to always having a girlfriend? How does she feel about her parents dying and the necessity of supporting her brother? How does she feel about her sister and the possibility that her own mood symptoms might intensify? How might the answers to these questions affect her decisions about having a child and maintaining her girlfriend? None of these questions will be fully answered during an initial evaluation.

Her Girlfriend and the Possibility of Having a Child

The initial evaluation can prepare Ms. Ingram for the therapeutic work necessary to decide whether she should remain in a relationship with her girlfriend and/or have a child. Both of these questions—like understanding the impact of her brother—do not lend themselves to quick, simple answers.

Dr. Vaughan (see section "Being Lesbian") discusses how Ms. Ingram's sexual development and orientation may impact her. In particular, she discusses how several themes are common reactions to growing up as a lesbian, including suppression and feelings of aloneness and difference. Such experiences are not, of course, universal, and so it would be important to explore Ms. Ingram's specific reactions and memories as well as how such thoughts and feelings might impact upon her experience within a relationship and as a mother. She may also wonder about her ability to be a good mother. Exploration of her specific concerns can be balanced by mentioning the research that indicates that children of same-sex couples develop similarly to other children (Bos et al. 2005; Tasker 2005). She may also have concerns that her child would inherit a developmental disability or bipolar disorder. Such an ongoing exploration might uncover issues that are not current, conscious concerns. As discussed by Dr. Person earlier in this chapter (see section "Love"), for example, Ms. Ingram's issues may not relate to her mood, her relationships, or her work difficulties, but to problems with dependency.

Her Job

As with questions related to her brother, sister, girlfriend, and possible child, the evaluating psychiatrist should not tell this otherwise-high-functioning woman whether she should quit her job and return to music. Evaluating the options out loud may help her decide, but it is likely that the therapist will only be able to help through an ongoing psychotherapy.

Treatment

The goal of the evaluation is a treatment recommendation, but in the case of Ms. Ingram, plans are clouded by diagnostic uncertainty. As discussed earlier, it is very important to get further information from Ms. Ingram so that her clinician can more accurately establish her diagnosis and thus choose the most appropriate treatment. A mood-stabilizing medication would likely be prescribed in the unlikely event that Ms. Ingram warranted a bipolar I diagnosis, but there is little data regarding the best first-line medication for bipolar II disorder, with some patients benefiting from an antidepressant and others from a mood stabilizer (see Suppes and Dennehy 2002 for a review). There are even fewer data for those patients with symptoms only of hypomania. Ms. Ingram's psychiatrist might prescribe an antidepressant medication for her depressive symptoms or a stimulant for her attentional difficulties, but neither has been well studied in people whose symptoms are subsyndromal. Further, both antidepressants and stimulants could induce a manic episode. Since Ms. Ingram has a family history of bipolar disorder, it would be especially important that her prescribing clinician monitor her very closely if she were to start either an antidepressant or stimulant. It would be possible to begin a stimulant or antidepressant in conjunction with a mood stabilizer, but there is no evidence that suggests that the combination would help her and significant evidence that such a combination could induce unpleasant side effects.

On the other hand, it appears that Ms. Ingram could greatly benefit from psychotherapy. Dr. Cabaniss (see section "Psychodynamic Psychotherapy") underlines the importance of establishing a diagnosis prior to embarking on treatment, and as is the case with medication selection, there are multiple types of available psychotherapies, each with different indications and limitations. The therapist should also know what the patient is looking for from psychotherapy. As is noted by Dr. Cabaniss, "many patients soon realize that their distress or dissatisfaction is about more than the presenting symptoms." Ms. Ingram appears curious about the relationships between various life events, her mood, and current interpersonal issues, and she may be well suited to a trial of psychodynamic psychotherapy. In the event that Ms. Ingram is diagnosed with bipolar disorder, there are several evidence-based psychotherapies, such as cognitive-behavioral therapy, family-focused therapy, interpersonal psychotherapy, and social rhythm therapy, that can be effective in conjunction with psychopharmacological treatments in maintaining stable mood and preventing relapse (see Miklowitz 2006 for a review).

Before any treatment is suggested, however, the clinician needs a more complete history and at least a tentative diagnosis. It would also be important for the evaluating psychiatrist to not agree to Ms. Ingram's request for immediate guidance; not only does the therapist not know the answers, but it is likely that the request reflects important dependency issues that belie her status as a "mistress of the universe." A more extended evaluation may well lead the patient to the decision that she could profit from a therapy that encourages greater understanding of her decisions, her relationships, and her self.

Summary Points

- Identification of symptom clusters is an important way to classify psychiatric illness, allowing for better research and more reliable treatment.

- Psychiatric symptoms exist on a spectrum so that very few behaviors, feelings, cognitions, perceptions, or experiences definitively separate the normal from the abnormal.

- Psychiatric evaluations often identify symptoms or clusters of symptoms that are subsyndromal or do not fit current classifications. Available treatment studies do not necessarily apply to these patients.

- Psychiatric evaluations often identify symptoms or clusters of symptoms that are not the patient's chief complaint. Treatment involves negotiation and awareness that many patients may not share that psychiatrist's particular values, priorities, or interests.

- Structured rating scales may help support diagnostic decisions and monitor response to treatment.

- Psychotherapy involves empathizing with the specific patient as well as recognizing likely developmental experiences.

- Psychotherapy requires making accurate diagnoses and setting specific goals.

Chapter 10

EXAM FAILURE AND GRACE JIN

Part A

GRACE JIN was a 23-year-old medical student who was referred to a psychiatrist by Student Health Services after she failed her midterm exam in Gross Anatomy. As she entered the room, the psychiatrist noticed that she was very well groomed in a conservative style. While she began the interview with inquiries as to confidentiality and whether or not she was crazy, she moved quickly to a detailed and fast-paced account of her feelings of absolute failure. She was panic stricken that she might have to repeat an academic year and was especially humiliated that her family and friends would discover that she was stupid and lazy. She had vague but troubling thoughts of being punished for bringing shame on her family.

Ms. Jin spent much of the first session describing her parents, who immigrated to this country when she was a child primarily so that she could receive a quality education and become a physician. She said she felt guilty and anxious most of the time, though her friends tended to describe her as perfect. She was aware that she never wanted her distress to show.

During the second evaluation session, the psychiatrist asked more specifically about the anxiety symptoms that the patient had mentioned in the prior session. The patient suddenly welled with tears, saying she had a horrible secret. She said that she spent hours staring at herself in the mirror, looking for imperfection.

In addition, she had been "a bit preoccupied" with having various diseases ever since a series of mild childhood illnesses, but medical school had intensified her concerns. Thus far, she had gone to Student Health for evaluation of psoriasis, Lyme disease, systemic lupus erythematosus, and a brain tumor. Evaluation tended to clear up her concern, but she then found a new disease over which to obsess. With each new disease, she anticipated that she would have to leave medical school and be taken care of at home.

The patient said that these worries had left her unable to sleep and unable to relax. While she said she would be interested in "talk therapy," she would rather avoid Western pharmacology.

Personal History

Ms. Jin was born in southern China, the eldest of three daughters. Her family immigrated to the United States when she was 4 years old. They moved to the Midwest, where her parents owned and operated the only Chinese restaurant in a small, rural town. Her aunt and uncle ran a similar restaurant 30 miles away. A straight-A student, Ms. Jin believed that she owed her academic effort to her parents, who had sacrificed their careers as teachers in China for her future. While her studiousness had been seen as a bit odd by her high school classmates, she was accepted by them at least partly because she had dated a star of the school's football team. This was barely tolerated by her parents, however, whose insistence that she date only Asian men was frustrated by the fact that the nearest Asian teenagers were 200 miles away.

While dating the football player, tolerating the criticism of her parents, working long hours at the family restaurant, watching out for her younger sisters, and leading a variety of extracurricular activities, Ms. Jin had secretly dated the high school's primary drug dealer, who she said was the only person who really excited her.

Her parents were pleased and proud when she went to a West Coast college that not only was famous but boasted a large number of young Chinese men. She had met her current boyfriend during her sophomore year. They fought about his irresponsibility and abuse of drugs and alcohol, but she believed that he was the perfect antidote to her seriousness. He was also her "cross to bear," saying that he was a "black-sheep Asian" who sported tattoos and had dropped out of college to pursue a career in music. Her parents knew of the relationship and did not approve. They repeatedly told her that her unemployed boyfriend would "ruin her life."

Throughout high school, college, and medical school, Ms. Jin had abstained from drugs, made excellent grades, and continued to volunteer frequently at a homeless shelter, edit school publications, and work as an emergency medical technician. She did not see these as choices and said she frequently felt unappreciated and worn out.

Personal Psychiatric History

The patient denied psychiatric problems aside from her "mirror obsession" that began when she was 10. At that time, she began to spend long periods staring at the uncontrollable jumpy movements of her face. After the movements disappeared, she focused on asymmetries and blemishes. She denied other obsessions or compulsions. She had no history of treatment.

Family Psychiatric History

None known, except that her younger sisters were both exceptional students who also planned to be doctors.

Medical History

The patient reported having had multiple colds and sore throats as a child. No serious illnesses.

Mental Status Exam

The patient was a trim, athletic, well-groomed young woman who was cooperative and eager to please. Her speech was rapid, crisp, and goal directed. She felt anxious, but her affect was full range and appropriate. She denied depression, suicidality, and psychotic symptoms. She was cognitively intact, and her insight and judgment appeared good.

Summary

Grace Jin was a 23-year-old medical student who was referred to an outpatient psychiatrist after she failed an exam. The first seven discussions will explore Ms. Jin's long-standing and acute reactions to stress and disappointment and will discuss treatment options. The discussion in the second half of the case will describe Ms. Jin's ongoing evaluation.

Discussions of the Case of Grace Jin, Part A

Interview of the Medical Student 382
  Scott J. Goldsmith, M.D.

Somatoform Disorders and Obsessionality. 387
  Brian A. Fallon, M.D.

Neurobiology of Obsessions 389
  Helen Blair Simpson, M.D., Ph.D.

Narcissistic Injury and Narcissistic Defenses. 393
  Nathan Kravis, M.D.

The First-Generation Asian American 398
  Sandra Park, M.D.

Complementary Medicine and Integrative Pharmacology . .402
  Richard P. Brown, M.D., and Patricia L. Gerbarg, M.D.

Mindfulness Meditation 405
  Susan Evans, Ph.D.

Part B 408

Interview of the Medical Student

Scott J. Goldsmith, M.D.

IMAGINE for a moment that, after a highly competitive search and many interviews, you are selected for a new job. You are told that your new career will be a humanitarian one—exciting, prestigious, and potentially lucrative.

When you arrive for work, however, you find that your task is to sit in a windowless room all day, listening to people speak in a made-up language. Each day, you are shown complicated lists, maps, and diagrams of strange objects in this foreign language, and then told to memorize them. You are forced to sit in a room full of dead bodies. You are told that you will not be paid for the first 4 years; instead; you will incur considerable debt.

As the job progresses, new rules are imposed. You are deprived of sleep. You are not given time to eat properly and exercise. You are required to appear calm while you cause people pain. You are told that people might die if you make an error as simple as not washing your hands properly.

To be honest, you were not sure you even wanted this job, but you certainly had to work very hard to get it. Perhaps you had an experience that made you think it would be rewarding. It certainly looked interesting in movies and on television, but you likely chose this career before you seriously considered other options. There is no good exit strategy, however, since leaving at this point would cost you your career, the respect of your family and friends, and your financial stability. This job is not all it was cracked up to be.

You are in medical school.

An astute psychiatrist can read just the first few words of this case presentation, "Grace Jin was a 23-year-old medical student," and begin to develop hypotheses about her. We would predict that she is a smart young woman under extraordinary pressure. We would assume that she, like all patients, is unique and that she has specific reasons for consulting a psychiatrist. We might also expect that her status as a medical student would lead to an especially thorough evaluation of the biological, psychological, and social aspects of her situation, but this final expectation is often not fulfilled. In my clinical experience running a mental health service for physicians in training, I have found that a student like Ms. Jin is likely to receive less-than-optimal care because of issues related to the psychiatrist's identifications, assumptions, and faulty recollections, any or all of which can sidetrack a thorough biopsychosocial evaluation.

The psychiatrist, by virtue of having finished medical school, will identify with Ms. Jin, and this leads to a number of common assumptions. For example, the psychiatrist might see a smart, well-groomed young student and assume that she is having the same sort of reaction to medical school that the psychiatrist has seen many times before (beginning, perhaps, with the psychiatrist's own reaction many years earlier). Such expectations can lead the therapist to assess Ms. Jin superficially, ignore her real concerns, and offer quick reassurance. Often, psychiatrists minimize and/or underdiagnose psychiatric illness among medical students, as well as other physicians and colleagues. In Ms. Jin's case, a casual dismissal of her concerns would likely lead to undertreatment and to a deepening sense of isolation.

A second consequence of a psychiatrist's identification with the medical student patient relates to the fact that many physicians appear to have a selective amnesia for the intensity of the stress of medical education and thereby minimize the role of medical education itself as a precipitant for psychiatric illness. In these cases, medical students who recognize and discuss the intensity of their experiences are often overdiagnosed with Axis II pathology or are labeled as masochistic, self-defeating complainers. In my experience, this is particularly true for students who were accepted to medical school based in large part on their nonscience backgrounds (e.g.,writers, artists). While these students may make excellent physicians, they may struggle during medical school, particularly during the preclinical, basic science years. We don't know Ms. Jin's specific academic background, but it is clear that she is overwhelmed and humiliated by her feelings of failure. A quick suggestion to accept academic mediocrity is unlikely to be helpful to any medical student, particularly one like Ms. Jin, who believes that her parents sacrificed their entire lives to allow their daughters to achieve.

An additional complication for Ms. Jin is that she is being evaluated by someone—a psychiatrist—who has evidently completed the very studies that she is finding difficult. While this may allow the psychiatrist to more fully understand her situation, it can also lead the patient to develop an early transferential mixture of envy, admiration, and rage—a reaction that can be fueled by statements that appear supportive but can be felt as empathic failures. For example, the psychiatrist might say, "It must be hard for you," which could be heard by Ms. Jin as "It must be hard for YOU; it wasn't for me." Since she describes her parents as intently focused on her success, Ms. Jin may find it hard to believe that the psychiatrist won't be similarly judgmental.

Psychiatrists treating medical students should also pay attention to a few common misguided assumptions. For example, the psychiatrist may too readily assume therapeutic sophistication in Ms. Jin, a young woman who may never have even met a therapist, much less know the basic rules of therapy. She may need confirmation, for example, that while the clinician may be employed by her medical school, the consultation is confidential. Further, she may worry that every behavior reflects psychopathology and that the therapist is able to read her mind. This concern that psychiatrists are in essence psychics is not uncommon, and while in Ms. Jin's case these concerns may eventually be fodder for interpretation, the creation of a comfortable alliance may require a more open and even didactic exchange of information than the psychiatrist might expect when working with someone as obviously bright as Ms. Jin.

The psychiatrist should not assume that Ms. Jin is unique in her concerns about medical school. Her fears of repeating an academic year, preoccupations with various medical illnesses, persistent anxiety, and insomnia are common among medical students and are not a priori pathological. I know of few colleagues who would relish the chance to revisit their first year of medical school. At the same time that medical school can undermine a student's confidence, it provides opportunities for real pride of achievement. The psychiatrist can fortify the patient's shaky self-esteem by warmly recognizing occasions when she mentions having mastered some basic science material or participated in such formative experiences as making a diagnosis, joining a code team, or counseling a patient and family during a crisis.

The psychiatrist should also recognize that the period after college and through one's 20s is a busy time and ideally includes completing a number of important life tasks. Challenges faced by Ms. Jin and her fellow students include, but are by no means limited to, separating from their families of origin, developing healthy intimate relationships, negotiating sexuality and sexual orientation, developing self-esteem that is not driven by external approval, and negotiating financial independence. In addition, most psychiatric disorders declare themselves in this age group. It is the reality that most medical students must navigate these challenges while undertaking the biological, psychological, and social stresses of training to be a physician.

Keeping these potential pitfalls in mind, the psychiatrist can more effectively perform a careful biopsychosocial evaluation that will take into consideration some of Ms. Jin's likely experiences. To begin with, she faces distinct biological stressors. In class all day, she will have limited exposure to sunlight, and little free time for recreation, exercise, socializing, and proper eating. During the weeks prior to examinations (and later, during clinical rotations), sleep hygiene may be particularly difficult, and Ms. Jin does complain of insomnia.

It is important to ask her about these stressors. Not only do such questions imply empathy with her situation, they can help develop a more complex understanding of the ways in which the experience of medical school has led to the onset or exacerbation of the symptoms that brought her to the consultation. Asking about stressors can easily lead to a discussion of what she does to deal with her uncomfortable feelings. It is not uncommon for medical students to use herbal supplements, prescription medications, alcohol, and/or street drugs in order to deal with stress, and Ms. Jin is more likely to reveal any substance use and abuse if she feels that the therapist understands her situation. While she has apparently denied drug use, she has been dating substance-abusing boyfriends since high school, and it would not be surprising if she were to hide drug abuse from a psychiatrist, particularly one who appeared not to understand her situation.

Ms. Jin presents with a variety of psychiatric symptoms that deserve thorough and tactful investigation, but it is also useful to recognize the psychological issues that are particularly common among medical students.

First-year medical students like Ms. Jin face heavy coursework, and they are also aware that failure to learn the material could hurt or even kill someone. As students spend more time on clinical rotations, they will need to effectively suppress the intense feelings of anger, sadness, and disgust that are routinely elicited by medical work. These feelings may be exacerbated in medical students who have significant personal experience with illness or death, as the posttraumatic aspects of these events are reactivated during the course of their education. They may also be particularly intense for Ms. Jin, who appears to be unusually anxious and who worries not only about getting illnesses but also about her own possible physical deformity.

Social stressors have been alluded to but deserve explicit attention. As we see with Ms. Jin, medical school isolates the student from friends and family, who, unless they too are physicians, cannot fully appreciate the engulfment of the medical school experience. In addition, medical students are expected to follow schedules created by the school and their clinical teams. Afforded little control, they are routinely prevented from taking care of personal and family crises, just as they are often required to miss holidays and important family events. The case report does not mention Ms. Jin's finances, but most medical students in the United States incur significant debt to pursue a career they chose many years earlier with little real experience. Adding insult to injury, supervising physicians often do not empathize with the plight of medical students but instead tend to shake their heads and ruefully repeat, "You cannot imagine how much harder this was in my day." This unhelpful intervention isolates students from mentors who might be otherwise able to offer support.

Medical school can be intense, harrowing, but also exhilarating, and the evaluating psychiatrist is in a unique position to help smooth this experience, particularly for students, like Ms. Jin, who equate happiness with academic success. Through simply asking about lifestyle issues (e.g., eating and sleeping), social supports, and outside interests, the psychiatrist can implicitly underline their importance. The clinician working with medical students may also need to demonstrate flexibility, as student schedules may preclude regularly scheduled sessions. Most importantly, Ms. Jin deserves the same good psychiatric evaluation and treatment as do all patients. By considering the unusual nature of the school experience, as well as likely transference and countertransference responses that can affect her treatment, the psychiatrist working with Ms. Jin will be best able to intervene at this critical juncture in her life. In the process the therapist can help Ms. Jin learn about herself, her symptoms, and the value of her chosen career.

Somatoform Disorders and Obsessionality

Brian A. Fallon, M.D.

AMONG a variety of concerns, Grace Jin has symptoms that point toward two of the somatoform disorders, hypochondriasis and body dysmorphic disorder. All of the somatoform disorders include physical concerns and/or complaints that are inadequately explained by a known medical condition. Diagnostic clarity is often frustrated by comorbidity, by the blurring of diagnostic boundaries, by the possibility of unusual medical presentations, and by the ubiquity of psychological issues (i.e., if a psychiatrist looks hard enough for a conflict, a conflict will generally be found). While the somatoform disorders have attracted the attention of such medical luminaries as Hippocrates, Galen, and Freud, they can also induce diagnostic frustration and therapeutic nihilism among clinicians. Nevertheless, an attentive, informed evaluation can help Ms. Jin as she tries to overcome an affliction that threatens to suck the pleasure out of her life.

Hypochondriasis

In some ways, Ms. Jin is unusual. Unlike other somatoform disorders, her possible diagnoses—hypochondriasis and body dysmorphic disorder—are associated with anxious obsessionality. While problematic, her complaints have not shut down her social and professional lives. She has agreed to see a psychiatrist. Other aspects of her presentation are more typical. Medical students do frequently worry that they have whatever disease they are studying, but their worries generally dissipate after a quick consultation with a friend or family member. Ms. Jin has gone to Student Health not once but four times for evaluation of four different diseases; this is not typical of a medical student. These obsessional worries do not calm her; she feels tortured. Such concerns could reflect hypochondriasis, in which intense, persistent obsessions about disease lead to compulsions to check with doctors—much as one sees with obsessive-compulsive disorder (OCD). To fit DSM criteria, these symptoms would need to persist off and on for at least 6 months and not respond adequately to reassurance.

On the other hand, repeated visits to student health could indicate a medical student who knows of no other way to seek help than to manifest her emotional distress in a physical way. Maybe it took four visits for the student health staff to finally get the message—"I need help"—and refer her to a psychiatrist—a possibility made more likely by her reluctance to reveal distress. Indeed, many aspects of this woman's history suggest that psychodynamic conflicts are major determinants of her behavior. Although persons with hypochondriasis tend to be harm avoidant, Ms. Jin had secretly dated her high school's biggest drug dealer and is currently living with an unemployed, substance-abusing musician. These features suggest that internal conflicts are motivating her seemingly poor choices. A clue may be found in her fantasy that her illness would force her to go home and be cared for by her family. Exploration of this fantasy would be an important way to understand her symptoms.

Body Dysmorphic Disorder

Ms. Jin's "horrible secret" is not her failed exam, her boyfriend, or her hypochondriacal concerns. Instead, she breaks into tears when she explains that the source of her anxiety is her need to stare into a mirror several hours each day. The intensity and duration of her self-observation points strongly at body dysmorphic disorder (BDD).

BDD typically emerges somewhat earlier than hypochondriasis, often in the mid-teens, and is seen in almost as many men as women. The extreme preoccupation with appearance negatively impacts on relationships, leading to social isolation and low marriage rates. BDD also has an impact on work and school. While Ms. Jin may have failed her exam for psychodynamic reasons, she may also have failed because her lengthy mirror rituals would have cut down on the time available to study. Further assessment should include uncovering the duration of her preoccupation with her appearance as well as exploring other behaviors which might accompany BDD, such as comparing, checking, grooming, camouflaging, and reassurance seeking. If she engages in a number of these activities, then behavioral treatments could be used to reduce the intensity and length of the rituals. Active exploration of related symptoms is important, since patients with BDD tend not to say anything if asked to say "whatever comes to mind." In fact, Ms. Jin's relative openness about her mirror checking is remarkable; BDD is generally hidden from friends, physicians, and therapists. It is also important to carefully evaluate her for commonly comorbid anxiety and mood disorders, such as OCD, social phobia, trichotillomania, and atypical depression.

Treatment

I would suggest an extended evaluation of perhaps 10 sessions during which her symptoms, feelings, and life situation would be explored. If the hypochondriasis and BDD start to dissipate, then I would recommend continuing the insight-oriented psychotherapy. If the BDD or hypochondriasis remains unchanged, then I would consider incorporating behavioral techniques such as graded exposure and response prevention. Cognitive-educational therapy for hypochondriasis has been manualized in a self-help format that has demonstrated efficacy (Barsky 2006). Cognitive-behavioral therapies have also been shown to help with BDD (Williams et al. 2006). A selective serotonin reuptake inhibitor can be quite helpful to patients with hypochondriasis or BDD (Fallon 2004). While Ms. Jin is reluctant to take Western medicines, her reluctance may subside once she advances in therapy. Most likely, a combination of strategies would be useful.

Ms. Jin obsesses about her health and appearance while engaging in behaviors that could place her health and appearance at risk. She is fear-ridden while also being assertive. After a lifetime of successes, she has become preoccupied with the belief that she is a failure. In short, this is a wonderfully interesting person to engage in therapy. I anticipate that Grace Jin will do well, as long as she continues in therapy and as long as the obsessional and ritualistic aspects of her life are addressed.

Neurobiology of Obsessions

Helen Blair Simpson, M.D., Ph.D.

GRACE Jin presents for treatment with multiple issues. One symptom that bothers her greatly is her "mirror obsession," calling it her "horrible secret." She reports spending hours staring at herself in the mirror, looking for bodily imperfections. She also reports being preoccupied with illness, always finding a new disease "over which to obsess." These "obsessions" cause her anxiety and insomnia.

Diagnosis

Does Grace have obsessive-compulsive disorder (OCD)? In DSM-IV-TR (American Psychiatric Association 2000), the obsessions of OCD are defined very specifically as "recurrent and persistent thoughts, impulses, or images that are experienced, at some time during the disturbance, as intrusive and inappropriate and that cause marked anxiety or distress." Thus, an obsession is not simply an excessive worry about a real-life problem; nor is it pleasurable. Grace has intrusive thoughts about imperfection and exaggerated fears about disease. These thoughts interfere with her functioning and cause her distress. Whether she has OCD is not clear from this description, however, for several reasons.

First, it is unusual for OCD patients to have obsessions without compulsions. Compulsions are repetitive behaviors (e.g., hand washing, ordering, checking) or mental acts (e.g., mental counting, repeating thoughts, mental reviewing) that the person feels driven to perform in response to an obsession or according to rigid rules. The aim of compulsions is to prevent a dreaded event or to reduce distress (e.g., washing after having the intrusive thought that one has touched something contaminated). One large study found that 96% of OCD patients had both obsessions and compulsions, and 80% had a mixture of behavioral and mental compulsions (Foa et al. 1995). Thus, obsessions in the absence of compulsions are rare in OCD.

Grace's time in front of the mirror sounds like a compulsion (e.g., visual and mental checking in response to intrusive fears of imperfection). She may also have compulsions related to her fears of illness (e.g., repetitively seeking medical evaluations to reassure herself that she is not ill). However, the case description does not provide sufficient details for us to be sure. If Grace is like many OCD patients, she will need careful questioning by an empathic clinician to clarify these symptoms. There are also likely to be additional manifestations of this "horrible secret" that she has yet to reveal.

Even with obsessions and compulsions, Grace may not have OCD. For example, spending hours in front of a mirror looking for imagined physical defects is typical of body dysmorphic disorder (BDD). If the obsessions or compulsions are restricted to appearance, then BDD is the more likely diagnosis. Of course, her obsessions also include concerns about medical illness, and this could be consistent with OCD. But excessive fear of a dread medical illness is also the hallmark of hypochondriasis.

The bottom line is that repetitive, intrusive, anxious thoughts can occur in various Axis I disorders, including OCD, BDD, hypochondriasis, posttraumatic stress disorder, and generalized anxiety disorder. On close examination, not all of these thoughts will be obsessions as defined by DSM-IV-TR, and obsessions by themselves are not diagnostic of OCD.

Neurobiology

Regardless of the Axis I diagnosis, Grace appears to have a brain that recurrently focuses on anxious thoughts. Studies have shown that up to 80% of the general population may experience intrusive, unpleasant, or unwanted thoughts and about 50% may engage in ritualistic behavior (Muris et al. 1997). An obsessional brain appears to be part of the human condition. Grace has more intrusive anxious thoughts than many people, however, and these recurrent thoughts disrupt her functioning.

What might be the etiology of such an excessive obsessional style? For example, does she obsess because of a genetic vulnerability, a developmental insult, a biological illness or toxin, an environmental event, or a cultural dilemma? In the case of OCD, there are case histories of new onset or exacerbation of OCD after many different etiological agents, including neurological lesions (e.g., stroke, head trauma, tumors), viral and bacterial illness, metabolic poisoning, and severe psychological trauma (Sasson et al. 2005; Simpson and Fallon 2000). OCD has also been shown to be highly familial in some cases, leading to the search for OCD genes (Hemmings and Stein 2006). In the case of Grace, one could speculate that her "multiple sore throats" as a child contributed to her obsessional brain, since there is an association between untreated streptococcal throat infections and OCD (Snider and Swedo 2004). However, as with most patients, it is hard to be sure which, if any, of these etiological agents is the culprit.

What might be the pathophysiology of such an excessive obsessional style? The assumption here is that any behavior (no matter its original cause) is mediated by the nervous system. Therefore, recurrent obsessing is evidence of a malfunctioning brain. Many studies have compared the brains of people with OCD with the brains of people without OCD. Studies using structural imaging (e.g., magnetic resonance imaging [MRI] or computed tomography [CT]) suggest that at least some OCD patients have abnormalities in the volume of their caudate nucleus. Studies of brain blood flow or metabolism have found that OCD is associated with hyperactivity in a brain circuit that includes the frontal lobes (specifically the orbitofrontal cortex), the basal ganglia (specifically the caudate nucleus), and the thalamus. This hyperactivity is increased when OCD symptoms are provoked compared with a resting state. Moreover, serotonin reuptake inhibitors (SRIs), the only medications proven effective for OCD, and cognitive-behavioral treatment, the only psychotherapy with demonstrated efficacy, decrease this hyperactivity in treatment responders. Together, these data have led to the idea that OCD is due to a hyperactive brain circuit that includes the orbitofrontal cortex, caudate nucleus, and thalamus. There are several different proposals for how this circuit may dysfunction. For example, one leading model proposes that OCD is due to an imbalance in the basal ganglia between the direct and indirect pathways resulting in thalamic disinhibition that then allows incoming stimuli excessive access to the cortex, leading to intrusive thoughts (Saxena et al. 2001).

With regard to the neurochemistry of OCD, it has been hypothesized for over 20 years that brain serotonergic dysfunction plays a role in the pathophysiology of OCD (Insel et al. 1985). This idea was originally based on the fact that SRIs are the only medications effective in OCD. However, SRIs might reduce OCD symptoms because they modulate other neurochemical systems that are defective, not because there is an abnormality in the serotonergic system. To date, brain imaging studies of the serotonergic system in OCD (Adams et al. 2005; Simpson et al. 2003) have led to inconsistent or unreplicated findings in small samples.

Other neurobiological systems have also been implicated in OCD. For example, it has been hypothesized that dopaminergic abnormalities exist in some OCD patients, based in part on clinical findings that antipsychotic medications augment SRI response in up to 50% of OCD patients (Dougherty et al. 2004). Studies of the brain dopaminergic system have also led to inconsistent or unreplicated findings in small samples (Denys et al. 2004). Rosenberg and colleagues found that glutamatergic compounds measured by magnetic resonance spectroscopy were increased in the caudate nucleus of SRI-naive children with OCD. These data led to hyperglutamatergic models of OCD and to speculation that OCD patients have abnormalities in glutamatergic-serotonergic neurotransmission in frontal-basal ganglia circuits (Carlsson 2000; Rosenberg and Keshavan 1998).

In summary, OCD has been associated with abnormalities in frontal basal ganglia circuits, but the precise functional abnormalities in OCD remain unclear. There are much more limited data for the etiology or pathophysiology of related disorders, such as BDD or hypochondriasis (Bartz and Hollander 2006). Whether all disorders involving intrusive anxious thoughts have hyperactivity in frontal-basal ganglia circuits is unclear and a source of ongoing scientific exploration.

Clinical Implications

Currently, there is little connection between the clinical care of a patient like Grace Jin and the neurobiological research just described. Treatment is based on the results of the clinical exam, not any direct examination of her brain. Contemplating how her brain is malfunctioning, however, may help with treatment planning. For example, if one conceptualizes her excessive obsessing as a manifestation of hyperactivity in frontal-basal ganglia circuits, one is more likely to eschew extended exploration of her intrusive thoughts in favor of an initial treatment goal of symptom relief through the use of such interventions as SRI medications and cognitive-behavioral therapy. Educating Grace about dysfunctional brain circuits may make Grace more receptive to pharmacotherapy. When she spends less time "obsessing," Grace may be more flexibly able to address such issues as her boyfriend, her family, her school, and herself.

Narcissistic Injury and Narcissistic Defenses

Nathan Kravis, M.D.

GRACE Jin experiences herself as struggling with what she feels to be the impossible expectations of her parents and her own need to be perfect. Her perfectionism serves to ward off panic-inducing fears of failure and shame that chronically threaten her sense of self-worth, for despite her high level of academic achievement and her high-octane industriousness, she worries that she will be revealed as stupid and lazy. In other words, she harbors intense feelings of fraudulence. These feelings fuel her anxiety and dysphoria as well as her fantasies of humiliation and punishment. They are usually masked by her rather grim determination to excel, but her failure on the anatomy exam punctures this fragile equilibrium and prompts her to seek treatment.

While an exam failure might safely be said to constitute a narcissistic injury for any medical student, it is clear that for Ms. Jin the stakes are especially high. Her panic and exaggerated fears of exposure and mortification show how she has relied upon academic performance to prop up a shaky self-esteem organized around parental approval. Pleasing her parents and garnering their praise and approval has become an increasingly fraught strategy for self-esteem maintenance as Ms. Jin moves into adulthood. Perhaps her parents' actual expectations have been distorted by Ms. Jin in the course of her internalization of them, so that now she has come to expect perfection of herself, and any evidence to the contrary occasions a massive disturbance of self-esteem. In any case, there are clear signs that Ms. Jin has been chafing under the strain of the impossible task she has assigned herself—namely, to be perfect and wonderful in every way imaginable.

Indeed, her defiant choices of disapproved boyfriends in high school (the football player, the drug dealer) and college (her substance-abusing current boyfriend) hint at the angry underbelly of the felt need to be perfect. Beneath her studious, obedient façade, Ms. Jin has secretly cultivated a rebellious persona, albeit mostly by proxy. Although her current boyfriend's irresponsible behavior bothers her, in choosing to be with him she vicariously enjoys his irresponsibility and hedonism, and this is her (so far unacknowledged) way of thumbing her nose at her parents, their values, and their traditions.

Perfectionism is a harsh taskmaster; it often engenders the enraged feeling that no one sufficiently understands how demanding and impossible one's life is, how hard one is striving to satisfy enormous expectations, and how pleasureless and draining this makes the experience of daily life. Ms. Jin's stated feelings of exhaustion and under-appreciation indicate that this may be true of her. Alongside the bitter feeling of being unappreciated, one often encounters the hidden grandiosity of martyrdom described by Cooper (1988) in his seminal work on the narcissistic-masochistic character.

Returning to Ms. Jin's presenting problem (the anatomy exam failure), one must wonder why such an accomplished student might stumble so conspicuously. Is she simply cracking under pressure, or has she unconsciously struck upon a way to declare her exhaustion with trying to maintain an unbroken record of success, a way to emancipate herself from the deadening treadmill of achievement that she can no longer pretend pleases her, a way to break free of the false self she has constructed and which now imprisons her? While failing an exam is humiliating, it represents a communication from the sane part of her who recognizes that her current modus operandi has become untenable. Her fantasy that she will be forced to leave medical school and be taken care of at home, while anxiety-ridden, also expresses the wish to cast off responsibility and, more importantly, to be able to feel lovable without having to earn love through the ceaseless performance of good deeds and spectacular academic feats.

Of course, in the broader context of being a 23-year-old medical student, Ms. Jin has entered a time of her life when setbacks, failures, and disappointments will likely come her way as never before, not just because medical training is arduous and replete with indignities and assaults on pride and self-esteem, but also because adult life itself is full of narcissistic injuries— abounding with, in Hamlet's famous phrase, "the slings and arrows of outrageous fortune" (*Hamlet* III,i,58). For this reason, narcissistic defenses are ubiquitous. Their deployment is not limited to people with narcissistic personality disorder, though they feature prominently in the repertoire of people with some degree of narcissistic pathology.

Narcissistic defenses include grandiosity, entitlement, haughty superiority, arrogant obliviousness, perfectionism, omnipotent control, idealization (of self or others), devaluation, and social withdrawal or self-sufficiency in the service of denying needing anything from anyone. Narcissistic defenses defend against feelings of inferiority, inadequacy, humiliation, shame, envy, and rage.

While she probably does not meet DSM diagnostic criteria for narcissistic personality disorder, Ms. Jin's heavy reliance on defenses such as perfectionism and idealization, her proneness to humiliation and shame, and her hidden rage about having to be so perfect all the time strongly suggest some degree of narcissistic disturbance. The "horrible secret" she feels ashamed to reveal in the second evaluation interview encapsulates such a disturbance and conveys a great deal of information about the nature of this disturbance. Her mirror gazing and her severe case of medical student hypochondria represent the awful trap of the narcissist: the constant accompaniment of the wish to be perfect is the anxious, shameful awareness of always falling short of this ideal. To the extent that Ms. Jin's lengthy sessions of skin inspection in front of the mirror metaphorically represent her ardent wish to be a perfect person with whom everyone will be pleased—and her dread of imperfection (which to her entails humiliation)—they also represent the reification of that metaphor into concrete behavior. In a classic paper, Reich (1960) observes that often people with narcissistic pathology have developed hypertrophied concerns with bodily intactness due to traumatic experiences (physical or psychological) in early childhood. Such people may defend against fears of bodily damage with a compensatory narcissistic erotization of their bodies. She postulates that narcissists tend toward hypochondria because excessive body narcissism and hypochondria are flip sides of the same coin.

This points to a broader consideration regarding people with narcissistic pathology, namely, their vulnerability to sudden oscillations in self-esteem and sudden shifts from admiration to contempt for others. The same aggressive competitiveness fueled by perfectionism and/or grandiosity is turned round upon the self in moments of narcissistic defeat, so that self-loathing supervenes and the self is experienced as castrated, damaged, or worthless. (This is another way of understanding the association of narcissism and hypochondria.) The dramatic plunge from prideful excellence to miserable self-loathing may contribute to the sense of fraudulence we have inferred in the case of Ms. Jin.

It is not at all uncommon for patients with narcissistic disturbances to seek treatment at a time of narcissistic injury. This is, obviously, a time of great stress. It is important to diagnose and appropriately treat any previously unrecognized major depression or dysthymic disorder. At the same time, the treating psychiatrist or psychotherapist must be prepared for bouts of intense dysphoria, sometimes attaining the pitch of suicidal despair, during the course of treatment as the patient's narcissistic defenses are examined and his or her reliance on retreats into perfectionism or grandiosity is challenged. At the moment of her initial evaluation, Ms. Jin appears more anxious than depressed. In fact, her mental status exam is noteworthy for the denial of depressed mood (despite the catastrophe that has just befallen her) and the impression she gives of being cooperative and eager to please. The discerning therapist will anticipate the emergence of hostile devaluation and contempt as Ms. Jin settles into treatment and begins to resent the perceived demand to be pleasing and compliant.

A huge problem for patients like Ms. Jin arises as treatment gets under way and the therapist presents himself or herself as a reliably attentive, thoughtful, trustworthy, and empathic interlocutor. This situation invites an upsurge in the longed-for yet feared dependence on a loving and caring object. In people with narcissistic disturbances, such dependence is feared because it tends to stimulate envy, and envy leads to interpersonal destructiveness (Kernberg 1975, 1984). Envy is destructive because it can lead someone to feel that he or she would rather spoil something good than have to bear watching someone else have it.

So narcissistic defenses are attempts to forestall aggressive and destructive responses toward those who are loving and helpful (e.g., the therapist) because such people make the narcissist feel humiliated and defeated by his or her own needs (Kernberg 1975)—hence the compensatory grandiosity and idealization of the self, including the omnipotent, controlling, destructive parts of the self. A very painful and crucial point in treatment is reached when the patient becomes aware of the therapist as a valuable external person and begins to experience conscious envy (Rosenfeld 1971). Facing the reality of being emotionally dependent on the therapist can lead to intense depression, even suicidality, and/or intense hatred and destructiveness, sometimes taking the form of self-destructive acting out (e.g., spoiling professional successes or personal relationships, or abruptly quitting therapy).

Prior to therapy, these patients have typically dealt with this struggle within themselves "by trying to get rid of their concern and love for their objects by killing [or shutting down] their loving dependent self and identifying themselves almost entirely with the destructive narcissistic part of the self which provides them with a sense of superiority and self-admiration" (Rosenfeld 1971, p. 174). To make true contact with the therapist threatens the patient with a weakening of this defensive armor of narcissistic omnipotent superiority. Hence, to change or to receive help is experienced as an attack.

The therapeutic task is to "help the patient to find and rescue the dependent sane part of the self from its trapped position inside the psychotic narcissistic structure" (Rosenfeld 1971, p. 175), as it is this sane part of him or her that can form a positive relationship with the therapist and with the rest of his or her world. Secondly, treatment aims to promote awareness of the split-off, omnipotent parts of the self that contain destructive, envious impulses that have, in effect, infantilized the patient and prevented him or her from growing up by leading him or her to spurn relationships that would be growth-promoting (Rosenfeld 1971). The patient needs to see how the effort to avert envy via retreats into grandiosity, perfectionism, or omnipotence end up being infantilizing and deadening.

We all fear the vulnerability and dependency of love to some extent. Insofar as the therapist represents a good object, any transference at all may be felt as a threatening form of dependency and may be resisted by mounting a bland, superficial friendliness as its substitute (Riviere 1936). Some patients insist that they have no transference whatsoever. This may be a way of denying the craving for a perfect object and avoiding the possibility of anxiety and fury about finding the therapist to be disappointingly ordinary. Ultimately, what these patients may fear most is the confrontation with the reality of what has been lost, missed, destroyed, or longed for and never had (Riviere 1936; Spillius 1993).

Even our most positive experiences of being loved—by lovers, parents, or therapists—include a sad, sometimes painful, and potentially embittering experience of being unknown or incompletely known. The wish for revenge is one available response to this (LaFarge 2006). In this sense, revenge may be said to be a by-product of love, since being loved is intrinsically inadequate as a narcissistically gratifying experience.

A person who unconsciously feels unlovable and inferior may try to project this inferiority onto someone toward whom he can then feel superior. He can then think of himself as legitimately attacking a bad object who deserves to be hated. Spillius refers to this as *impenitent envy*—envy without guilt or responsibility. In such cases defenses serve not only to maintain a sense of grievance but also to evade the painful acknowledgment that one desperately wants a good object but does not have or has not had one. Feeling perpetual grievance and blame, however miserable, is less painful than mourning the loss of relationships one wishes one had had (Spillius 1993). Feeling aggrieved can thereby become an important form of narcissistic defense, especially for the narcissistic-masochistic character (Cooper 1988).

The terrible quandary faced by people with significant narcissistic disturbances is that their envy stunts their growth and constricts their personalities.

Envy leading to attacks on the goodness of the object can block or thwart learning from experience and getting anything new or good from the object world (Rosenfeld 1971). While sometimes narcissistic defenses—particularly idealization, omnipotent control, and narcissistic withdrawal into self-sufficiency—are attempts at forestalling destructive attacks on good objects, they are nevertheless deadening (Ogden 1995).

Successfully treating such persons involves helping them integrate their own destructiveness (Kernberg 1975); facilitating their mourning the missed, lost, and/or squandered opportunities rather than preserving them as organizing grievances (Spillius 1993); and prodding them to cope with the narcissistic vulnerability of love and dependence, with all its attendant risks of hurt and disappointment. The therapist, too, must guard against emotional withdrawal in the face of the devaluing attacks that so often accompany these therapeutic tasks (Kernberg 1975).

The First-Generation Asian American

Sandra Park, M.D.

INTERPRETING the impact of culture in the Grace Jin vignette is inherently problematic. Doing so risks perpetuating Asian stereotypes and ignoring the vast heterogeneity within the Chinese culture. Nevertheless, culture informs one's ideals and values, and attention must be paid in order to gain a three-dimensional understanding of the patient. The cultural formulation as outlined in an appendix of DSM-IV-TR (American Psychiatric Association 2000) seeks to understand how culture influences the individual: her cultural/ethnic identity; her symptoms; her environment; the therapeutic relationship; and overall care.

Grace Jin identifies herself as a first-generation Chinese American. Her *cultural identity,* which may be partly unconscious, is manifested in how she has chosen to incorporate the norms, customs, and beliefs of her Asian and

American backgrounds. Her bicultural identity begins with her name. Having immigrated to the United States at age 4, she or her parents chose her first name to better assimilate into the dominant culture. Assimilating to America is a source of tension for Ms. Jin. Like many children of immigrants, Ms. Jin experiences opposing pressures: to succeed in the United States while remaining rooted in traditional Asian ways (Uba 1994). Ms. Jin's studiousness and pursuit of a medical career are in line with the expectations of many immigrant families whose central reason for immigration was to create better opportunities for the children. Ms. Jin experiences much ambivalence about being an obedient daughter, however, evident in her choosing boyfriends who clash with her parents' ideas of a suitable mate.

Ms. Jin's *ethnic identity*—the attitudes she has about her cultural group, attitudes that organize her view of herself and others—is influenced by how she is received. Given the visible racial differences between herself and the community in which she grew up, she would likely be seen as different regardless of her wishes to assimilate. While not explicit in the case discussion, her experiences with prejudice and racism would be of interest to the therapist, as these may have resulted in feelings such as anger, shame, self-hatred, or pride.

Another area of exploration would be Ms. Jin's experiences emigrating from China. Immigration involves the real separation from one's country, family, and culture, but it also represents a symbolic separation from the earliest objects—as illustrated by phrases such as "mother country" or "fatherland" (Lijtmaer 2001). As such, emigration has been likened to other developmental landmarks such as Mahler's separation-individuation phase and Blos's second individuation of adolescence. Akhtar (1995, 1999) termed immigration a "third individuation," to further distinguish it from other phases. These processes have in common the separation from one's primary objects with an ensuing restructuring of identity. Inherent in the separation process is loss and mourning. What one loses are not just things external to oneself, such as family, friends, and customs, but also a part of the self that is tied to the native country (Grinberg and Grinberg 1989). Additionally, when one's values are no longer held in esteem by society, this can also result in a loss of pride. In that way immigration has been described as a potential narcissistic injury. The loss of language carries additional significance. Entering into an environment in which one does not understand the native tongue can cause the newcomer to feel excluded, isolated, and regressed. It is not surprising, then, that immigration is often experienced as a psychic trauma (Gonzalez et al. 1999).

While the questions might not be explicitly asked, the therapist may be curious if Ms. Jin had memories of the original move from China. What were the losses and gains? Had there been a drop in the family's socioeconomic status when the parents transitioned from being teachers in China to running a restaurant in the United States? Did she lose her parents' emotional support as they struggled to adapt to America themselves? How well did her parents speak English? If Ms. Jin was thrust into the role of their translator and liaison with the outside world, how did this affect her?

While she has, overall, thrived in the United States, Ms. Jin has not completely resolved the dilemma of how to straddle multiple cultures and vacillates in her desire to belong. As expected by her parents, she is a dutiful daughter, a studious medical student, and the girlfriend of an Asian man. That same boyfriend is, however, an unemployed drug abuser who represents her "dark side." This difficulty in integrating her Asian and American sides is evident in her fear that her therapist may prescribe her "Western pharmacology." Like her choice of boyfriends, her view toward medication is multidetermined. It may reflect a preference for Chinese medicine or a fear of side effects that are especially prevalent in Asians because of dosing schedules that do not take into account genetic differences in metabolism. Her hesitation might signify her fear of being labeled a psychiatric patient. It may also reflect an inability to integrate her ethnic identity with her budding identity as an American physician. Such concerns do not necessarily need to be discussed with the patient, but an understanding of them can inform the discussion, particularly if medications might be useful.

Culture can not only inform our understanding of the patient but also explicate her symptoms. For example, Ms. Jin seems to have been influenced by Asian attitudes, such as the focus on shame and an emphasis on emotional restraint. Shame is often described as a fear of "losing face." One can speculate that Ms. Jin's early mirror preoccupation is a symbolic representation of her fear of losing face. Because many Asians value emotional reserve, psychiatric distress is often expressed somatically rather than affectively; physical complaints may be a face-saving means of receiving help (Kleinman 1982). Ms. Jin manages her feelings by exhibiting an outward appearance of "perfection," despite her inner experience of anxiety and guilt.

Although Ms. Jin's traits may be culturally syntonic, she still experiences anxiety and guilt, possibly because she views Asian and American values in opposition. One goal of therapy would be to help Ms. Jin become more aware of both the cultural conflict between American and Asian values, as well as her own intrapsychic conflict. While some symptoms may be normal within one cultural context, these same symptoms may be deemed pathologic by the culture of origin. One would wonder if Ms. Jin's severe anxiety and perfectionism reflected not only her family's and subculture's desire for success but also her own excessive interpretation of this desire.

The environment plays an important role in the psychological functioning of an immigrant. The Jin family left China and entered a community without an appreciable Asian presence. This move likely impacted the family structure. Immigrating at the age of 4 as the eldest child, Ms. Jin probably assimilated to American society more quickly than her parents and may have acted as translator and negotiator with the outside world, reversing traditional family roles (Uba 1994). This role might have contributed to her sense of competence, importance, and resentment. Additionally, Ms. Jin may have seen her parents as ineffectual, which could have been a source of disappointment, shame, anger, or guilt.

The therapeutic relationship is also affected by cultural issues. While many Asians believe that it is noble to hide their true feelings, they would feel especially ashamed of criticizing their parents because of filial piety. This feeling is likely to conflict with the view of the typical American therapist, who values emotional expressivity. The therapist risks pathologizing what may be culturally syntonic, particularly if these characteristics clash with American therapeutic ideals (Cabaniss et al. 1994).

In working with culturally dissimilar patients, therapists should be aware of countertransference attitudes. Therapists of different cultural backgrounds may feel culturally superior, pitying, or aggressive toward the patient, or avoid learning about the patient's culture. Another pitfall is focusing too much on the patient's culture, which risks making the patient feel understood solely along the lines of his or her difference, rather than as an individual. A therapist who shares a background with the patient may not have resolved his or her own cultural conflicts and may be judgmental toward the patient—for example, "If I've overcome such hardships, what's wrong with my patient that he or she can't, too?" (Ton and Lim 2006). And a therapist may overidentify with the patient and become overzealous in the treatment, develop blind spots by assuming cultural similarities, or become detached for fear of being overly involved (Comas-Diaz and Jacobsen 1991, cited in Ton and Lim 2006).

A culturally informed treatment enables both the therapist and Ms. Jin to understand how culture has shaped her psychology. As Ms. Jin elaborates her symptoms, she can tease apart her various struggles: the conflict between cultures, the tensions between her and her intimates, and the internal battles that have caused her distress. The therapist can facilitate the integration of Ms. Jin's multicultural identities and enable Ms. Jin to resume the process of identity formation and consolidation.

Complementary Medicine and Integrative Pharmacology

Richard P. Brown, M.D.
Patricia L. Gerbarg, M.D.

GRACE Jin is a good candidate for complementary medicine and integrative pharmacology. Although stressed and anxious, she probably does not have a major mood disorder. While she worries about developing illnesses and examines her body in the mirror looking for imperfections, it is unlikely that she has a somatoform disorder. She may have obsessive traits but does not appear to have obsessive-compulsive disorder. Ms. Jin's initial evaluation should include an investigation into discrete psychiatric syndromes, but it seems most likely that her debilitating levels of stress are caused by a combination of her own high expectations and her inability to soothe herself. A variety of herbs and complementary treatments have been shown to reduce such stress and increase the capacity for joy and happiness.

Ms. Jin's refusal of "Western pharmacology" does not necessarily reflect conflict or avoidance, and it is certainly not unusual. While conventional synthetic psychotropic drugs are widely prescribed, they tend to cause side effects such as weight gain and sexual dysfunction, contributing to the high incidence of nonadherence. Over one-third of the prescriptions for psychotropic medications are never filled, while of those that are filled, most are taken incorrectly. Even when taken properly, these medications only partially improve the overall quality of life. People do not only want to reduce anxiety and depression; they want to feel an enhanced sense of joy, a reduced vulnerability to relapse, and a greater sense of resilience. This would be particularly true of Ms. Jin, who has just begun an educational process in which she will be required to function at a high level intellectually while under prolonged mental and physical stress.

Herbs and complementary treatments constitute the primary form of medical care in many parts of the world, where they are not viewed as "alternative." There are many herbal medications that may positively impact mental health, and several have been shown to be effective in replicated clinical trials. As with Western pharmacology, treatment selection depends on the diagnosis. If, for example, the focus of Ms. Jin's treatment is her tendency to feel stress as a bodily sensation, then she might be diagnosed with a somatoform disorder. In that case, the clinician might recommend *St. John's wort,* a gentle but often effective herbal treatment that has been shown in a recent placebo-controlled, double-blind study to reduce the symptoms of somatoform disorder in patients without depression (Muller et al. 2004). St. John's wort was as well tolerated as the placebo in that study and has generally been well tolerated at moderate dosages. At dosages above 900 mg/day, it produces side effects similar to those caused by the selective serotonin reuptake inhibitors (SSRIs).

Multiple clinical trials have demonstrated St. John's wort's effectiveness in depression. As with some other treatments that are not controlled by the U.S. Food and Drug Administration (FDA), some brands of St. John's wort do not contain replicable amounts of the active ingredient. For this reason, it is important to use trusted brands. In Germany, where St. John's wort is the most frequently prescribed antidepressant (fluoxetine is second), a panel of experts approved one brand, Kira, that is available over-the-counter in the United States.

S-adenosylmethionine (SAM-e) is at least as effective as St. John's wort in the treatment of depression. SAM-e is a natural metabolite that has been shown to be as effective as prescription antidepressants for mild to severe depression in more than 30 controlled clinical trials. It does not cause weight gain or sexual dysfunction and has shown no adverse interactions with other medications (Brown et al. 2008). As is the case with other antidepressants, high doses of either of these medications could induce mania in a small subset of patients.

If Ms. Jin does not have a somatoform disorder or depression, then she might be viewed as having anxiety or a stress disorder. Several herbs have been demonstrated to reduce stress without inducing side effects. For example, *Rhodiola rosea* has been studied extensively in the former Soviet Union and Sweden for treatment of posttraumatic stress disorder. It not only reduces stress and anxiety but also improves brain function and academic performance in university and high school students taking exams (Brown et al. 2002, 2004). Ms. Jin complained of being "unable to sleep and unable to relax," and insomnia is a frequent component of both depression and anxiety. Two herbs are widely used to improve sleep. *Valerian* has been used for hundreds of years in Europe to relieve insomnia. Eight recent studies have studied valerian, but all have been methodologically flawed. *Lavender aromatherapy* is not only helpful with insomnia but is safe for use during pregnancy.

In addition to our usual diagnostic categories, we would evaluate this patient's stress response system. Composed of the sympathetic nervous system (SNS) and hypothalamic-pituitary-adrenal axis (HPA), the stress response system includes an activation part that allows us to approach rewards and an inhibitory part that helps us avoid punishment or things that we do not like. It appears that Ms. Jin is overly activated in regard to both aspects of this "fight or flight" response, as if she were a driver with one foot on the brake and the other on the accelerator. This stress response system is counterbalanced by the parasympathetic system (PNS), whose main pathway is the vagus nerve. The PNS is the part of the autonomic nervous system that soothes, repairs, recharges, and restores energy. It is also crucial for social bonding, trust, and acceptance. It appears that Ms. Jin has learned neither how to stabilize the SNS components that are out of balance nor how to activate the underfunctioning PNS.

One of the most effective ways to address this imbalance is through a series of breathing exercises and movements that are taught within yoga. Breathing techniques specifically calm and balance the SNS and activate the PNS. While yoga has been practiced for thousands of years, it is only now being systematically studied for depression, posttraumatic stress disorder, and other medical conditions associated with stress and anxiety. While Westerners tend to view yoga as esoteric, yoga in its native lands is viewed both as a path to Enlightenment and a practical way to feel better (Brown and Gerbarg 2005a, 2005b; Gerbarg and Brown 2005).

Some yoga principles might be discussed directly with Ms. Jin. For example, she might benefit from the simple yoga adage that expectation reduces the joy in life. The therapist might help her explore her expectations of herself as well as her parents' expectations of her. This might enable her to address these expectations in less anxious and more productive ways. In the course of learning yoga breathing, some people see more clearly what they need to do to balance their life. Instead of making self-destructive choices in relationships, for example, they shift their priorities from excess excitement and overstimulation toward peacefulness and stability.

Biofeedback combined with yoga breathing can also be quite helpful for certain kinds of anxiety. In both, the central goal is the acquisition of enhanced self-regulation. Biofeedback is uniquely poised to take advantage of the fact that the PNS is modulated via the vagus nerve and can be measured by increased heart rate variability. Through the use of some basic breathing techniques, a home computer, and readily available software programs (see, e.g., www.heartmath.com), fingertip sensors can assess heart rate variability and help the patient attain a state of deep relaxation.

Biofeedback and yoga breathing can be used to improve emotional regulation and cognition. While this work can be done alone, many people profit from the enhanced social contact that is brought about through a multidimensional program with weekly group practices. In the case of Ms. Jin, she has long felt like an outsider and is now living in a city far from friends and family. Her local supports appear to be a competitive medical school social system and a problematic boyfriend. Joining a yoga course would provide the infrastructure for a regular practice and a social group that might serve as an oasis of peace and acceptance.

In regard to specific suggestions for Ms. Jin, we would recommend *R. rosea* (such as Rosavin Plus, Arctic Root, Energy Kare, or Rhodax brands) as a calming yet energizing, resilience-enhancing tonic. The dose would start at 150 mg taken 30 minutes before breakfast. The dosage would be gradually increased as tolerated to a maximum of 300 mg in the morning plus 150 mg 30 minutes before lunch. We would teach her a simple form of yoga breathing (e.g., Ujjayi, or alternate nostril breathing) in the office; this breathing tends to have immediate calming effects. We would also outline a daily home breath practice and suggest that she pursue a yoga routine. These are not so much suggestions as negotiations, since Ms. Jin's preferences are vital to the success of the treatment.

Complementary and alternative treatments empower the patient to use natural tools to enhance internal self-regulation. Since they do not stigmatize the patient as defective, such interventions can be especially well suited to people who are sensitive to stigma and/or who do not carry a formal psychiatric diagnosis. Further, they tend to lack the sorts of side effects that bedevil almost all psychiatric medications. Many psychiatrists do not know much about herbs, meditation techniques, and bodily exercises such as yoga. Nevertheless, their effectiveness, coupled with the limitations of Western pharmacology, have led such practices to becoming well known to patients who seek to improve their mental health outside of traditional medicine.

Mindfulness Meditation

Susan Evans, Ph.D.

GRACE Jin suffers from worry. She worries about the future and the past and relentlessly responds to nonexistent threats. She might warrant a number of possible DSM-IV-TR diagnoses and psychoanalytic formulations, and she might respond to many types of therapy. Regardless of her specific diagnosis or eventual treatment, however, meditation may be an effective way for her to become more relaxed.

While sometimes marginalized in the West as being overly esoteric or "Eastern," various forms of meditation are taught and practiced within virtually every cultural and religious tradition. Some techniques focus on a preselected object, like a mantra or a rosary, while others focus on physical sensations or the breath. Regardless of the focus, meditation typically involves concentrated, nonjudgmental attention. Meditation might be especially helpful to Ms. Jin, since focusing on the present moment might diminish her anxiety and improve her adaptive responses (Borkovec et al. 1999). It might also make her more "mindful."

What is mindfulness? It may be best defined as moment-to-moment nonjudgmental awareness that is cultivated by paying attention in a particular way, on purpose, to the present moment. Mindfulness practice promotes increased awareness of our bodies, thoughts, emotions, and behaviors and leads to increased perspective and clarity in the moment. Originating within Buddhism, mindful meditation helps the practitioner reach a state of "bare attention" (Thera 1972). This focus on careful observation hints at the importance of wakefulness, as illustrated in the following anecdote: When asked by his followers if he was God, Buddha would reply, "No, I'm awake." This answer underlines that meditation is not mysterious or mystical but rather a pursuit of an understanding of one's own mental processes. As such, it does not conflict with Western religions. Further, it overlaps significantly with multiple types of psychotherapy, including psychoanalysis. Like many skills, mindfulness meditation requires regular effort and discipline.

Hundreds of clinical studies have demonstrated the usefulness of meditation, and these studies have become increasingly rigorous and increasingly targeted at specific psychiatric populations. The best studied of these techniques is *mindfulness-based meditation stress reduction* (MBSR), a treatment that is done in small groups and features a variety of relaxation techniques, including meditation. It has been used and tested in medical centers, as well as within schools, prisons, athletic programs, and the workplace. Meditation may reduce anxiety in people who lack a psychiatric diagnosis as well as in persons with anxiety disorders (Kabat-Zinn et al. 1994). Not only did MBSR acutely reduce symptoms in that study, the patients maintained their anxiety reductions and their meditation practices at 3-year follow up (Miller et al. 1995). More recent studies have demonstrated the effectiveness of MBSR for a host of physical problems (e.g., fibromyalgia, psoriasis, pain) and psychiatric disorders (e.g., depression, anxiety), as well as in a variety of populations, including medical students.

If Ms. Jin were to explore MBSR, she would learn how to observe her thoughts and feelings with less judgment, reactivity, and identification. Her fears and anxiety would be increasingly experienced as passing, transient events that do not necessarily reflect reality. In addition to these cognitive and emotional changes, meditation can induce a state of physical relaxation. Long noted by meditation practitioners, this "relaxation response" induces a physiological state of quietude characterized by a decrease in heart rate, blood pressure, respiration, and metabolic rate (Benson 1975). Such an effect would be especially useful in someone like Ms. Jin, who appears to suffer from autonomic arousal, edginess, and insomnia that are all associated with worry and anxiety.

MBSR classes typically meet for 8 consecutive weeks, and the classes are 2.5 hours in length. Classes make use of sitting meditation, body scan meditation, and hatha yoga. In sitting meditation, Ms. Jin would be instructed to comfortably sit and use her breath as an anchor to focus her attention in the present moment. The instruction may be, "Bring your attention to your breath, noticing it perhaps at your nostrils or your belly. Every time you notice your mind wandering off the breath (which it inevitably will do since this is the nature of our minds), without judging yourself in any way, bring your attention back to your breath. If your mind wanders off a thousand times, bring it back a thousand times." *Body scan meditation* involves focusing the attention on each of the different parts of the body. It is systematic in that the client moves through the various regions of the body in a particular order. For example, Ms. Jin may be instructed to bring her attention to the toes of the left foot, becoming aware of the big toe, the little toe, and all the toes in between. Gradually her attention would shift from the toes to the foot, ankle, lower calf, and so forth. A third aspect of MBSR classes would be devoted to *hatha yoga,* and Ms. Jin would be asked to focus on her breath while nonjudgmentally observing her sensations, thoughts, and feelings. Depending on her yoga prowess (and the prowess of her neighbors), yoga might induce Ms. Jin into feelings of frustration, discomfort, pride, and envy. For someone who is competitive and perfectionistic, the adjunctive use of yoga can be an excellent way to practice nonjudgmental observation.

Clients taking the MBSR class are expected to practice the mindfulness practices on their own for 45 minutes, 6 days each week. This is a significant commitment, and so it would be useful for Ms. Jin and the clinician to discuss her willingness to devote the effort and time to the program. Prior experience with meditation and yoga might help her adjust to the required discipline and might also point to ways in which she would be likely to have difficulty. Ms. Jin has demonstrated a long-standing ability to maintain a schedule, has already said that she would prefer to avoid Western pharmacology, and would desperately like to reduce her level of anxiety and worry. A course of meditation might fit her very well.

Part B

GRACE JIN and the consulting psychiatrist agreed to extend the evaluation in order to assess the issues and conflicts that might be upsetting her. During the third and fourth sessions, she discussed her worries about school, her relationships with friends and family, and her views of herself. Ms. Jin described ongoing anxiety and obsessionality. She described feeling comfortable as a helper who was constantly tutoring and counseling her classmates and younger sisters, but she realized that she often ended up being disappointed by their response to her efforts.

The patient presented to the fifth session in a tank top with a noticeable barbed wire tattoo around her left biceps. She said she saw herself as something of a paradox in that she was generally seen as perfect but that her father would likely have a stroke if he saw the tattoo. The patient then wondered aloud if the tattoo could ever be removed, "or would it be a permanent mark of rebellion?" She noted that she was a bit confused by her relationship with her boyfriend, who she felt connected with her "dark side." He was often upset that her efforts to help others took time away from him, and she believed that he was a selfish brat. She said that her friends wondered why she would date an unemployed musician who abused alcohol and cocaine, but she liked the fact that he was exciting and lived in a different, more dangerous subculture. She had not told her parents that he had moved in with her and that she was supporting him through her student loans.

She began the following session by saying, with a smile, "While I don't think it will be helpful, I know that patients are supposed to bring in dreams, and so I've got one for you." In the dream, she was lost in a very strange place and wanted to find her way back to a classroom. Ghosts kept jumping out at her. One accused her of being a whore. She looked down and saw bugs on her skin. A man appeared but seemed uninterested in helping her. When asked for any thoughts about the dream, she remembered a story of her parents' life in China, where people were poor and the rice had been infested with bugs. She recalled that her parents believed that their ancestors sometimes came back as ghosts. Then she said: "Is this getting us anywhere? I didn't come here to talk about dreams. I just want to pass my exams."

At the same time that Ms. Jin was expressing her opinion about the relevance of dream analysis, the therapist was silently associating to the dream, particularly linking her parents (the ghostly ancestors), the hard times in China (the bugs), and her freedoms (the whore). The therapist said, "You try to meet the expectations of your parents and boyfriend, and that's exhausting." Ms. Jin stared at the therapist and quietly said, "They aren't the problem. If we're going to start blaming people, perhaps we could look at your inability to say anything helpful." She then said, "And now, I suppose you'll just want to give me some medications or something." The therapist responded, "Looks like your parents and boyfriend aren't the only ones who bring you down. Perhaps some of those same feelings are transferred onto me." Ms. Jin blushed and lapsed into silence. After a few moments, she quietly apologized and looked to the ground.

Summary

Grace Jin initially presented with feelings of anxiety and humiliation after having failed to pass a midterm exam. An extended evaluation led to an exploration of long-standing personality issues. The following discussions focus on psychodynamic technique, psychoanalytic theory, and treatment selection.

Discussions of the
Case of Grace Jin, Part B

Therapeutic Zeal 410
  Roy Schafer, Ph.D.

Empathy. 413
  Eve Leeman, M.D.

Self Psychology 416
  Jeffrey K. Halpern, M.D., and Sharone Ornstein, M.D.

The Kohut/Kernberg Controversy .421
  Nathan Kravis, M.D.

Evidence-Based Psychotherapy 426
  Andrew J. Gerber, M.D., Ph.D.

The Self-Defeating Patient. 431
  Arnold M. Cooper, M.D.

Overview of an Evaluation 434
  Robert Michels, M.D.

Summary Points 437

Therapeutic Zeal

Roy Schafer, Ph.D.

THERAPEUTIC zeal is the covering term for all those instances in which a psychotherapist tries too hard to get beneficial results. Here, "too hard" means putting pressure on the patient to change for the better and not rarely to change rapidly or dramatically. In these instances, the patient has the last word on how much is too much; therapeutic zeal makes it plain to the patient that he or she is being used by the therapist to gratify the therapist's narcissistic strivings. Such zeal activates deep feelings of having been used by others—particularly parents—and is a common source of heightened sensitivity and grievance in therapy. In response to the therapist's demands for reassuring signs of her or his own effectiveness, the patient might bring about a stalemate by becoming unresponsive or by making meaningless and obstructive shows of dependence, gratitude, and compliance. In the worst case, the result might be exacerbation of the presenting complaints or the patient's quitting treatment.

Therapeutic zeal indicates a lack of empathy—specifically empathy for how difficult it is to achieve significant change in one's way of living. The patient must cope with so much anxiety, shame, and guilt before that kind of change can begin. Dynamic psychotherapy is not aimed at promoting this change through direct reassurance and advice; rather, its aim is to develop insight into the unconscious emotional basis of symptoms and character difficulties. This insight frees the patient to venture into the challenging areas of change and, over time, helps stabilize the beneficial consequences of doing so.

Developing genuine insight cannot be hurried. Dynamic psychotherapy requires of the patient much self-confrontation and self-revelation to a relative stranger—the psychotherapist. It takes time and effortful understanding to develop trust in this stranger. The zealous psychotherapist is blind to this problem and manifests a lack of empathy that works against developing trust. This therapy requires of the therapist a high degree of patience, acceptance, curiosity, and a readiness to hear the patient out so as to get to understand her or his way of seeing thing. It also requires the ability to tolerate stretches of ambiguity, unknowingness, repetition, and self-justification. Finally, the therapist must maintain poise in the face of the patient's doubts and criticisms about the method and the therapist. The psychotherapist who is too fixed on the goals of treatment is no longer "in the moment," is no longer a good listener, and has become too zealous. Paradoxically, overattentiveness to the goals of treatment does not facilitate reaching those goals.

In contrast, the therapist who is consistently patient, accepting, and curious is showing how little she or he wants to dominate the patient or observe him or her "from on high" as a specimen of humanity to be classified and manipulated. By developing the patient's confidence in these ways, the therapist earns the right to be a partner in working out understanding and defining desirable routes of change. On the therapist's part, nothing has been decided in advance except to do responsible and responsive work; the approach is two-sided. In contrast, the approach dominated by therapeutic zeal is one-sided; its authoritarian tone discourages genuine change for the better.

Today, there are many pressures on therapists to get quick or dramatic results. These pressures inhere in limited staff and facilities; heavy caseloads; limits of time and frequency imposed by insurance companies; the impatience of patients owing to their other occupational, familial, and educational responsibilities; and patients' understandably defensive wishes to reach their personal goals without undergoing the pains of working out their core problems. Neither the times nor the make-up of the human personality favor extensive explorations of the internal world.

Not to be overlooked in this regard are the personal pressures that spring not from circumstance or the patient's needs but from the therapist's personality. Being human, too, therapists have their own doubts about themselves, some more than others. They might doubt their basic goodness. They might lack confidence in their ability to understand. They might over-identify with their patients by projecting their own needs and fears into them and then, through their zeal, act out their wish to cure themselves; and self-cure might imply curing people whose personal development and current lives they have taken into themselves as aspects of their self-image.

Therapeutic zeal is expressed in a number of ways, some of them quite obvious, others subtle. A therapeutic manner too self-assured and controlling is a dead giveaway. Other obvious ways include getting annoyed or openly frustrated with patients who do not change in the way the therapist desires; "blaming" the patient by vindictively attributing lack of results to more severe pathology than was initially assumed; or overusing such terms as *passive aggressive* and *poorly motivated*. A shade less obvious, except to the seasoned practitioner, is flooding the patient with speculative interpretations before much is known about the patient's inner life and before the patient has begun to settle into the relationship. Less obvious is addressing the patient's problems in ways that demand an unreasonable amount of self-tolerance and emotional readiness for change.

The scenario with Grace Jin represents an example of the therapist expecting too much from the patient, particularly in the final interchange. Ms. Jin has brought in a dream, which may reflect her growing confidence in the therapist as well as her desire to be seen as a "good patient." While she wonders if this is getting them anywhere, the dream seems to have provoked a series of associations in the therapist that may have fanned the flames of therapeutic zeal: ancestral ghosts may be parents who limit her freedom and emphasize the importance of duty, for example, while the uninterested man may be the therapist (regardless of the therapist's actual gender). The dream leads the enthusiastic therapist to assert that the expectations of her parents lead to exhaustion, which prompts an irritated denial from the patient that her parents are to blame. The therapist responds to her anger by asserting that her feelings for her parents and boyfriend have been "transferred" onto the therapist. The patient's response to this "interpretation" is an anxious silence and, after a pause, an apology. It is not known how things proceed from this point, but it may be that she was aware of feeling angry at a therapist who had ignored her feelings. It may be that she has powerful protective feelings toward her parents and boyfriend and is not ready to criticize them. It may be that she has tendencies toward self-abasement and idealization of her therapist and is simply not ready to be treated as a coworker in the therapeutic project. These possibilities—and others—await further inquiry. We do know, however, that Ms. Jin's silence and irritation are signs that she is asking her therapist to curb his or her therapeutic zeal.

Instances of pushing ahead of the patient in this zealous way are neither rare nor disastrous. As this anecdote shows, they can instruct the therapist as to the best pace for this patient's progress. Impatience only sets both of them back. The therapist's getting too excited by what seems to be a sign of progress is a sign that the therapist is feeling too much in need of reassuring signs of progress and so is likely to try, often unknowingly, to force the patient to "get better." In this respect, as in many others, doing dynamic therapy is a balancing act for the therapist: too much and too little are as common as getting it right. The thing is to learn from each instance.

Empathy

Eve Leeman, M.D.

ESTABLISHING an empathic connection is the central task of the initial phase of therapy and is critical to therapeutic success. The development of such a connection does not follow a particular template, but varies among patients and therapists and changes over the course of treatment. The case of Grace Jin illustrates some potential threats to this alliance, and how therapeutic flexibility can maximize the likelihood of a good outcome. Seeking psychiatric help conjures many difficult emotions; the psychiatrist's first job is to listen carefully without rushing to interpret or advise, and to calmly encourage the patient to tell her story.

Many patients who begin treatment have significant ambivalence. Some may have been prompted to come by others, perhaps by another doctor, a parent, a child, a spouse, or a friend, or, in Ms. Jin's case, by the University Health Services. While she may appreciate their concern, she may also feel coerced and skeptical about whether a psychiatrist can help. Like many people, Ms. Jin may be hopeful that treatment will make her feel better, but she may also be embarrassed about seeking help, or afraid that she will be perceived as mentally ill. She may also worry that she will be rejected for being too healthy or otherwise undeserving or that the psychiatrist will misunderstand her or be incompetent and waste her time and money.

Ms. Jin's Chinese parents probably have no familiarity with the process or potential benefits of psychotherapy, and Ms. Jin, who has adopted her parents' model of hard work and ambition, is likely terrified that seeking psychiatric help is a sign of weakness. She has already been gravely humiliated by failing an exam, and she fears that she will never live up to her parents' expectations. She anticipates criticism from the therapist, much as she feels berated by her parents and herself.

Yet Ms. Jin expresses an interest in "talk therapy" in spite of her misgivings. In the midst of such ambivalence, the therapist can help to deepen the alliance by normalizing and validating the patient's experience. When Ms. Jin asks whether she is "crazy," for example, the therapist might respond by suggesting that anyone under the pressure of medical school might benefit from talking to someone, implicitly disavowing the notion that she is mentally ill. Ms. Jin feels panicky about being revealed as a failure, so the therapist might start by focusing on her strengths. It is often not helpful or necessary to make a diagnosis early on. Rather, the therapist ought to establish an empathic framework for treatment, reiterating the real concerns that the patient has expressed. These supportive strategies help to elicit the patient's cooperation in defining the therapeutic task as one of helping her to realize the fruits of her obvious capabilities in a way that makes her happier and more in charge of her own life.

Ms. Jin feels that her relationships have required that she fulfill demands in order to be loved. Many people who seek psychotherapy feel similarly, and this may present in the transference, as when Ms. Jin suggests that the therapist has excessive expectations of her. Taking her complaint seriously, the therapist can acknowledge that the comment sounded critical; after all, the therapist isn't perfect. The therapist can praise the patient for expressing her feelings directly, assuring her that this is a harbinger of therapeutic success.

Ms. Jin also expresses mixed feelings about her boyfriend, tempting the therapist to judge her relationship as self-defeating. Refrain. Psychiatrists cannot make accurate predictions about relationships or career choices, and should not pretend to have access to such wisdom, even if patients seem to want advice. Relationships are complicated and fluid, and people, including therapists, change dramatically depending upon whom they are relating to. Nothing is objective, and Ms. Jin's emotional state impacts her boyfriend's behavior; their relationship may evolve as she changes, and she may describe him very differently in a later interview.

It is far more effective to respond to ambivalence, whether about relationships, careers, or whatever, by drawing out both sides of the patient's quandary, empathizing with her longing for the positives and her frustration with the negatives. Don't take sides; try instead to adhere to the old psychiatric maxim: "Don't just do something, sit there." If the patient feels the therapist truly resonates with her dilemma, she is much more likely to articulate her concerns. While Ms. Jin's boyfriend has obvious liabilities, the therapist might also explore the attributes that the patient finds attractive. Ms. Jin does not like her self image as a perfect nerd, for example, and so her boyfriend may expose her to a wild, creative, rebellious side of life. As treatment develops, Ms. Jin may learn to participate in alternative culture without having to suffer her boyfriend's derision, or pay his bills, but she needs to reach this conclusion herself. Again, the goal is to help Ms. Jin learn to trust her own decision-making ability and to figure out what is most likely to make her happy.

The therapeutic posture must be one of empathy, even though the patient may resist since she has little empathy for herself. The psychiatrist's position as a medical school graduate might bring out competitive feelings in any patient, particularly a medical student, but these can be diffused by sharing small personal failures on the path to graduation. By demonstrating how different the practice of medicine is from memorizing anatomy details, the psychiatrist also provides a living example that Ms. Jin's choice of medicine as a career does not negate the possibility that she can be herself.

For this patient, or anyone who is punishingly self-critical, the psychiatrist can serve as a model of a non-obsessive approach, highlighting her own small imperfections. For example, the therapist can acknowledge occasional lateness, or delayed phone calls, implying that perfection is unnecessary for a successful career in medicine. Similarly, the therapist might share an interest in a movie or book the patient mentions, demonstrating that a medical career can be rewarding without being all-consuming.

While Ms. Jin deserves a thorough psychiatric evaluation, the therapist should maintain a balanced, nonjudgmental approach that allows for the possibility that her anxiety symptoms reflect her harsh self-criticism rather than a psychiatric disorder. Further, an excessive emphasis on her symptoms might encourage her to regress, eliciting a more dependent, ill side of her character instead of mobilizing her strengths.

This is an important general point. The therapist must help Ms. Jin learn to trust her own judgment. Rather than undermine Ms. Jin's decisions, the therapist should make it clear that the agenda of therapy is not predetermined but rather evolves with the patient's sense of what matters. The patient's knowledge and experience is crucial to a thorough understanding of her dilemma, and while the therapist may have general knowledge and experience, the patient is the expert in her own particulars.

The discussion of medication can be done with the same philosophic approach. Psychiatric trial data show a significant placebo response in almost all psychiatric treatments; in fact, nonspecific factors are more consistently helpful across clinical trials than any specific drug or operationalized therapy response. Pharmacological interventions can be enormously helpful to patients, but how patients feel about taking medicine hugely affects how well the medicine works.

Ms. Jin says she does not want to try Western medicine, and it is never a good idea to sacrifice the alliance by insisting. Even though pharmacology has become a mainstay of psychiatric practice, the efficacy of medication treatment still leaves much to be desired. Moreover, studies show that 25%–50% of patients choose not to follow our medication recommendations. When a patient is ambivalent about medications, it is more helpful to empathize with her uncertainty than to engage in a power struggle. Not only does insistence on medications often prove fruitless, a power struggle is likely to reduce the effectiveness of the nonspecific factors that are often as effective as the suggested medication. Further, insistence can undermine the therapeutic alliance, the potential for empathy, and the likelihood that Ms. Jin will learn to advocate for her own happiness.

Self Psychology

Jeffrey K. Halpern, M.D.
Sharone Ornstein, M.D.

THE self psychological approach centers upon a sustained effort to understand the patient's subjective experience. Developed over the past 50 years, self psychology emphasizes two theoretical concepts that differentiate it from other psychotherapeutic schools. The first is the elaboration of two particular transference paradigms that predictably develop during the treatment of people with narcissistic disorders. The second is a view that narcissism is a normal developmental process and a driving force and not primarily pathological or defensive. How do these concepts apply to Grace Jin?

As Ms. Jin tells us her story, we begin to assemble details of her life. We note her hypertrophied search for perfection, her dread of failure (and her actual failure of her Gross Anatomy exam); her intense preoccupation with shame, humiliation, and imperfection; her fear that she is crazy; her engrossment before her reflection in the mirror; her hypochondriacal perturbations; and her "secret life," which she describes as both exciting and her cross to bear. We note characteristics of a narcissistic personality disorder with obsessional and masochistic features, and somatoform disorder. We want to deepen this descriptive approach by paying closer attention to Ms. Jin's experience of her symptoms and especially to her experiences of the therapist.

Ms. Jin's therapist, in reporting this case, has attempted to conceal himself (or herself). We have no direct disclosures about his reactions to the patient or assessment of the patient's feelings toward him. The case report has been written from the viewpoint of a dimly omniscient, objective, and anonymous narrator. We might infer that the therapist's conscious or unconscious theories indicate that personal disclosures are not relevant, or that the therapist's feelings toward the patient should be "analyzed away." Perhaps the therapist is using this theoretical stance to distance himself from an uneasy identification with this younger colleague. From our theoretical viewpoint, crucial data are missing. We would have written the case from the perspective of a particular therapist's effort to enter into Ms. Jin's experiential world and her responses to the therapist's efforts.

This effort is at the core of the self psychological approach; it is the empathic perspective. It is important to distinguish between our ordinary empathy and our psychotherapeutic empathy. Ordinary empathy is an immediate, sporadic, and intuitive capacity for recognizing what another is experiencing. Psychotherapeutic empathy is a prolonged, reflective, and sometimes effortful immersion in the subjective experiences of another. Psychotherapeutic empathy comprises a complex cognitive process informed by experience, information, and theoretical perspectives. Psychotherapeutic empathy is a commitment to the patient's perspective. Instead of simply recognizing our own strong reactions to being the target of the patient's fantasies and emotions, we try to develop an empathetic understanding of what it feels like to experience those fantasies and emotions (i.e., to be the subject of those experiences) (Schwaber 1981). In addition, we distinguish empathic listening from the communication of our understanding to the patient. Empathy is a method for listening to the patient—a commitment to a perspective—not an intervention. We can then make interventions from within the patient's perspective.

Although Ms. Jin's therapist does not report the case from inside the patient's experience as a novelist might, we begin to imagine her experience: she immediately inquires about confidentiality, and we sense her "paranoia" and her fear of shame. She asks if she is crazy, and we sense our authority and her need for reassurance. Despite her mortification and secretiveness, she urgently describes her feelings of absolute failure; her use of "absolute" suggests a world of the highest standards and ambitions that if unmet will lead to her downfall as defective, "stupid and lazy." The possibilities for disappointing her family especially haunt her. She tells us her parents left China for the good of their children. Although she intimates that she and her parents are deeply attached and dependent upon one another, there is no hint of affection in her account. She conveys the intractable obligation she feels toward her parents, and we wonder about her parents; intelligent, frustrated in the pursuit of their own ambitions, living vicariously through their daughter, and needing her to be and perform for them in specific ways. Ms. Jin's therapist has elicited a history and listened attentively, and we imagine the patient feels relief and hope. We suspect that she is beginning to need the therapist to be and to perform in specific ways for her.

In the next session, Ms. Jin reveals that she spends hours staring at herself in the mirror, not admiring and pining at her image as Narcissus did in myth, but gazing apprehensively for imperfections and asymmetries. Her narcissism manifests less as blatant grandiosity and obliviousness than as diffidence and painful sensitivity to potential shame. We think that in scrutinizing herself (her entire body?) in her reflection, she does more than wistfully criticize her features: in seeking perfection in the mirror she evokes a

frustrated need to display herself with pride and without reserve, and to experience recognition, validation, and admiration for a much larger horizon
of self experience than her parents would countenance. As part of her hypochondriacal concerns, about diseases that disfigure the body or damage the
mind, she envisions dropping out of medical school to be nursed for her imperfections at home, a regressive but reparative hope.

Telling another person the disparate facets of her life is a novel occurrence for her. She discloses her attraction to black-sheep men whom she
finds both thrilling and a source of guilt and shame. It seems to us a significant moment when she displays to her therapist her barbed wire tattoo, an
imperfection she fears would mortify her parents. Her interest in tattoos is a
flag she hoists against her fears of disfiguring imperfections, partly reaction
formation against bodily blemishes and partly rebellion against the parental
demands for perfect performance. What she calls her rebellious and dark side
appears to be restitutive of a larger self experience. She has not been able to
openly confront or disappoint her parents. The boyfriends and tattoo are sur-
reptitious expressions of anger at their demands and an ambivalent attempt
to establish more autonomy. This dark side, mostly sexual and sadomasoch-
istic in nature, is enlivening for her because her imperfect and unaccepted
self experiences are seen and enjoyed by her boyfriend, who, to her relief, is
unlikely to esteem her academic attainments. There is much the therapist
does not yet know or understand, but attentive listening and clarifying without judging or arguing her experiential reality leads us to anticipate the be-
ginnings of a mirroring selfobject transference. What does this mean?

Selfobject is a concept developed by Heinz Kohut to delineate the particular function that the therapist serves for patients struggling with unresolved
narcissistic needs and wishes. In other words, the therapist performs selfobject functions for Ms. Jin when his presence, action, or expression promotes,
stabilizes, restores, or enlivens Ms. Jin's self experience. The therapist as a separate individual is not experientially important to Ms. Jin. Indeed, the therapist—or rather the function the therapist serves—is felt to be part of the self,
and therefore the term *selfobject* is used rather than self and object. As the
therapy proceeds, Ms. Jin's experiences of her therapist will reflect an amal-
gamation of her past efforts to elicit selfobject responsiveness, especially from
her parents, as well as efforts to guard against frustration and disappointment
in these endeavors. Her experiences will also begin to organize around her
hopes of obtaining these functions anew from her therapist. This organization
of Ms. Jin's experience in the treatment constitutes a *selfobject transference.*

Kohut originally described two types of selfobject transferences, *mirroring* and *idealizing,* which reflect a developmental point of view that is intrinsic to self psychology. (Subsequently, other types of selfobject transferences
have been described.) Every child requires recognition, affirmation, and val-

idation of himself and others—experiences that make grandiose, omnipotent, and entitled claims. Optimally, when the child is frustrated in his omnipotent assumptions, the parent helps him navigate his disappointments. If the parent's response is excessively stimulating of the child's grandiosity (especially if the response is in the service of the parent's own thwarted ambitions) or if the response is insistently critical of the child's displays of pride, then the gradual maturation of grandiosity into healthy and realistic pride, confidence, and ambition is disturbed. In therapy a mirroring transference may then unfold in which the patient experiences the therapist as responding, or failing to respond, to the patient's needs for recognition, affirmation, and validation. In the mirror transference's most archaic form, the patient demands recognition of a grandiose self but also fears this recognition because he dreads repetitions of past humiliations. With maturation the patient does not tyrannically and rigidly require a selfobject to feel a sense of pride, confidence, and a firm sense of self.

Concurrent with the child's grandiose sense of himself, the child needs to idealize significant people in his life in order to participate vicariously with their greater strength and other admired qualities. Optimally, the child is gradually disappointed with the idealized figure, and archaic idealizations are replaced by mature values and ideals that give a sense of direction to his life. Conversely, if the child is too traumatically disappointed in this need he will lack the perseverance, enthusiasm, and purpose that come from having a sense of personal values and ideals. When such a person comes to therapy, an idealizing (selfobject) transference may unfold in which the therapist is experienced as responding, and at times failing to respond, to the patient's need for protection and enhancement through participation in the idealized qualities of the therapist. With progress in the treatment, the patient does not relentlessly require a selfobject to feel enthusiasm in the pursuit of goals and ideals. It should be noted that a self psychological approach differentiates idealization as a defense from idealization that represents a developmental need.

We predict that in Ms. Jin's treatment, the predominant transference to unfold will be a mirror transference, largely because we speculate that it is likely that she would have idealized her hardworking, intelligent, and devoted parents. They appear, however, less likely to have provided adequate mirroring, requiring instead that she become an extension of their own selfobject needs. This would have led them to selectively and problematically mirror aspects of her self experience and performance.

Like free association or evenly hovering attention, sustained empathic immersion is frequently observed in the breach. Our wandering attention and intrusive thoughts and feelings that disrupt our focus on the patient's subjective experience are openings to understanding. For example, while listening to Ms. Jin, we may find ourselves identifying not with her self-sacrificing excitement when she is with her boyfriend but with what it might be like to be her parent. Or her sadistic boyfriend. We may feel frightened by our identification with her and her self-defeating behavior in medical school. She draws us into identifications and roles that vividly suggest how others respond to her and how she elicits characteristic patterns of interactions. It becomes necessary and effortful for us to work our way back to Ms. Jin, the subject of the experiences, retaining and using what we have learned from these breaches in our empathic immersion.

Let us assume that, like her therapist in the vignette, we say to Ms. Jin, "You try to meet the expectations of your parents and boyfriend, and that's exhausting." She turns distant and cold. She is indignant that we indict her relationship to her parents and boyfriend and insists we are not helpful. Suddenly, she is embarrassed and apologizes. We are puzzled. Was it not our intention to be encouraging; to say don't be too hard on yourself? We realize that we did not understand how she would hear our intervention.

We would observe the disruption and try with Ms. Jin to reconstruct what just happened between us. This may take time, and Ms. Jin will experience our efforts to reflect nondefensively and without imputation. We speculate that such an exploration with Ms. Jin will reveal that she felt our intervention as injurious to her belief in the vitality, prestige, and potency she accords to doing it all. She has been a good and hardworking patient but she is disappointed in our reception of her performance: we have not admired or believed in her ability to do it all. By withdrawing contemptuously, she protects this treasured, perfect, and grandiose self. Equally important, by placing her parents and boyfriend together, our intervention dismisses in one patronizing sweep, the troubling, exciting, imperfect, and unintegrated dark side of her self experience that she has been revealing to us and thought we understood. In our phrasing of the intervention, we are also dismissing the depth of her attachment to her parents and their attachment to her while ultimately siding with their dictates about a medical career. It misses entirely what she means when she says that her boyfriend is the only one who really understands and cares about her. Perhaps her apology reflects a Chinese cultural attitude toward authority as well as a masochistic bid to declare in effect: look at me, see what a good daughter I am. In her submissive apology, she may unconsciously gain control over disappointment and shame by turning it into a masochistic pleasure. Our intervention was well intentioned, but it seems to have recapitulated an early experience in which she presented herself to be admired and validated only to find that her parents responded to her in a way that reflected their own needs.

These early interactions are consistent with the development of a mirroring selfobject transference, in which Ms. Jin reveals her need to be admired and known—fundamental needs of her grandiose self. The therapeutic intervention reflects, then, a retraumatization that will likely lead to increased resistance to a further unfolding of the mirroring selfobject transference. Such a lapse is not, however, fatal to the treatment. Continued efforts to understand with Ms. Jin this selfobject failure and her responses to it can allow the expression of further selfobject needs and therefore to a deepening of the treatment and a more mature sense of pride, confidence, and resilience.

We hope to have illustrated how the self psychological approach to the patient is guided by sustained empathic immersion in the patient's subjective experience. "Objective reality" is important, as is countertransference, but a core task for the therapist is the effortful return from these positions to an understanding of the patient's subjective experience. We view this perspective as essential in the treatment of narcissistic disorders. The concept of selfobject transference and the view that narcissism is a developmental process and driving force are essential pole stars in our efforts at empathic understanding.

The Kohut/Kernberg Controversy

Nathan Kravis, M.D.

BEGINNING in the 1970s an important controversy arose in psychoanalytic circles regarding the conceptualization and treatment of narcissistic character pathology. While there is now a vast literature with scores of contributors participating in this controversy, its chief protagonists have been Heinz Kohut (1913–1982) and Otto Kernberg (b. 1928).

Kohut was the originator of *self psychology*. His two major works were his books *The Analysis of the Self* (1971) and *The Restoration of the Self* (1977). A classically trained psychoanalyst, Kohut, by mid-career, had become increasingly attuned to the impersonal yet attached way some patients related to him, seeing in this not an avoidance of oedipal-level conflicts around love and hate (i.e., not ambivalence), but a craving for an omnipotent, idealizable object and/or a need for the therapist to supply certain mirroring experiences.

Kohut began to view patients who made use of him in this seemingly somewhat impersonal way as people who were not avoiding conflicts over closeness but who were elaborating in the transference one of two early childhood constellations that he came to call *selfobject transferences*. (In self psychology parlance a *selfobject* is an object used for inner self-maintenance. A selfobject is not an autonomous other, but an object needed for self-cohesion—an object that fulfils one's need to be admired and affirmed, as well as the need to have people to look up to and feel connected with.) Kohut rejected DSM-style diagnosis via criteria sets of symptoms and traits in favor of diagnosis by the type of transference manifest in treatment. He described two types of selfobject transferences—the mirror and the idealizing—reflecting two hypothesized developmental lines (Kohut 1971, 1977; Kohut and Wolf 1978; Ornstein 1978).

The *mirror transference* centers on Kohut's concept of the *grandiose self*. In Kohut's developmental schema, the grandiose self is a normal early psychic structure that, with appropriate maternal responses of admiration and approval, develops into healthy and realistic self-esteem, accompanied by the capacity to enjoy the exercise of one's capabilities. In the absence, deficiency, or abrupt cessation of these needed maternal responses, the patient becomes fixated at the level of the grandiose self or its archaic, regressive forms. This will manifest itself in treatment by the activation of the mirror transference (or one of its more archaic subtypes—the *twinship* or *merger selfobject transferences*).

The second developmental line postulated by Kohut is organized around the idealized object. The need for an idealizable parental object represents a primary developmental need, a step along the path leading from archaic idealizations to (via their transformation and internalization) the formation of healthy ideals and the capacity for empathy, creativity, humor, and wisdom. In the absence or precipitous loss in childhood of such an object, fixation upon the idealized parental object or its archaic, regressive forms will ensue and will be seen in subsequent treatment of an adult as the idealizing selfobject transference.

From Kohut's perspective, treatment will reveal and consist of the vicissitudes of these two types of transferences and their underlying genetic constellations. The self psychologically oriented therapist allows these selfobject transferences to unfold, reactivating the need for cohesiveness sought by the grandiose self or the desired union with the idealized object. The inevitable frustrations and disappointments of the treatment situation, including behavior by the therapist experienced by the patient as an empathic lapse, will evoke fragmentation experiences, with shame and narcissistic rage as their markers. Working through will involve restoring continuity and cohesiveness by understanding the dynamics of these disruptions with special attention to the therapist's role in maintaining the patient's narcissistic equilibrium. Once this has been accomplished, patient and therapist work toward a reconstruction of the original narcissistic trauma presumed to be of etiologic significance. With repeated cycling through such fragmentation/restoration sequences, patient and therapist have the opportunity to see how restoration is achieved and what light this sheds on the dynamics of the therapist's role in the patient's maintenance of self-cohesion and self-esteem, and on the origins of the problems in this area. The patient then has the opportunity to assume for himself functions earlier assigned to the selfobject-analyst, and thus, through such "transmuting internalizations" (Kohut 1971), to acquire these functions as permanent psychic structures.

The final interaction between Grace Jin and her therapist could be taken as an example of just such a disruption. A self psychologically oriented therapist would want to focus with Ms. Jin on how his comment and her overall experience of describing her dream to him disappointed and angered her, leading her into a shameful retreat and an apology she knows is unnecessary. Her contempt and dejection would be understood as her characteristic way of handling feeling misunderstood.

From a self psychological perspective, the goals of treatment include shame reduction (with consequent reduction in narcissistic rage), increased self-cohesion, enhanced ability to pursue one's own goals and values, an enhanced ability to seek and maintain relationships with better differentiated selfobjects, decreased reliance on archaic selfobjects, and, via transmuting internalization, an enhanced ability to assume for oneself the self-esteem–maintaining functions previously assigned to the selfobject-therapist.

In contrast to Kohut, Kernberg believes that narcissistic pathology does not stem from *arrested* development, but rather from a *pathological* development in which ego and superego strivings are poorly differentiated and object relations are pathological. The problem is not just a lack of internalization of normal, idealized ego and superego forerunners, but an active distortion of them together with a pathological devaluation of external objects. In other words, it's a matter of not just the absence of certain psychic structures (due to hypothesized developmental arrest), but a pathological development of earlier structures such that normal ones cannot develop later (Kernberg 1975).

Kernberg adopted Kohut's term *grandiose self* as an apt clinical moniker, but whereas Kohut saw the grandiose self as a normal developmental structure, Kernberg conceptualizes the grandiose self as a pathological structure whose persistence in adulthood is the hallmark of narcissistic pathology. In Kernberg's view, the grandiose self reflects the pathological condensation of ideal self, ideal object, and actual self in the setting of basically intact ego boundaries and reality testing but with prominent reliance on the more "primitive" defenses clustered around splitting (projection, projective identification, idealization, and devaluation). Kernberg regards narcissistic personality disorder as a variant of borderline personality organization, with the pathological grandiose self as a stabilizing psychic structure that allows for relatively intact ego functioning and surface adaptation in the presence of poorly integrated self and object representations. Such integration is, for Kernberg, a basic developmental task that, if not achieved, will lead to excessive reliance on splitting persisting into adulthood. Splitting explains the coexistence of haughty grandiosity and inferiority and shyness in the same personality (Kernberg 1975).

Building on the work of Klein (1957), Rosenfeld (1971), and others, Kernberg identifies chronic and intense envy as the cardinal feature of narcissistic personality disorder. Clinically, the grandiose self permits denial of dependence on the therapist, which helps keep envy and narcissistic rage (as well as fear and guilt secondary to this rage) at bay, but does not satisfy the underlying "desperate longing for a loving relationship that will not be destroyed by hatred" (Kernberg 1975, p. 274). Kernberg views Kohut's mirror and idealizing transferences as the alternating activation of different components of the pathological grandiose self. What Kohut described as a mirror transference, Kernberg regards as a projective identification in which the patient projects the grandiose self onto the therapist and then attempts via omnipotent control to have the therapist "follow exactly what is required in order to maintain the projection and to avoid the emergence of the analyst as an independent, autonomous object" (Kernberg 1975, p. 278). Likewise, from Kernberg's perspective, idealization of the therapist, rather than promoting healing, represents the projection of the grandiose self onto the therapist and defends against envy, humiliation, and rage (unlike higher-level idealization which defends against guilt over hostility and aggression).

Although the grandiose self stabilizes the personality by permitting denial of dependence on others, thereby protecting against narcissistic rage and envy, it also leads to the ongoing devaluation of others and warps object relations accordingly. In treatment, the grandiose self is utilized in the transference to avoid the emergence of the split-off, dissociated, repressed, or projected "bad'"self—bad because felt to be weak, needy, or babyish (Kernberg 1984). During periods of negative transference, the therapist should expect an oscillating identification of the self or the therapist with the previously split-off "bad" self and object representations (Kernberg 1975).

Kohut viewed hostile aggression as arising secondary to empathic lapses by the parents in childhood and by the therapist in the treatment situation. As noted earlier, he handled shame and narcissistic rage as the byproducts of fragmentation experiences. Kernberg, by contrast, sees aggression as primary and evident particularly in the patient's envy and as often leading the patient to launch attacks on the therapist's basic goodness. From his perspective, neglecting or deferring the interpretation of hostilely tinged negative transference is unempathic and contraindicated because it can lead to an augmentation of the patient's fear of his own aggression and destructiveness and therefore courts the risk of escalating the patient (Kernberg 1975).

It can be supportive to show the patient how narcissistic defenses against rage and contempt are also efforts to preserve the therapist as a good object (Kernberg 1975). During stretches of therapy in which the patient complains that "nothing is happening," or that the dialogue is irrelevant and useless, the therapist should consider the possibility of an unconscious need to destroy or undo the good that has actually been done, or the good the patient is now receiving (Kernberg 1975). This may reflect an inability to depend on the therapist as a maternal or paternal figure as well as the envy aroused by demonstrations of the therapist's capacity to be giving and creative.

A therapist working primarily with this approach might point out the way in which Ms. Jin, after dutifully offering her report of the dream, immediately feels the need to denounce it by saying, "Is this getting us anywhere? I didn't come here to talk about dreams." Her sweeping disdain for the therapist, loudly proclaimed in her sense of the therapist's "inability to say anything helpful," would also be commented upon—not for the purpose of disputation, but in an effort to show Ms. Jin her apparent need to wrap the gift of the dream in feelings of bitter denunciation and contempt. Is this her way of trying to repudiate the desire to please the therapist?

From a Kernbergian perspective, the primary goal of treatment is to promote and enhance the integration of good and bad self and object representations. As treatment advances, the narcissistic patient is gradually better able to experience the therapist as someone who can tolerate hostile aggression without either retaliating or being destroyed by it. Such experiences will promote the taming of narcissistic rage and envy, and an enhanced capacity for guilt and gratitude attendant upon the acknowledgement of one's own aggressive and destructive tendencies. This optimally leads to an enhanced capacity to depend appropriately on others, with gradual internalization of the therapist as a good object (Kernberg 1984).

Some commentators on the Kohut/Kernberg controversy have speculated that these two towering figures in American psychiatry have actually been describing (and theorizing about) different though slightly overlapping clinical populations. As Gabbard (2005) has noted, the DSM diagnostic criteria for narcissistic personality disorder describe the arrogant, grandiose, interpersonally exploitative, "noisy" narcissist, but not the shy, covertly grandiose, hypersensitive (perhaps slightly paranoid) narcissist who shuns attention in order to avoid feeling slighted and humiliated. Of course, these are not necessarily pure types. But in much of the literature on narcissism, one sees a tendency toward dichotomization: Kernberg's envious, oblivious, greedy, grandiose, aggressive narcissist versus Kohut's more vulnerable, hypervigilant, "covert" narcissist prone to self-fragmentation experiences (Gabbard 2005). But contributors from both camps would likely agree on the central clinical phenomenology of narcissistic pathology—particularly in individuals who seek treatment, for these are people whose lives are marred by their inability to love (or, more broadly, by the compromised quality of their object relations). The capacities to love, empathize, experience genuine interest and concern in others, tolerate ambivalence in long-term relationships, and acknowledge one's own contributions to interpersonal difficulties—all of which characterize health—are problem areas in persons with narcissistic personality disorder (Gabbard 2005).

Evidence-Based Psychotherapy

Andrew J. Gerber, M.D., Ph.D.

FOR as long as psychotherapy, in its various forms, has been in existence, practitioners and recipients have debated whether it is more of a science or an art. The consensus of contemporary academic psychiatry and psychology is that while there may be some aspects of therapeutic technique and process that will always defy precise description, there is *enough* that can be objectively described and studied to warrant including it in our list of science-based treatments. Though empirical research on psychotherapy dates back almost 100 years, there has been an explosion of such studies in the past two decades, yielding information that is helpful in choosing which therapy to recommend for which patients and even in shedding light on when in the treatment certain aspects of treatment are most effective.

The case of Grace Jin illustrates the complexity of an individual patient ~sentation, yet also provides us with details that allow us to use the avail-
. evidence base for psychotherapy. As Ms. Jin is no doubt learning in

medical school, even patients with the most straightforward and well-understood nonpsychiatric disorders, such as appendicitis or myocardial infarction, present with infinite variety. The job of a good physician or medical student is to elaborate a differential diagnosis based on the most important presenting signs and symptoms, and then, as the differential is narrowed down, identify the treatments believed to be helpful for these diagnoses, as suggested by available scientific evidence.

Ms. Jin presents with acute symptoms of anxiety and depression, as well as long-term difficulties with relationships, work, motivation, defenses, and self-image, all of which relate to what we usually refer to as personality or character. Psychotherapy research has something to tell us about each of these. Anxiety and depression are among the most well-researched diagnoses in the psychotherapy research literature. Starting in the mid 1990s, the clinical psychology division of the American Psychological Association established a set of standard criteria for *empirically validated treatments* (EVTs) (Chambless et al. 1998). In order to be considered an EVT, a therapy must 1) have been shown to be better than placebo or as good or better than an established treatment in a group-design study or large case series, 2) be well described in a treatment manual, 3) have been studied in well-characterized patient populations, and 4) have been studied in this way by at least two different investigatory teams.

According to the aforementioned criteria, *cognitive-behavioral therapy* (CBT) is listed as an EVT for panic disorder and generalized anxiety disorder; *exposure treatment* for agoraphobia, specific phobia, and obsessive-compulsive disorder (OCD); and *stress inoculation training* for coping with stressors. For depression, *behavior therapy, cognitive therapy* (CT), and *interpersonal therapy* (IPT) are listed as EVTs (Chambless et al. 1998). Each of these designations is based on rigorously executed and replicated trials of psychotherapy for specific patient populations. While Ms. Jin's presentation and differential diagnosis do not match neatly with any of these studies, her symptoms of anxiety and depression undoubtedly do match with the symptoms of some of the patients in these studies, and the existing evidence suggests that one or more of these EVTs may be helpful for her. In addition, while Ms. Jin appears to prefer psychotherapy to medications, she is also a medical student who is likely to appreciate scientific evidence. When the clinician is negotiating a treatment plan with her, it might be useful to point out that psychotherapy alone is often as effective as medication in the treatment of mild to moderate depression, though the combination of psychotherapy and medication is usually best (Hollon et al. 2002).

The identification of EVTs opens up many large and important questions about how best to conduct psychotherapy studies and then most usefully apply the results to individual patients. First, it is worthwhile to differentiate studies of *efficacy*—in which patient samples and treatments are made as homogeneous and "pure" as possible—from those of *effectiveness,* where psychotherapy and its recipients are studied in a heterogeneous "real-world" situation. By decreasing heterogeneity, efficacy studies are more likely to find differences between contrasting groups (e.g., a population of patients with major depression and no comorbidities undergoing a carefully manualized version of CBT as compared with a similar population who remain on a wait list with no treatment at all), but at the expense of limiting the generalizability of their findings to the wider world of practitioners. Meanwhile, effectiveness studies are more generalizable, but the findings are often complicated by the comorbidities inherent in their study populations. A well-informed consumer of the psychotherapy research literature absorbs data from both types of studies and applies them to the case at hand.

An additional complicating factor in integrating the psychotherapy literature stems from the fact that the majority of comparative outcome trials find no difference in the effect of competing active treatments (Luborsky et al. 1975; Rosenzweig 1936). Saul Rosenzweig (1936) went on to compare this observation to a scene in *Alice in Wonderland* in which the Dodo Bird, after overseeing an unusual race, declared, "Everybody has won and all must have prizes." To this day, most of the studies that find differences between groups are comparing one or more active treatments against a nontreatment (e.g., a wait-list control, treatment-as-usual, or a treatment specifically designed to be missing an important ingredient).

This problem of interpreting the literature is compounded by an "allegiance effect" whereby the psychotherapy preferred by the study's main author is usually found to be more effective than its competitors (Luborsky et al. 1999). Interpreters of this finding divide into two camps. In the first are those who believe that most psychotherapies achieve the same effects because their differences are superficial and patient improvement is truly driven by a set of "common factors," including the patient–therapist relationship, the benefit of having an expert help form a logical narrative of the patient's problems, and the positive effect of the patient believing that he or she is doing something to solve his or her difficulties (Frank 1988). The other camp argues that the Dodo Bird effect is the result of outcome trials with insufficient sample sizes and a lack of sophistication in subdividing patients and techniques into groups that would show meaningful differences.

Evidence is mounting that more sophisticated psychotherapy trials that take into consideration both the details of the therapy (i.e., the process) and the results (i.e., the outcome) can tease out differential treatment effects. Several retrospective analyses indicate that patients with an *anaclitic* style of ¬ression—characterized by prominent dependency needs, disruptions of personal relatedness, and the use of avoidant defenses—benefit more from psychotherapies with supportive and structured elements. Meanwhile, patients with *introjective* depression—such as people like Ms. Jin who use more obsessional defenses and whose problems tend to relate to self-definition, autonomy, and self-worth—have better outcomes with exploratory, unstructured treatments such as four-times-a-week psychoanalysis (Blatt 1992).

Another recent finding with important implications for psychotherapy recommendations and future research is that the psychotherapy category into which a patient has been assigned may not reveal the nature of the active elements of the treatment. Ablon and Jones (1998) found, in a retrospective analysis of a major depression treatment study comparing CBT and IPT, that the extent to which treatment *in either group* matched a prototype of psychodynamic psychotherapy (characterized by exploration and emphasis on the patient-therapist relationship) was the best predictor of patient outcome. Thus, the widely reported finding that CBT and IPT were equally effective masked a more interesting result: that use of certain techniques in both therapies made an important difference for the patient (Ablon and Jones 1998). Ms. Jin's therapist would do well to have training in multiple forms of psychotherapy and to know which techniques were likely to be most useful for the patient.

Ms. Jin's therapist senses that by staying with the patient and listening empathically, a useful therapeutic alliance will form. Though this may seem obvious, the history of medicine and psychiatry is littered with treatments that seemed intuitive at the time but later turned out to be ineffective or even harmful when studied systematically. In this case, however, common knowledge appears to be correct: researchers have demonstrated that the therapeutic alliance is one of the most reliable and robust predictors of good therapeutic outcome. Researchers have also found that exploratory interventions—in which a therapist points out unconscious and/or historical roots of current problems, particularly with regard to the patient-therapist relationship—are most useful when done in the context of a good relationship. These findings might remind Ms. Jin's therapist of the importance of tact and timing; it would be useful for the therapist to defer commenting on Ms. Jin's dream, for example, or quickly pointing out the negative aspects of people she loves. Even if insightful and accurate, therapeutic comments that are premature or frightening not only may be ineffective but could permanently rupture their relationship.

Psychodynamic psychotherapy and psychoanalysis have suffered recently in the eyes of consumers, trainees, insurance companies, and research funding agencies from the reputation that they lack an evidence base and thus deserve to be replaced by newer, better-researched treatments such as CBT, behavior therapy, and IPT. While it is certainly true that psychoanalytic treatments have less of a research culture and a shorter research history than competing therapies, it is easily forgotten that empirical research in psychoanalytic treatments dates back to 1917 and that empirical research into psychoanalytic treatments faces challenges that shorter, more well-defined treatments do not (Fonagy et al. 2001). Westen and others have argued that the standard of the *randomized controlled trial* (RCT), while useful in some ways, unfairly biases the research literature, and particularly the selection of EVTs, against psychodynamic treatments to the detriment of our knowledge and patient care (Westen et al. 2004). RCTs of psychotherapy may offer misleading results because they favor measurement of short-term symptom change in noncomorbid populations. Real patients, such as Ms. Jin, and therapists are interested in more than the short-term symptom change that may reflect the natural course of disease and/or the presence of common factors. Ms. Jin and most therapists are interested in long-term shifts in character structure and personality that make for a more free and enjoyable life. These are harder, though not impossible, to measure (Shedler and Westen 2004). In addition, addressing these issues requires a flexibility on the part of the clinician that often defies a treatment manual and "adherence" to a single therapeutic model.

The most progressive emerging model of psychotherapy research and its relationship to good patient care conceptualizes a "hierarchy of evidence" whereby professionals and their patients can take into consideration a wide range of data, each viewed through the lens of its benefits and limitations (Gabbard et al. 2002). RCTs sit atop this hierarchy in that they adhere to a rigorous empirical standard, but they lack the flexibility to adequately represent longer term and more in-depth treatments of heterogeneous populations. Open trials, which do not randomize, are more applicable to some patient populations and treatments but are more vulnerable to confounding variables. Pre-post trials, looking only at a single group of patients over time, and case series, consisting of a compilation of individual reports, help tease out more complicated situations and may be more useful for the clinician seeking to understand a specific case, though they are less able to tease out large scale differences. The therapist who works with Ms. Jin is most likely to be effective by carefully synthesizing and incorporating these different types of psychotherapy research.

The Self-Defeating Patient

Arnold M. Cooper, M.D.

GRACE Jin presents the apparent puzzle of an intelligent, well-educated young woman charged with realizing the ambitions of her family, who unpredictably fails a first-year medical student course. She responds to this failure with panic, humiliation, and impending punishment. Her history reveals a childhood of high expectations in which she helped with the family business and cared for the younger sisters. She has mild obsessive-compulsive symptoms and recurring hypochondriasis, recently severe enough to interfere with sleep and relaxation. Although the family is referred to several times, there is no mention of any affectionate bond between her and any other family member or among any of the family. One is left, perhaps unfairly, with the impression that her parents, preoccupied with survival and success in their adoptive land, had little time for play and affection with their oldest child.

Ms. Jin has, at least since high school, presented two apparently different personalities. She is a good girl who works hard and helps her parents, but she has long carried on a secret life of dating drug-dealing substance abusers, whom she finds exciting. In an obvious ironic obedience to her parents who told her to date an Asian man in contrast to the Caucasians of her high school years, she picked a "black sheep Asian," a tattooed, alcoholic drug abuser. In effect, she seem unconsciously to be saying, "you said I should date an Asian, so I am dating an Asian. What more could you ask of me?" thereby ridiculing the demands made of her.

It is easy to see her as a post-teenager in rebellion against straight-laced, demanding parents. But there are many forms of rebellion, and one of the questions raised by Ms. Jin is why her rebellion takes such self-destructive forms—flunking a course, picking boyfriends whom she supports and are potentially dangerous, and getting a tattoo of which she is ashamed.

In her first dream she refers to feeling lost, bad (a whore), and trying to find her way back to a classroom, with a man who is not interested in helping her. The therapist suggests that she is exhausted by her parents' expectations. She emphatically rejects the suggestion that her parents and boyfriend might be to blame and reproaches the therapist for his failings, revealing her angry expectation that he is not really interested in her personally, but will force medication on her—perhaps an early transference indication that she expects the therapist to be exactly like her parents. It is clear that Ms. Jin is not about to yield to expressions of kindness, sympathy, or what to the therapist might seem empathic. It also seems clear that the therapist is avoiding acknowledging hostile transference manifestations.

The sparse clinical evidence does not allow for a definitive psychodynamic understanding of Ms. Jin, but in the interest of demonstrating one formulation among several, I will take the liberty of focusing one-sidedly on her narcissistic-masochistic propensities. From that point of view, Ms. Jin is rebelling against demanding, seemingly unaffectionate parents through a series of self-destructive activities. Given her apparent intelligence and capacities, she could rebel in ways that might not damage her—for example, follow a different career, find an appropriate Caucasian boyfriend, and so forth. Instead, her rebellions include dating "exciting" men and getting tattoos, activities that she finds unacceptable and that lead her to feeling dependent, guilty, and humiliated—the exact feelings that would emerge if she submitted to parental demands. What seems like rebelliousness should perhaps more precisely be seen as pseudo-rebellion, since every one of her "rebellious" acts forces her further into guilt and dependency, failing to liberate her. In flunking a medical student course that she could easily pass, she again puts herself at the mercy of authority, and to her it makes little difference whether it is her parents, the school administration, or the student health service.

Within a few sessions, Ms. Jin begins to experience the therapist as an extension of her parents—unresponsive to her and her needs, self-centered, applying formulaic solutions to her rather than sharing personal deep interest. The therapist, perhaps already powerfully influenced by her angry coldness, responds to her the way her parents have responded—he wants her to be good and do well—but he has not yet heard what it might be that she desires—and at this point she undoubtedly does not know herself.

The tattoo may be of some interest. In addition to whatever it represents as a fashion, barbed wire is an explicitly cruel way of keeping unwanted creatures in their place. One guess is that her barbed wire tattoo expresses her sense of being unwanted, unloved, and helplessly imprisoned. In short, this woman of talents uses none of them to gain the freedom she allegedly wants, but uses all her capacities to further reduce herself to helplessness.

How to explain such behavior? One possibility for at least a subset of these patients is that they are experts at snatching defeat from the jaws of victory. While seemingly frustrating, such behavior creates a secret satisfaction. Their aim in life is no longer the expectable one of these patients' achieving independence and pleasure but the neurotic one of demonstrating that they are victimized and tortured. Feeling that they cannot control the outside world or their own fate, humiliated by their helplessness, dependency, and need for love that is not available, they adopt a defensive policy that guarantees some sense of mastery. They unconsciously provoke failure, disappointment, and reproach, thus demonstrating that they control their world, which is exactly as they know it to be—cruel, unloving, and unreliable. Secretly, unconsciously, they derive some variety of satisfaction or pleasure by controlling their own self-damage, predicting the negative outcome of their actions, and being able to frustrate the claims of parents. They then hide the guilty secret of their angry self-damaging behaviors, and, instead, experience conscious guilt and remorse over the "pseudo-aggression" of their rebellious behavior and superficial but unsuccessful efforts at reparation.

The therapist should expect that Ms. Jin will resort to the most imaginative strategies for defeating the efforts of the therapist, demonstrating that he is uncaring, that she is beyond repair, that she suffers from illnesses that were never before seen by mankind, that so-called nice people are untrustworthy, and that "bad people" are more reliable because they don't pretend to be good.

Ms. Jin obviously has many strengths, including her intelligence and her capacity for hard work. In addition, she has a long-standing capacity to form attachments, even if these relationships tend to be self-destructive. A therapist will need to try to enlist her in the battle with her harsh superego with which she is eager to cooperate, and to help her to understand that what she is really guilty of is self-destructive behavior; she has damaged no one as much as herself.

One might predict that treatment will be neither brief nor easy, but successful. Ms. Jin has countered a deep narcissistic injury with masochistic behaviors that include failure, self-abasement, and humiliation. Her sense of being attacked and her methods of counterattack will manifest themselves in therapy. The therapist has already had a taste of Ms. Jin's sarcasm. Her response to obvious aspects of her first dream hints at a deep-seated belief that no one is genuinely interested in her. Her powerful claim is that everyone has used her and that no one has ever loved her. She will do her best to prove that this is true in the treatment. She is facing deep sadness in acknowledging the depth of her disappointment in her family, the pain of feeling so unloved and unappreciated, and the bitter anger that she has so far expressed in self-damaging behaviors. It will be the therapist's task to help her to begin to think about herself—a task she has avoided—and to confront painful aspects of her self against which she has spent a lifetime building narcissistic-masochistic defenses that help her disavow her deep feelings of hurt, worthlessness, and resentment. Steering through the temptations to be too helpful to this wonderful young woman and too angry at her endless provocations and her resistance to receiving help is the job of the therapist.

Overview of an Evaluation

Robert Michels, M.D.

GRACE Jin, the person, goes to the Student Health Service. They refer her to a psychiatrist (we are not told what that means, to her or to them). The psychiatrist meets with her, and, together, they will construct Grace Jin, the patient. There are, as always, many options involved—what they will make central, what they will view as subordinate, and what will remain out of their awareness. Ms. Jin is a woman, a medical student, Chinese, an immigrant, a young adult; is highly intelligent, rebellious, high achieving, sexual, seductive, anxious, somatically symptomatic, obsessional, substance abusing; has just failed an examination; is preoccupied with examining her body, is ashamed of that preoccupation, wants help, fears help; and has just met the therapist and, at least for the moment, may be more concerned with figuring out what the therapist and the therapy are all about than with learning about herself. Each of these is a possible focus of the treatment. We know little about the therapist (and perhaps are being invited to imagine ourselves in her or his place). However, this lack of knowledge about the therapist raises more difficulties as the story evolves, because in reality such stories evolve in interaction with a therapist who participates in the process. Thus, for example, a strategy of emphasizing reassurance, based on Ms. Jin's considerable assets and adaptive talents, will lead to a quite different patient than one of focusing on her symptoms, on her narcissistic-masochistic character structure, or on the immediate transference–countertransference constellation.

In many ways the task of writing a discussion of a case such as this is the opposite of the clinical task of working with such a patient. Every clinician approaches a new patient with both memories and desires—favorite theories, knowledge of the literature, personal experiences, countertransference predispositions, and the like. However, good clinicians are open minded. They take in the patient, and the richness and complexity of a real person pushes their memories and desires, their theories and prejudices, to the background. We are all familiar with the frequent experience of clinicians who seem to differ sharply in theory or writing but are much more similar when they discuss a real patient in depth. Here we have a brief and somewhat ambiguous account, one designed to bring the clinician's favorite theories and anticipatory set to the foreground, in bold relief, rather than replacing them with the multifaceted reality of an actual patient. Such a case presentation is similar to the psychoanalytic practice of reducing the reminders of reality so that the patient's fantasies will be all the more vivid.

Our discussants approach Ms. Jin from a variety of perspectives. Some emphasize the patient herself and particularly her psychopathology, somatoform disorders, and obsessionalism; others her narcissistic and masochistic psychodynamics; others her sociocultural contexts (medical student, first-generation American); still others emphasize the transference–countertransference constellation (the empathic connection and therapeutic zeal). Finally, several discuss the implications of their perspective for strategies of treatment: self-psychology, meditation, complementary medicine and evidence-based psychotherapy. Each of these perspectives is potentially relevant. One of the most difficult tasks in clinical work is for the clinician to select which perspective to employ and then fit it to the patient, the clinician, the problem, and the setting. One of the most important principles in clinical work is that any selection should always be tentative—to be assessed, evaluated, and possibly changed or reformulated. The clinician who always approaches patients with the same perspective, or who, once embarked on a treatment program, is unable to reassess or modify it, is at best limited and at worst dangerous. There are many ways to start thinking about Ms. Jin, but a clinician must be open to rethinking, particularly if the initial approach founders. There are many clues that most, perhaps all, approaches here are likely to founder! The patient does not match a simple formula that might generate an algorithm for what to do. Many patients do match such templates, and comprehensive assessments may then add little of value. It is reasonable to defer them in such situations, but here we do not have that luxury. There are prominent Axis I, Axis II, and situational issues, and the diagnosis is not clear.

Ms. Jin has secrets; she hides things—boyfriends, drugs, a tattoo, the fact she examines her body—and this predicts that she will also keep secrets from her therapist. The therapist wants to know more and decides to "extend the evaluation." The patient responds, dutifully, with a dream. Dreams are valuable, not only in psychotherapy but also in evaluations; they often reveal things that might otherwise be hidden, not only from the therapist but from the patient as well. Seeing a therapist is an emotionally charged event, and dreams that are recounted during an evaluation are often about that evaluation. She dreams of being lost in a strange place (the evaluation) and wanting to get back to a classroom (school), but being distracted by ghosts (family, the past), by being called a whore (guilt, anticipation of disapproval for her sexuality), and by experiencing bugs on her skin (her symptoms). A man (the therapist) is not interested in helping. She associates to the ghosts, the past, and the bugs, but not to being called a whore or to the unhelpful man (the therapist and the evaluation). The therapist responds with supportive reassurance, and she replies by criticizing him directly, but then gives up—"You'll just want to give me some medication." He responds with an accurate but formal and unempathic response—it's only transference. She recognizes that he has backed away and blushingly apologizes. The story stops at this critical junction; the evaluation has come to an end. An error such as this could have been corrected easily if the therapist recognized what had happened and was able to discuss it; patients forgive errors that do not reveal malevolence.

The clinician's next task is to share the understanding he has developed in the evaluation with the patient; discuss the plausible options, including their advantages and disadvantages; offer advice (if he has some and can deal with the inevitable transference complications); and then conduct the treatment or refer the patient to someone else who can. There are many issues in selecting an approach—"external" factors (time, money, availability); the patient's diagnosis, pathology, and character; the therapist's competence and interest; and the patient's preferences. The way in which the therapist handles this discussion is likely to have a powerful influence on any therapy that follows, the patient's attitude toward therapy and therapists in general, and her attitude toward future therapy.

Several of the discussants emphasize the powerful impact of the doctor–patient relationship—the therapeutic alliance, the transference–countertransference constellation (I am using these terms as overlapping categories)—in shaping the treatment and determining the outcome. The initial hints are not all promising. Whom does the doctor represent—her parents, the medical school, the dominant culture, or none of the above? Who is the therapist in reality—a trainee or a graduate? Younger or older? Male or female? European, Asian, or other? The patient has lived most of her life as feeling marginalized, an outsider. Can she use the treatment as a safe place to talk, or is she once again an outsider, appropriately mistrustful of an alien ritual. Many studies have suggested that success or failure in negotiating the initial relationship is highly correlated with the ultimate success of the treatment.

Opportunities for countertransference abound (they always abound). Each of her identities—Chinese, a woman, an immigrant, a medical student— invites the therapist's fantasies and projections. Furthermore she actively elicits them. She is provocative and seductive and displays a pattern of what one discussant terms "ironic compliance." Of course, countertransferential responses such as these are not inherently bad. In fact they can be major tools of therapy if used appropriately. For that to happen, they must first be recognized and studied—subjects of interest rather than subjects of avoidance.

From this point there are many ways that the story might continue. Symptomatic treatment is unlikely to solve many of her problems, although it might offer relief and an opportunity to develop a stronger bond to her therapist. Her predisposition to shame and humiliation is likely to make her wary of treatment, but her pain and aloneness may lead her to it. If she becomes involved, the options may become clarified. Support, symptom relief, and time may lead to a therapy that can explore the deeper roots of her difficulties. Nothing in the presentation suggests that such treatment is impossible; but nothing suggests that it is likely to be easy.

Summary Points

- Otherwise healthy people may present to psychiatrists because they are dealing with unusually difficult stressors. They often rebound quickly.

- People with obvious strengths can have Axis I disorders. Their strengths may lead to underdiagnosis and undertreatment.

- Research into psychiatric treatments relies on robust diagnoses. When the diagnoses are uncertain, treatment selection relies on multiple types of data.

- People develop unconscious defenses against assaults on their pride and self-esteem. These defenses can lead to isolation, rigidity, and unhappiness.

- Self-damaging activities can lead to unconscious gratification.

- Symptoms can be reduced by interventions that are nonverbal (e.g., yoga and meditation), that use words as adjunctive (e.g., pharmacology), and that focus almost entirely on words and meaning (psychoanalytic therapy).

- Psychotherapy can be scientifically researched.

- Psychiatric listening is structured by the therapist's theories and assumptions.

- Overzealous interpretations damage the alliance.

- There are many ways for therapy to go wrong.

- There are many ways for therapy to go right.

Chapter 1:
Double Depression and James Avery

DEPRESSION

Gualtieri CT, Johnson LG, Benedict KB: Neurocognition in depression: patients on and off medication versus healthy comparison subjects. J Neuropsychiatry Clin Neurosci 18:217–225, 2006

Keller MB, Klien DN, Hirschfeld RMA, et al: Results of the DSM-IV mood disorders field trial. Am J Psychiatry 152:843–849, 1995

Kennedy N, Abbott R, Paykel ES: Longitudinal syndromal symptoms after severe depression: 10-year follow-up study. Br J Psychiatry 184:330–336, 2004

Kessler RC, McGonagle KA, Zhao S, et al: Lifetime and 12-month prevalence of DSM-III-R psychiatric disorders in the United States: results for the National Comorbidity Survey. Arch Gen Psychiatry 51:8–19, 1994

Miller DK, Malmstrom MS, Joshi S, et al: Clinically relevant levels of depression in community-dwelling middle-aged African Americans. J Am Geriatr Soc 52:741–748, 2004

Weissman MM, Livingston B, Leaf J, et al: Affective disorders, in Psychiatric Disorders in America: The Epidemiologic Catchment Area Study. Edited by Robins LN, Regier DA. New York, Free Press, 1991, p 53

Wells KB, Stewart A, Hays RD, et al: The functioning and well-being of depressed patients: results from the Medical Outcomes Study. JAMA 262:914–919, 1989

Williams DR, Gonzalez HM, Neighbors H, et al: Prevalence and distribution of major depressive disorder in African Americans, Caribbean blacks, and non-Hispanic whites: results from the National Survey of American Life. Arch Gen Psychiatry 64:305–315, 2007

SUICIDE

Beck AT, Steer RA, Kovacs M, et al: Hopelessness and eventual suicide: a 10-year prospective study of patients hospitalized with suicidal ideation. Am J Psychiatry 142:559–563, 1985

Beck AT, Brown G, Berchick RJ, et al: Relationship between hopelessness and ultimate suicide: a replication with psychiatric outpatients. Am J Psychiatry 147:190–195, 1990

Bostwick JM, Pankratz VS: Affective disorders and suicide risk: a reexamination. Am J Psychiatry 157:1925–1932, 2000

Busch KA, Fawcett J, Jacobs DG: Clinical correlates of inpatient suicide. J Clin Psychiatry 64:14–19, 2003

Fawcett J, Scheftner WA, Fogg L, et al: Time-related predictors of suicide in major affective disorder. Am J Psychiatry 47:1189–1194, 1990

Harris EC, Barraclough B: Suicide as an outcome for mental disorders: a meta-analysis. Br J Psychiatry 170:205–228, 1997

Hayward L, Zubrick SR, Silburn S: Blood alcohol levels in suicide cases. J Epidemiol Community Health 46:256–260, 1992

Kposowa AJ: Unemployment and suicide: a cohort analysis of social factors predicting suicide in the US National Longitudinal Mortality Study. Psychol Med 31:127–138, 2001

Luoma JB, Pearson JL: Suicide and marital status in United States, 1991–1996: is widowhood a risk factor? Am J Public Health 92:1518–1522, 2002

Marzuk PM, Tardiff K, Hirsch CS: The epidemiology of murder-suicide. JAMA 267:3179–3183, 1992

Marzuk PM, Hartwell N, Leon AC, et al: Executive functioning in depressed patients with suicidal ideation. Acta Psychiatr Scand 112:294–301, 2005

Neeleman J, Halpern D, Leon D, et al: Tolerance of suicide, religion and suicide rates: an ecological and individual study in 19 Western countries. Psychol Med 27:1165–1171, 1997

Robins E, Murphy GE, Wilkinson RH, et al: Some clinical considerations in the prevention of suicide based on a study of 134 successful suicides. Am J Public Health 49:888–899, 1959

THE PSYCHODYNAMIC FORMULATION

Alliance of Psychoanalytic Organizations: Psychodynamic Diagnostic Manual (PDM). Silver Spring, MD, Alliance of Psychoanalytic Organizations, 2006

American Psychiatric Association: Diagnostic and Statistical Manual of Mental Disorders, 4th Edition. Washington, DC, American Psychiatric Association, 1994

Brenner I: Psychic Trauma: Dynamics, Symptoms, and Treatment. Oxford, UK, Rowman & Littlefield, 2004

Krupnick JL, Sotsky SM, Simmens S, et al: The role of the therapeutic alliance in psychotherapy and pharmacotherapy outcome: findings in the National Institute of Mental Health Treatment of Depression Collaborative Research Program. J Consult Clin Psychol 64:532–539, 1996

Lister EG, Auchincloss EL, Cooper AM: The psychodynamic formulation, in Psychodynamic Concepts in General Psychiatry. Edited by Schwartz HJ, Bleiberg E, Weissman SH. Washington, DC, American Psychiatric Press, 1995, pp 13–25

Westen D, Novotny CM, Thompson-Brenner H: The empirical status of empirically supported psychotherapies: assumptions, findings, and reporting in controlled clinical trials. Psychol Bull 130:631–663, 2004

THE INTERVIEW OF THE DEPRESSED PATIENT

Beck AT: Depression: Clinical, Experimental, and Theoretical Aspects. New York, Harper & Row, 1967

Carlat D: The Psychiatric Interview: A Practical Guide, 2nd Edition. Philadelphia, PA, Lippincott Williams & Wilkins, 2005

MacKinnon RA, Michels R, Buckley P: The Psychiatric Interview in Clinical Practice, 2nd Edition. Washington, DC, American Psychiatric Publishing, 2006

Reiser DE, Schroder AK: Patient Interviewing: The Human Dimension. Baltimore, MD, Williams & Wilkins, 1980

Shea SC: Psychiatric Interviewing: The Art of Understanding. Philadelphia, PA, WB Saunders, 1988

Sullivan HS: The Psychiatric Interview. New York, WW Norton, 1970

THE AFRICAN AMERICAN PATIENT

Altman N: The Analyst in the Inner City: Race, Class, and Culture Through a Psychoanalytic Lens, Vol 3. Hillsdale, NJ, Analytic Press, 1995

Boyd-Franklin N: Black Families in Therapy: Understanding the African American Experience, 2nd Edition. New York, Guilford, 2003

Gladwell M: Blink: The Power of Thinking Without Thinking. New York, Little, Brown, 2000

Guthrie RV: Even the Rat Was White: A Historical View of Psychology. New York, Harper & Row, 1976

Jones RL (ed): Black Psychology, 4th Edition. Hampton, VA, Cobb & Henry Publishing, 2004

Parham T, Ajanu A, White JL: The Psychology of Blacks: An African Centered Perspective. Upper Saddle River, NJ, Pearson Education, 1999

Smith H, Leary K (eds): Race, culture, and ethnicity in the consulting room. Psychoanal Q 75(1), 2006

Staples R: Black Masculinity: The Black Male's Role in American Society. San Francisco, CA, Black Scholar Press, 1990

NEUROBIOLOGY OF STRESS

Arendt T, Stieler J, Strijkstra AM, et al: Reversible paired helical filament-like phosphorylation of tau is an adaptive process associated with neuronal plasticity in hibernating animals. J Neurosci 23:6972–6981, 2003

Cameron HA, McKay RDG: Adult neurogenesis produces a large pool of new granule cells in the dentate gyrus. J Comp Neurol 435:406–417, 2001

Conrad CD, Magarinos AM, LeDoux JE, et al: Repeated restraint stress facilitates fear conditioning independently of causing hippocampal CA3 dendritic atrophy. Behav Neurosci 113:902–913, 1999

Convit A, Wolf OT, Tarshish C, et al: Reduced glucose tolerance is associated with poor memory performance and hippocampal atrophy among normal elderly. Proc Natl Acad Sci U S A 100:2019–2022, 2003

Driessen M, Herrmann J, Stahl K, et al: Magnetic resonance imaging volumes of the hippocampus and the amygdala in women with borderline personality disorder and early traumatization. Arch Gen Psychiatry 57:1115–1122, 2000

Frodl T, Meisenzahl EM, Zetzsche T, et al: Larger amygdala volumes in first depressive episode as compared to recurrent major depression and healthy control subjects. Biol Psychiatry 53:338–344, 2003

Liston C, Miller MM, Goldwater DS, et al: Stress-induced alterations in prefrontal cortical dendritic morphology predict selective impairments in perceptual attentional set-shifting. J Neurosci 26:7870–7874, 2006

MacQueen GM, Campbell S, McEwen BS, et al: Course of illness, hippocampal function, and hippocampal volume in major depression. Proc Natl Acad Sci U S A 100:1387–1392, 2003

McEwen BS: Protective and damaging effects of stress mediators. N Engl J Med 338:171–179, 1998

McEwen BS: Stress and hippocampal plasticity. Annu Rev Neurosci 22:105–122, 1999

McEwen BS, Stellar E: Stress and the individual: mechanisms leading to disease. Arch Intern Med 153:2093–2101, 1993

McEwen BS, Wingfield JC: The concept of allostasis in biology and biomedicine. Horm Behav 43:2–15, 2003

Nesse RM: Is depression an adaptation? Arch Gen Psychiatry 57:14–20, 2000

Pawlak R, Rao BS, Melchor JP, et al: Tissue plasminogen activator and plasminogen mediate stress-induced decline of neuronal and cognitive functions in the mouse hippocampus. Proc Natl Acad Sci U S A 102:18201–18206, 2005

Pitman RK: Hippocampal diminution in PTSD: more (or less?) than meets the eye. Hippocampus 11:73–74, 2001

Popov VI, Bocharova LS, Bragin AG: Repeated changes of dendritic morphology in the hippocampus of ground squirrels in the course of hibernation. Neuroscience 48:45–51, 1992

Radley JJ, Rocher AB, Miller M, et al: Repeated stress induces dendritic spine loss in the rat medial prefrontal cortex. Cerebral Cortex 16:313–320, 2005

Sapolsky RM, Romero LM, Munck AU: How do glucocorticoids influence stress responses? Integrating permissive, suppressive, stimulatory, and preparative actions. Endocrine Rev 21:55–89, 2000

Sheline YI, Gado MH, Kraemer HC: Untreated depression and hippocampal volume loss. Am J Psychiatry 160:1516–1518, 2003

Sterling P, Eyer J: Allostasis: a new paradigm to explain arousal pathology, in Handbook of Life Stress, Cognition, and Health. Edited by Fisher S, Reason J. New York, Wiley, 1988, pp 629–640

Thayer JF, Lane RD: A model of neurovisceral integration in emotion regulation and dysregulation. J Affect Disord 61:201–216, 2000

Vermetten E, Vythilingam M, Southwick SM, et al: Long-term treatment with paroxetine increases verbal declarative memory and hippocampal volume in posttraumatic stress disorder. Biol Psychiatry 54:693–702, 2003

Vyas A, Mitra R, Rao BS, et al: Chronic stress induces contrasting patterns of dendritic remodeling in hippocampal and amygdaloid neurons. J Neurosci 22:6810–6818, 2002

WHAT IS PSYCHIATRY?

Berrios G: The History of Mental Symptoms. Cambridge, UK, Cambridge University Press, 1996

Berrios G, Porter R (eds): The History of Clinical Psychiatry. London, Atholone Press, 1995

Clarke E, Jacyna LS: Nineteenth Century Origins of Neuroscientific Concepts. Berkeley, University of California Press, 1987

Makari G: Revolution in Mind: The Creation of Psychoanalysis. New York, HarperCollins, 2008

Shorter E: A Historical Dictionary of Psychiatry. Oxford, UK, Oxford University Press, 2005, pp 232–233

INPATIENT PSYCHIATRY

Beck AT, Rush AJ, Shaw BF, et al: Cognitive Therapy of Depression. New York: Guilford, 1979

Gunderson JG: Principles and Practice of Milieu Therapy. New York, Jason Aronson, 1983

Linehan MM: Cognitive-Behavioral Treatment of Borderline Personality Disorder. New York: Guilford, 1993

Menninger WW: Role of the psychiatric hospital in the treatment of mental illness, in Kaplan and Sadock's Comprehensive Textbook of Psychiatry, 8th Edition, Vol 2. Edited by Sadock BJ, Sadock VA. Philadelphia, Lippincott Williams & Wilkins, 2005, pp 3210–3218

Munich RL, Gabbard GO (section eds): Hospital psychiatry, in American Psychiatric Press Review of Psychiatry, Vol 11. Edited by Tasman A, Riba MB. Washington, DC, American Psychiatric Press, 1992, pp 499–603

Sederer LI, Rothschild AJ: Acute Care Psychiatry: Diagnosis and Treatment. Williams & Wilkins, 1997

PSYCHOPHARMACOLOGY OF DEPRESSION

Agency for Health Care Policy and Research: Depression in Primary Care, Vol 2: Treatment of Major Depression (AHCPR Publ No 93-0551). Rockville, MD, U.S. Department of Health and Human Services, 1993

Malhotra AK, Murphy GM, Kennedy JL: Pharmacogenetics of psychotropic drug response. Am J Psychiatry 161:780–796, 2004

Quitkin FM: Depression with atypical features: diagnostic validity, prevalence, and treatment. Prim Care Companion J Clin Psychiatry 4:94–99, 2002

Thase ME, Entsuah AR, Rudolph RL: Remission rates during treatment with venlafaxine or selective serotonin reuptake inhibitors. Br J Psychiatry 178:234–241, 2001

Trivedi MH, Fava M, Wiesnewski S, et al: Medication augmentation after the failure of SSRIs for depression. N Engl J Med 354:1243–1252, 2006

PHARMACOGENOMICS

Glatt CE, Reus VI: Pharmacogenetics of monoamine transporters. Pharmacogenomics 4:583–596, 2003

Kirchheiner J, Klein C, Meineke I, et al: Bupropion and 4-OH-bupropion pharmacokinetics in relation to genetic polymorphisms in CYP2B6. Pharmacogenetics 13:619–626, 2003

Kirchheiner J, Nickchen K, Bauer M, et al: Pharmacogenetics of antidepressants and antipsychotics: the contribution of allelic variations to the phenotype of drug response. Mol Psychiatry 9:442–473, 2004

Lesch KP, Bengel D, Heils A, et al: Association of anxiety-related traits with a polymorphism in the serotonin transporter gene regulatory region. Science 274:1527–1531, 1996

BRAIN STIMULATION AND NEUROMODULATION

American Psychiatric Association, Task Force on Electroconvulsive Therapy: The Practice of Electroconvulsive Therapy: Recommendations for Treatment, Training, and Privileging. Washington, DC, American Psychiatric Association, 2001

Lisanby SH (ed): Brain Stimulation in Psychiatric Treatment. Review of Psychiatry, Vol 23. Oldham JO, Riba MB, Series Editors. Washington, DC, American Psychiatric Publishing, 2004

Lisanby SH, Luber B, Schlaepfer TE, et al: Safety and feasibility of magnetic seizure therapy (MST) in major depression: randomized within-subject comparison with electroconvulsive therapy. Neuropsychopharmacology 28:1852–1865, 2003

Mantovani A, Lisanby SH: Transcranial magnetic stimulation in the treatment of depression, in Transcranial Magnetic Stimulation in Clinical Psychiatry. Edited by George MS, Belmaker RH. Washington, DC, American Psychiatric Publishing, 2007, pp 113–152

Wassermann EM, Lisanby SH: Therapeutic application of repetitive transcranial magnetic stimulation: a review. Clin Neurophysiol 112:1367–1377, 2001

Wassermann EM, Epstein CM, Ziemann U, et al (eds): Oxford Handbook of Transcranial Stimulation. New York, Oxford University Press, 2008

SUPPORTIVE PSYCHOTHERAPY

Aviram RB, Hellerstein DJ, Gerson J, et al: Adapting supportive psychotherapy for individuals with borderline personality disorder who self-injure or attempt suicide. J Psychiatr Pract 10:145–155, 2004

Hellerstein DJ, Pinsker H, Rosenthal RN, et al: Supportive therapy as the treatment model of choice. J Psychother Pract Res 3:300–306, 1994

Novalis RN, Rojcewicz SJ, Peele R: Clinical Manual of Supportive Psychotherapy. Washington, DC, American Psychiatric Press, 1993

Pinsker H: A Primer of Supportive Psychotherapy. Hillsdale, NJ, Analytic Press, 1997

Winston A, Rosenthal RN, Pinsker H: Introduction to Supportive Psychotherapy (Core Competencies in Psychotherapy). Washington, DC, American Psychiatric Publishing, 2004

COUPLES THERAPY

Gottman JM: What Predicts Divorce? Hillsdale, NJ, Lawrence Erlbaum, 1994

Gottman JM: Why Marriages Succeed or Fail. New York, Simon & Schuster, 1994

Gottman JM: The Marriage Clinic. New York, WW Norton, 1999

Gurman AS, Jacobson NS (eds): Clinical Handbook of Couple Therapy. New York, Guilford, 2002

Minuchin S: Families and Family Therapy. Cambridge, MA, Harvard University Press, 1974

Saer C: Marriage Contracts and Couple Therapy. New York, Brunner-Routledge, 1976

OVERVIEW OF DOUBLE DEPRESSION

Gelenberg AJ, Trivedi MH, Rush AJ, et al: Randomized, placebo-controlled trial of nefazodone maintenance treatment in preventing recurrence in chronic depression. Biol Psychiatry 54:806–817, 2003

Keller MB, McCullough JP, Klein DN, et al: A comparison of nefazodone, the cognitive behavioral-analysis system of psychotherapy, and their combination for the treatment of chronic depression. N Engl J Med 342:1462–1470, 2000

Klein DN, Santiago NJ, Vivian D, et al: Cognitive Behavioral Analysis System of Psychotherapy as a maintenance treatment for chronic depression. J Consult Clin Psychol 72:631–638, 2004

Kocsis JH, Friedman RA, Markowitz JC, et al: Maintenance therapy for chronic depression: a controlled clinical trial of desipramine. Arch Gen Psychiatry 53:769–774, 1996

Kocsis JH, Schatzberg A, Rush AJ, et al: Psychosocial outcomes following long-term, double-blind treatment of chronic depression with sertraline vs placebo. Arch Gen Psychiatry 59:723–728, 2002

McCullough JP: Treatment for Chronic Depression: Cognitive Behavioral Analysis System of Psychotherapy (CBASP). New York, Guilford, 2000

Schatzberg AF, Rush AJ, Arnow BA, et al: Chronic depression: medication (nefazodone) or psychotherapy (CBASP) is effective when the other is not. Arch Gen Psychiatry 62:513–520, 2005

Thase ME, Rush AJ, Howland RH, et al: Double-blind switch study of imipramine or sertraline treatment of antidepressant-resistant chronic depression. Arch Gen Psychiatry 59:233–239, 2002

Chapter 2:
Geriatric Depression and Peter Burke

CAPACITY

Alexopoulos GS, Borson S, Cuthbert BN, et al: Assessment of late life depression. Biol Psychiatry 52:164–174, 2002

Appelbaum PS, Grisso T: Assessing patients' capacities to consent to treatment. N Engl J Med 319:1635–1638, 1988

Cavanagh SR, Shin LM, Karamouz N, et al: Psychiatric and emotional sequelae of surgical amputation. Psychosomatics 47:459–464, 2006

Cooper AM, Michels R: The psychodynamic formulation: its purpose, structure, and clinical application. Am J Psychiatry 144:543–550, 1987

MacKinnon RA, Michels R, Buckley PJ: The hospitalized patient. in The Psychiatric Interview in Clinical Practice, 2nd Edition. Washington DC, American Psychiatric Publishing, 2006, pp 505–520

Rosenberg PB, Johnston D, Lyketsos CG: A clinical approach to mild cognitive impairment. Am J Psychiatry 163:1884–1889, 2006

Viederman M, Perry SW: Use of psychodynamic life narrative in the treatment of depression in the physically ill. Gen Hosp Psychiatry 3:177–185, 1980

THE PSYCHIATRIC ATTITUDE

Greene P, Kane D, Christ GH, et al: FDNY Crisis Counseling: Innovative Responses to 9/11 Firefighters, Families, and Communities. New York, Wiley, 2006

Halberstam D: Firehouse. Hyperion, New York, 2002

Perry S, Viederman M: Adaptation of residents to consultation-liaison psychiatry, I: working with the physically ill. Gen Hosp Psychiatry 3:141–147, 1981

Viederman M: The Therapeutic Consultation: Finding the Patient. Am J Psychother 60:153–159, 2006

DEPRESSION AND MEDICAL ILLNESS

American Psychiatric Association: Diagnostic and Statistical Manual of Mental Disorders, Fourth Edition. Washington, DC, American Psychiatric Association, 1994

Breitbart W, Heller KS: Reframing hope: meaning-centered care for patients near the end of life. J Palliat Med 6:979–988, 2003

Glassman AH, O'Connor CM, Califf RM, et al: Sertraline treatment of major depression in patients with acute MI or unstable angina. JAMA 288:701–709, 2002

Glassman AH, Bigger JTJ, Gaffney M, et al: Onset of major depression associated with acute coronary syndromes: relationship of onset, major depressive disorder history, and episode severity to sertraline benefit. Arch Gen Psychiatry 63:283–288, 2006

Hance MR, Carney M, Freedland KE, et al: Depression in patients with coronary heart disease. Gen Hosp Psychiatry 18:61–65, 1996

Kahana RJ, Bibring GL: Personality types in medical management, in Psychiatry and Medical Practice in a General Hospital. Edited by Zinberg N. New York, International Universities Press, 1964, pp 108–123

Koszycki D, Lafontaine S, Frasure-Smith N, et al: An open-label trial of interpersonal psychotherapy in depressed patients with coronary disease. Psychosomatics 45:319–324, 2004

Lesperance FN, Frasure-Smith N, Talajic M: Major depression before and after myocardial infarction: its nature and consequences. Psychosom Med 58:99–110, 1996

Rodin GM, Nolan RP, Katz MR: Depression, in The American Psychiatric Publishing Textbook of Psychosomatic Medicine. Edited by Levenson JL. Washington, DC, American Psychiatric Publishing, 2005, pp 193–217

Schulz R, Beach SR, Ives DG, et al: Association between depression and mortality in older adults. Arch Intern Med 160:1761–1768, 2000

Viederman M, Perry SW: Use of a psychodynamic life narrative in the treatment of depression in the physically ill. Gen Hosp Psychiatry 3:177–185, 1980

Weissman MM, Markowitz JC: Comprehensive Guide to Interpersonal Psychotherapy. New York, Basic Books, 2000

Writing Committee for the ENRICHD Investigators: Effects of treating depression and low perceived social support on clinical events after myocardial infarction: the Enhancing Recovery in Coronary Heart Disease Patients (ENRICHD) randomized trial. JAMA 289:3106–3116, 2003

NEUROTROPHINS

Chao MV: Neurotrophins and their receptors: a convergence point for many signaling pathways. Nature Rev Neurosci 4:299–309, 2003

Chen K, Nishimura MC, Armanini MP, et al: Disruption of a single allele of the nerve growth factor gene results in atrophy of basal forebrain cholinergic neurons and memory deficits. J Neurosci 17:7288–7296, 1997

Chen ZY, Jing D, Bath KG, et al: Genetic variant BDNF (Val66Met) polymorphism alters anxiety-related behavior. Science 314:140–143, 2006

Egan MF, Kojima M, Callicott JH, et al: The BDNF val66met polymorphism affects activity-dependent secretion of BDNF and human memory and hippocampal function. Cell 112:257–269, 2003

Huang E, Reichardt L: Trk receptors: roles in neuronal signal transduction. Ann Rev Biochem 72:609–642, 2003

Lee FS, Kim AH, Khursigara G, et al: The uniqueness of being a neurotrophin receptor. Curr Opin Neurobiol 11:281, 2001

Levi-Montalcini R: The nerve growth factor: thirty-five years later. Science 237:1154–1162, 2001

Roux P, Barker P: Neurotrophin signaling through the p75 neurotrophin receptor. Prog Neurobiol 67:203–233, 2002

TESTING AT THE BEDSIDE

Beck AT, Steer RA, Brown GK: Beck Depression Inventory–II. Manual. San Antonio, TX, Psychological Corporation, 1996

Blessed G, Tomlinson BE, Roth M: The association between quantitative measures of dementia and of senile changes in the cerebral grey matter of elderly subjects. Br J Psychiatry 114:797–811, 1968

Brink TL, Yesavage JA, Lum O, et al: Screening tests for geriatric depression. Clin Gerontol 1:37–43, 1982

Butcher JN, Dahlstrom WG, Graham JR, et al: Manual for the Restandardized Minnesota Multiphasic Personality Inventory: MMPI-2. Minneapolis, University of Minnesota Press, 1989

Chochinov HM, Wilson KG, Enns M, et al: "Are you depressed?" Screening for depression in the terminally ill. Am J Psychiatry 154:674–676, 1997

Folstein MF, Folstein SE, Fanjang G: Mini-Mental State Examination: User's Guide. Odessa, FL, Psychological Assessment Resources, 2001

Hamilton M: Development of a rating scale for primary depressive illness. Br J Soc Clin Psychol 6:278–296, 1967

Jurica PJ, Leitten CL, Mattis S: Dementia Rating Scale–2 (DRS-2) Professional Manual. Odessa, FL, Psychological Assessment Resources, 2002

Kiernan RJ, Mueller J, Langston JW: Cognistat (Neurobehavioral Cognitive State Examination). Lutz, FL, Psychological Assessment Resources, 1995

Lezak MD, Howieson DB, Loring DW: Neuropsychological Assessment, 4th Edition. New York, Oxford University Press, 2004

Mason BJ, Kocsis JH, Leon AC, et al: Measurement of severity and treatment response in dysthymia. Psychiatric Annals 23:625–631, 1993

Morey LC: Personality Assessment Inventory: Professional Manual. Odessa, FL, Psychological Assessment Resources, 1991

Randolph C, Tierney MC, Mohr E, et al: The Repeatable Battery for the Assessment of Neuropsychological Status (RBANS): preliminary clinical validity. J Clin Exp Neuropsychol 20:310–319, 1998

Rosen WG, Mohs RC, Davis KL: A new rating scale of Alzheimer's disease. Am J Psychiatry 141:1351–1364, 1984

Samton JB, Ferrando SJ, Sanelli P, et al: The Clock Drawing Test: diagnostic, functional, and neuroimaging correlates in older patients evaluated in the consultation-liaison setting. J Neuropsychiatry Clin Neurosci 17:533–540, 2005

Wechsler D: Wechsler Adult Intelligence Scale–III. San Antonio, TX, The Psychological Corporation, 1997

Yesavage JA, Brink TL, Rose TL, et al: Development and validation of a geriatric screening scale: a preliminary report. J Psychiatr Res 17:37–49, 1982–1983

Zung WWK: A self-rating depression scale: Arch Gen Psychiatry 16:543–547, 1967

INTERPERSONAL PSYCHOTHERAPY

Hamilton M: A rating scale for depression. J Neurol Neurosurg Psychiatry 25:56–62, 1960

Koszycki D, Lafontaine S, Frasure-Smith N, et al: An open-label trial of interpersonal psychotherapy in depressed patients with coronary disease. Psychosomatics 45:319–324, 2004

Markowitz JC: Interpersonal Psychotherapy for Dysthymic Disorder. Washington, DC, American Psychiatric Press, 1998

Markowitz JC, Swartz HA: Case formulation in interpersonal psychotherapy of depression, in Handbook of Psychotherapy Case Formulation, 2nd Edition. Edited by Eells TD. New York, Guilford, 2007, pp 221–250

Markowitz JC, Kocsis JH, Fishman B, et al: Treatment of HIV-positive patients with depressive symptoms. Arch Gen Psychiatry 55:452–457, 1998

Parsons T: Illness and the role of the physician: a sociological perspective. Am J Orthopsychiatry 21:452–460, 1951

Reynolds CF, Frank E, Perel JM, et al: Nortriptyline and interpersonal psychotherapy as maintenance therapies for recurrent depression: a randomized controlled trial in patients older than 59 years. JAMA 281:39–45, 1999

Reynolds CF III, Dew MA, Pollock BG, et al: Maintenance treatment of major depression in old age. N Engl J Med 354:1130–1138, 2006

Schulberg HC, Block MR, Madonia MJ, et al: Treating major depression in primary care practice: eight-month clinical outcomes. Arch Gen Psychiatry 53:913–919, 1996

Weissman MM, Markowitz JC, Klerman GL: Comprehensive Guide to Interpersonal Psychotherapy. New York, Basic Books, 2000

Weissman MM, Markowitz JC, Klerman GL: A Clinician's Quick Guide to Interpersonal Psychotherapy. New York, Oxford University Press, 2007

OVERVIEW OF GERIATRIC DEPRESSION

Alexopoulos GS: Depression in the elderly. Lancet 365:1961–1970, 2005

Alexopoulos GS, Meyers BS, Young RC, et al: The course of geriatric depression with "reversible dementia": a controlled study. Am J Psychiatry 150:1693–1699, 1993

Alexopoulos GS, Meyers BS, Young RC, et al: The "vascular depression" hypothesis. Arch Gen Psychiatry 54:915–922, 1997

Alexopoulos GS, Katz IR, Reynolds CF, et al: The Expert Consensus Guideline Series. Pharmacotherapy of geriatric depression. Postgrad Med (Special Report), October 2001

Alexopoulos GS, Borson S, Cuthbert BN, et al: Assessment of late-life depression. Biol Psychiatry 52:164–174, 2002

Alexopoulos GS, Raue P, Arean P: Problem-solving therapy in geriatric depression with executive dysfunction. Am J Geriatr Psychiatry 11:46–52, 2003

Alexopoulos GS, Kiosses N, Heo M, et al: Executive dysfunction and the course of geriatric depression. Biol Psychiatry 58:204–210, 2005

Davidson KW, Kupfer DJ, Bigger JT, et al: National Heart, Lung and Blood Institute Work Group. Assessment and treatment of depression in patients with cardiovascular disease. National Heart, Lung, and Blood Institute Working Group Report. Psychosom Med 68:645–650, 2006

Duman RS, Heninger GR, Nestler EJ: A molecular and cellular theory of depression. Arch Gen Psychiatry 54:597–606, 1997

Golden CJ: The Stroop Color and Word Test (Manual). Chicago, IL, Stoetling, 1978

Mattis S: Dementia Rating Scale. Odessa, FL, Psychological Assessment Resources, 1989

Peterson JC, Charlson ME, Williams-Russo P, et al: New postoperative depressive symptoms and long-term cardiac outcomes after coronary artery bypass surgery. Am J Geriatr Psychiatry 10:192–198, 2002

Chapter 3:
Mood Instability and Amy Cahill

MOOD INSTABILITY

American Psychiatric Association: Diagnostic and Statistical Manual of Mental Disorders. Washington, DC, American Psychiatric Association, 2000

Berk M, Berk L, Castle D: A collaborative approach to the treatment alliance in bipolar disorder. Bipolar Disord 6:504–518, 2006

Colom F, Vieta E, Tacchi MJ, et al: Identifying and improving non-adherence in bipolar disorders. Bipolar Disord 7 (suppl 5):24–31, 2005

Goodwin FK, Jamison KR: Suicide, in Manic-Depressive Illness. New York. Oxford University Press, 1990, pp 227–244

Grant BF, Stinson FS, Hasin DS, et al: Prevalence, correlates, and comorbidity of bipolar I disorder and Axis I and II disorders: results from the National Epidemiologic Survey on Alcohol and Related Conditions. J Clin Psychiatry 66:1205–1215, 2005

Hawton K, Sutton L, Haw C, et al: Suicide and attempted suicide in bipolar disorder: a systematic review of risk factors. J Clin Psychiatry 66:693–704, 2005

Kessler RC, Borges G, Walters EE: Prevalence of and risk factors for lifetime suicide attempts in the National Comorbidity Survey. Arch Gen Psychiatry 56:617–626, 1999

Rucci P, Frank E, Kostelnik B, et al: Suicide attempts in patients with bipolar I disorder during acute and maintenance phases of intensive treatment with pharmacotherapy and adjunctive psychotherapy. Am J Psychiatry 159:1160–1164, 2002

Trivedi MH, Fava M, Wisniewski SR, et al: Medication augmentation after the failure of SSRIs for depression. N Engl J Med 354:1243–1252, 2006

BORDERLINE PERSONALITY ORGANIZATION

Clarkin JF, Yeomans FE, Kernberg OF: Psychotherapy for Borderline Personality: Focusing on Object Relations. Washington DC, American Psychiatric Press, 2006

Jacobson E: The Self and the Object World. New York, International Universities Press, 1964

Kernberg OF: Borderline personality organization. J Am Psychoanal Assoc 15:641–685, 1967

Kernberg OF: Internal World and External Reality: Object Relations Theory Applied. New York, Jason Aronson, 1980

Klein M: Envy and Gratitude, a Study of Unconscious Sources. New York, Basic Books, 1957

Yeomans FE, Selzer MA, Clarkin JF: Treating the Borderline Patient: A Contract-Based Approach. New York, Basic Books, 1992

AXIS I AND AXIS II

American Psychiatric Association: Diagnostic and Statistical Manual of Mental Disorders, 4th Edition. Washington, DC, American Psychiatric Association, 1994

Benazzi F: A continuity between bipolar II depression and major depressive disorder? Prog Neuropsychopharmacol Biol Psychiatry 30:1043–1050, 2006

Clarkin JF, Posner M: Defining the mechanisms of borderline personality disorder. Psychopathology 38:58–63, 2005

Gunderson JG, Weinberg I, Daversa M, et al: Descriptive and longitudinal observations on the relationship of borderline personality disorder and bipolar disorder. Am J Psychiatry 163:1173–1178, 2006

Roth A, Fonagy P: What Works for Whom? A Critical Review of Psychotherapy Research, 2nd Edition. New York, Guilford, 2005

Skodol AE, Oldham JM, Bender DS, et al:: Dimensional representations of DSM-IV personality disorders: relationships to functional impairment. Am J Psychiatry 162:1919–1925, 2005

Stone MH: Relationship of borderline personality disorder and bipolar disorder. Am J Psychiatry 163:1126–1128, 2006

EATING DISORDERS

Halmi KA: The Multimodal Treatment of Eating Disorders. World Psychiatry 4:69–73, 2005

Halmi KA, Agras WS, Crow S, et al: Predictors of treatment acceptance and completion in anorexia nervosa. Arch Gen Psychiatry 62:776–781, 2005

Maj M, Halmi K, Lopez-Ibor JJ, et al (eds): Eating Disorders. Chichester, England, Wiley, 2003

DIALECTICAL BEHAVIOR THERAPY

Aviram RB, Brodsky BS, Stanley B: Borderline personality disorder, stigma, and treatment implications. Harv Rev Psychiatry 14:249–256, 2006

Brodsky BS, Stanley B: Dialectical behavior therapy for borderline personality disorder. Psychiatr Annals 32:347–356, 2002

Brodsky BS, Groves SA, Oquendo MA, et al: Interpersonal precipitants and suicide attempts in borderline personality disorder. J Suicide Life-Threat Behav 36:313–322, 2006

Gunderson JG, Ridolfi M: Borderline personality disorder: suicidality and self-mutilation. Ann N Y Acad Sci 932:61–77, 2001

Linehan MM: Cognitive Behavioral Treatment of Borderline Personality Disorder. New York, Guilford, 1993a

Linehan MM: Skills Training Manual for Treating Borderline Personality Disorder. New York, Guilford, 1993b

Stanley B, Brodsky BS: Dialectical behavior therapy, in The American Psychiatric Publishing Textbook of Personality Disorders. Edited by Oldham JO, Skodol AE, Bender DS. Washington, DC, American Psychiatric Publishing, 2005a, pp 307–320

Stanley B, Brodsky BS: Suicidal and self-injurious behavior in borderline personality disorder: the self-regulation action model, in Understanding and Treating Borderline Personality Disorder: A Guide for Professionals and Families. Edited by Gunderson JG, Hoffman PD. American Psychiatric Publishing, Washington, DC, 2005b, pp 43–63

Stanley B, Gameroff MJ, Michalsen V, et al: Are suicide attempters who self-mutilate a unique population? Am J Psychiatry 158:427–432, 2001

RISK MANAGEMENT

Appelbaum PS, Gutheil TG: Clinical Handbook of Psychiatry and the Law, 4th Edition. Philadelphia, PA, Lippincott. 2006, pp 157–161

Gutheil TG: Paranoia and progress notes: a guide to forensically informed psychiatric record keeping. Hosp Community Psychiatry 31:479–482, 1980

Gutheil TG, Hilliard JT: Don't write me down: legal clinical and risk management aspects of patients requests that therapists not keep notes or records. Am J Psychother 55:157–165, 2001

Mattson M: Quality indicators, in Textbook of Hospital Psychiatry. Edited by Sharfstein S. Washington, DC, American Psychiatric Publishing, 2008

Practice guideline for the assessment and treatment of patients with suicidal behaviors. Am J Psychiatry 160 (11, suppl):1–60, 2003; see pp 27–28, 30–33

Work Group on Psychiatric Evaluation; American Psychiatric Association Steering Committee on Practice Guidelines: Psychiatric evaluation of adults, 2nd edition. American Psychiatric Association. Am J Psychiatry 163 (6, suppl):3–36, 2006; see pp 4–5

PHARMACOLOGY OF MOOD INSTABILITY

Practice guideline for the treatment of patients with bipolar disorder (revision). Am J Psychiatry 159 (4, suppl):1–50, 2002

Practice guideline for the treatment of patients with borderline personality. American Psychiatric Association. Am J Psychiatry 158 (10, suppl):1–52, 2001

Treatment of patients with eating disorders, third edition. Am J Psychiatry 163 (7, suppl):4–54, 2006

OVERVIEW OF MOOD INSTABILITY

Cutler JL: Therapeutic settings, in Psychiatry. Edited by Cutler JL, Marcus ER. Philadelphia, PA, WB Saunders, 1999, pp 270–273

Feinstein RE: Suicide and violence, in Psychiatry. Edited by Cutler JL, Marcus ER. Philadelphia, PA, WB Saunders, 1999, pp 201–220

Gabbard GO: Psychodynamic Psychiatry in Clinical Practice, 4th Edition. Washington, DC, American Psychiatric Publishing, 2005, pp 427–482

Kernberg OF: Severe Personality Disorders: Psychotherapeutic Strategies. New Haven, CT, Yale University Press, 1984, pp 27–51

MacKinnon RA, Michels R, Buckley PJ: The Psychiatric Interview in Clinical Practice, 2nd Edition. Washington, DC, American Psychiatric Press, 2006, pp 325–352, 481–504

Magill CA: The boundary between borderline personality disorder and bipolar disorder: current concepts and challenges. Can J Psychiatry 49:551–556, 2004

Shea SC: Psychiatric Interviewing: The Art of Understanding, 2nd Edition. Philadelphia, PA, WB Saunders, 1998, pp 341–442

Stone MH: Relationship of borderline personality disorder and bipolar disorder. Am J Psychiatry 163:1126–1128, 2006

Zimmerman M, Mattia JI: Axis I diagnostic comorbidity and borderline personality disorder. Compr Psychiatry 40:245–252, 1999

Chapter 4:
Schizophrenia and Anthony Da Piazza

SCHIZOPHRENIA

Andreasen NC, Olsen S: Negative vs positive schizophrenia: definition and validation. Arch Gen Psychiatry 39:789–794, 1982

Bateson G, Jackson DD, Haley J, et al: Toward a theory of schizophrenia. Behav Sci 1:251–264, 1956

Bebbington P, Kuipers L: The predictive utility of expressed emotion in schizophrenia: an aggregate analysis. Psychol Med 24:707–718, 1994 [erratum in Psychol Med 25:215, 1995]

Bleuler E: Dementia Praecox; or, the Group of Schizophrenias (1911). Translated by Joseph Zinkin; foreword by Nolan D, Lewis C. New York, International Universities Press, 1950

Buchanan RW, Carpenter WT: Domains of psychopathology: an approach to the reduction of heterogeneity in schizophrenia. J Nerv Ment Dis 182:193–204, 1994

Carpenter WT Jr, Strauss JS, Muleh S: Are there pathognomonic symptoms in schizophrenia? An empiric investigation of Schneider's first-rank symptoms. Arch Gen Psychiatry 28:847–852, 1973

Green MF, Kern RS, Braff DL, et al: Neurocognitive deficits and functional outcome in schizophrenia: are we measuring the "right stuff"? Schizophr Bull 26:119–136, 2000

Hegarty JD, Baldessarini RJ, Tohen M, et al: One hundred years of schizophrenia: a meta-analysis of the outcome literature. Am J Psychiatry 151:1409–1416, 1994

Kraepelin E: Dementia Praecox and Paraphrenia (1919). Translated by Barclay RM. Edited by Robertson GM. Huntington, NY, Krieger, 1971

Mortensen PB, Pedersen CB, Westergaard T, et al: Effects of family history and place and season of birth on the risk of schizophrenia. N Engl J Med 340:603–608, 1999

Parker G: Re-searching the schizophrenogenic mother. J Nerv Ment Dis 170:452–462, 1982

Schneider K: Clinical Psychopathology. Translated by Hamilton MW. Preface by Anderson EW. New York, Grune & Stratton, 1959

Shirzadi AA, Ghaemi SN: Side effects of atypical antipsychotics: extrapyramidal symptoms and the metabolic syndrome. Harv Rev Psychiatry 14:152–164, 2006

VIOLENCE AND SCHIZOPHRENIA

Alpert JE, Spillmann MK: Psychotherapeutic approaches to aggressive and violent patients. Psychiatr Clin North Am 20:453–472, 1997

Citrome L: The psychopharmacology of violence with emphasis on schizophrenia, Part 1: acute treatment. J Clin Psychiatry 68:163–164, 2007a

Citrome L The psychopharmacology of violence with emphasis on schizophrenia, Part 2: long-term treatment. J Clin Psychiatry 68:331–332, 2007b

Foley SR, Kelly BD, Clarke M, et al: Incidence and clinical correlates of aggression and violence at presentation in patients with first episode psychosis. Schizophr Res 72:161–168, 2005

Gregg L, Barrowclough C, Haddock G: Reasons for increased substance use in psychosis. Clin Psychol Rev 27:494–510, 2007

Hucker S: Psychiatric aspects of risk assessment (2005). Available at: http://www.forensicpsychiatry.ca/risk/assessment.htm. Accessed August 12, 2007.

Naudts K, Hodgins S: Schizophrenia and violence: a search for neurobiological correlates. Current Opinion in Psychiatry 19:533–538, 2006

Simons RI, Tardiff K (eds): Textbook of Violence Assessment and Management. Washington, DC, American Psychiatric Publishing, 2008

Soyka M, Graz C., Bottlender R, et al: Clinical correlates of later violence and criminal offences in schizophrenia. Schizophr Res 94:89–98, 2007

Torrey EF: Violence and schizophrenia. Schizophr Res 88:3–4, 2006

Vevera J, Hubbard A, Vesely A, et al: Violent behaviour in schizophrenia. Br J Psychiatry 187:426–430, 2005

SCHIZOPHRENIA AND BRAIN CIRCUITRY: A NEUROIMAGING PERSPECTIVE

Blakemore SJ, Wolpert DM, Frith CD: Abnormalities in the awareness of action. Trends Cogn Sci 6:237–242, 2002

Callicott JH, Bertolino A, Mattay VS, et al: Physiological dysfunction of the dorsolateral prefrontal cortex in schizophrenia revisited. Cereb Cortex 10:1078–1092, 2000

Cummings JL, Mega MS: Neuropsychiatry and Behavioral Neuroscience. New York, Oxford University Press, 2003

Epstein J, Stern E, Silbersweig D: Mesolimbic activity associated with psychosis in schizophrenia: symptom-specific PET studies. Ann N Y Acad Sci 877:562–574, 1999

Friston KJ, Frith CD: Schizophrenia: a disconnection syndrome? Clin Neurosci 3:89–97, 1995

Gaitatzis A, Trimble MR, Sander JW: The psychiatric comorbidity of epilepsy. Acta Neurol Scand 110:207–220, 2004

Grace AA: Gating of information flow within the limbic system and the pathophysiology of schizophrenia. Brain Res Brain Res Rev 31:330–341, 2000

Harrison PJ: The neuropathology of schizophrenia: a critical review of the data and their interpretation. Brain 122 (pt 4):593–624, 1999

Heimer L, Alheid GF, de Olmos JS, et al: The accumbens: beyond the core-shell dichotomy. J Neuropsychiatry Clin Neurosci 9:354–381, 1997

Holt DJ, Kunkel L, Weiss AP, et al: Increased medial temporal lobe activation during the passive viewing of emotional and neutral facial expressions in schizophrenia. Schizophr Res 82:153–162, 2006

Kapur S: Psychosis as a state of aberrant salience: a framework linking biology, phenomenology, and pharmacology in schizophrenia. Am J Psychiatry 160:13–23, 2003

Kubicki M, Westin CF, McCarley RW, et al: The application of DTI to investigate white matter abnormalities in schizophrenia. Ann N Y Acad Sci 1064:134–148, 2005

Liddle PF: The symptoms of chronic schizophrenia: a reexamination of the positive-negative dichotomy. Br J Psychiatry 151:145–151, 1987

Liddle PF, Friston KJ, Frith CD, et al: Patterns of cerebral blood flow in schizophrenia. Br J Psychiatry 160:179–186, 1992

Lipska BK, Weinberger DR: To model a psychiatric disorder in animals: schizophrenia as a reality test. Neuropsychopharmacology 23:223–239, 2000

Roth BL, Sheffler D, Potkin SG: Atypical antipsychotic drug actions: unitary or multiple mechanisms for "atypicality"? Clin Neurosci Res 3:108–117, 2003

Silbersweig DA, Stern E, Frith C, et al: A functional neuroanatomy of hallucinations in schizophrenia. Nature 378:176–179, 1995

Taylor SF, Phan KL, Britton JC, et al: Neural response to emotional salience in schizophrenia. Neuropsychopharmacology 30:984–995, 2005

Weinberger DR, Berman KF, Suddath R, et al: Evidence of dysfunction of a prefrontal-limbic network in schizophrenia: a magnetic resonance imaging and regional cerebral blood flow study of discordant monozygotic twins. Am J Psychiatry 149:890–897, 1992

Weinberger DR, Egan MF, Bertolino A, et al: Prefrontal neurons and the genetics of schizophrenia. Biol Psychiatry 50:825–844, 2001

Wright IC, Rabe-Hesketh S, Woodruff PW, et al: Meta-analysis of regional brain volumes in schizophrenia. Am J Psychiatry 157:16–25, 2000

PSYCHODYNAMICS OF PSYCHOSIS

Fromm-Reichmann F: Principles of Intensive Psychotherapy. Chicago, IL, University of Chicago Press, 1950

Frosch J: The Psychotic Process. Madison, CT, International Universities Press, 1983

Gabbard G: Psychodynamic Psychiatry in Clinical Practice, 4th Edition. Washington, DC, American Psychiatric Publishing, 2005

Marcus ER: Psychosis and Near Psychosis: Ego Function, Symbol Structure, Treatment, 2nd Edition. Madison, CT, International Universities Press, 2003

OUTSIDER ART

Cardinal R: Outsider Art. New York, Praeger, 1972

Dubuffet J: L'Art Brut Préferé aux Arts Culturels. Paris, Rene Drouin, 1949

Kris E: Psychoanalytic Explorations in Art. New York, International Universities Press, 1952

MacGregor J: The Discovery of the Art of the Insane. Princeton, NJ, Princeton University Press, 1989

Prinzhorn H: The Artistry of the Mentally Ill (1922). New York, Praeger, 1972

PHARMACOLOGY OF SCHIZOPHRENIA

Amador X, David AS: Insight and Psychosis. New York, Oxford University Press, 1998

Freedman R: The choice of antipsychotic drugs for schizophrenia. N Engl J Med 353:1286–1288, 2005

Lieberman JA, Stroup TS, McEvoy JP: Effectiveness of antipsychotic drugs in patients with schizophrenia. N Engl J Med 353:1209–1223, 2005

Lindenmayer JP, Khan A: Psychopathology, in The American Psychiatric Publishing Textbook of Schizophrenia. Edited by Lieberman JA, Stroup TS, Perkins DO. Washington, DC, American Psychiatric Publishing, 2006, pp 187–221

McEvoy JP, Lieberman JA, Stroup TS: Effectiveness of clozapine versus olanzapine, quetiapine, and risperidone in patients with chronic schizophrenia who did not respond to prior atypical antipsychotic treatment. Am J Psychiatry 163:600–610, 2006

Robinson DG, Woerner MG, Delman HM, Kane JM: Pharmacological treatments for first-episode schizophrenia. Schizophr Bull 31:705–722, 2005

Stroup TS, Kraus JE, Marder SR: Pharmacotherapies, in The American Psychiatric Publishing Textbook of Schizophrenia. Edited by Lieberman JA, Stroup TS, Perkins DO. Washington, DC, American Psychiatric Publishing, 2006a, pp 303–325

Stroup TS, Lieberman JA, McEvoy JP: Effectiveness of olanzapine, quetiapine, risperidone, and ziprasidone in patients with chronic schizophrenia following discontinuation of a previous atypical antipsychotic. Am J Psychiatry 163:611–622, 2006b

COGNITIVE-BEHAVIORAL THERAPY

Beck AT, Rector NA: Cognitive therapy of schizophrenia. Am J Psychother 54:291–300, 2000

Bentall R: Madness Explained: Psychosis and Human Nature. New York, Penguin, 2003

Chadwick PDJ, Birchwood MJ, Trower P: Cognitive Therapy for Delusions, Voices and Paranoia. Chichester, UK, Wiley, 1996

Chadwick PDJ, Sambrooke S, Rasch S, et al: Challenging the omnipotence of voices: group cognitive therapy for voices. Behav Res Ther 38:993–1003, 2000

Fowler D, Garety P, Kuipers E: Cognitive Behavior Threrapy for Psychosis: Theory and Practice. New York, Wiley, 1995

Gaudiano BA: Cognitive behavior therapies for psychotic disorders: current empirical status and future directions. Clin Psychol 12:33–50, 2005

Gumley A, Matthias S: Staying Well After Psychosis: A Cognitive Interpersonal Approach to Recovery and Relapse Prevention. New York, Wiley, 2006

Kingdom D, Turkington D: Cognitive Therapy of Schizophrenia. New York, Guilford, 2005

Landa Y, Silverstein SM, Schwartz F, et al: Group CBT for delusions: helping patients improve reality testing. Journal of Contemporary Psychotherapy 36:9–17, 2006

Morrison PA, Renton JC, Dunn H, et al: Cognitive Therapy for Psychosis. A Formulation–Based Approach. New York, Brunner-Routledge, 2004

Nelson H: Cognitive Behavioral Therapy with Schizophrenia. A Practice Manual. Cheltenham, UK, Stanley Thornes, 1997

Zubin J, Spring B: Vulnerability: a new view on schizophrenia. J Abnorm Psychol 86:103–126, 1977

COMPREHENSIVE HEALTHCARE

American Diabetes Association, American Psychiatric Association, American Association of Clinical Endocrinologists, North American Association for the Study of Obesity: Consensus development conference on antipsychotic drugs and obesity and diabetes. Diabetes Care 27:596–601, 2004

Berkowitz RI, Fabricatore AN: Obesity, psychiatric status, and psychiatric medications. Psychiatr Clin North Am 28:39–54, 2005

Casey DE: Metabolic issues and cardiovascular disease in patients with psychiatric disorders. Am J Med 118 (suppl 2):155–225, 2005

Katon W, Unutzer J, Fan M, et al: Cost-effectiveness and net benefit of enhanced treatment of depression for older adults with diabetes and depression. Diabetes Care 29:265–270, 2006

McEvoy JP, Meyer JM, Goff DC, et al: Prevalence of the metabolic syndrome in patients with schizophrenia: baseline results from the Clinical Antipsychotic Trial of Intervention Effectiveness (CATIE) schizophrenia trial and comparison with national estimates from NHANES III. Schizophr Res 80:19–32, 2005

Nasrallah HA, Meyer JM, Goff DC, et al: Low rates of treatment for hypertension, dyslipidemia, and diabetes in schizophrenia: data from CATIE schizophrenia trial sample at baseline. Schizophr Res 86:15-22, 2006

Newcomer JW, Nasrallah HA, Loebel AD: The Atypical Antipsychotics Therapy and Metabolic Issues national survey: practical patterns and knowledge of psychiatrists. J Clin Psychopharm 24 (5, suppl 1):S1–S6, 2004

RECOVERY

Corrigan PW: Recovery from schizophrenia and the role of evidence-based psychosocial interventions. Expert Review of Neurotherapeutics 6:993–1004, 2006

McGurk SR, Mueser KT, Pascaris A: Cognitive training and supported employment for persons with severe mental illness: one-year results from a randomized controlled trial. Schizophr Bull 31:898–909, 2005

Nasrallah HA, Lasser R: Improving patient outcomes in schizophrenia: achieving remission. J Psychopharmacol 20 (suppl 6):S57–S61, 2006

Ralph RO, Corrigan PW (eds): Recovery in Mental Illness. Washington, DC, American Psychological Press, 2005

Shepherd M, Watt D, Falloon I, et al: The natural history of schizophrenia: a five year follow up study of outcome and prediction in a representative sample of schizophrenics. Psychol Med Monogr Suppl 15:1–46, 1989

HOMELESSNESS AND SOCIAL HISTORY

Cohen CI: Overcoming social amnesia: the role for a social perspective in psychiatric research and practice. Psychiatr Serv 51:72–78, 2000

Estroff SE: Making It Crazy. Berkeley, University of California Press, 1981

Geertz C: The Interpretation of Cultures. New York, Basic, 1973

Hogan MF: Transmittal letter to the President. Interim Report to the President 2002. New Freedom Commission on Mental Health, 2002

Hopper K: Commentary: on the transformation of the moral economy of care, Cult Med Psychiatry 25:473–484, 2001

Hopper K, Baxter E, Cox S: Not making it crazy: some remarks on the young homeless patient in New York City, in The Young Adult Chronic Patient (New Directions for Mental Health Services 14). Edited by Pepper B, Ryglewicz H, 1982, pp 33–42

Laing RD: The Divided Self. London, Tavistock, 1959

Laing RD: The Politics of Experience. London, Tavistock, 1967

Lamb HR (ed): The Homeless Mentally Ill. Washington, DC, American Psychiatric Press, 1984

O'Hara A: Housing for people with mental illness: update of a report to the President's New Freedom Commission. Psychiatr Serv 58:907–913, 2007

Trilling L: Sincerity and Authenticity. Cambridge, MA, Harvard University Press, 1972

Tsemberis S, Eisenberg RF: Pathways to housing: supported housing for street dwelling individuals with psychiatric disabilities, Psychiatr Serv 51:487–493, 2000

OVERVIEW OF SCHIZOPHRENIA

Abi-Dargham A, Rodenhiser J, Printz D, et al: Increased baseline occupancy of D2 receptors by dopamine in schizophrenia. Proc Natl Acad Sci U S A 97:8104–8109, 2000

Bleuler E: Dementia Praecox; or, the Group of Schizophrenias (1911). Translated by Joseph Zinkin; foreword by Nolan D, Lewis C. New York, International Universities Press, 1950

Keefe RS, Silva SG, Perkins DO, et al: The effects of atypical antipsychotic drugs on neurocognitive impairment in schizophrenia: a review and meta-analysis. Schizophr Bull 25:201–222, 1999

Krystal JH, Abi-Dargham A, Larvelle M, et al: Pharmacologic models of psychoses, in Neurobiology of Mental Illness. Edited by Charney DS, Nestler E. New York, Oxford University Press, 2004, pp 214–224

Winokur G, Tsuang MT: The Natural History of Mania, Depression, and Schizophrenia. Washington, DC, American Psychiatric Press, 1996

Chapter 5:
Terminal Illness and Dorothy Ewing

DELIRIUM

Armstrong SC, Cozza KL, Watanabe KS: The misdiagnosis of delirium. Psychosomatics. 38:433–439, 1997

Breitbart W, Gibson C, Tremblay A: The delirium experience: delirium recall and delirium-related distress in hospitalized cancer patients. Psychosomatics 43:183–194, 2002

Folstein MF, Folstein SE, McHugh PR: "Mini-Mental State": a practical method for grading the cognitive state of patients for the clinician. J Psychiatr Res 12:189–195, 1975

Inouye SK, Bogardus ST, Charpentier PA, et al: A multicomponent intervention to prevent delirium in hospitalized older patients. N Engl J Med 340:669–676, 1999

Macleod AD: Delirium: the clinical concept. Palliat Support Care 4:305–312, 2006

Samton JB, Ferrando SJ, Sanelli P, et al: The Clock Drawing Test: diagnostic, functional, and neuroimaging correlates in older patients evaluated in the consultation-liaison setting. J Neuropsychiatry Clin Neurosci 17:533–540, 2005

Trzepacz PT, Meagher DJ: Delirium, in The American Psychiatric Publishing Textbook of Psychosomatic Medicine. Edited by Levenson JL. Washington, DC, American Psychiatric Publishing, 2005, pp 91–130

PAIN AND SUBSTANCE ABUSE

Massie MJ, Holland JC: The cancer patient with pain: psychiatric complications and their management. J Pain Symptom Manage 7:99–109, 1992

Passik SD, Kirsh KL, McDonald MV, et al: A pilot survey of aberrant drug-taking attitudes and behaviors in samples of cancer and AIDS patients. J Pain Symptom Manage 19:274–286, 2000

Passik SD, Kirsh KL, Donaghy K, et al: Pain and aberrant drug-related behaviors in medically ill patients with and without histories of substance abuse. Clin J Pain 22:173–181, 2006

Weissman DE, Haddox JD: Opioid pseudoaddiction—an iatrogenic syndrome. Pain 36:363–366, 1989

THE PSYCHODYNAMIC CONSULTATION

Beecher HK: Pain in men wounded in battle. Ann Surg 123:95–105, 1946

Erikson EH: Identity and the Life Cycle (Psychological Issues, Vol 1, No 1). New York, International Universities Press, 1959

Viederman M: The psychodynamic life narrative: a psychotherapeutic intervention useful in crisis situations. Psychiatry 46:236–246, 1983

WORKING WITH THE FAMILY

Baider L, Cooper CI, De-Nour A: Cancer and the Family, 2nd Edition. Chichester, UK, Wiley, 2000

Harding R, Higginson I: What is the best way to help caregivers in cancer and palliative care? A systematic literature review of interventions and their effectiveness. Palliat Med 17:63–74, 2003

Kato PM, Mann T: A synthesis of psychological interventions for the bereaved. Clin Psychol Rev 19:275–296, 1999

Kissane DW, Bloch S: Family Focused Grief Therapy. Maidenhead, Berkshire, UK, Open University Press, 2002

Kissane DW, Bloch S, McKenzie M, et al: Family grief therapy: a preliminary account of a new model to promote healthy family functioning during palliative care and bereavement. Psycho-oncology 7:14–25, 1998

Kissane DW, McKenzie M, Bloch S, et al: Family focused grief therapy: a randomized controlled trial in palliative care and bereavement. Am J Psychiatry 163:1208–1218, 2006

THE DIFFICULT PATIENT

Groves J: Taking care of the hateful patient. N Engl J Med 298:883–887, 1978

Groves MA, Muskin PR: Psychological responses to illness, in The American Psychiatric Publishing Textbook of Psychosomatic Medicine. Edited by Levenson JL. Washington, DC, American Psychiatric Publishing, 2005, pp 67–90

Kahana RJ, Bibring GL: Personality types in medical management, in Psychiatry and Medical Practice in a General Hospital. Edited by Zinberg N. New York, International Universities Press, 1964, pp 108–123

Lipowski ZJ: Review of consultation psychiatry and psychosomatic medicine, I: general principles. Psychosom Med 29:153–171, 1967

Marks RM, Sachar EJ: Undertreatment of medical inpatients with narcotic analgesics. Ann Intern Med 78:173–181, 1973

Muskin PR: The medical hospital, in Psychodynamic Concepts in General Psychiatry. Edited by Schwartz HJ. Washington, DC, American Psychiatric Press, 1995, pp 69–88

Muskin PR, Haase EK: Personality disorders, in Textbook of Primary Care Medicine, 3rd Edition. Noble J, Editor-in-Chief. St Louis, MO, CV Mosby, 2001, pp 458–464

GENETIC COUNSELING

Antoniou A, Pharoah PD, Narod S: Average risk of breast and ovarian cancer associated with BRCA1 or BRCA2 mutations detected in case series unselected for family history: a combined analysis of 22 studies. Am J Hum Genet 72:1117–1130, 2003

Friebel TM, Domchek SM, Neuhausen SL, et al: Bilateral prophylactic oophorectomy and bilateral prophylactic mastectomy in a prospective cohort of unaffected BRCA1 and BRCA2 mutation carriers. Clin Breast Cancer 7:875–882, 2007

Garber JE, Offit K: Hereditary cancer predisposition syndromes. J Clin Oncol 23:276–292, 2005

King MC, Marks JH, Mandell JB: Breast and ovarian cancer risks due to inherited mutations in BRCA1 and BRCA2. Science 302:643–646, 2003

Massie MJ, Greenberg DB: Oncology, in The American Psychiatric Publishing Textbook of Psychosomatic Medicine. Edited by Levenson JL. Washington, DC, American Psychiatric Publishing, 2005, pp 517–534

Narod SA, Offit K: Prevention and management of hereditary breast cancer. J Clin Oncol 23:1656–1663, 2005

Offit K, Thom P: Ethical and legal aspects of cancer genetic testing. Semin Oncol 34:435–443, 2007

Payne DK, Biggs C, Tran KN, et al: Women's regrets after bilateral prophylactic mastectomy. Ann Surg Oncol 7:150–154, 2000

Rebbeck TR, Lynch HT, Neuhausen SL, et al: Prophylactic oophorectomy in carriers of BRCA1 or BRCA2 mutations. N Engl J Med 346:1616–1622, 2002

Rebbeck TR, Friebel T, Lynch HT, et al: Bilateral prophylactic mastectomy reduces breast cancer risk in BRCA1 and BRCA2 mutation carriers: the PROSE study. J Clin Oncol 22:1055–1062, 2004

Robson M, Offit K: Clinical practice: management of an inherited predisposition to breast cancer. N Engl J Med 357:154–162, 2007

Smith KL, Robson ME: Update on hereditary breast cancer. Curr Oncol Rep 8:14–21, 2006

SPIRITUALITY

Baumeister RF (ed): Religion and psychology. Special Issue. Psychological Inquiry 13(3), 2002

Breitbart W, Gibson C, Poppito S, et al: Psychotherapeutic interventions at the end of life: a focus on meaning and spirituality. Can J Psychiatry 49:366–372, 2004

Fehring R, Miller J, Shaw C: Spiritual well-being, religiosity, hope, depression, and other mood states in elderly people coping with cancer. Oncol Nurs Forum 24:663–671, 1997

Josephson AM, Larson DB, Juthani N: What's happening in psychiatry regarding spirituality? Psychiatric Annals 30:533–541, 1999

Kearney M, Mount B: Spiritual care of the dying patient, in Handbook of Psychiatry in Palliative Medicine. Edited by Chochinov H, Breitbart W. New York, Oxford University Press, 2000, pp 357–373

McClain CS, Rosenfeld B, Breitbart W: Effect of spiritual well-being on end-of-life despair in terminally ill cancer patients. Lancet 361:1603–1607, 2003

McClain-Jacobson C, Rosenfeld B, Kosinski A, et al: Belief in an afterlife, spiritual well-being, and end-of-life despair in patients with advanced cancer. Gen Hosp Psychiatry 26:484–486, 2004

Nelson CJ, Rosenfeld B, Breitbart W, et al: Spirituality, religion, and depression in the terminally ill. Psychosomatics 43:213–220, 2002

Pargament K, Smith B, Koenig H, et al: Patterns of positive and negative religious coping with major life stressors. Journal for the Scientific Study of Religion 37:710–724, 1998

Sloan RP, Bagiella E, Powell T: Religion, spirituality, and medicine. Lancet 353:664–667, 1999

Viederman M: The psychodynamic life narrative: a psychotherapeutic intervention useful in crisis situations. Psychiatry 46:236–246, 1983

MEANING-CENTERED THERAPY

Breitbart W: Spirituality and meaning in supportive care: spirituality- and meaning-centered group psychotherapy interventions in advanced cancer. Support Care Cancer 10:272–280, 2002

Breitbart W, Gibson C, Poppito SR, et al: Psychotherapeutic interventions at the end of life: a focus on meaning and spirituality. Can J Psychiatry 49:366–372, 2004

Frankl VF: Man's Search for Meaning. 4th Edition. New York, Simon & Schuster, 1959

Frankl VF: The Will to Meaning. 2nd Edition. New York, Penguin, 1969

Greenstein M, Breitbart W: Cancer and the experience of meaning: a group psychotherapy program for people with cancer. Am J Psychother 54:486–500, 2000

Griffiths C, Norton L, Wagstaff G, et al: Existential concerns in late stage cancer. Eur J Oncol Nurs 6:243–246, 2002

Strang P: Existential consequences of unrelieved cancer pain. Palliat Med 11:299–305, 1997

Strang P: Cancer pain: a provoker of emotional, social and existential distress. Acta Oncol 37:641–644, 1998

Strang P, Strang S, Hultborn R, et al: Existential pain—an entity, a provocation, or a challenge? J Pain Symptom Manage 27:241–250, 2004

Yalom ID: Existential Psychotherapy. New York, Basic Books, 1980

THE DOCTOR–PATIENT RELATIONSHIP

Danis M, Southerland LI, Garrett JM, et al: A prospective study of advance directives for life-sustaining care. N Engl J Med 324:882–888, 1991

Danis M, Federman D, Fins JJ, et al: Incorporating palliative care into critical care education: principles, challenges, and opportunities. Crit Care Med 27:2005–2013, 1999

Fins JJ: From contract to covenant in advance care planning. J Law Med Ethics 27:46–51, 1999

Fins JJ: From indifference to goodness. Journal of Religion and Health 35:245–254, 1996

Fins JJ. Breaking the silence: futility, fear and anger, in Futility: Decisions Near the End of Life, Vol 7. Newton, MA, Education Development Center, 1997, pp 26–27

Fins JJ: A Palliative Ethic of Care: Clinical Wisdom at Life's End. Sudbury, MA, Jones & Bartlett, 2006

Fins JJ, Nilson EG: An approach to educating residents about palliative care and clinical ethics. Acad Med 75:662–665, 2000

Fins JJ, Solomon MZ: Communication in intensive care settings: the challenge of futility disputes. Crit Care Med 29(suppl):N10–N15, 2001

Fins JJ, Bacchetta MD, Miller FG: Clinical pragmatism: a method of moral problem solving. Kennedy Institute of Ethics Journal 7:129–145, 1997

Fins JJ, Miller FG, Acres CA, et al: End-of-life decision-making in the hospital: current practices and future prospects. J Pain Symptom Manage 17:6–15, 1999

Fins JJ, Gentilesco BJ, Carver A, et al: Reflective practice and palliative care education: a clerkship responds to the informal and hidden curriculum. Acad Med 78:307–312, 2003

Fins JJ, Maltby BS, Friedmann E, et al: Contracts, covenants and advance care planning: an empirical study of the moral obligations of patient and proxy. J Pain Symptom Manage 29:55–68, 2005

Haupt BJ: Characteristics of hospice care discharges and their length of service: United States, 2000. Vital Health Stat 13(154):1–36, 2003

Hoyer T: A History of the Medicare hospice benefit. Hosp Journal 13:61–69, 1998

Institute of Medicine: To Err is Human. Edited by Kohn LT, Corrigan JM, Donaldson MS. Washington, DC, National Academy Press, 2002

Miller SC, Kinzbrunner B, Pettit P, et al: How does the timing of hospice referral influence hospice care in the last days of life? J Am Geriatr Soc 51:798–806, 2003

Stevens R: In Sickness and in Wealth: American Hospitals in the Twentieth Century. Baltmore, MD, Johns Hopkins Press, 1999

Wagner GS, Cebe B, Rozear MP (eds): What This Patient Needs Is a Doctor. Durham, NC, Carolina Academic Press, 1978

Wanzer SH, Adelstein SJ, Cranford RE, et al: The physician's responsibility toward hopelessly ill patients. N Engl Med 310:955–999, 1984

OVERVIEW OF HOSPITAL PSYCHODYNAMICS

Bion WR: Experiences in Groups and Other Papers. New York, Basic Books, 1961

Engel GL: The need for a new medical model: a challenge for biomedicine. Science 196:129–136, 1977

Erikson E: Childhood and Society, 2nd Edition. New York, WW Norton, 1963

Fonagy P: Attachment Theory and Psychoanalysis. New York, Other Press, 1993

James H: The middle years (1893), in The Portable Henry James. Edited by Auchard J. New York, Penguin, 2004

Kissane DW, Bloch S: Family Focused Grief Therapy. Maidenhead, Berkshire, UK, Open University Press, 2002

Klein M: Contributions to Psycho-analysis 1921–1945. London, Hogarth Press, 1948

Kubler-Ross E: On Death and Dying. London, Routledge, 1973

MacKinnon RA, Michels R, Buckley J: The hospitalized patient, in The Psychiatric Interview in Clinical Practice, 2nd Edition. Washington, DC, American Psychiatric Publishing, 2006, pp 505–520

Vaillant G: Adaptation to Life. Boston, MA, Little, Brown, 1977

Chapter 6:
Agitation and Stephen Franken

EVALUATING AN EMERGENCY PATIENT

MacKinnon RA, Michels R, Buckley PJ: The emergency patient, in The Psychiatric Interview in Clinical Practice, 2nd Edition. Washington, DC, American Psychiatric Publishing, 2006, pp 481–520

STIMULANT ABUSE

Gorski TT: An overview of the twelve steps, in Understanding the Twelve Steps: An Interpretation and Guide for Recovering People. New York, Fireside, 1989, pp 31–41

Kalivas PW, Volkow ND: The neural basis of addiction: a pathology of motivation and choice. Am J Psychiatry 162:1403–1413, 2005

Khantzian EJ: The self-medication hypothesis of addictive disorders, in Treating Addiction as a Human Process. Northvale, NJ, Jason Aronson, 1999, pp 165–179

Kosten TR, O'Connor PG: Management of drug and alcohol withdrawal. N Engl J Med 348:1786–1795, 2003

Leschner AI: Science-based views of drug addiction and its treatment. JAMA 282:1314–1316, 1999

Levounis P, Ruggiero JS: Outpatient management of crystal methamphetamine dependence among gay and bisexual men: how can it be done? Prim Psychiatry 13:75–80, 2006

Marlatt GA: Basic principles and strategies of harm reduction, in Harm Reduction: Pragmatic Strategies for Managing High-Risk Behaviors. New York, Guilford, 1998, pp 49–66

Marlowe A: Addiction, in How to Stop Time: Heroin From A to Z. New York, Anchor Books, 2000, pp 9–10

Miller WR, Rollnick S: Why do people change? in Motivational Interviewing: Preparing People for Change, 2nd Edition. New York, Guilford, 2002, pp 3–12

Nunes EV, Levin FR: Treatment of depression in patients with alcohol and other drug dependence: a meta-analysis. JAMA 291:1887–1896, 2004

Olsen P, Levounis P: Sober Siblings: How to Help Your Alcoholic Brother or Sister—and Not Lose Yourself. New York, Da Capo, 2008

Rosenthal RN, Levounis P: Polysubstance use, abuse, and dependence, in Clinical Textbook of Addictive Disorders, 3rd Edition. Edited by Frances RJ, Miller SI, Mack AH. New York, Guilford, 2005, pp 245–270

Vocci FJ, Acri J, Elkashef A: Medication development for addictive disorders: the state of the science. Am J Psychiatry 162:1432–1440, 2005

CONSULTATION-LIAISON PSYCHIATRY

MacKinnon R, Michels RA, Buckley PJ: The hospitalized patient, in The Psychiatric Interview in Clinical Practice, 2nd Edition. Washington, DC, American Psychiatric Publishing, 2006, pp 505–520

Smith FA, Querques J, Levenson JL, et al: Psychiatric assessment and consultation, in The American Psychiatric Publishing Textbook of Psychosomatic Medicine. Edited by Levenson JL. Washington, DC, American Psychiatric Publishing, 2005, pp 3–14

Perry S, Viederman M: Adaptation of residents to Consultation-Liaison Psychiatry, I: working with the physically ill. Gen Hosp Psychiatry 3:141–147, 1981

Perry S, Viederman M: Adaptation of residents to Consultation-Liaison Psychiatry, II: working with the non-psychiatric staff. Gen Hosp Psychiatry 3:149–156, 1981

INFORMED CONSENT

Bayer R, Fairchild AL: Changing the paradigm for HIV testing—the end of exceptionalism. N Engl J Med 355:647–649, 2006

Berg JW, Appelbaum PS, Lidz CW, et al: Informed Consent: Legal Theory and Clinical Practice, 2nd Edition. New York, Oxford University Press, 2001

Faden RR, Beauchamp TL: A History and Theory of Informed Consent. New York, Oxford University Press, 1986

Schloendorff v Society of New York Hospital, 211 NY 125, 105 NE 92 (1914)

Salgo v Leland-Stanford Jr University Board of Trustees, 154 CalApp 2d 560, 317 P2d 170 (CalApp 1957)

HIV AND AIDS

Centers for Disease Control and Prevention: HIV and AIDS—United States, 1981–2001. MMWR Morb Mortal Wkly Rep 50:430–434, 2001a

Centers for Disease Control and Prevention: HIV Prevention Strategic Plan Through 2005. Atlanta, GA, Centers for Disease Control and Prevention, January 2001b

Chang L, Ernst T, Leonido-Yee M, et al: Highly active antiretroviral therapy reverses brain metabolite abnormalities in mild HIV dementia. Neurology 53:782–789, 1999

Crone C, Gabriel GM: Comprehensive review of hepatitis C for psychiatrists: risks, screening, diagnosis, treatment, and interferon-based therapy complications. J Psychiatr Pract 9:93–110, 2003

Ferrando SJ, Lyketsos CG: Psychiatric comorbidities in medically ill patients with HIV/AIDS, in Psychiatric Aspects of HIV/AIDS. Edited by Ruiz P, Fernandez F. Philadelphia, PA, Lippincott Williams & Wilkins, 2006, pp 198–211

Ferrando SJ, Tiamson-Kassab MLA: HIV disease, in Psychosomatic Medicine. Edited by Blumenfield M, Strain JJ. Philadelphia, PA, Lippincott Williams & Wilkins, 2006, pp 277–296

Ferrando S, van Gorp W, McElhiney M, et al: Highly active antiretroviral treatment (HAART) in HIV infection: benefits for neuropsychological function. AIDS 12:F65–F70, 1998

Ferrando SJ, Rabkin JG, van Gorp WG, et al: Longitudinal improvement in psychomotor processing speed is associated with potent combination antiretroviral therapy in HIV-1 infection. J Neuropsychiatry Clin Neurosci 15:208–214, 2003

Filippi C, Sze G, Farber SJ, et al: Regression of HIV encephalopathy and basal ganglia signal intensity abnormality at MR imaging in patients with AIDS after the initiation of protease inhibitor therapy. Radiology 206:491–498, 1998

Gisslen M, Hagberg L, Svennerholm B, et al: HIV-1 RNA is not detectable in the cerebrospinal fluid during antiretroviral combination therapy. AIDS 11:1194, 1997

Hinkin CH, Hardy DJ, Mason KL, et al: Medication adherence in HIV-infected adults: effect of patient age, cognitive status and substance abuse. AIDS 1 (suppl 18):19–25, 2004

Letendre SL, McCutchan JA, Childers ME, et al: Enhancing antiretroviral therapy for human immunodeficiency virus cognitive disorders. Ann Neurol 56:416–423, 2004

Marra CM, Lockhart D, Zunt JR, et al: Changes in CSF and plasma HIV-1 RNA and cognition after starting potent antiretroviral therapy. Neurology 60:1388–1390, 2003

Ryan EL, Morgello S, Isaacs K, et al: Neuropsychiatric impact of hepatitis C on advanced HIV. Neurology 62:957–962, 2004

Sacktor N, Lyles RH, Skolasky R, et al: HIV-associated neurologic disease incidence changes. Multicenter AIDS Cohort Study, 1990–1998. Neurology 56:257–260, 2001

St. Louis ME, Rauch KJ, Petersen LR, et al: Seroprevalence rates of human immunodeficiency virus infection at sentinel hospitals in the United States. The Sentinel Hospital Surveillance Group. N Engl J Med 323:213–218, 1990

Tozzi V, Balestra P, Galgani S, et al: Positive and sustained effects of highly active antiretroviral therapy on HIV-1-associated neurocognitive impairment. AIDS 13:1889–1897, 1999

van Gorp WG, Rabkin JG, Ferrando SJ, et al: Neuropsychiatric predictors of return to work in HIV/AIDS. J Int Neuropsychol Soc 13:80–89, 2007

Wilkie FL, Goodkin K, Eisdorfer C, et al: Mild cognitive impairment and risk of mortality in HIV-1 infection. J Neuropsychiatry Clin Neurosci 10:125–132, 1998

INTERNALIZED HOMOPHOBIA

Friedman RC: Male Homosexuality: A Contemporary Psychoanalytic Perspective. New Haven, CT, Yale University Press, 1988

Friedman RC: The issue of homosexuality in psychoanalysis, in Identity, Gender and Sexuality 150 years After Freud. London, International Psychoanalytic Association, 2006, pp 79–97

Friedman RC, Downey JI: Special Article: Homosexuality. N Engl J Med 331:923–930, 1994

Friedman RC, Downey JI: Sexual Orientation and Psychoanalysis: Sexual Science and Clinical Practice. New York, Columbia University Press, 2002

Herek G: Heterosexism and homophobia, in Textbook of Homosexuality and Mental Health. Edited by Cabaj RP, Stein T. Washington, DC, American Psychiatric Press, 1996, pp 101–113

Kessler RC, Berglund P, Demler O, et al: Lifetime prevalence and age-of-onset distributions of DSM-IV disorders in the National Comorbidity Survey Replication. Arch Gen Psychiatry 62:593–602, 2005

Laumann EO, Gagnon JH, Michael RT, et al: The Social Organization of Sexuality: Sexual Practices in the United States. Chicago, IL, University of Chicago Press, 1994

Malyon A: Psychotherapeutic implications of internalized homophobia in gay men. J Homosex 7:59–69, 1982

Weinberg GH: Society and the Healthy Homosexual. New York, St Martin's Press, 1972

SEXUALITY AND SEXUAL DYSFUNCTION

Asboe D, Catalan J, Mandalia S, et al: Sexual dysfunction in HIV-positive men is multi-factorial: a study of prevalence and associated factors. AIDS Care 19:955–965, 2007

Collazos E, Martinez E, Mayo J, et al: Sexual dysfunction in HIV-infected patients treated with highly active antiretroviral therapy. J Acquire Immune Defic Syndr 31:322–326, 2002

Levine SB, Risen CB, Althof SE: Handbook of Clinical Sexuality for Mental Health Professionals. New York, Brunner/Routledge, 2003

Taylor MJ: Strategies for managing antidepressant-induced sexual dysfunction: a review. Curr Psychiatry Rep 8:431–436, 2006

JEKYLL AND HYDE

Beattie HJ: A Fairbairnian analysis of Robert Louis Stevenson's Strange Case of Dr Jekyll and Mr Hyde, in Fairbairn, Then and Now. Edited by Skolnick NJ, Scharff DE. Hillsdale, NJ, Analytic Press, 1998, pp 197–211

Beattie HJ: Father and son: the origins of Strange Case of Dr Jekyll and Mr Hyde. Psychoanal Study Child 56:317–360, 2001

Stevenson RL: The Strange Case of Dr Jekyll and Mr Hyde and Other Tales of Terror. Edited by Mighall R. London, Penguin, 2002

Stevenson RL: Strange Case of Dr Jekyll and Mr Hyde (Norton Critical Edition). Edited by Linehan K. New York, WW Norton, 2003

PSYCHOTHERAPY SELECTION

De Jonghe F, Rijnierse P, Janssen R: Psychoanalytic supportive therapy. J Am Psychoanal Assoc 42:421–446, 1994

Dewald P: Psychotherapy: A Dynamic Approach. New York, Basic Books, 1971

Douglas CJ: Teaching supportive psychotherapy to psychiatric residents. Am J Psychiatry 165:445–452, 2008

Modell A: The "holding environment" and the therapeutic action of psychoanalysis. J Am Psychoanal Assoc 24:285–307, 1976

Perry S, Frances A, Klar H, et al: Selection criteria for individual dynamic psychotherapies. Psychiatr Q 55:3–16, 1983

Pine F: Supportive psychotherapy: a psychoanalytic perspective. Psychiatric Annals 16:526–529, 1986

Schlesinger HJ: Diagnosis and prescription for psychotherapy. Bull Menninger Clin 33:269–278, 1969

Winnicott DW: Psychiatric disorders in terms of infantile maturational processes, in The Maturational Processes and the Facilitating Environment. New York, International Universities Press, 1965, pp 230–241

OVERVIEW OF CONNECTION

Center for Substance Abuse Treatment: Enhancing Motivation for Change in Substance Abuse Treatment. Treatment Improvement Protocol (TIP) Series 35 (DHHS Publ SMA 03-3811). Rockville, MD, Substance Abuse and Mental Health Services Administration, 1999

Cournos F: Parental death in childhood: theory and therapy. Journal of Practical Psychiatry and Behavioral Health 5:336–345, 1999

Dumaret AC: Adult outcome of children reared for long term periods in foster families. Child Abuse Neglect 21:911–927, 1997

Kessler RC, Davis CD, Kendler KS: Childhood adversity and adult psychiatric disorder in the US National Comorbidity Survey. Psychol Med 27:1101–1119, 1997

Pilowsky DJ: Psychopathology among children placed in family foster care. Psychiatr Serv 46:906–910, 1995

Practice guideline for the treatment of patients with HIV/AIDS. Work Group on HIV/AIDS. American Psychiatric Association. Am J Psychiatry 157 (11, suppl):1–62, 2000

Chapter 7:
Adolescent Bereavement and Amelia Gutierrez

AN ETHICAL DILEMMA

Appelbaum PS: Depressed? Get out!: dealing with suicidal students on college campuses. Psychiatr Serv 57:914–916, 2006

Capriccioso R: Counseling crisis. Inside Higher Ed, March 13, 2006. Available at: http://insidehighered.com/news/2006/03/13/counseling. Accessed June 29, 2006.

Lake P, Tribbensee N: The emerging crisis of college student suicide: law and policy responses to serious forms of self-inflicted injury. Stetson Law Review 32:125–157, 2002

Pavela G: Questions and Answers on College Student Suicide: A Law and Policy Perspective. Ashville, NC, College Administration Publications, 2006

Schieszler v Ferrum College, 236 F.Supp.2d 602 (W.D. Va. 2002)

Shin v Massachusetts Institute of Technology, 19 Mass. L. Rep. 570 (Middle-sex Super. Ct. 2005)

ADOLESCENT BEREAVEMENT

American Psychiatric Association: Diagnostic and Statistical Manual of Mental Disorders, 4th Edition, Text Revision. Washington, DC, American Psychiatric Association, 2000

Brent DA, Moritz G, Bridge J, et al: Long-term impact of exposure to suicide: a three-year controlled follow-up. J Am Acad Child Adolesc Psychiatry 35:646–653, 1996

Cerel J, Fristad MA, Verducci J, et al: Childhood bereavement: psychopathology in the 2 years postparental death. J Am Acad Child Adolesc Psychiatry 45:681–690, 2006

Cohen JA, Mannarino AP, Knudsen K: Treating childhood traumatic grief: a pilot study. J Am Acad Child Adolesc Psychiatry 43:1225–1233, 2004

Pfeffer CR, Jiang H, Kakuma T, et al: Group intervention for children bereaved by the suicide of a relative. J Am Acad Child Adolesc Psychiatry 41:505–513, 2002

Pfeffer CR, Altemus M, Heo M, et al: Salivary cortisol and psychopathology in children bereaved by the September 11, 2001 terror attacks. Biol Psychiatry 61:957–965, 2007

Prigerson HG, Bierhals, AJ, Kasi SV, et al: Complicated grief as a distinct disorder from bereavement-related depression and anxiety: a replication study. Am J Psychiatry 153:1484–1488, 1996

SUICIDE

Arango V, Underwood MD, Gubbi AV, et al: Localized alterations in pre- and postsynaptic serotonin binding sites in the ventrolateral prefrontal cortex of suicide victims. Brain Res 688:121–133, 1995

Coryell W: DST abnormality as a predictor of course in major depression. J Affect Disord 19:163–169, 1990

Malone KM, Ellis SP, Currier D, et al: Platelet 5-HT2A receptor subresponsivity and lethality of attempted suicide in depressed inpatients. Int J Neuropsychopharmacol 10:335–343, 2007

Mann JJ: Neurobiology of suicidal behaviour. Nat Rev Neurosci 4:819–828, 2003

Mann JJ, Arango V: Neurobiology of suicidal behavior, in The Harvard Medical School Guide to Suicide Assessment and Intervention. Edited by Jacobs DG. San Francisco, Jossey-Bass, 1999

Mann JJ, Huang YY, Underwood MD, et al: A serotonin transporter gene promoter polymorphism (5-HTTLPR) and prefrontal cortical binding in major depression and suicide. Arch Gen Psychiatry 57:729–738, 2000

Mann JJ, Currier D, Stanley B, et al: Can biological tests assist prediction of suicide in mood disorders? Int J Neuropsychopharmacol 9:465–474, 2006

Pandey GN, Dwivedi Y, Pandey SC, et al: Low phosphoinositide-specific phospholipase C activity and expression of phospholipase C beta1 protein in the prefrontal cortex of teenage suicide subjects. Am J Psychiatry 156:1895–1901, 1999

INTERVIEW OF THE ADOLESCENT

Dulcan MK, Martini RD, Lake M: Evaluation and treatment planning, in Concise Guide to Child and Adolescent Psychiatry, 3rd Edition. Washington, DC, American Psychiatric Publishing, 2003, pp 7–21

King RA, Schowalter JE: The clinical interview of the adolescent, in The American Psychiatric Publishing Textbook of Child and Adolescent Psychiatry, 3rd Edition. Edited by Wiener JM, Dulcan MK. Washington, DC, American Psychiatric Publishing, 2004, pp 113–116

Weissman S, Sylvester C: Observation, interview and mental status assessment: puberty, adolescents and young adults, in Handbook of Child and Adolescent Psychiatry, Vol 5: Clinical Assessment and Intervention Planning. Edited by Noshpitz JD. New York, Wiley, 1998, pp 210–215

PSYCHOLOGICAL IMPACT OF DISLOCATION

Bowlby J: Separation: Anxiety and Anger. New York, Basic Books, 1973

Engel GL: The clinical application of the biopsychosocial model. Am J Psychiatry 137:535–544, 1980

Fogelson RM: Downtown: Its Rise and Fall, 1880–1950. New Haven, CT, Yale University Press, 2001

Fullilove M: Psychiatric implications of displacement: contributions from the psychology of place. Am J Psychiatry 153:1516–1523, 1996

Fullilove MT: The House of Joshua: Meditations on Family and Place. Lincoln, University of Nebraska Press, 1999

Fullilove M: Root Shock: How Tearing Up City Neighborhoods Hurts America and What We Can Do About It. New York, Ballantine/One World, 2004

Robins A, Fullilove FM, Myers RE, et al: Hillscapes: Envisioning a Healthy Urban Habitat. Pittsburgh, University of Pittsburgh Graduate School of Public Health, 1999

THE DOMINICAN PATIENT

Canino IA, Gonzalez NM: Socio-cultural issues in adolescent development, in Textbook of Adolescent Psychiatry. Edited by Rosner L. London, Arnold, 2003, pp 165–170

Canino IA, Spurlock J: Culturally Diverse Children and Adolescents: Assessment, Diagnosis, and Treatment. New York, Guilford, 2000

Hacket R, Hacket L: Child psychiatry across cultures. International Review of Psychiatry 11:225–235, 1999

Hernandez R, Rivera-Batiz F: Dominicans in the United States: A Socioeconomic Profile, 2000 (Dominican Research Monographs). New York, CUNY Dominican Studies Institute, 2003

Koss-Chiono J, Vargas LA: Working With Latino Youth: Culture, Development, and Context. San Francisco, CA, Jossey-Bass, 1999

Lewis-Fernandez R, Kleinman A: Cultural psychiatry: theoretical, clinical, and research issues. Psychiatr Clin North Am 18:433–448, 1995

Mezzich JE, Kleinman A, Fabrega H, et al (eds): Culture and Psychiatric Diagnosis: A DSM-IV Perspective. Washington, DC, American Psychiatric Press, 1996

Phinney JS, Rotheram MJ (eds): Children's Ethnic Socialization: Pluralism and Development. Newbury Park, CA, Sage, 1986

Rubio-Stipec M, Canino I, Hsiao-Rei M, et al: Cultural factors influencing the selection, use, and interpretation of psychiatric measures, in Handbook of Psychiatric Measures, 2nd Edition. Edited by Rush AJ, First MB, Blacker D. Washington, DC, American Psychiatric Publishing, 2008, pp 23–32

Spencer MB, Dornbusch SM, Mont-Reynauld R: Challenges in studying minority youth, in At the Threshold: The Developing Adolescent. Edited by Feldman SS, Elliot GR. Cambridge, MA, Harvard University Press, 1990, pp 123–146

Tseng WS: Culture and society, in Handbook of Cultural Psychiatry. San Diego, CA, Academic Press, 2001, pp 23–37

Vazquez CI: Dominicans, in The Latino Psychiatric Patient: Assessment and Treatment. Edited by Lopez AG, Carrillo E. Washington, DC, American Psychiatric Press, 2001, pp 87–96

Vazquez CI: Dominican families, in Ethnicity and Family Therapy, 3rd Edition. Edited by McGoldrick M, Giordano J, Garcia N. New York, Guilford, 2005, pp 216–228

VIRGINIA WOOLF: ON BEING ILL

Dalsimer K: Female Adolescence: Psychoanalytic Reflections on Literature. New Haven, CT, Yale University Press, 1986

Dalsimer K: Virginia Woolf: Becoming a Writer. New Haven, CT, Yale University Press, 2001

Woolf V: On being ill (1926), in The Essays of Virginia Woolf, Vol 4. Edited by McNeillie A. London, Hogarth Press, 1994, pp 317–329

Woolf V: The Letters of Virginia Woolf, Vols 1–6. Edited by Nicolson N, Trautman J. London, Hogarth Press, 1975–1980

Woolf V: The Diaries of Virginia Woolf, Vols 1–5. Edited by Bell AO. New York, Harcourt Brace Jovanovich, 1977–1984

Woolf V: Moments of Being, 2nd Edition. Edited by Schulkind J. New York, Harvest Books/Harcourt Brace, 1985

NEUROBIOLOGY OF ATTACHMENT

Cameron NM, Champagne FA, Carine P, et al: The programming of individual differences in defensive responses and reproductive strategies in the rat through variations in maternal care. Neurosci Biobehav Rev 29:843–865, 2005

Carpenter LL, Carvalho JP, Tyrka AR, et al: Decreased adrenocorticotropic hormone and cortisol responses to stress in healthy adults reporting significant childhood maltreatment. Biol Psychiatry 62:1080–1087, 2007

Freud S: Mourning and melancholia (1917[1915]), in Standard Edition of the Complete Psychological Works of Sigmund Freud, Vol 14. Translated and edited by Strachey J. London, Hogarth Press, 1957, pp 237–260

Harkness KL, Bruce AE, Lumley MN: The role of childhood abuse and neglect in the sensitization to stressful life events in adolescent depression. J Abnorm Psychol 115:730–741, 2006

Harlow HF, Zimmerman RR: Affectional responses in the infant monkey: orphaned baby monkeys develop a strong and persistent attachment to inanimate surrogate mothers. Science 130:421–432, 1959

Hofer MA: Studies on how early maternal separation produces behavioral change in young rats. Psychosom Med 37:245–264, 1975

Hofer MA: Multiple regulators of ultrasonic vocalization in the infant rat. Psychoneuroendocrinology 21:203–217, 1996

Lindemann E: Symptomatology and management of acute grief. Am J Psychiatry 101:141–148, 1944

Masson J, Darmon M, Conjard A, et al: Mice lacking brain/kidney phosphate–activated glutaminase (GLS1) have impaired glutamatergic synaptic transmission, altered breathing, disorganized goal-directed behavior and die shortly after birth. J Neurosci 26:4660–4671, 2006

Polan HJ, Hofer MA: Psychobiological origins of infant attachment and its role in development, in Handbook of Attachment: Theory, Research, and Clinical Applications, 2nd Edition. Edited by Cassidy J, Shaver PR. New York, Guilford, 2008

Polan HJ, Milano D, Eljuga L, et al: Development of rats' maternally-directed orienting from birth to day 2. Dev Psychobiol 40:81–103, 2002

Spitz R: Hospitalism: an inquiry into the genesis of psychiatric conditions in early childhood. Psychoanal Study Child 1:53–74, 1945

Widom CS, DuMont K, Czaja SJ: A prospective investigation of major depressive disorder and comorbidity in abused and neglected children grown up. Arch Gen Psychiatry 64:49–56, 2007

PHARMACOLOGY OF ADOLESCENT DEPRESSION

Brent DA: Antidepressants and pediatric depression: the risk of doing nothing. N Engl J Med 351:1598–1601, 2004

Emslie GJ, Rush AJ, Weinberg WA, et al: A double-blind, randomized, placebo-controlled trial of fluoxetine in children and adolescents with depression. Arch Gen Psychiatry 54:1031–1037, 1997

Emslie GJ, Heiligenstein JH, Wagner KD, et al: Fluoxetine for acute treatment of depression in children and adolescents: a placebo-controlled, randomized clinical trial. J Am Acad Child Adolesc Psychiatry 41:1205–1215, 2002

Hammad TA, Laughren T, Racoosin J: Suicidality in pediatric patients treated with antidepressant drugs. Arch Gen Psychiatry 63:332–339, 2006

Hugher CW, Emslie GJ, Crismon ML, et al: The Texas Children's Medication Algorithm Project: report of the Texas Consensus Conference Panel on Medication Treatment of Childhood Major Depression. J Am Acad Child Adolesc Psychiatry 38:1442–1454, 1999

Jick H, Kaye JA, Jick SS: Antidepressants and the risk of suicidal behaviors. JAMA 292:338–343, 2004

Leon AC, Marzuk PM, Tardiff K, et al: Antidepressants and youth suicide in New York City, 1999–2002. J Am Acad Child Adolesc Psychiatry 45:1054–1058, 2006

March J, Silva S, Petrycki S, et al, Treatment for Adolescents With Depression Study (TADS) Team: Fluoxetine, cognitive-behavioral therapy, and their combination for adolescents with depression: Treatment for Adolescents With Depression Study (TADS) randomized controlled trial. JAMA 292:807–820, 2004

Olfson M, Shaffer D, Marcus SV, et al: Relationship between antidepressant medication treatment and suicide in adolescents. Arch Gen Psychiatry 60:978–982, 2003

Wagner KD, Ambrosini P, Rynn M, et al: Efficacy of sertraline in the treatment of children and adolescents with major depressive disorder: two randomized controlled trials. JAMA 290:1033–1041, 2003

INTERPERSONAL PSYCHOTHERAPY

American Academy of Child and Adolescent Psychiatry: Practice parameters for the assessment and treatment of children and adolescents with depressive disorders. J Am Acad Child Adolesc Psychiatry 37 (suppl 10):63S–83S, 1998

Bowlby J: Attachment and Loss, Vol 3: Loss: Sadness and Depression. London, Hogarth Press/Institute of Psychoanalysis, 1980, pp 265–433

Frank E, Kupfer DJ, Perel JM, et al: Three-year outcomes for maintenance therapies in recurrent depression. Arch Gen Psychiatry 47:1093–1099, 1990

Kumar G, Pepe D, Steer RA: Adolescent psychiatric inpatients' self-reported reasons for cutting themselves. J Nerv Ment Dis 192:830–836, 2005

Mufson L, Weissman MM, Moreau D, et al: The efficacy of interpersonal psychotherapy for depressed adolescents. Arch Gen Psychiatry 56:573–579, 1999

Mufson L, Dorta KP, Moreau D, et al: Interpersonal Psychotherapy for Depressed Adolescents, 2nd Edition. New York, Guilford, 2004a

Mufson L, Dorta KP, Wickramaratne P, et al: A randomized effectiveness trial of interpersonal psychotherapy for depressed adolescents. Arch General Psychiatry 61:577–584, 2004b

Raphael B: Anatomy of Bereavement. New York, Basic Books, 1983

Rosselló J, Bernal G: The efficacy of cognitive-behavioral and interpersonal treatments for depression in Puerto Rican adolescents. J Consult Clin Psychol 67:734–745, 1999

Weissman MM, Markowitz, JC, Klerman GL: Comprehensive Guide to Interpersonal Psychotherapy. New York, Basic Books, 2000

PSYCHODYNAMICS OF DEPRESSION

Abraham K: Notes on the psycho-analytical investigation and treatment of manic depressive insanity and allied conditions (1911), in Selected Papers on Psycho-analysis. London, Hogarth Press, 1927, pp 137–156

Bibring E: The mechanics of depression, in Affective Disorders: Psychoanalytic Contributions to Their Study. Edited by Greenacre P. New York, International Universities Press, 1953, pp 13–48

Busch FN, Rudden MG, Shapiro T: Psychodynamic Treatment of Depression. Washington, DC, American Psychiatric Press, 2004

Freud S: Mourning and melancholia (1917[1915]), in Standard Edition of the Complete Psychological Works of Sigmund Freud, Vol 14. Translated and edited by Strachey J. London, Hogarth Press, 1957, pp 237–260

Jacobson E: Depression: Comparative Studies of Normal, Neurotic, and Psychotic Conditions. New York, International Universities Press, 1971

Rado S: The problem of melancholia. Int J Psychoanal 9:420–438, 1928

OVERVIEW OF ADOLESCENT BEREAVEMENT

Bowlby J: Attachment and Loss, Vol 1. New York, Basic Books, 1969

Breaking Away. Film, 20th Century Fox. Peter Yates, Dir., 1979

Erikson E: Identity and the Life Cycle (1950). New York, WW Norton, 1994

Roth P: Letting Go. New York, Vintage, 1962

Shapiro T: Normalization in adolescence. J Am Psychoanal Assoc 56:123–146, 2008

Chapter 8:
Anxiety and Sophia Hastings

ANXIETY DISORDERS

Mannuzza S, Schneier FR, Chapman TF, et al: Generalized social phobia: reliability and validity. Arch Gen Psychiatry 52:230–237, 1995

Schneier FR, Johnson J, Horning CD, et al: Social phobia: comorbidity and morbidity in an epidemiologic sample. Arch Gen Psychiatry 49:282–288, 1992

Turner S, Beidel DC, Townsley RM: Social phobia: a comparison of specific and generalized subtypes and avoidant personality disorder. J Abnorm Psychol 101:326–331, 1992

ALCOHOL ABUSE

Alcoholics Anonymous World Services: Living Sober. New York, Alcoholics Anonymous World Services, 1998

American Psychiatric Association: Diagnostic and Statistical Manual of Mental Disorders, 4th Edition. Washington, DC, American Psychiatric Association, 1994

Bouza C, Angeles M, Muñoz A, et al: Efficacy and safety of naltrexone and acamprosate in the treatment of alcohol dependence: a systematic review. Addiction 99(7):267–280, 2005

DiClemente CC: Addiction and Change: How Addictions Develop and Addicted People Recover. New York, Guilford, 2003

Khantzian EJ: The self-medication hypothesis of substance abuse disorders: a reconsideration and recent applications. Harv Rev Psychiatry 4:231–244, 1997

Khantzian EJ, Mack JE: How AA works and why it's important for clinicians to understand. J Subst Abuse Treat 2:77–92, 1994

Lowinson J, Ruiz P, Millman RB, et al (eds): Substance Abuse: A Comprehensive Textbook. Philadelphia, PA, Lippincott Williams & Wilkins, 2005

Miller WR, Rollnick S: Motivational Interviewing: Preparing People for Change, 2nd Edition. New York, Guilford, 2002

NEUROBIOLOGY OF ALCOHOL

Davis KM, Wu JY: Role of glutamatergic and GABAergic systems in alcoholism. J Biomed Sci 8(1):7–19, 2001

Herrera DG, Yague AG, Johnsen-Soriano S, et al: Selective impairment of hippocampal neurogenesis by chronic alcoholism: protective effects of an antioxidant. Proc Natl Acad Sci U S A 100:7919–7924, 2003

Kumar S, Kralic JE, Alturaihi H, et al: Chronic ethanol consumption enhances internalization of $alpha_1$ subunit–containing $GABA_A$ receptors in cerebral cortex. J Neurochem 86:700–708, 2003

Kumar SR, Fleming L, Morrow AL: Ethanol regulation of gamma–aminobutyric acid A receptors: genomic and nongenomic mechanisms. Pharmacol Ther 101:211–226, 2004

Narahashi T, Kuriyama K, Illes P, et al: Neuroreceptors and ion channels as targets of alcohol. Alcohol Clin Exp Res 25 (5 suppl ISBRA):182S–188S, 2001

Nevo I, Hamon M: Neurotransmitter and neuromodulatory mechanisms involved in alcohol abuse and alcoholism. Neurochem Int 26:305–336, 1995 (discussion 337–342)

Rammes G, Mahal B, Putzke J, et al: The anti-craving compound acamprosate acts as a weak NMDA-receptor antagonist, but modulates NMDA-receptor subunit expression similar to memantine and MK-801. Neuropharmacology 40:749–760, 2001

Santarelli L, Saxe M, Gross C, et al: Requirement of hippocampal neurogenesis for the behavioral effects of antidepressants. Science 301:805–809, 2003

Tan CY, Weaver DF: Molecular pathogenesis of alcohol withdrawal seizures: the modified lipid-protein interaction mechanism. Seizure 6:255–274, 1997

PHARMACOLOGY OF ANXIETY

Blanco C, Schneier FR, Schmidt A, et al: Pharmacological treatment of social anxiety disorder: a meta-analysis. Depress Anxiety 18:29–40, 2003

Davidson JRT, Potts N, Richichi E, et al: Treatment of social phobia with clonazepam and placebo. J Clin Psychopharmacol 13:423–428, 1993

Kushner MG, Abrams K, Thuras P, et al: Follow-up study of anxiety disorder and alcohol dependence in comorbid alcoholism treatment patients. Alcohol Clin Exp Res 29:1432–1443, 2005

Liebowitz MR, Gelenberg AJ, Munjack D: Venlafaxine extended release vs placebo and paroxetine in social anxiety disorder. Arch Gen Psychiatry 62:190–198, 2005

Schneier FR: Social anxiety disorder. N Engl J Med 355:1029–1036, 2006

Stein DJ, Ipser JC, van Balkom AJ. Pharmacotherapy for social anxiety disorder. Cochrane Database of Systematic Reviews 2004, Issue 4, Article No: CD001206. DOI: 10.1002/14651858.CD001206.pub2

Stein MB, Goldin PR, Sareen J, et al: Increased amygdala activation to angry and contemptuous faces in generalized social phobia. Arch Gen Psychiatry 59:1027–1034, 2002

COGNITIVE-BEHAVIORAL THERAPY

Beck AT, Rush, AJ, Shaw BF, et al: Cognitive Therapy of Depression. New York, Guilford, 1979

Beck J: Cognitive Therapy: Basics and Beyond. New York, Guilford, 1995

Butler A, Chapman JE, Forman EM, et al: The empirical status of cognitive-behavioral therapy: a review of meta-analysis. Clin Psychol Rev 26:17–31, 2006

Evans S, Ferrando S, Findler M, et al: Mindfulness-based cognitive therapy for generalized anxiety disorder. J Anxiety Disord 22:716–721, 2008

Haby MM, Donnelly M, Corry J, et al: Cognitive behavioural therapy for depression, panic disorder and generalized anxiety disorder: a meta-regression of factors that may predict outcome. Aust NZ J Psychiatry 40:9–19, 2006

PANIC-FOCUSED PSYCHODYNAMIC PSYCHOTHERAPY

American Psychiatric Association: Diagnostic and Statistical Manual of Mental Disorders, 4th Edition, Text Revision. Washington, DC, American Psychiatric Association, 2000

Busch FN, Milrod BL: Psychodynamic theory and treatment of social anxiety disorder, in Social Anxiety Disorder. Edited by Bandelow B, Stein DJ. New York, Marcel Dekker, 2004, pp 251–265

Busch FN, Cooper AM, Klerman GL, et al: Neurophysiological, cognitive-behavioral and psychoanalytic approaches to panic disorder: toward an integration. Psychoanalytic Inquiry 11:316–332, 1991

Busch FN, Shear MK, Cooper AM, et al: An empirical study of defense mechanisms in panic disorder. J Nerv Ment Dis 183:299–303, 1995

Milrod BL, Busch FN, Cooper AM, et al: Manual of Panic-Focused Psychodynamic Psychotherapy. Washington, DC, American Psychiatric Press, 1997

Milrod B, Busch F, Leon A, et al: An open trial of psychodynamic psychotherapy for panic disorder—a pilot study. Am J Psychiatry 157:1878–1880, 2000

Milrod B, Busch F, Leon AC, et al: A pilot open trial of brief psychodynamic psychotherapy for panic disorder. J Psychother Prac Res 10:1–7, 2001

Milrod B, Leon AC, Busch F, et al: A randomized controlled clinical trial of psychoanalytic psychotherapy for panic disorder. Am J Psychiatry 164:265–272, 2007

Shear MK, Cooper AM, Klerman GL, et al: A psychodynamic model of panic disorder. Am J Psychiatry 150:859–866, 1993

Wiborg IM, Dahl AA: Does brief dynamic psychotherapy reduce the relapse rate of panic disorder? Arch Gen Psychiatry 53:689–694, 1996

AFTER EFFECTS OF SEXUAL ABUSE

American Psychiatric Association: Diagnostic and Statistical Manual of Mental Disorders, 4th Edition, Text Revision. Washington, DC, American Psychiatric Association, 2000

Anda RF, Whitfield CL, Felitti VJ, et al: Adverse childhood experiences, alcoholic parents, and later risk of alcoholism and depression. Psychiatr Serv 53:1001–1009, 2002

Breuer J, Freud S: Studies on hysteria (1893–1895), in Standard Edition of the Complete Psychological Works of Sigmund Freud, Vol 2. Translated and edited by Strachey J. London, Hogarth Press, 1955, pp 1–319

Fairbairn WRD: Psychological Studies of the Personality. London, Routledge & Kegan Paul, 1952

Freud S: Remembering, repeating and working-through (further recommendations on the technique of psycho-analysis II) (1914), in Standard Edition of the Complete Psychological Works of Sigmund Freud, Vol 12. Translated and edited by Strachey J. London, Hogarth Press, 1958, pp 145–156

Herman JL: Trauma and Recovery. New York, Basic Books, 1992

Najavits LM: Seeking Safety: A Treatment Manual for PTSD and Substance Abuse. New York, Guilford, 2002

Person EP, Klar H: Establishing trauma: the difficulty distinguishing between memories and fantasies. J Am Psychoanal Assoc 42:1055–1081, 1994

Schechter DS, Brunelli SA, Cunningham N, et al: Mother-daughter relationships and child sexual abuse: a pilot study of 35 dyads. Bull Menninger Clin 66:39–60, 2002

van der Kolk BA, Roth S, Pelcovitz D, et al: Disorders of extreme stress: the empirical foundation of a complex adaptation to trauma. J Trauma Stress 18:389–399, 2005

Williams LM: Recall of childhood trauma: a prospective study of women's memories of child sexual abuse. J Consult Clin Psychol 62:1167–1176, 1994

Zanarini MC, Frankenburg FR, Dubo ED, et al: Axis I comorbidity of borderline personality disorder. Am J Psychiatry 155:1733–1739, 1998

Zanarini MC, Frankenburg FR, Hennen J, et al: Prediction of the 10-year course of borderline personality disorder. Am J Psychiatry 163:827–832, 2006

OVERVIEW OF COUNTERTRANSFERENCE

Bowlby J: A Secure Base: Parent-Child Attachment and Healthy Human Development. New York, Basic Books, 1988

Fairbairn WRD: An Object-Relations Theory of the Personality. New York, Basic Books, 1952

Gabbard G: Miscarriages of psychoanalytic treatment with suicidal patients. Int J Psychoanal 84:249–261, 2003

MacKinnon RA, Michaels R, Buckley PJ: The traumatized patient, in The Psychiatric Interview in Clinical Practice, 2nd Edition. Washington, DC, American Psychiatric Publishing, 2006, pp 315–323

Shengold L: Soul Murder. New Haven, CT, Yale University Press, 1989

Chapter 9:
Hypomania and Jennifer Ingram

ATTENTION DEFICIT

American Academy of Child and Adolescent Psychiatry: Practice parameter for the use of stimulant medications in the treatment of children, adolescents, and adults. J Am Acad Child Adolesc Psychiatry 41 (suppl 2):26–49, 2002

American Psychiatric Association: Diagnostic and Statistical Manual of Mental Disorders, 4th Edition, Text Revision. Washington, DC, American Psychiatric Association, 2000

Barkley RA: Genetics of childhood disorders: ADHD, Part 1: the executive functions and ADHD. J Am Acad Child Adolesc Psychiatry 39:1064–1068, 2000

Barkley RA (ed): Attention-Deficit Hyperactivity Disorder: A Handbook for Diagnosis and Treatment, 3rd Edition. New York, Guilford, 2006

Barkley RA, Fischer M, Smallish L, et al: Does the treatment of attention-deficit/hyperactivity disorder with stimulants contribute to drug use/abuse? A 13-year prospective study. Pediatrics 111:97–109, 2003

Biederman J, Faraone SV, Spencer T, et al: Patterns of psychiatric comorbidity: cognition, and psychosocial functioning in adults with attention deficit hyperactivity disorder. Am J Psychiatry 150:1792–1798, 1993

Doyle BB: Understanding and Treating Adults With Attention Deficit Hyperactivity Disorder. Washington, DC, American Psychiatric Publishing, 2006

Fan J, Fossella J, Sommer T, et al: Mapping the genetic variation of executive attention onto brain activity. Proc Natl Acad Sci U S A 100:7406–7411, 2003

Fossella J, Sommer T, Fan J, et al: Assessing the molecular genetics of attention networks. BMC Neurosci 3:14, 2002

Jensen PS, Hinshaw SP, Swanson JM, et al: Findings from the NIMH Multimodal Treatment Study of ADHD (MTA): implications and applications for primary care providers. Devel Behav Pediatr 2:60–73, 2001

Murphy KR, Gordon M: Assessment of adults with ADHD, in Attention-Deficit Hyperactivity Disorder: A Handbook for Diagnosis and Treatment, 3rd Edition. Edited by Barkley RA. New York, Guilford, 2006, pp 425–452

Paule MG, Rowland AS, Ferguson SA, et al: Attention-deficit/hyperactivity disorder: characteristics, interventions, models. Neurotoxicol Teratol 22:631–651, 2000

Rowland AS, Lesesne CA, Abramowitz, AJ: The epidemiology of attention-deficit/hyperactivity disorder: a public health view. Mental Health and Developmental Disabilities Research Reviews 8:162–170, 2002

Taylor EW, Keltner NL: Messy purse girls: adult females and ADHD. Perspect Psychiatr Care 38:69–72, 2002

Wasserman RC, Kelleher KJ, Bocian A, et al: Identification of attentional and hyperactivity problems in primary care: a report from pediatric research in office settings and the ambulatory sentinel practice network. Pediatrics 103(3):E38, 1999

Wilens TE, Faraone SV, Biederman J, et al: Does stimulant therapy of attention-deficit/hyperactivity disorder beget later substance abuse? A meta-analytic review of the literature. Pediatrics 111:179–185, 2003

BIPOLAR DISORDER

Bizzari J, Sbrana A, Ravani L, et al: The spectrum of substance abuse in bipolar disorder: reasons for use, sensation seeking and substance sensitivity. Bipolar Disord 9:213–220, 2007

Cermakian N, Boivin D: A molecular perspective of human circadian rhythm disorders. Brain Res Brain Res Rev 42:204–220, 2003

Gheaemi NS, Ko J, Goodwin FK: The bipolar spectrum of the antidepressant view of the world. J Psychiatr Pract 7:287–297, 2001

Goodwin FK, Jamison KR: Manic Depressive Illness. New York, Oxford University Press, 1990

Mansour HA, Monk TH, Nimgaonkar VL: Circadian genes and bipolar disorder. Ann Med 37 (3):196–205, 2005

McClung C: Circadian genes, rhythms and the biology of mood disorders. Pharmacol Ther 114:222–232, 2007

Post RM: Kindling and sensitization as models for affective episode recurrence, cyclicity, and tolerance phenomena. Neurosci Biobehav Rev 31:858873, 2007

Roybal K, Theobold D, Graham A, et al: Mania-like behavior induced by disruption of CLOCK. Proc Natl Acad Sci USA 104:6406–6411, 2007

Sachs G, Nirenberg A, Clabrese J, et al: Effectivenesss of adjunctive antidepressant treatment for bipolar disorder. N Engl J Med 356:1711–1722, 2007

Simon N, Pollack M, Fischmann D, et al: Complicated grief and its correlates in patients with bipolar disorder. J Clin Psychiatry 66:1105–1110, 2005

Smith L, Cornelius V, Bell A, et al: Effectiveness of mood stabilizers and antipsychotics in the maintenance phase of bipolar disorder: a systematic review of randomized controlled trials. Bipolar Disord 9:394–412, 2007

Suppes T, Dennehy E, Hirschfeld R, et al: The Texas Implementation of Medication Algorithms: update to the algorithms of bipolar I disorder. J Clin Psychiatry 66:870–886, 2005

Yerevanian B, Koek R, Mintz J: Bipolar pharmacotherapy and suicidal behavior, Part I: lithium, divalproex and carbamazepine. J Affect Disord 103(1–3, July 12):5–11, 2007 (Epub)

BIPOLAR SPECTRUM DISORDER

Akiskal HS, Pinto O: The evolving bipolar spectrum prototypes I, II, III and IV. Psychiatr Clin N Am 22:518–534, 1999

Baldessarini RJ, Tondon L, Hennen J: Lithium treatment and suicide risk in major affective disorders: update and new findings. J Clin Psychiatry 64(suppl 5):44–52, 2003

Clayton PJ, Pitts FN, Winokur G: Affective disorder, IV: mania. Compr Psychiatry 6:313–322, 1965

Coke RG, Kruger S, Shugar G: Comparative evaluation of two self-report mania rating scales. Biol Psychiatry 40:279–283, 1996

Frank E (ed): Treating Bipolar Disorder: A Clinician's Guide to Interpersonal and Social Rhythm Therapy. New York, Guilford, 2005

Goodwin F, Jamison KR: Manic Depressive Illness, 2nd Edition. New York, Oxford University Press, 2007

Klerman GL: The classification of bipolar disorders. Psychiatric Annals 17:13–17, 1987

McHugh P, Slavney PR: The Perspectives of Psychiatry, 2nd Edition. Baltimore, MD, Johns Hopkins University Press, 1998

Miller MN, Miller BE: Premenstrual exacerbations of mood disorders. Psychopharmacol Bull 35(3):135–149, 2001

Nierenberg AA, Miyahara S, Spencer T, et al: Clinical and diagnostic implications of lifetime attention-deficit/hyperactivity disorder comorbidity in adults with bipolar disorder: data from the first 1000 STEP-BD participants. Biol Psychiatry 57:1467–1473, 2005

Ross RG: Psychotic and manic-like symptoms during stimulant treatment of attention deficit hyperactivity disorder. Am J Psychiatry 163:1149–1152, 2006

Young RC, Biggs JT, Ziegler VE, et al: A rating scale for mania: reliability, validity, and sensitivity. Br J Psychiatry 133:429–435, 1978

PREMENSTRUAL DYSPHORIA

American Psychiatric Association: Diagnostic and Statistical Manual of Mental Disorders, 4th Edition, Text Revision. Washington, DC, American Psychiatric Association, 2000

Endicott J, Nee J, Harrison W: Daily Record of Severity of Problems (DRSP): reliability and validity. Arch Womens Ment Health 9:41–49, 2006

Eriksson O, Backstrom T, Stridsberg M, et al: Differential response to estrogen challenge test in women with and without premenstrual dysphoria. Psychoneuroendocrinology 31:415–427, 2005

Freeman E: Premenstrual syndrome and premenstrual dysphoric disorder: definitions and diagnosis. Psychoneuroendocrinology 28 (suppl 3):25–37, 2003

Freeman E, Schweizer E, Rickels K: Personality factors in women with premenstrual sydrome. Psychosomatic Med 57:453–459, 1995

Freeman E, DeRubeis R, Rickels K: Reliability and validity of a daily diary for premenstrual syndrome. Psychiatry Res 65:97–106, 1996

Freeman E, Sondheimer S, Sammel M, et al: A preliminary study of luteal phase versus symptom-onset dosing with escitalopram for premenstrual dysphoric disorder. J Clin Psychiatry 66:769–773, 2005

Halbreich U, Borenstein J, Pearlstein T, et al: The prevalence, impairment, impact and burden of premenstrual dysphoric disorder (PMS/PMDD). Psychoneuroendocrinology 28 (suppl 3):1–24, 2003

Mortola JF, Girton L, Beck L, et al: Diagnosis of premenstrual syndrome by a simple prospective and reliable instrument: the Calandar of Premenstrual Experiences. Obstet Gynecol 76:302–307, 1990

Pearlstein T, Frank E, Rivera-Tovar A, et al: Prevalence of Axis I and Axis II disorders in women with late luteal phase dysphoric disorder. J Affect Disord 20:129–134, 1990

Schmidt PJ, Nieman LK, Danaceau MA, et al: Differential behavioral effects of gonadal steroids in women with and in those without premenstrual syndrome. N Engl J Med 338:209–216, 1998

Wittchen HU, Becker E, Lieb R, et al: Prevalence, incidence and stability of premenstrual dysphoric disorder in the community. Psychol Med 32:119–132, 2002

World Health Organization: International Classification of Diseases, 10th Revision. Geneva, World Health Organization, 1992

SLEEP

Barbini B, Benedetti F, Colombo C, et al: Dark therapy for mania: a pilot study. Bipolar Disord 7:98–101, 2005

Benedetti F, Barbini B, Fulgosi MC, et al: Combined total sleep deprivation and light therapy in the treatment of drug-resistant bipolar depression: acute response and long-term remission rates. J Clin Psychiatry 66:1535–1540, 2005

Lam RW, Carter D, Misri S, et al: A controlled study of light therapy in women with late luteal phase dysphoric disorder. Psychiatry Res 86:185–192, 1999

Leibenluft E, Turner EH, Feldman-Naim S, et al: Light therapy in patients with rapid cycling bipolar disorder: preliminary results. Psychopharmacol Bull 31:705–710, 1995

Rybak YE, McNeely HE, Mackenzie B, et al: An open trial of light therapy in adult attention deficit hyperactivity disorder. J Clin Psychiatry 67:1527–1535, 2006

Sit D, Wisner KL, Hanusa BH, et al: Light therapy for bipolar disorder: a case series in women. Bipolar Disord 9:918–927, 2007

Terman M: Light on sleep, in Sleep Science: Integrating Basic Research and Clinical Practice. Edited by Schwartz WJ. Basel, Switzerland, S Karger, 1997, pp 229–249

Terman M, Terman JS: Light therapy for seasonal and nonseasonal depression: efficacy, protocol, safety, and side effects. CNS Spectr 10:647–663, 2005

Williams JBW, Terman M: Structured Interview Guide for the Hamilton Depression Rating Scale With Atypical Depression Supplement (SIGH-ADS). New York, New York State Psychiatric Institute, 2003

Wirz-Justice A, Quinto C, Cajochen C, et al: A rapid-cycling bipolar patient treated with long nights, bed rest, and light. Biol Psychiatry 45:1075–1077, 1999

Wirz-Justice A, Benedetti F, Berger M, et al: Chronotherapeutics (light and wake therapy) in affective disorders. Psychol Med 35:939–944, 2005

AUTISM'S EFFECT ON THE FAMILY

Frith U (ed): Autism and Asperger's Syndrome. Cambridge, UK, Cambridge University Press, 1991

Glasberg B: The development of siblings' understanding of autistic spectrum disorders. J Autism Devel Disord 30:143–156, 2000

Kanner L: Autistic disturbances of affective contact. Nervous Child 2:217–250, 1943

Stainton T, Besser H: The positive impact of children with an intellectual disability on the family. Journal of Intellectual and Developmental Disability 23:57–70, 1998

Verte S, Roeyers H, Buysse A: Behavioral problems, social competence and self-concept in siblings of children with autism. Child Care Health Dev 29:193–205, 2003

Wing L: Asperger's syndrome: a clinical account. Psychol Med 22:115–129, 1981

CREATIVITY AND MENTAL ILLNESS

Andreasen NC: Creativity and mental illness: prevalence rates in writers and their first-degree relatives. Am J Psychiatry 144:1288–1292, 1987

Becker G: The Mad Genius Controversy: A Study in the Sociology of Deviance. Beverly Hills, CA, Sage, 1978

Frosch WA: Moods, madness, and music, I: major affective disease and musical creativity. Compr Psychiatry 28:315–322, 1987

Frosch WA: Creativity: is there a worm in the apple? J R Soc Med 88:506–508, 1996

Greenacre P: The childhood of ten artists: libidinal phase development and giftedness. Psychoanal Study Child 12:47–72, 1957

Hyslop TB: The Great Abnormals. London, Philip Allan, 1925

Jamison KR: Mood disorders and patterns of creativity in British writers and artists. Psychiatry 52:125–134, 1989

Jamison KR: Touched With Fire: Manic Depressive Illness and the Artistic Temperament. New York, Free Press, 1993

Nisbet JF: The Insanity of Genius, and the General Inequality of Human Faculty Physiologically Considered, 4th Edition. London, Grant Richards, 1900

Schildkraut JJ, Hirschfeld AJ, Murphy BM: Mind and mood in modern art, II: depressive disorders, spirituality, and early deaths in the abstract expressionist artists of the New York School. Am J Psychiatry 151:482–488, 1994

Trilling L: Art and neurosis, in The Liberal Imagination. Garden City, NY, Doubleday, 1957, pp 155–175

BEING LESBIAN

Auchincloss EL, Vaughan SC: Psychoanalysis and homosexuality. J Am Psychoanal Assoc 49:1157–1186, 2001

Burch B: Between women: the mother-daughter romance and homoerotic transference in psychotherapy. Psychoanalytic Psychology 13:475–494, 1996

D'Ercole A, Drescher J (eds): Uncoupling Convention: Psychoanalytic Approaches to Same-Sex Couples and Families. Hillsdale, NJ, Analytic Press, 2004

Deutsch L: Out of the closet and on to the couch: a psychoanalytic exploration of lesbian development, in Lesbians and Psychoanalysis: Revolutions in Theory and Practice. Edited by Glassgold JM, Iasenza ES. New York, Free Press, 1995, pp 19–37

Downey JI: Review of lesbian identity and contemporary psychotherapy: a framework for clinical practice. J Am Acad Psychoanal Dyn Psychiatry 34:561–563, 2006

Downey J, Friedman R: Internalized homophobia in lesbian relationships. J Am Acad Psychoanal 23:435–447, 1995

Erikson E: Identity and the Life Cycle. New York, International Universities Press, 1959

Glassgold JM, Iasenza S (eds): Lesbians, Feminism, and Psychoanalysis: The Second Wave. Binghamton, NY, Harrington Park Press/Haworth Press, 2004

Glazer D: Lesbian mothers: a foot in two worlds, in Sexualities Lost and Found: Lesbians, Psychoanalysis, and Culture. Edited by Gould E, Kiersky S. Madison, CT, International Universities Press, 2001, pp 247–257

Phillips SH, Richardson J, Vaughan SC: Sexual orientation and psychotherapy, in Oxford Textbook of Psychotherapy. Edited by Gabbard GO, Beck JS, Holmes J. New York, Oxford University Press, 2005, pp 302–308

Vaughan S: Psychoanalytic and biological perspectives on lesbian patients: why developmental themes are more important in psychotherapy. Harv Rev Psychiatry 6(3):160–164, 1998

LOVE

Faderman L: Odd Girls and Twilight Lovers: A History of Lesbian Life in Twentieth Century America. New York, Columbia University Press, 1992

Friedrich O: The Grave of Alice B Toklas, in The Grave of Alice B Toklas and Other Reports From the Past. New York, International Publishing, 1989, pp 1–43

Keefer BP, Kelly R: Female adolescence: difficult for heterosexual girls, hazardous for lesbians, in Rethinking Psychoanalysis and the Homosexualities. Edited by Winer JA, Anderson JW, Dohler BJ, et al. Hillsdale, NJ, Analytic Press, 2002, pp 243–252

Miller PY, Fowlkes MR: Social and behavioral constructions of female sexuality, in Women, Sex, and Sexuality. Edited by Stimpson CP, Person ES. Chicago, IL, University of Chicago Press, 1980, pp 256–273

Person ES: Something borrowed: how mutual influences among gays, lesbians, bisexuals, and straights changed women's lives and psychoanalytic theories, in The Annual of Psychoanalysis. Hillsdale, NJ, Analytic Press, 2004, pp 81–98

Person ES: Dreams of Love and Fateful Encounters: The Power of Romantic Passion. Washington, DC, American Psychiatric Publishing, 2007

Rich A: Compulsory heterosexuality and lesbian existence, in Women, Sex, and Sexuality. Edited by Stimpson CP, Person ES. Chicago, IL, University of Chicago Press, 1980, pp 62–91

PSYCHODYNAMIC PSYCHOTHERAPY

Caligor E, Kernberg O, Clarkin J: Handbook of Dynamic Psychotherapy for Higher Level Personality Pathology. Washington, DC, American Psychiatric Publishing, 2007

Gabbard G: Long-Term Psychodynamic Psychotherapy. Washington, DC, American Psychiatric Publishing, 2004

Gabbard G: Psychodynamic Psychiatry in Clinical Practice, 4th Edition. Washington, DC, American Psychiatric Publishing, 2005

MacKinnon RA, Michels R, Buckley PJ: The Psychiatric Interview in Clinical Practice, 2nd Edition. Washington, DC, American Psychiatric Publishing, 2006

Winston A, Rosenthal R, Pinsker H: Introduction to Supportive Psychotherapy. Washington, DC, American Psychiatric Publishing, 2004

OVERVIEW OF HYPOMANIA

Akiskal HS, Pinto O: The evolving bipolar spectrum: prototypes I, II, III, and IV. Psychiatr Clin N Am 22:517–534, 1999

American Psychiatric Association: Diagnostic and Statistical Manual of Mental Disorders, Fourth Edition, Text Revision. Washington, DC, American Psychiatric Association, 2000

Angst J, Gamma A, Benazzi F, et al: Toward a redefinition of subthreshold bipolarity: epidemiology and proposed criteria for bipolar II, minor bipolar disorders and hypomania. J Affect Disord 73:133–146, 2003

Beck AT, Ward CH, Mendelson M, et al: An inventory for measuring depression. Arch Gen Psychiatry 4:561–571, 1961

Bos HM, van Balen F, van den Boom DC: Lesbian families and family functioning: an overview. Patient Educ Couns 559:263–275, 2005

Brown TE: Brown Attention-Deficit Disorders Scales: Manual. San Antonio, TX, Psychological Corporation, 1996

Conners CK, Erhardt D, Sparrow EP: Conners' Adult ADHD Rating Scales: Technical Manual. New York, Multi-Health Systems, 1999

Faraone SV, Biederman J, Spencer T, et al: Diagnosing adult attention deficit hyperactivity disorder: are late onset and subthreshold diagnoses valid? Am J Psychiatry 163:1720–1729, 2006

Golombok S, Perry B, Burston A, et al: Children with lesbian parents: a community study. Dev Psychol 39:20–33, 2003

Kessler RC, Adler L, Barkley R, et al: The prevalence and correlates of adult ADHD in the United States: results from the National Comorbidity Survey Replication. Am J Psychiatry 163:716–723, 2006

McGough JJ, Barkley RA: Diagnostic controversies in adult attention deficit hyperactivity disorder. Am J Psychiatry 161:1948–1956, 2004

Miklowitz DJ: A review of evidence-based psychosocial interventions for bipolar disorder. J Clin Psychiatry 67 (suppl 11):28–33, 2006

Murphy K, Barkley RA: Prevalence of DSM-IV symptoms of ADHD in adult licensed drivers: implications for clinical diagnosis. J Atten Disord 1:147–161, 1996

Patterson CJ: Children of lesbian and gay families. Child Dev 63:1025–1042, 1992

Practice guideline for the treatment of patients with bipolar disorder (revision). Am J Psychiatry 159 (4, suppl):1–50, 2002

Suppes T, Dennehy EB: Evidence-based long-term treatment of bipolar II disorder. J Clin Psychiatry 63:29–33, 2002

Tasker F: Lesbian mothers, gay fathers, and their children: a review. J Dev Behav Pediatr 26:224–240, 2005

Wainright JL, Russell ST, Patterson CJ: Psychosocial adjustment, school outcomes, and romantic relationships of adolescents with same-sex parents. Child Dev 75:1886–1898, 2004

Ward MF, Wender PH, Reimherr FW: The Wender Utah Rating Scale: an aid in the retrospective diagnosis of childhood attention-deficit hyperactivity disorder. Am J Psychiatry 150:885–890, 1993

Wender EH: Attention-deficit hyperactivity disorders in adolescence. J Dev Behav Pediatr 16:192–195, 1995

Young RC, Briggs JT, Ziegler VE, et al: A rating scale for mania: reliability, validity, and sensitivity. Br J Psychiatry 133:429–435, 1978

Chapter 10:
Exam Failure and Grace Jin

INTERVIEW OF THE MEDICAL STUDENT

Chandavarkar U, Azzam A, Mathews CA: Anxiety symptoms and perceived performance in medical students. Depress Anxiety 24:103–111, 2006

Dyrbye LN, Thomas MR, Shanafelt TD: Medical student distress: causes, consequences, and proposed solutions. Mayo Clin Proc 80:1613–1622, 2005

Dyrbye L, Thomas M, Shanafelt T: Systematic review of depression, anxiety, and other indicators of psychological distress among U.S. and Canadian medical students. Acad Med 81:354–373, 2006

Levine RE, Litwins SD, Frye AW: An evaluation of depressed mood in two classes of medical students. Acad Psychiatry 30:235–237, 2006

Tjia J, Givens JL, Shea JA: Factors associated with undertreatment of medical student depression. J Am Coll Health 53:219–224, 2005

Tyssen R, Vaglum P, Gronvold NT, et al: Suicidal ideation among medical students and young physicians: a nationwide and prospective study of prevalence and predictors. J Affect Disord 64:69–79, 2001

SOMATOFORM DISORDERS AND OBSESSIONALITY

Barsky AJ: Stop Being Your Symptoms and Start Being Yourself. New York, HarperCollins, 2006

Fallon BA: Pharmacotherapy of somatoform disorders. J Psychosom Res 56:455–460, 2004

Williams J, Hadjistavropoulos T, Sharpe D: A meta-analysis of psychologic and pharmacologic treatments of body dysmorphic disorder. Behav Res Ther 44:99–111, 2006

NEUROBIOLOGY OF OBSESSIONS

Adams KH, Hansen ES, Pinborg LH, et al: Patients with obsessive-compulsive disorder have increased 5-HT$_{2A}$ receptor binding in the caudate nuclei. Int J Neuropsychopharmacol 8:391–401, 2005

American Psychiatric Association: Diagnostic and Statistical Manual of Mental Disorders, 4th Edition, Text Revision. Washington, DC, American Psychiatric Association, 2000

Bartz JA, Hollander E: Is obsessive-compulsive disorder an anxiety disorder? Prog Neuropsychopharmacol Biol Psychiatry 30:338–352, 2006

Carlsson ML: On the role of cortical glutamate in obsessive-compulsive disorder and attention-deficit hyperactivity disorder, two phenomenologically antithetical conditions. Acta Psychiatr Scand 102:401–413, 2000

Denys D, Zohar J, Westenberg HG: The role of dopamine in obsessive-compulsive disorder: preclinical and clinical evidence. J Clin Psychiatry 65 (suppl 14):11–17, 2004

Dougherty DD, Rauch SL, Jenike MA: Pharmacotherapy for obsessive-compulsive disorder. J Clin Psychol 60:1195–1202, 2004

Foa EB, Kozak MJ, Goodman WK, et al: DSM-IV field trial: obsessive-compulsive disorder. Am J Psychiatry 152:90–96, 1995

Hemmings SM, Stein DJ: The current status of association studies in obsessive-compulsive disorder. Psychiatr Clin North Am 29:411–444, 2006

Insel TR, Mueller EA, Alterman I, et al: Obsessive-compulsive disorder and serotonin: is there a connection? Biol Psychiatry 20:1174–1188, 1985

Muris P, Merckelbach H, Clavan M: Abnormal and normal compulsions. Behav Res Ther 35:249–252, 1997

Rosenberg DR, Keshavan MS: Toward a neurodevelopmental model of obsessive-compulsive disorder. Biol Psychiatry 43:623–640, 1998

Sasson Y, Dekel S, Nacasch N, et al: Posttraumatic obsessive-compulsive disorder: a case series. Psychiatry Res 135:145–152, 2005

Saxena S, Bota RG, Brody AL: Brain-behavior relationships in obsessive-compulsive disorder. Semin Clin Neuropsychiatry 6:82–101, 2001

Simpson HB, Fallon BA: Obsessive-compulsive disorder: an overview. J Psychiatr Pract 6:3–17, 2000

Simpson HB, Lombardo I, Slifstein M, et al: Serotonin transporters in obsessive-compulsive disorder: a positron emission tomography study with [^{11}C]McN 5652. Biol Psychiatry 54:1414–1421, 2003

Snider LA, Swedo SE: PANDAS: current status and directions for research. Mol Psychiatry 9:900–907, 2004

NARCISSISTIC INJURY AND NARCISSISTIC DEFENSES

Cooper AM: The narcissistic-masochistic character, in Masochism: Current Psychoanalytic Perspectives. Edited by Glick RA, Meyers DI. Hillsdale, NJ, Analytic Press, 1988, pp 117–138

Kernberg OF: Borderline Conditions and Pathological Narcissism. New York, Jason Aronson, 1975

Kernberg OF: Severe Personality Disorders: Psychotherapeutic Strategies. New Haven, CT, Yale University Press, 1984

LaFarge L: The wish for revenge. Psychoanal Q 75:447–475, 2006

Ogden T: Analyzing forms of aliveness and deadness of the transference-countertransference. Int J Psychoanal 76:695–709, 1995

Reich A: Pathologic forms of self-esteem regulation (1960), in Psychoanalytic Contributions. New York, International Universities Press, 1973, pp 88–311

Riviere J: A contribution to the analysis of the negative therapeutic reaction. Int J Psychoanal 17:304–320, 1936

Rosenfeld H: A clinical approach to the psychoanalytic theory of the life and death instincts: an investigation into the aggressive aspects of narcissism. Int J Psychoanal 52:169–178, 1971

Spillius EB: Varieties of envious experience (1993), in The Contemporary Kleinians of London. Edited by Schafer R. Madison, CT, International Universities Press, 1997, pp 143–170

THE FIRST-GENERATION ASIAN AMERICAN

Akhtar S: A third individuation: immigration, identity, and the psychoanalytic process. J Am Psychoanal Assoc 43:1051–1084, 1995

Akhtar S: Immigration and Identity: Turmoil, Treatment, and Transformation. Hillsdale, NJ, Jason Aronson, 1999

American Psychiatric Association: Diagnostic and Statistical Manual of Mental Disorders, 4th Edition, Text Revision. Washington, DC, American Psychiatric Association, 2000

Cabaniss DL, Oquendo MA, Singer MB: The impact of psychoanalytic values on transference and countertransference. J Am Acad Psychoanal 22:609–621, 1994

Comas-Diaz L, Jacobsen FM: Ethnocultural transference and countertransference in the therapeutic dyad. Am J Orthopsychiatry 61:392–402, 1991

Garza-Guerrero AC: Culture shock: its mourning and the vicissitudes of identity. J Am Psychoanal Assoc 22:408–429, 1974

Gonzalez EA, Natale RA, Pimentel C, et al: The narcissistic injury and psychopathology of migration: the case of a Nicaraguan man. Journal of Contemporary Psychotherapy 29:185–194, 1999

Grinberg L, Grinberg R: Psychoanalytic Perspectives on Migration and Exile. New Haven, CT, Yale University Press, 1989

Group for the Advancement of Psychiatry: Cultural Assessment in Clinical Psychiatry. Washington, DC, American Psychiatric Publishing, 2002

Kleinman A: Neurasthenia and depression: a study of somatization and culture in China. Cult Med Psychiatry 6:117–190, 1982

Lijtmaer RM: Splitting and nostalgia in recent immigrants: psychodynamic considerations. J Am Acad Psychoanal 29:427–438, 2001

Marlin O: Special issues in the analytic treatment of immigrants and refugees. Issues in Psychoanalytic Psychology 16:7–16, 1994

Pedersen S: Psychopathological reactions to extreme social displacements (refugee neuroses). Psychoanal Rev 36:344–354, 1949

Phinney JS: Ethnic identity in adolescents and adults: review of research. Psychol Bull 180:499–514, 1990

Phinney JS: When we talk about American ethnic groups, what do we mean? Am Psychol 51:918–927, 1996

Tang NM: Some psychoanalytic implications of Chinese philosophy and child-rearing practices. Psychoanal Study Child 47:371–389, 1992

Ton H, Lim RF: The assessment of culturally diverse individuals, in Clinical Manual of Cultural Psychiatry. Edited by Lim RF. Washington, DC, American Psychiatric Publishing, 2006, pp 3–31

Uba L: Asian Americans: Personality Patterns, Identity, and Mental Health. New York, Guilford, 1994

COMPLEMENTARY MEDICINE AND INTEGRATIVE PHARMACOLOGY

Brown RP, Gerbarg PL: Integrative psychopharmacology: a practical approach to herbs and nutrients in psychiatry, in Complementary and Alternative Medicine and Psychiatry (Review of Psychiatry Series, Vol 19, No 1; Series Editors Oldham JO, Riba MB). Edited by Muskin PR. Washington, DC, American Psychiatric Press, 2000, pp 1–66

Brown RP, Gerberg PL: Sudarshan Kriya yogic breathing in the treatment of stress, anxiety, and depression, Part I: neurophysiologic model. J Altern Complement Med 11:189–201, 2005a

Brown RP, Gerbarg PL: Sudarshan Kriya Yogic breathing in the treatment of stress, anxiety, and depression, Part II: clinical applications and guidelines. J Altern Complement Med 11:711–717, 2005b

Brown RP, Gerbarg PL, Ramazanov Z: A phythomedical review of Rhodiola rosea. Herbalgram 56:40–62, 2002

Brown RP, Gerbarg PL, Muskin PR: Alternative treatments in psychiatry (Chapter 104), in Psychiatry, 2nd Edition. Edited by Tasman A, Kay J, Lieberman J. London, Wiley, 2003, pp 2147–2183

Brown RP, Gerbarg PL, Graham B: The Rhodiola Revolution. New York, Rodale Press, 2004

Brown RP, Gerbarg PL, Muskin PR: How to Use Herbs, Nutrients, and Yoga in Mental Health Care. New York, WW Norton, 2008

Gerbarg PG, Brown RP: Yoga: a breath of relief for Hurricane Katrina refugees. Current Psychiatry 4:55–67, 2005

Muller T, Mannel M, Murck, H, et al: Treatment of somatoform disorders with St John's wort: a randomized, double-blind and placebo-controlled trial. Psychosom Med 66:538–547, 2004

MINDFULNESS MEDITATION

Barlow D: Anxiety and Its Disorders: The Nature and Treatment of Anxiety and Panic. New York, Guilford, 1988

Benson H: The Relaxation Response. New York, Avon Books, 1975

Borkovec TD, Hazlett-Stevens H, Diaz ML: The role of positive beliefs about worry in generalized anxiety disorder and its treatment. Clin Psychol Psychother 6:126–138, 1999

Deatherage G: The clinical use of "mindfulness" meditation techniques in short term psychotherapy. Journal of Transpersonal Psychology 7:133–143, 1975

Kabat-Zinn J, Massion AO, Kristeller J, et al: Wherever You Go There You Are: Mindfulness Meditation in Everyday Life. New York, Hyperion, 1994

Lenderking WR, Santorelli SF: Effectiveness of a meditation-based stress reduction program in the treatment of anxiety disorders. Am J Psychiatry 149:936–953, 1992

Miller J, Fletcher K, Kabat-Zinn J: Three-year follow-up and clinical implications of a mindfulness-based stress reduction intervention in the treatment of anxiety disorders. Gen Hosp Psychiatry 17:192–200, 1995

Thera N: The Power of Mindfulness. San Francisco, CA, Unity Press, 1972

Young JE, Klosko JS: Reinventing Your Life. New York, Plume, 1994

EMPATHY

Ackerman SJ, Hilsenroth MJ: A review of therapist characteristics and techniques positively impacting the therapeutic alliance. Clin Psychol Rev 23:1–33, 2003

Gunderson JG, Najavits LM, Leonhard C, et al: Ontogeny of the therapeutic alliance in borderline patients. Psychother Res 7:301–309, 1997

Horvath AO, Greenberg LS (eds): The Working Alliance: Theory, Research and Practice. New York, Wiley, 1994

Horvath AO, Luborsky L: The role of the therapeutic alliance in psychotherapy. J Consult Clin Psychol 61:561–573, 1993

Krupnick JL, Sotsky SM, Simmens S, et al: The role of the therapeutic alliance in psychotherapy and pharmacotherapy outcome: findings in the National Institute of Mental Health Treatment of Depression Collaborative Research Program. J Consult Clin Psychol 64:532–539, 1996

Leeman E: The costs of compliance. J Am Acad Psychoanal Dyn Psychiatry 35:179–187, 2007

Leeman E, Leeman S: Neuronal metaphors: probing neurobiology for psychodynamic meaning. J Am Acad Psychoanal Dyn Psychiatry 32:645–659, 2004

SELF PSYCHOLOGY

Kohut H: The Analysis of the Self. New York, International Universities Press, 1971

Kohut H: Thoughts on narcissism and narcissistic rage. Psychoanal Study Child 27:360–400, 1972

Kohut H: The Restoration of the Self. New York, International Universities Press, 1977

Kohut H: How Does Analysis Cure? Edited by Goldberg A. London, University of Chicago Press, 1984

Ornstein A: Selfobject transferences and the process of working through. Progress in Self Psychology 6:41–58, 1990

Ornstein PH: Remarks on the central position of empathy in psychoanalysis. Bull Assoc Psychoanal Med 18:95–108, 1979

Mollon P: Releasing the Self: the Healing Legacy of Heinz Kohut. London, Whurr Publishers, 2001

Schwaber E: Narcissism, self psychology, and the listening perspective. Annual of Psychoanalysis 9:115–131, 1981

Siegel A: Heinz Kohut and the Psychology of the Self. London, Routledge, 1996

Teicholz J: Kohut, Loewald, and the Postmoderns: A Comparative Study of Self and Relationship. Hillsdale, NJ, Analytic Press, 1999

THE KOHUT/KERNBERG CONTROVERSY

Gabbard G: Cluster B personality disorders: narcissistic, in Psychodynamic Psychiatry in Clinical Practice, 4th Edition. Washington, DC, American Psychiatric Publishing, 2005, pp 483–512

Kernberg OF: Borderline Conditions and Pathological Narcissism. New York, Jason Aronson, 1975

Kernberg OF: Severe Personality Disorders: Psychotherapeutic Strategies. New Haven, CT, Yale University Press, 1984

Klein M: Envy and gratitude (1957), in Envy and Gratitude and Other Works (The Writings of Melanie Klein, Vol 3). New York, Free Press, 1975, pp 176–235

Kohut H: The Analysis of the Self: A Systematic Approach to the Psychoanalytic Treatment of Narcissistic Personality Disorders. New York, International Universities Press, 1971

Kohut H: The Restoration of the Self. Madison, CT, International Universities Press, 1977

Kohut H, Wolf ES: The disorders of the self and their treatment: an outline. Int J Psychoanal 59:413–425, 1978

Ornstein PH: The evolution of Heinz Kohut's psychoanalytic psychology of the self, in The Search for the Self: Selected Writings of Heinz Kohut, 1950–1978, Vol 1. New York, International Universities Press, 1978, pp 1–106

Ronningstam EF (ed): Disorders of Narcissism: Diagnostic, Clinical, and Empirical Implications. Washington, DC, American Psychiatric Press, 1998

Rosenfeld H: A clinical approach to the psychoanalytic theory of the life and death instincts: an investigation into the aggressive aspects of narcissism. Int J Psychoanal 52:169–178, 1971

EVIDENCE-BASED PSYCHOTHERAPY

Ablon S, Jones EE: How expert clinicians' prototypes of an ideal treatment correlate with outcome in psychodynamic and cognitive-behavioral therapy. Psychother Res 8:71–83, 1998

Blatt SJ: The differential effect of psychotherapy and psychoanalysis with anaclitic and introjective patients: the Menninger Psychotherapy Research Project revisited. J Am Psychoanal Assoc 40:691–724, 1992

Chambless DL, Baker M, Baucom DH, et al: Update on empirically validated therapies II. Clin Psychol 51:3–16, 1998

Fonagy P, Jones EE, Kächele H, et al: An Open Door Review of Outcome Studies in Psychoanalysis. London, International Psychoanalytic Association, 2001

Frank JD: Specific and non-specific factors in psychotherapy. Curr Opin Psychiatry 1:289–292, 1988

Gabbard GO, Gunderson JG, Fonagy P: The place of psychoanalytic treatments within psychiatry. Arch Gen Psychiatry 59:505–510, 2002

Hollon SD, Thase ME, Markowitz JC: Treatment and prevention of depression. Psychological Sciences in the Public Interest 3(2):39–77, 2002

Lambert MJ, Bergin AE: The effectiveness of psychotherapy, in Handbook of Psychotherapy and Behavior Change. Edited by Bergin AE, Garfield SL. New York, Wiley, 1994, pp 143–189

Luborsky L, Singer B, Luborsky L: Comparative studies of psychotherapies. Arch Gen Psychiatry 32:995–1008, 1975

Luborsky L, Diguer L, Seligman DA, et al: The researcher's own therapy allegiances: a "wild card" in comparisons of treatment efficacy. Clinical Psychology: Science and Practice 6:95–106, 1999

Rosenzweig S: Some implicit common factors in diverse methods in psychotherapy. Am J Orthopsychiatry 6:412–415, 1936

Shedler J, Westen D: Refining personality disorder diagnosis: integrating science and practice. Am J Psychiatry 161:1350–1365, 2004

Westen D, Novotny CM, Thompson-Brenner H: The empirical status of empirically supported psychotherapies: assumptions, findings, and reporting in controlled clinical trials. Psychol Bull 130:631–663, 2004

THE SELF-DEFEATING PATIENT

Cooper AM: The narcissistic-masochistic character, in Masochism: Current Psychoanalytic Perspectives. Edited by Glick RA, Meyers DI. Hillsdale, NJ, Analytic Press, 1988, pp 117–138

Cooper AM: The Quiet Revolution in American Psychoanalysis: Selected Papers of Arnold M Cooper. Edited by Auchincloss EL. New York, Brunner/Routledge, 2005

SUBJECT INDEX

*Page numbers printed in **boldface** type refer to tables or figures.*

AA (Alcoholics Anonymous), 228, 309, 323
Abstinence
    alcohol abuse and, 308, 311, 323
    psychiatric attitude and, 67, 69
Acamprosate, **229**, 309
ACC (anterior cingulate cortex), and schizophrenia, 143
Access to care, for geriatric depression, 85–86
ACT (assertive community treatment), 164–165
Actigraphy, 355–356
Activity programming, 140
Acute brain syndrome, 178
Adaptive families, 188
Adaptive plasticity, and stress, 25, 26–27, 48
ADAS (Alzheimer Disease Assessment Scale), 80
ADHD. *See* Attention-deficit/ hyperactivity disorder (ADHD)
Adjustment disorder, 89
Adolescence. *See also* Adolescent bereavement; Age; Age at onset
    autism and, 359
    onset of symptoms in bipolar disorder and borderline personality disorder, 98
    psychopharmacology for depression in, 286–289
    safety and depression in, 290
Adolescent bereavement
    case description, 264–267
    cultural issues, 276–279
    ethical dilemma, 261–264

    initial presentation, 257–258
    interpersonal psychotherapy, 289–292
    interviews, 269–272
    mental status exam, 259
    neurobiology of attachment, 283–286
    personal history, 258
    personal psychiatric history, 259
    psychodynamics of depression, 292–296
    psychological impact of dislocation, 273–276
    psychopharmacology, 286–289
    suicidal ideation, 267–269
    summary of case, 296–298
    Virginia Woolf's use of metaphor for, 280–283
Adrenal steroids, and stress, 26
Adults. *See also* Age; Age at onset
    diagnosis of ADHD in, 342, 374, 375
    treatment refusal in case of geriatric depression and children as, 64
Affect, and schizophrenia, 133
Affective dysregulation, and borderline personality disorder, 122
African Americans
    double depression and, 21–24
    pharmacogenetics and, 40
    social support and depressive symptoms in, 8
Age, and coping style, 265. *See also* Adolescence; Adolescent bereavement; Adults; Age at onset; Childhood trauma; Geriatric depression

Age at onset. *See also* Age
   bipolar disorder and borderline
      personality disorder, 98
   schizophrenia and, 135
Aggression, and Kohut/Kernberg
   controversy, 424–425
Agitation
   consultation-liaison psychiatry,
      233–235
   evaluation of emergency patient,
      219–225, 248
   HIV/AIDS and, 230–231, 239–243,
      252, 255
   informed consent, 235–239
   initial presentation, 213–214
   internalized homophobia, 243–246
   Jekyll and Hyde as metaphor,
      249–251
   management of multiple patients in
      emergency department,
      215–219
   mental status exam, 231–232
   personal history, 231
   personal psychiatric history, 231
   psychotherapy selection, 251–254
   sexuality and sexual dysfunction,
      246–248
   substance abuse, 223, **224,**
      225–232, 233–235, 239–254
   summary of case, 254–256
Agreeableness, as dimension of
   personality, 108
AIDS. *See* HIV/AIDS
Akathisia, and antipsychotics, 152–153
Alcohol abuse. *See also* Substance
   abuse
   anxiety and, 300, 303, 304,
      305–312, 330
   geriatric depression and, 68
   neurobiology of, 310–312
   stages of change in, **306**
Alcoholics Anonymous (AA), 228, 309,
   323
Alexithymia, 6
Allostasis, 25

Alogia, 133
Alzheimer Disease Assessment Scale
   (ADAS), 80
Alzheimer's disease
   chronic depression as risk factor for,
      91
   differential diagnosis of dementia
      and, 80
   neurotrophins and, 75
American Diabetes Association, 160
American Psychiatric Association, 160,
   167
American Psychological Association,
   427
American With Disabilities Act, 263
Amphetamines
   agitation and abuse of, 223, **224,**
      226, **227,** 228
   attention-deficit/hyperactivity
      disorder and, 344
   mood instability and, 122, 123
Amygdala, and stress, 26–27
Anaclitic depression, 284
Anger, and psychodynamics of
   depression, 293, 295, 296
Anhedonia, 6, 133
Animal models
   of attachment, 284–286
   of depression, 74
   of stress, 26, 27–28
Anonymity, as psychoanalytic
   principle, 67, 69
Anorexia nervosa, 109, 110
Anosognosia, 152
Anterior cingulate cortex (ACC), and
   schizophrenia, 143
Anticipatory guidance, and supportive
   psychotherapy, 48
Antidepressants. *See also* Selective
   serotonin reuptake inhibitors;
   Tricyclic antidepressants
   attention-deficit/hyperactivity
      disorder and, 344
   brain changes in depression and, 28
   depression in medically ill and, 72

double depression and, 35–38, 54,
56
geriatric depression and, 89
hypomania and, 377
suicidality in adolescents and, 287
Antipsychotics. *See also* Atypical
antipsychotics; Second-generation
antipsychotics
agitation and, 230
delirium and, 177
geriatric depression and, 90
mood instability and, 123
schizophrenia and, 152–153,
154–155
Antisocial personality disorder, 343
Anxiety. *See also* Anxiety disorders
alcohol abuse, 300, 303, 304,
305–312, 330
cognitive-behavioral therapy,
315–319
countertransference, 332–336
double depression, 19
exam failure, 427
family psychiatric history, 301
initial case presentation, 299–300
mental status exam, 301
panic-focused psychodynamic
psychotherapy, 319–327
personal history, 300
personal psychiatric history, 300
psychopharmacology, 313–315
sexual abuse, 328–336
terminal illness, 192
Anxiety cycle, 323–324
Anxiety disorders. *See also* Anxiety
adults with ADHD and, 343
diagnosis of, 302–304
meditation and, 406
Apathy, and schizophrenia, 133
Aripiprazole, 153
Aristotle, 360
Art, and schizophrenia, 149–151
Asian Americans, and cultural issues,
398–401
Asperger, Hans, 358

Asperger's syndrome, 339, 357, 358, 359
Assertive community treatment (ACT),
164–165
Assessment, of suicide risk in case of
double depression, 9–12. *See also*
Diagnosis; Evaluation
Atomoxetine, 344
Attachment, neurobiology of, 283–286
Attention-deficit/hyperactivity disorder
(ADHD), and case study of
hypomania, 337, 341–345, 350,
356, 366, 373–374, 375
Attitudinal sources of meaning, **202,**
203
Atypical antipsychotics. *See also*
Antipsychotics
anxiety and, 308
bipolar disorder and, 348
schizophrenia and, 153
Atypical depression, 35
Autism, 338, 357–360
Autonomy
capacity and, 63, 64, 65
informed consent and, 235
Avoidant personality disorder, 303
Avolition, and schizophrenia, 133

Balint, Michael, 146
Basal ganglia, and obsessive-
compulsive disorder, 392
BDD (body dysmorphic disorder), 388,
389, 390, 395
BDI-II (Beck Depression Inventory–II),
80
BDNF (brain-derived neurotrophic
factor), and depression, 74, 75–76
Beautiful Mind, A (film), 135
Beck Depression Inventory-II (BDI-II),
80
Bedside testing, and geriatric
depression, 76–81
Behavioral analysis, and dialectical
behavior therapy, 114
Behavioral desensitization, and anxiety,
316

Behavior therapy, for depression, 427.
   See also Breathing techniques;
   Cognitive-behavioral therapy;
   Relaxation techniques
Beneficence
   capacity and, 63, 64, 65
   informed consent and, 236
Benzodiazepines
   anxiety and, 308, 314–315
   double depression and, 35
   PTSD symptoms and, 330
   schizophrenia and, 140
   terminal illness and delirium, 177
Benztropine
   agitation and, 214, 221
   schizophrenia and, 130, 155
Bereavement. *See also* Adolescent
   bereavement; Grief; Loss
   definition of, 264
   geriatric depression and, 82
Best interests standard, and capacity, 64
Biofeedback, 404
Bion, Wilfred, 209, 210
Bio-psycho-social-spiritual approach,
   to terminally ill patient, 209
Biopsychosocial evaluation, of agitation
   and substance abuse, 248
Biopsychosocial variables, and double
   depression in African American
   patient, 21
Bipolar depression, 347
Bipolar disorder. *See also* Hypomania
   comorbidity of adult ADHD and,
      375
   diagnosis in case of mood
      instability, 96–99, 118, 125
   differential diagnosis of double
      depression, 7
   DSM distinction between Axis I and
      II disorders, 106–108
   family psychiatric history in case of
      hypomania, 339–340, 345–348
   misdiagnosis of borderline
      personality disorder as, 99
   mood disorders and, 374–375

Bipolar I disorder, 346, 349, 377
Bipolar II disorder, 349, 377
Blessed Dementia Scale, 80
Bleuler, Eugen, 133, 134, 169
BMI (body mass index), 110
Body, and chronic depression, 28.
   See also Mind–body problem
Body dysmorphic disorder (BDD), 388,
   389, 390, 395
Body mass index (BMI), 110
Body scan meditation, 407
Borderline personality disorder (BPD)
   diagnosis in case of mood
      instability, 96–99, 118, 125
   dialectical behavior therapy for,
      113
   DSM distinction between Axis I and
      II disorders, 106–108
   psychopharmacology and, 121–122
   suicide attempts and, 114–115
Borderline personality organization
   (BPO), and mood instability,
   99–105
Boundary violations, 335
BPD. *See* Borderline personality
   disorder (BPD)
BPO (borderline personality
   organization), and mood
   instability, 99–105
Brain. *See also* Neurobiology
   adaptive plasticity and, 26–27
   alcohol abuse and, 312
   delirium and metabolism of, 176
   electroconvulsive therapy and
      stimulation of, 41–45
   neuroimaging studies of
      schizophrenia and, 141–145
   obsessive-compulsive disorder and,
      391–392
   stimulant abuse and, 228
Brain-derived neurotrophic factor
   (BDNF), and depression, 74,
   75–76
Breast cancer, 173, 179, 194, 195
Breathing techniques, 404, 405

Breuer, J., 329
Buddhism, 406
Bulimia nervosa, 109, 110, 122
Bulimic cycle, 110, **111**
Buprenorphine, **229**
Bupropion
    adolescent bereavement and, 288
    attention-deficit/hyperactivity
        disorder and, 344
    double depression and, 36, 37, 40
    eating disorders and, 122
    seizure disorders and, 36, 122
    sexual dysfunction and, 248
    substance dependence and, **229**
Buspirone, 288

c-AMP response element binding factor
    (CREB), 74
Cancer. *See also* Breast cancer; Terminal
    illness
    family medical history, 174
    genetic counseling and, 194–196
    terminal illness and, 179, 180
Capacity
    geriatric depression and refusal of
        treatment, 63–67, 68, 91
    informed consent and, 237
Carbamazepine, 348
Catecholamines, and stress, 25
CA3 pyramidal neurons, and stress,
    26
Caudate nucleus, and obsessive-
    compulsive disorder, 391
CBASP (Cognitive Behavioral Analysis
    System of Psychotherapy), 55–56
CDT. *See* Clock drawing test (CDT)
Centers for Disease Control and
    Prevention (CDC), 238
Central nervous system (CNS), and
    HIV, 241
Character traits, and difficult patient,
    193–194
Chart notes, 234–235. *See also*
    Documentation
Childhood trauma, 255, 304

Children. *See also* Age; Childhood
    trauma
    autism and, 359–360
    of same-sex couples, 376
Chlorpromazine, 153
Circadian rhythms, and bipolar
    disorder, 347
Clock drawing test (CDT)
    double depression and, 4, 10, 28
    geriatric depression and, 61, 64, 65,
        77, 80
    mood stability and, 95
    terminal illness and, 177
Clock genes, 347
Clomipramine, 322
Clonazepam
    anxiety and, 314, 323, 324, 332
    mood stability and, 94, 122–123
Closeness circle, 290
Clozapine, and schizophrenia, 140,
    154, 155, 160
CNS (central nervous system), and
    HIV, 241
Cocaine
    agitation and, 223, **224**, 225, 226,
        227, 228, 230, 234
    PTSD symptoms and, 330
Cognistat, 80
Cognitive Behavioral Analysis System
    of Psychotherapy (CBASP),
    55–56
Cognitive-behavioral therapy
    adolescent bereavement and, 267
    adults with attention-deficit/
        hyperactivity disorder and,
        344
    anxiety and, 315–319, 324
    for eating disorders, 111–112
    empirically validated treatments
        and, 427
    major depression and, 429
    medically ill depressed patient and,
        72
    schizophrenia and, 140, 156–159,
        164

Cognitive deficits. *See also* Cognitive-perceptual symptoms
  double depression and, 7, 8, 44
  geriatric depression and, 63–64, 77–80, 90
  schizophrenia and, 134, 170
Cognitive-educational therapy, for hypochondriasis, 389
Cognitive-perceptual symptoms, and borderline personality disorder, 122
Cognitive restructuring, and anxiety, 316
Cognitive therapy, and empirically validated treatments for depression, 427. *See also* Cognitive-behavioral therapy
Colon cancer, 195, 196
Combined treatment, for double depression, 56
Comorbidity
  of adult ADHD and bipolar disorder, 375
  of bipolar and borderline personality disorders, 107
  of substance abuse and PTSD, 330
Complementary medicine, and exam failure, 402–405
Compliance, and schizophrenia, 163. *See also* Nonadherence
Complicated bereavement, 82, 265, 266, 267
Comprehensive health care, and schizophrenia, 159–162
Compulsions, and obsessive-compulsive disorder, 390
Confidentiality, and adolescent bereavement, 270–271
Conflict, borderline patients and internal, 103
Conscientiousness, as dimension of personality, 107
Consultation-liaison psychiatry
  for agitation and substance abuse, 233–235
  terminal illness and, 206–207

Consumer movement, 165
Contingency management, 117, 229
Continuity of care, for geriatric depression, 86–87
Coordination of care, for geriatric depression, 87–88
Coping
  developmental age and, 265
  terminal illness and, 199
Cornell Dysthymia Rating Scale, 81
Coronary artery disease, and depression, 71, 72
Cortisol, and stress, 28
Countertransference. *See also* Therapeutic alliance; Transference
  adolescent bereavement and, 269, 272
  anxiety and, 326, 332–336
  couples therapy for double depression and, 53
  exam failure in medical student and, 401, 421, 434, 435, 436
  mood instability and, 125, 127
  terminal illness and difficult patient, 190
Couples therapy, and double depression, 49–53
Creative sources of meaning, **202,** 203
Creativity, and mental illness, 360–362
CREB (c-AMP response element binding factor), 74
Crystal methamphetamine, 225–226, **227,** 228, 230, 234
Culture
  African American patients and, 21–22, 23
  Asian American patients and, 398–401
  Dominican patients and, 276–279
  lesbianism and, 364
Cushing's syndrome, 28
Cyclothymia, 349
Cytochrome P450 (CYP), 39–40

Dark therapy, 356
Day treatment programs, 34

DBS (deep brain stimulation), 43, 44, 45

DBT (dialectical behavior therapy), for mood instability, 113–117

Death, and terminal illness, 185

Declaration of Helsinki, 236

Deep brain stimulation (DBS), 43, 44, 45

Defenses
anxiety and, 320–321, 324
borderline personality organization and, 102–103
exam failure in medical student and narcissistic, 393–398, 425
hypomania and, 365–366
mood instability and, 125
psychodynamics of depression and, 294

Delirium
agitation, substance abuse, and HIV infection, 233, 234, 241, 242, 252
post-ECT, 44
terminal illness and, 175–178, 181–183, 187, 189

Delusions
differentiating religious belief from, 199
geriatric depression and, 89–90
psychosis and, 134
schizophrenia and, 163

Dementia
comorbid HIV and hepatitis C, 242
delirium and, 177
geriatric depression and, 80, 90–91

Dementia praecox, 133, 346

Dementia Rating Scale (DRS), 80, 90

Denial
anxiety and, 320, 325
eating disorders and, 109, 112
hypomania and, 365

Dentate gyrus–CA3 system, and stress, 26

Dependence, and narcissistic disturbances, 396

Dependency, and hypomania, 368

Depression. *See also* Double depression; Geriatric depression; Major depression
Alzheimer's disease and chronic, 91
combined therapy for treatment-resistant, 56
exam failure and, 427
hypomania and, 368
neurotrophins and pathophysiology of, 73–74
psychodynamics of, 292–296
psychopharmacology for adolescents and, 286–289
psychotherapy and anaclitic style of, 428–429
rating scales for, 80–81
sleep disruptions and, 347
underdiagnosis of in minority groups, 23

Depression cycle, **295**

Depressive neurosis, 54

Depressive personality disorder, 16, 55

Depressive triad, 19–20

Devaluation
borderline personality organization and, 102–103
depression and, 294, 295

Development, and cultural issues, 278–279

Dextroamphetamine, 94

Diabetes
double depression and, 1, 3, 28, 44
geriatric depression and, 59, 61, 72
schizophrenia and, 161

Diagnosis. *See also* Assessment; Differential diagnosis; Evaluation
of adult ADHD, 342–343, 374
of agitation, 221
of anxiety disorders, 302–304
of bipolar spectrum disorders, 347
of delirium, 175–176
of double depression, 33
exam failure in medical student and, 390

Diagnosis (*continued*)
  misdiagnosis of borderline
    personality disorder as bipolar
    disorder, 99
  of mood instability, 96–99
  of schizophrenia, 169
  underdiagnosis of depression in
    minority groups, 23
  underdiagnosis of psychiatric illness
    in medical students, 383
Dialectical behavior therapy (DBT), for
  mood instability, 113–117
Diary of Anne Frank, 281
Diazepam, 35
Differential diagnosis. *See also* Diagnosis
  bipolar disorder and, 350
  delirium in case of terminal illness
    and, 175
  of HIV-associated neuropsychiatric
    disturbances, **240**
Difficult patient, and terminal illness,
  190–194
Disclosure, and informed consent,
  236–237
Dislocation, adolescent bereavement and
  psychological impact of, 273–276
Disorganized symptoms, of
  schizophrenia, 133, 141
Dissociation, and traumatic memories,
  330, 331, 334
Disulfiram, **229,** 309
DLPFC (dorsolateral prefrontal cortex),
  and schizophrenia, 142–143
DNR (Do Not Resuscitate) paperwork,
  205
Doctor–patient relationship. *See also*
  Therapeutic alliance
  management of suicidal patient and,
    12
  terminal illness and, 204–207
Documentation. *See also* Chart notes
  suicidality in case of double
    depression and, 13–14
  suicide risk in case of mood stability
    and, 119–120

Dominican Republic, and culture in
  case of adolescent bereavement,
  276–279
Do Not Resuscitate (DNR) paperwork,
  205
Dopamine system
  models of schizophrenia and, 170, 171
  obsessive-compulsive disorder and,
    392
Dorsolateral prefrontal cortex
  (DLPFC), and schizophrenia,
  142–143
Double depression
  African American patients and,
    21–24
  couples therapy and, 49–53
  definition of psychiatry and, 29–32
  electroconvulsive therapy, 40–45
  family psychiatric history, 3
  geriatric depression and, 90
  initial presentation, 1–2
  inpatient psychiatry, 32–34
  interviews, 18–21
  medical history, 3
  mental status exam, 3–4, 10
  neurobiology of stress and, 24–29
  personal history, 2–3
  personal psychiatric history, 3
  pharmacogenomics and, 35, 38–40
  psychodynamic formulation and,
    14–17
  psychopharmacology, 34–38, 54–55
  suicide attempts, 1, 8, 9–14, 43–44
  summary of case, 53–57
  supportive psychotherapy, 45–49
  symptoms and evaluation, 5–9
Dreams, and exam failure in medical
  student, 408–409, 412, 431, 433,
  435–436
Drospirenone, 354
DRS (Dementia Rating Scale), 80, 90
Drug–drug interactions, and geriatric
  depression, 87
Drug seeking, and pain medications,
  182

DSM system, and distinction between Axis I and Axis II, 106–108
DSM-IV
  borderline personality disorder and, 100
  eating disorders and, 109
  premenstrual dysphoric disorder and, 352
DSM-IV-TR
  attention-deficit/hyperactivity disorder and, 343–344
  bipolar spectrum disorders and, 346
  borderline personality disorder and, 97
  cultural formulation in, 398
  duration of bereavement and, 266
  manic episode and, 97
  obsessive-compulsive disorder and, 390
  posttraumatic stress disorder and, 328
  premenstrual dysphoric disorder and, **352**
DTR (*Dysfunctional Thought Record, The*), 317
Dubuffet, Jean, 149
Duloxetine, 36
Duration, of symptoms of depression, 7
Dusk-to-dawn simulation, and light therapy, 356–357
Dyads, and object relations theory, 100, 333–334
Dysfunctional Thought Record, The (DTR), 317
Dysthymia, 6, 10, 55
Dysthymic disorder, 54, 82

Eating disorders, and mood instability, 108–113, 122
ECT. *See* Electroconvulsive therapy (ECT)
EEG (electroencephalogram), and delirium, 177
Efference copy, and frontal cortex, 144

Efficacy, and studies of treatment effectiveness, 428
Ego, and psychodynamic therapy, 146, 372. *See also* Superego
Electroconvulsive therapy (ECT)
  BDNF transcription and, 74
  double depression and, 40–45
  treatment-resistant depression and, 73
Electroencephalogram (EEG), and delirium, 177
Electronic medical records, 87
Emergency room (ER). *See also* Psychiatric emergency department
  mood instability and, 93–94, 113–117, 124–127
  schizophrenia and, 129
Emotionally disturbed person, 213, 220, 250
Empathy
  interview with double depression patient and, 20–21
  psychotherapy for exam failure in medical student and, 410, 413–415, 417
Empirically validated treatments (EVTs), 427, 430
Endocrinological derangements, and HIV infection, 242
Engel, George, 31, 273
Environment
  development of depression and, 7–8
  inpatient psychiatry and, 32
Envy, and narcissistic disturbances, 397–398, 424–425
Epidemiology. *See* Prevalence
Epilepsy, and prevalence of psychoses, 143
Epinephrine, **227**
EPS (extrapyramidal signs and symptoms), 152
ER. *See* Emergency room (ER)
Erectile dysfunction, 246, 247–248
Erikson, Erik, 208, 296, 363–364

Ethics
  consultation and, 206–207
  schools and expulsion of students
    with suicidal ideation,
    261–264
Ethnic identity, 399
Euthymia, 48, 71
Evaluation. *See also* Assessment;
  Diagnosis
  of agitation in emergency patient,
    219–225, 248
  exam failure in medical student and
    extended, 408–409
Evidence-based psychotherapy, and
  exam failure in medical student,
  426–430
EVTs (empirically validated treatments), 427, 430
Exam failure
  complementary medicine and
    integrative pharmacology,
    402–405
  cultural issues for Asian Americans,
    398–401
  diagnosis and, 390
  empathy in psychotherapy,
    413–415, 417
  evidence-based psychotherapy,
    426–430
  extended evaluation, 408–409
  initial presentation, 379–380
  interviews, 382–386
  Kohut/Kernberg controversy,
    421–426
  mental status exam, 381
  mindfulness meditation, 405–407
  narcissistic injury and defenses,
    393–398
  neurobiology of obsessions,
    391–393
  obsessive-compulsive disorder, 390,
    391
  personal history, 380
  personal psychiatric history, 381
  self-defeating patient, 431–433

self psychology, 416–421
somatoform disorders and
  obsessionality, 387–389
summary of case, 434–437
therapeutic zeal and, 410–412
Existential psychiatry, 167
Existential suffering, and pain of
  terminal illness, 200–203
Experiential sources of meaning, **202,**
  203
Exposure treatment, 427
Extrapyramidal signs and symptoms
  (EPS), 152
Extraversion, and dimensions of
  personality, 107
Extrinsic religiosity, 197

False submission, and hospitalization,
  117
Familial pattern, of cancer, 194
Family. *See also* Family medical history;
  Family psychiatric history; Family
  therapy; Parents
  autism and, 357–360
  coordination of care for geriatric
    depression and, 88
  cultural issues and patient from
    Dominican Republic, 277, 278
  difficult patient and, 192
  eating disorders and, 112
  genetic counseling for cancer and,
    194–196
  meetings of, 187–188
  terminal illness and, 186–190, 192,
    210–211
Family focused grief therapy (FFGT),
  189
Family medical history, and terminal
  illness case, 174
Family psychiatric history
  anxiety and, 301
  double depression and, 3
  geriatric depression and, 61
  hypomania and, 339–340, 375–376
  schizophrenia and, 131

Family therapy, for schizophrenia, 164
FDA (Food and Drug Administration), 41, 42, 121, **229**, 286, 288, 344
FFGT (family focused grief therapy), 189
FGAs. *See* First-generation antipsychotics (FGAs)
Filial attachment, 284
First-generation antipsychotics (FGAs), and schizophrenia, 153. *See also* Antipsychotics
Five Factor Model, and personality dimensions, 107–108
Fluoxetine
depression in adolescents and, 286–287, 288
double depression and, 2, 35, 36
eating disorders and, 112
mood instability and, 94, 122, 123
Focal brain stimulation, 41
Focused therapy, and double depression, 11, 55–56
Food and Drug Administration (FDA), 41, 42, 121, **229**, 286, 288, 344
Formulation, and cognitive-behavioral therapy, 157–158
Frank, Anne, 281
Frankl, Victor, 201
Freud, Sigmund, 136, 146, 283, 293, 329, 369
Frontotemporal networks, and schizophrenia, 144
Functional impairment, and double depression, 7

GABA (gamma-aminobutyric acid), 310–312
Gabapentin, 315
gamma-aminobutyric acid (GABA), 310–312
Gender, and diagnosis of ADHD, 343
Gender identity, 244
Gender roles, and culture, 277, 278
Genetic counseling, and cancer, 194–196

Genetics. *See also* Pharmacogenomics
attachment and, 285
family history of depression and, 7
neurotrophins and, 75–76
obsessive-compulsive disorder and, 391
schizophrenia and, 136
Geriatric depression
bedside testing and, 76–81
capacity and, 63–67, 91
family psychiatric history, 61
initial presentation, 59–60
interpersonal psychotherapy, 81–84
medical history, 61
medical illness, 70–73
mental status exam, 61
neurotrophins, 73–76
personal history, 60–61
personal psychiatric history, 61
psychiatric attitude, 67–70
service delivery, 85–88
summary of case, 88–91
Geriatric Depression Scale, 81
Glucocorticoids, and stress, 25
Glucose regulation, and stress, 28
Glutamatergic model, of schizophrenia, 170–171
Glutamatergic-serotonergic neurotransmission, and obsessive-compulsive disorder, 392
Graded hierarchy, and anxiety, **318**, 324
Grandiosity, and exam failure in medical student, 395, 396, 397, 419
Green, Michael, 134
Greenacre, Phyllis, 360
Grief. *See also* Adolescent bereavement; Bereavement; Loss
definition of, 264
geriatric depression and, 82
terminal illness and, 189
Group therapy, and dialectical behavior therapy, 114

HAART (highly active antiretroviral therapy), 241–242

HAD (HIV-associated dementia), 241

Hallucinations, and schizophrenia, 156, 157

Haloperidol
agitation and, 214, 221
schizophrenia and, 130, 136, 152, 154, 155, 160

Hamilton Rating Scale for Depression (Ham-D), 80–81, 83, 84, 355

Harm reduction model, and substance abuse, 228

Hatha yoga, 407

Health care. *See also* Medical conditions; Medical history
proxies for decision making on, 64, 205–206
schizophrenia and comprehensive, 159–162
status of patient and, 192–193
training of physicians and, 204–205, 206

Healthy families, 210–211

Heart disease, and depression, 71–72

Heinroth, Johann Christian August, 29–30

Hepatitis C, and substance abuse, 242

Herbal medications, 402–403

Highly active antiretroviral therapy (HAART), 241–242

Hippocampus
depression and, 74
schizophrenia and, 143–144
stress and, 26, 27, 28

Hippocrates, 121

Historical sources of meaning, **202**

HIV/AIDS, and agitation, 230–231, 238–243, 248, 252, 255

HIV-associated dementia (HAD), 241

HIV-associated minor cognitive motor disorder (MCMD), 241

Home health care, and geriatric depression, 86

Homelessness, and schizophrenia, 165–168

Homosexuality
agitation and substance abuse, 230, 235, 243–248
hypomania and, 338, 342, 362–369, 376

Hopefulness, and recovery from schizophrenia, 162

Hopelessness, as risk factor for suicide, 10

Hospice care, 206

Hospitalist movement, 206

Hospitalization
for eating disorders, 109, 110
management of suicidal patients and, 12
mood instability and, 117, 126
schizophrenia and, 163
terminal illness and psychodynamics of, 207–212

Hostile families, 188, 210, 211

HPA. *See* Hypothalamic-pituitary-adrenal (HPA) axis

Hyperactive delirium, 177

Hyperglutamatergic model, of obsessive-compulsive disorder, 392

Hypertension, and double depression case, 1, 3, 36, 44

Hypoactive delirium, 177

Hypochondriasis, and exam failure in medical student, 387–388, 389, 395, 431

Hypomania
attention deficit disorder, 337, 341–345
bipolar spectrum disorders, 345–351
creativity and mental illness, 360–362
family psychiatric history, 339–340, 357–360, 375–376
initial presentation, 337–339
lesbianism, 338, 342, 362–369, 376

mental status exam, 340, 349
personal history, 339
personal psychiatric history, 339
premenstrual dysphoria, 350,
    352–354
psychodynamic psychotherapy,
    369–372
sleep disruptions, 354–357
summary of case, 373–378
Hypothalamic-pituitary-adrenal (HPA)
    axis
complicated bereavement and, 266
stress response system and, 268,
    403
Hypothalamus, and bipolar disorder,
    347
Hypothyroidism, 7
Hysteresis, 274

ICU psychosis, 178
Idealization
    borderline personality organization
        and, 102–103
    depression and, 294, 295
    exam failure in medical student and,
        395, 396, 418–419, 422, 424
Identity
    Asian American patient and cultural
        or ethnic, 398–399
    borderline personality organization
        and diffusion of, 102, 103
    homosexuality and, 245
Imipramine, 54, 315
Immigration, and restructuring of
    identity, 399, 400–401
Implied consent, 238
Impulsive–behavioral dyscontrol, and
    borderline personality disorder,
    122
Impulsivity, and borderline personality
    disorder, 108
Incident pain, 182, 183
Informed consent, and agitation in
    psychiatric emergency
    department, 235–239

Inpatient psychiatry, and double
    depression, 32–34. *See also*
    Hospitalization
Insight-oriented psychotherapy, and
    exam failure in medical student,
    389, 410–415
Insomnia, and depression in medically
    ill, 71. *See also* Sleep
Interdisciplinary treatment, and
    inpatient psychiatry, 33
Internal State Scale, 350
Interpersonal deficits, 82
Interpersonal inventory, 83, 290
Interpersonal psychotherapy (IPT)
    adolescent bereavement and,
        289–292
    bipolar disorder and, 351
    empirically validated treatments for
        depression and, 427
    geriatric depression and, 81–84
    major depression and, 429
    medically ill depressed patient and,
        72
Interviews. *See also* Motivational
    interviewing
    adolescent bereavement and, 269–
        272
    agitation in psychiatric emergency
        department and, 220–221, 223
    double depression and, 18–21
    exam failure in medical school
        student and, 382–386
Intoxication, and stimulant abuse,
    225–226
Intrinsic religiosity, 197
Introjective depression, 429
IPT. *See* Interpersonal psychotherapy
    (IPT)
Irony, as psychoanalytic concept, 70

Jackson, John Hughlings, 30
James, Henry, 209

Kanner, Leo, 357, 358
Kernberg, Otto, 421–426

Klein, Melanie, 146, 209–210
Kohut, Heinz, 418, 421–426
Kraepelin, Emil, 31, 133, 134, 136, 168, 169, 346
Kubler-Ross, Elisabeth, 208

Laboratory tests, and extent of alcohol abuse, 306
Lamotrigine, 348
Lavender aromatherapy, 403
Legal issues. *See* Capacity; Informed consent; Malpractice
Lesbianism. *See* Homosexuality
Life events, and interpersonal psychotherapy approach to depression, 82
Life inventory, and terminal illness, 208–209
Life narrative, and terminal illness, 185
Light therapy, and sleep disruptions, 356–357
Lithium
adolescent bereavement and, 288
bipolar disorder and, 347–348
Locke, John, 342
Lorazepam
agitation and, 214, 221
anxiety and, 315
Loss. *See also* Bereavement; Grief
early intervention to prevent psychopathology, 267
forced displacement and, 276

Magnetic resonance imaging (MRI), 42
Magnetic seizure therapy (MST), 42–43, 45
Maintenance treatment, and interpersonal psychotherapy for geriatric depression, 84
Major depression
diagnosis of, 55
medical illness in geriatric patient and, 70, 71, 82, 89

treatment studies comparing cognitive-behavioral and interpersonal psychotherapy for, 429
Major depressive disorder, 6
Malpractice
difficult patient and, 192
documentation of suicide risk and, 119–120
Management, of suicidal patient, 12–13
MAOIs. *See* Monoamine oxidase inhibitors (MAOIs)
Marriage, and couples therapy in case of double depression, 49–53
Maturation, and adolescent bereavement, 296
MBSR (mindfulness-based meditation stress reduction), 405–407
MCMD. *See* HIV-associated minor cognitive motor disorder (MCMD)
Meaning-centered therapy, and terminal illness, 200–203
Medial prefrontal cortex, and stress, 27
Medial temporal lobe, and schizophrenia, 143–144, 145
Medical conditions. *See also* Cancer; Diabetes; Health care; HIV/AIDS; Medical history; Terminal illness; Treatment refusal
agitation in psychiatric emergency department and, 221, 223
geriatric depression and, 70–73
psychosis and, 134
rates of in schizophrenia patients, 160
Medical history. *See also* Family medical history; Medical conditions
double depression and, 3
geriatric depression and, 61
terminal illness and, 174
Medical school, and exam failure in student, 382–386, 414–415
Medicare, 206

Medications. *See also* Psychopharmacology
  geriatric depression in medically ill
    patient and, 87–88
  HIV/AIDS and, 241–242
  substance dependence and, **229**
Meditation, and exam failure in
  medical student, 405–407
Meet-and-greet, and psychiatric
  emergency department, 218
Mental status exam
  adolescent bereavement and, 259
  agitation and, 231–232
  anxiety and, 301
  double depression and, 3–4, 10
  exam failure and, 381, 396
  geriatric depression and, 61
  hypomania and, 340, 349
  mood stability and, 95
  schizophrenia and, 131
  terminal illness and, 174, 180
Metabolic encephalopathy, 178
Methadone, **229**
Methylphenidate, 344
Meyer, Adolph, 31
Mind–body problem, in development
  of psychiatry, 30
Mindfulness-based meditation stress
  reduction (MBSR), 405–407
Mini-Mental State Examination (MMSE)
  double depression and, 4, 10, 28, 44
  geriatric depression and, 61, 64, 65,
    77, **78–79**, 80
  hypomania and, 350
  mood stability and, 95
  terminal illness and, 177, 180
Minnesota Multiphasic Personality
  Inventory, 81
Mirroring, and selfobject transference,
  418–419, 422
Mirtazapine, 288
MMSE. *See* Mini-Mental State
  Examination (MMSE)
Modafinil, 226, 344
Moderation management, and
  substance abuse, 228

Monoamine oxidase inhibitors
  (MAOIs)
  adolescent bereavement and, 288
  attention-deficit/hyperactivity
    disorder and, 344
  BDNF transcription and, 74
  mood instability and, 122
  social anxiety and, 315
Monoamine system, and stress, 24
Mood disorders, in adults with ADHD,
  343, 374
Mood instability
  borderline personality organization,
    99–105
  diagnosis in case of, 96–99
  dialectical behavior therapy and,
    113–117
  DSM distinction between Axis I and
    Axis II, 106–108
  eating disorders, 108–113
  initial presentation, 93–94
  mental status exam, 95
  personal history, 94
  personal psychiatric history, 95
  psychopharmacology and, 121–124
  risk management, 118–120
  suicide threats, 93, 95, 103, 105,
    107, 114–115, 117, 118–120,
    125–126
  summary of case, 124–127
Mood stabilizers. *See also* Lithium
  bipolar disorder and, 348
  eating disorders and, 112
  schizophrenia and, 155
Morphine, 182–183
Mortality, and depression in medically
  ill, 72
Motivational interviewing
  anxiety and alcohol abuse, 307
  schizophrenia and, 163, 164
  substance abuse and, 228–229
Mourning, and attachment, 283
MRI (magnetic resonance imaging), 42
MST (magnetic seizure therapy),
  42–43, 45

Naltrexone, **229**, 309
NAMI (National Alliance on Mental
    Illness), 162, 165
Narcissism and narcissistic personality
    disorder, and exam failure in
    medical student, 393–398, 416,
    421, 423, 424, 425–426, 433
Nash, John, 135
National Alliance on Mental Illness
    (NAMI), 162, 165
National Comorbidity Study, 375
National Institute of Mental Health, 56
Nature–nurture question, 30–31
Negative expressed emotion, and
    schizophrenia, 135
Negative feedback strategies, and
    schizophrenia, 140
Negative symptoms, of schizophrenia,
    133–134
Nerve growth factor (NGF), 74–75
Neurobiology. *See also* Brain;
    Neurotransmitters
    of attachment, 283–286
    of obsessions, 391–393
    of schizophrenia, 141–145
    of stress, 24–29
    of violent behavior in
        schizophrenia, 139
Neurogenesis, and alcohol abuse, 312
Neuroimaging, and brain circuitry in
    schizophrenia, 141–145
Neuroleptic malignant syndrome, 176
Neurological disorders, and secondary
    depression, 71
Neuromodulation, and
    electroconvulsive therapy, 41
Neuropsychiatric complications, of
    HIV/AIDS, 240, 241
Neuroticism
    dimensions of personality and, 107,
        108
    geriatric depression and, 76
Neurotransmitters. *See also* Dopamine
    system; Serotonin system
    alcohol abuse and, 310

obsessive-compulsive disorder and,
    392
Neurotrophins, and geriatric
    depression, 73–76
Neutrality
    adolescent bereavement and, 270
    as psychoanalytic principle, 67, 68
New York, and psychiatric disorders in
    homeless populations, 167
NGF (nerve growth factor), 74–75
Nicotine, **229**
NMDA (*N*-methyl-D-aspartate), 310–312
Nonadherence. *See also* Compliance
    double depression and, 36
    medications for geriatric depression
        and, 87
Norepinephrine, **227**
Nuremberg Code, 236

Objective reality, and self psychology,
    421
Object relations theory
    anxiety and sexual abuse, 333–334
    borderline personality organization
        and, 100
    hospital-based psychotherapies and,
        207
Obsessions and obsessionality, and
    exam failure in medical student,
    387–389, 391–393
Obsessive-compulsive disorder (OCD),
    and exam failure in medical
    student, 390, 391
Olanzapine
    mood instability and, 112
    schizophrenia and, 154
Opioids, and terminal illness, 176, 177,
    179, 182
Oral contraceptives, and premenstrual
    dysphoric disorder, 353, 354
Orbitofrontal cortex, and obsessive-
    compulsive disorder, 391
Outsider art, 149–151
Ovarian cancer, 195, 196
Oxycodone, 182–183

Pain and pain medications, and
terminal illness, 177, 178–179,
181–183, 184, 191–192, 200–203
Palliative care, and terminal illness,
186
Panic
anxiety and attacks of, 303, 313
panic cycle, **317**
psychodynamic psychotherapy for,
319–327
Paranoid-type schizophrenia, 169–170
Parasympathetic nervous system, and
stress, 25, 404
Parents, traumatic grief and death of,
266. *See also* Family
Paroxetine, 314
Partial hospitalization, 34
Passive aggression, 294
Patient history. *See* Family psychiatric
history; Medical history; Personal
history; Personal psychiatric
history
Patient types, and evaluation in
psychiatric emergency
department, **222–223**
Pattern recognition, and agitation,
222–223
PDD (pervasive developmental
disorder), 357–359
Psychiatric emergency department
(PED)
Perfectionism, and exam failure in
medical student, 393–394, 395,
396, 397
Peripheral vascular disease, and
geriatric depression, 61, 89
Personal history
adolescent bereavement and, 258
agitation and, 231
anxiety and, 300
double depression and, 2–3
exam failure and, 380
geriatric depression and, 60–61
hypomania and, 339
mood stability and, 94

schizophrenia and, 130
terminal illness and, 173
Personality. *See also* Personality
disorders; Split personality
borderline personality organization
and, 100–103
Five Factor Model of dimensions,
107–108
internalized homophobia and, 244
rating scales and, 81
Personality Assessment Inventory, 81
Personality disorders
differential diagnosis of double
depression and, 7, 54
overlapping diagnoses of major
depression, substance abuse,
and, 10
Personal psychiatric history
adolescent bereavement and, 259
agitation and, 231
anxiety and, 300
double depression and, 3
exam failure and, 381
geriatric depression and, 61
hypomania and, 339
mood stability and, 95
schizophrenia and, 130
Pervasive developmental disorder
(PDD), 357–359
PET (positron emission tomography),
141
Pharmacodynamics, 39
Pharmacogenomics, and double
depression, 35, 38–40
Pharmacokinetics, 38–39
Place, sense of, 273–274, 275
PMDD (premenstrual dysphoric
disorder), 350, 352–354, 356,
375
PMS (premenstrual syndrome), 352,
353, 375
Police, and psychiatric emergency
department, 213, 217, 219–220
Polymorphisms, and
pharmacogenetics, 39

Polypharmacy
  bipolar disorder and borderline
    personality disorder, 98
  terminal illness and, 176
Positive symptoms, of schizophrenia,
  133
Positron emission tomography (PET),
  141
Posttraumatic stress disorder (PTSD)
  anxiety and alcohol abuse, 304, 313,
    328–329, 331
  comorbidity with substance abuse,
    330
  traumatic grief and, 265–266
Prefrontal cortex
  schizophrenia and, 142–143
  stress and, 27
Pregabalin, 315
Premenstrual dysphoric disorder
  (PMDD), 350, 352–354, 356, 375
Premenstrual syndrome (PMS), 352,
  353, 375
Prevalence
  of bipolar spectrum disorders, 346
  of depression in general population,
    6
  of depression in medically ill, 71
  of HIV infection, 240
  of premenstrual dysphoric disorder,
    353
  of psychosis in epilepsy patients,
    143
  of violence in schizophrenia, 138
Primary prevention, of cancer, 195
Prinzhorn, Hans, 149–150, 151
Problem list, and cognitive-behavioral
  therapy for schizophrenia, **158**
Problem-solving therapy, for geriatric
  depression, 90
Prodrome, and schizophrenia, 135
Prostate cancer, 195, 196
Proxy, and medical decisions, 64,
  205–206
Pseudo-addiction, 182
Pseudodementia, 91

Psychiatric attitude, and geriatric
  depression, 67–70
Psychiatric emergency department
  (PED). *See also* Emergency room
  case of agitation and, 213–214
  evaluation of patients in, 219–225
  management of multiple patients in,
    215–219
Psychiatry, definition of, 29–32
Psychodynamic(s) and psychodynamic
  therapy
  anxiety and panic-focused, 319–327
  consultation in case of terminal
    illness and, 183–186
  depression in adolescents and,
    292–296
  depression in medically ill and, 72
  formulation of double depression
    and, 14–17
  hospitals and terminal illness,
    207–212
  hypomania and, 369–372, 377–378
  psychosis and, 146–148
Psychodynamic Diagnostic Manual
  (Alliance of Psychoanalytic
  Organizations 2006), 16
Psychoeducation
  adults with attention-deficit/
    hyperactivity disorder and, 345
  anxiety disorders and, 315–316
  delirium in case of terminal illness
    and, 178
  double depression and, 37
  genetic counseling for cancer and, 195
Psychomotor poverty, and
  schizophrenia, 141
Psychopharmacology. *See also*
  Antidepressants; Antipsychotics;
  Medications; Mood stabilizers;
  Polypharmacy; Side effects
  anxiety and, 313–315
  Asian American patients and
    cultural issues, 400
  complementary medicine and
    integrative, 402–405

depression in adolescents and, 286–289

double depression and, 34–38, 54–55

eating disorders and, 112

management of suicidality and, 13

mood instability and, 121–124

schizophrenia and, 130, 139–140, 151–155

substance abuse and, 229

Psychosis

pharmacologic models of, 170–171

psychodynamics of, 146–148

schizophrenia and, 134

Psychosocial interventions, for delirium in terminal illness case, 178

Psychotherapy. *See also* Cognitive-behavioral therapy; Dialectical behavior therapy; Insight-oriented psychotherapy; Interpersonal psychotherapy; Meaning-centered therapy; Psychodynamic(s) and psychodynamic therapy; Supportive psychotherapy

adults with attention-deficit/hyperactivity disorder and, 344

anxiety and alcohol abuse, 308

exam failure in medical student and evidence-based, 426–430

hospital-based, 207–212

for medically ill depressed patient, 72

schizophrenia and, 140

selection of methods in case of agitation and substance abuse, 251–254

Psychotic depression, 89–90

PTSD. *See* Posttraumatic stress disorder (PTSD)

Quetiapine, 308, 324

Racism, and African American patients, 22–23

Rainman (film), 359

Randomized controlled trial (RCT), 430

Rapid neuroleptization, of antipsychotics, 154

RBANS (Repeatable Battery for the Assessment of Neuropsychological Status), 80

RCT (randomized controlled trial), 430

Reaction formation

adolescent bereavement and, 294

anxiety and, 320, 325

Reactive oxygen species (ROS), 312

Reality distortion, and schizophrenia, 141, 143

Reasonable person standard, 236–237

Recovery, from schizophrenia, 162–165

Rehabilitation, and geriatric depression, 84, 87

Rehabilitation Act, Section 504, 263

Reil, Johann Christian, 29–30

Relapse

cognitive-behavioral therapy for schizophrenia and prevention of, 159

electroconvulsive therapy and prevention of in double depression, 44

recovery from schizophrenia and, 163

substance abuse and, 228–230

Relaxation techniques, and anxiety, 316, 324

Religion. *See also* Buddhism; Spirituality

African American patients and, 23

Dominican patients and, 277, 278

homophobia and, 245

risk factors for suicide and, 10

terminal illness and, 197, **198**, 199

Remission, and antidepressants, 35

Repeatable Battery for the Assessment of Neuropsychological Status (RBANS), 80

Repression, and defense mechanisms, 320, 325, 365

Response rate, to antidepressants, 35
Restraints, and agitation in psychiatric
   emergency department, 221
Rhodiola rosea, 403
Risk factors
   for suicide, 9–10, 126
   for violence in schizophrenia, 138
Risk management, for mood stability,
   118–120
Risperidone
   mood instability and, 94, 122, 123
   schizophrenia and, 154
Role playing
   interpersonal psychotherapy and,
     290–291
   social anxiety and, 318
Role transitions, and interpersonal
   psychotherapy, 82, 289, 291.
   See also Gender roles
ROS (reactive oxygen species), 312

SAD (social anxiety disorder), 303, 315
S-adenosylmethionine (SAM-e), 403
Safety
   delirium and, 177
   depressed adolescents and, 290
   double depression and suicide, 9, 12
   psychiatric emergency department
     and, 216, 220
   violence in schizophrenia patients
     and, 138
SAM-e (*S*-adenosylmethionine), 403
St. John's wort, 403
Salgo v. Stanford University (1957), 236
Schelling, Friedrich, 29
Schizophrenia
   autism and, 358
   cognitive-behavioral therapy,
     156–159, 164
   comprehensive health care, 159–162
   diagnostic concept and description
     of, 133–137
   family psychiatric history, 131
   homelessness and social history,
     165–168

initial presentation, 129
mental status exam, 131
neuroimaging and brain circuitry,
   141–145
outsider art, 149–151
personal history, 130
personal psychiatric history,
   130
psychodynamics of psychosis and,
   146–148
psychopharmacology, 130,
   139–140, 151–155
recovery from, 162–165
substance abuse, 130, 134, 135,
   138–139, 167
summary of case, 168–172
violence and, 130, 135, 137–140
Schloendorff v. Society of New York
   Hospital (1914), 236
Schneider, Kurt, 133, 134
Schools, and expulsion of students
   with suicidal ideation, 261–264
Schumann, Robert, 361
SCN (suprachiasmatic nucleus), and
   bipolar disorder, 347
Seasonal affective disorder, 357
Secondary prevention, of cancer, 196
Second-generation antipsychotics
   (SGAs). *See also* Antipsychotics
   mood instability and, 123
   schizophrenia and, 153, 154–155
Selective serotonin reuptake inhibitors
   (SSRIs)
   adolescent bereavement and, 288
   anxiety and alcohol abuse, 308,
     313–314, 315
   BDNF transcription and, 74
   hypochondriasis or body
     dysmorphic disorder and,
     389
   mood instability and, 122
   obsessive-compulsive disorders and,
     391
   premenstrual dysphoric disorder
     and, 354

Self
borderline personality organization
and, 101–102, **104,** 105
Kohut's concept of grandiose, 422,
423–424
Self-criticism, and psychodynamics of
depression, 293–294, 295
Self-defeating patient, and exam failure
in medical student, 431–433
Self-empowerment, and recovery from
schizophrenia, 162
Self-esteem
double depression and, 47
exam failure and, 393–394
Self-injurious behavior. *See also* Suicide
and suicidal ideation
adolescent bereavement and, 259,
268, 272, 292, 295
bipolar disorder and, 107
borderline personality disorder and,
107, 114–115
mood instability and, 116–117
Self-medication hypothesis, and
substance abuse, 139
Selfobject, and transference, 418–421, 422
Self-portraits, and case study of
schizophrenia, 150, 164
Self-psychology, and exam failure in
medical student, 416–421
Self-report(s), about sleep, 355
Self-Report Manic Inventory, 350
Serotonin-norepinephrine reuptake
inhibitors (SNRIs)
anxiety and, 314, 315
BDNF transcription and, 74
eating disorders and, 112
mood stability and, 122
Serotonin syndrome, 176
Serotonin system
obsessive-compulsive disorder and,
392
pharmacodynamics and, 39
schizophrenia and, 170, 171
suicidal behavior and abnormalities
in, 268, 269

Sertraline
anxiety and, 323, 324
depression in adolescents and, 287
depression in medically ill and, 72
double depression and, 2, 36, 54
Service delivery, and geriatric
depression, 85–88
Severity of illness, and inpatient
psychiatry, 32
Sexual abuse, and anxiety, 326, 327,
328–336
Sexual fantasies, 244, 245
Sexuality. *See also* Homosexuality
adolescent bereavement and,
271–272, 297
agitation and substance abuse,
246–248
couples therapy for double
depression and, 52
hypomania and relationships,
366–369
safe sex and, 245–246
SGAs. *See* Second-generation
antipsychotics (SGAs)
Shame, and cultural issues, 400
Sick role, and interpersonal
psychotherapy, 83, 290
Side effects, of pharmacology
of antipsychotics, 152–153
bupropion and, 36, 40
HAART medications and, 242
Sign-out, from psychiatric emergency
department, 216–218
Sildenafil, 248
Single-nucleotide polymorphism
(SNP), and genetics of depression,
75–76
Sliding scale of capacity, 65
Skills training group, 114
Sleep. *See also* Insomnia
depression and disruptions of,
347
hypomania and, 338, 346–347,
354–357, 375
Sleep polysomnography, 356

SNP (single-nucleotide polymor-
  phism), and genetics of depres-
  sion, 75–76
SNRIs. *See* Serotonin-norepinephrine
  reuptake inhibitors (SNRIs)
SNS (sympathetic nervous system),
  and stress response, 403, 404
Social anxiety disorder (SAD), 303, 315
Social history, and schizophrenia,
  165–168
Social networks, and forced
  displacement, 273, 274
Social phobia, 303
Social rhythm therapy, 351
Social skills training, 318
Social support, and depressive
  symptoms in African Americans, 8
Somatization, and anxiety, 320
Somatoform disorders, and exam
  failure in medical student,
  387–389, 402, 416
Sources of meaning, and meaning-
  centered therapy, **202**
Spirituality. *See also* Religion
  recovery from schizophrenia and,
  162
  terminal illness and, 197–199
Split personality, and Jekyll and Hyde
  as metaphor, 249–251
Splitting
  borderline personality organization
  and, 101–102
  Kohut's concept of grandiose self
  and, 424
SPT. *See* Supportive psychotherapy
  (SPT)
SSRIs. *See* Selective serotonin reuptake
  inhibitors (SSRIs)
Stevens, Rosemary, 206
Stevenson, Robert Louis, 249–251
Still, George, 342
Stimulant abuse, 225–232
Stress. *See also* Life events
  exam failure in medical student and,
  384, 385, 386, 402, 403–404

neurobiology of, 24–29
psychiatric admission and, 34
schizophrenia and, 156
Stress inoculation training, 427
Stroop Color-Word Test, 90
Substance abuse. *See also* Alcohol
  abuse
  adolescent bereavement and, 271
  adults with ADHD and, 343
  agitation in psychiatric emergency
    department and, 223, **224,**
    225–232, 233–235, 239–254
  comorbidity with PTSD, 330
  double depression and, 6–7, 10
  exam failure in medical student and,
    385
  HIV/AIDS and, 239–243
  informed consent and, 235–239
  pain medications for terminal
    illness and, 181–183
  schizophrenia and, 130, 134, 135,
    138–139, 167
Substance use–associated hypomania,
  349
Subthreshold symptoms, of
  schizophrenia, 163–164
Suggestion, in psychoanalysis, 68
Suicide and suicidal ideation. *See also*
  Self-injurious behavior
  adolescent bereavement and,
    267–269, 295
  antidepressants for adolescents and,
    287
  bipolar disorder and, 347, 351
  borderline personality disorder and,
    114–115
  double depression and, 1, 8, 9–14,
    43–44
  mood instability and, 93, 95, 103,
    105, 107, 114–115, 117,
    118–120, 125–126
  schizophrenia and rates of, 160
  schools and expulsion of students,
    261–264
Sullen families, 188–189, 210, 211

Superego, and object relations theory, 103

Supportive psychotherapy (SPT)
agitation, substance abuse, and HIV infection, 253–254
double depression and, 45–49
treatment of suicidality and, 13

Suprachiasmatic nucleus (SCN), and bipolar disorder, 347

Sympathetic nervous system (SNS), and stress response, 403, 404

Sympathomimetic drugs, **227**

Symptom attribution, and diagnosis of depression in medically ill, 71

Tactfulness, and interviews, 20

Tadalafil, 248

Tardive dyskinesia (TD), 136, 152

TCAs. *See* Tricyclic antidepressants (TCAs)

tDCS (transcranial direct current stimulation), 43

Terminal illness
delirium and, 175–178, 181–183, 187, 189
difficult patient, 190–194
doctor–patient relationship, 204–207
family and, 186–190, 192, 210–211
family medical history, 174
hospital psychodynamics, 207–212
initial presentation of case, 173
meaning-centered therapy, 200–203
medical history, 174
mental status exam, 174, 180
personal history, 173
psychodynamic consultation, 183–186
spirituality and, 197–199

Termination, of interpersonal psychotherapy for geriatric depression, 84

Texas Children's Medication Algorithm Project, 288

TFP (transference-focused psychotherapy), 103–105

Thalamus, and obsessive-compulsive disorder, 391–392

Therapeutic alliance. *See also* Countertransference; Doctor–patient relationship; Transference
agitation, substance abuse, and HIV infection, 253
anxiety and alcohol abuse, 304, 305, 333
double depression and, 14, 17, 37, 46
exam failure in medical school student, 384, 401, 410–415, 429, 436
geriatric depression and, 65–66, 69
schizophrenia and, 140, 146–147, 156–157, 159
terminal illness and, 209

Therapeutic privilege, 238

Thyroid hormone, and augmentation of SSRIs, 288

TMS (transcranial magnetic stimulation), 42, 43, 44, 45

Topiramate, 112

Toxicology screen, and agitation, 223, **224,** 225

Transcranial direct current stimulation (tDCS), 43

Transcranial magnetic stimulation (TMS), 42, 43, 44, 45

Transference. *See also* Countertransference; Therapeutic alliance
adolescent bereavement and, 269
anxiety and, 325
concept of selfobject and, 418–421, 422
exam failure in medical school student, 384, 397, 418–421, 432, 435, 436
experience of self in borderline personality organization and, **104**

Transference-focused psychotherapy (TFP), 103–105

Trauma, transgenerational transmission of, 255

Traumatic grief, 265–266

Treatment factors, and inpatient psychiatry, 32

Treatment goals, and cognitive-behavioral therapy for schizophrenia, **158**

Treatment refusal
difficult patient and, 191
geriatric depression and, 59–60, 63, 65, 88–89

Triage, in psychiatric emergency department, 218–219

Tricyclic antidepressants (TCAs). *See also* Antidepressants
adolescent bereavement and, 288
attention-deficit/hyperactivity disorder and, 344
cardiac disease and, 36
mood instability and, 122
pediatric patients and, 287
social anxiety and, 315

Trilling, Lionel, 360

Tuskegee Syphilis Experiment, 22

Twelve-step programs, for substance abuse, 228, 308, 309

Unipolar mania, 349

Urban renewal, impact of on social networks, 273, 274, 275

Vagal nerve stimulation (VNS), 42, 44, 45

Vaillant, George, 208

Valerian, 403

Valproate, 348

Valproic acid, and mood instability, 94, 122, 123

Values, and cultural issues, 400

Vardenafil, 248

Varenicline, **229**

Vascular disease, and geriatric depression, 89, 90

Venlafaxine, 36, 112, 288
adolescent bereavement and, 288
anxiety and, 315
double depression and, 36
mood instability and, 112

Ventral striatum, and schizophrenia, 145

Violence, and schizophrenia, 130, 135, 137–140. *See also* Self-injurious behavior; Suicide and suicidal ideation

VNS (vagal nerve stimulation), 42, 44, 45

Voluntariness, and informed consent, 237

WAIS-III (Wechsler Adult Intelligence Scale–III), 80

Web sites, and adults with ADHD, 345

Wechsler Adult Intelligence Scale–III (WAIS-III), 80

Wing, Lorna, 358

Withdrawal
alcohol abuse, 305
stimulant abuse, 226

Wolf, Hugo, 361

Woolf, Virginia, 280–283

Worst case scenario, and psychiatric emergency department, **217**

Wundt, Wilhelm, 30

Yaz-24, 354

Yoga, 404–405, 407

Young Mania Rating Scale, 350

Zolpidem, 94, 122, 123

Zung Self-Rating Depression Scale, 81

INDEX OF CASES BY DIAGNOSTIC CONCEPTS

Adjustment disorder
  Peter Burke, 67, 69
  Sophia Hastings, 308, 311, 323
Adolescent bereavement
  Amelia Gutierrez, 257–298
Agitation
  Stephen Franken, 213–256
Alcohol abuse. *See also* Substance abuse
  Peter Burke, 68
  Sophia Hastings, 300, 303, 304, 305–312, 330
Alexithymia
  James Avery, 6
Anaclitic depression
  Amelia Gutierrez, 284
Anorexia nervosa. *See also* Eating disorders
  Amy Cahill, 109, 110
Antisocial personality disorder
  Jennifer Ingram, 343
Anxiety. *See also* Anxiety disorders
  James Avery, 19
  Dorothy Ewing, 192
  Sophia Hastings, 299–300, 301, 303, 304, 305–336
  Grace Jin, 427
Anxiety disorders. *See also* Anxiety
  Sophia Hastings, 302–304
  Jennifer Ingram, 343
  Grace Jin, 406
Asperger's syndrome
  Jennifer Ingram, 339, 357, 358, 359
Attention-deficit/hyperactivity disorder (ADHD)
  Jennifer Ingram, 337, 341–345, 350, 356, 366, 373–374, 375

Atypical depression
  James Avery, 35
Avoidant personality disorder
  Sophia Hastings, 303

Bipolar depression
  Jennifer Ingram, 347
Bipolar disorder. *See also* Bipolar I disorder; Bipolar II disorder
  James Avery, 7
  Amy Cahill, 96–99, 106–108, 118, 125
  Jennifer Ingram, 339–340, 345–348, 374–375
Bipolar I disorder
  Jennifer Ingram, 346, 349, 377
Bipolar II disorder
  Jennifer Ingram, 349, 377
Body dysmorphic disorder (BDD)
  Grace Jin, 388, 389, 390, 395
Borderline personality disorder (BPD)
  Amy Cahill, 96–99, 106–108, 113, 114–115, 118, 121–122, 125
Borderline personality organization (BPO)
  Amy Cahill, 99–105
Bulimia nervosa. *See also* Eating disorders
  Amy Cahill, 109, 110, 122

Cyclothymia
  Jennifer Ingram, 349

Delirium
  James Avery, 44
  Dorothy Ewing, 175–178, 181–183, 187, 189
  Stephen Franken, 233, 234, 241, 242, 252

Delusions
  Peter Burke, 89–90
  Anthony Da Piazza, 134, 163
  Dorothy Ewing, 199
Dementia. *See* HIV-associated
  dementia; Pseudodementia
Depression. *See also* Anaclitic
  depression; Atypical depression;
  Bipolar depression; Double
  depression; Geriatric depression;
  Introjective depression; Major
  depression; Psychotic depression
  James Avery, 23, 56
  Peter Burke, 73–74, 80–81, 91
  Amelia Gutierrez, 286–289,
    292–296
  Jennifer Ingram, 347, 368
  Grace Jin, 427, 428–429
Depressive neurosis
  James Avery, 54
Depressive personality disorder
  James Avery, 16, 55
Dissociation
  Sophia Hastings, 330, 331, 334
Double depression
  James Avery, 1–57
  Peter Burke, 90
Dysthymia. *See also* Dysthymic
  disorder
  James Avery, 6, 10, 55
Dysthymic disorder. *See also* Dysthymia
  James Avery, 54
  Peter Burke, 82

Eating disorders. *See also* Anorexia
  nervosa; Bulimia nervosa
  Amy Cahill, 108–113, 122
Euthymia
  James Avery, 48
  Peter Burke, 71
Exam failure
  Grace Jin, 379–437

Geriatric depression
  Peter Burke, 59–92

Hallucinations
  Anthony Da Piazza, 156, 157
HIV-associated dementia (HAD)
  Stephen Franken, 241
Hyperactive and hypoactive delirium
  Dorothy Ewing, 177
Hypochondriasis
  Grace Jin, 387–388, 389, 395,
    431
Hypomania
  Jennifer Ingram, 337–378
Hysteresis
  Amelia Gutierrez, 274

ICU psychosis
  Dorothy Ewing, 178
Introjective depression
  Grace Jin, 429

Major depression. *See also* Major
  depressive disorder
  James Avery, 55
  Peter Burke, 70, 71, 82, 89
  Grace Jin, 429
Major depressive disorder. *See also*
  Major depression
  James Avery, 6
Mania. *See* Hypomania
Mood disorders
  Jennifer Ingram, 343, 374
Mood instability
  Amy Cahill, 93–127

Narcissistic personality disorder
  Grace Jin, 393–398, 416, 421, 423,
    424, 425–426, 433

Obsessive-compulsive disorder
  Grace Jin, 390, 391

Panic
  Sophia Hastings, 303, 313, 317,
    319–327
Paranoid-type schizophrenia
  Anthony Da Piazza, 169–170

Personality disorders. *See also*
Antisocial personality disorder;
Depressive personality disorder;
Narcissistic personality disorder
James Avery, 7, 10, 54
Pervasive developmental disorder
(PDD)
Jennifer Ingram, 357–359
Posttraumatic stress disorder (PTSD)
Amelia Gutierrez, 265–266
Sophia Hastings, 304, 313,
328–329, 330, 331
Premenstrual dysphoric disorder
(PMDD)
Jennifer Ingram, 350, 352–354, 356,
375
Premenstrual syndrome (PMS)
Jennifer Ingram, 352, 353, 375
Pseudodementia
Peter Burke, 91
Psychosis
Anthony Da Piazza, 134, 146–148,
170–171
Psychotic depression
Peter Burke, 89–90

Schizophrenia. *See also* Paranoid-type
schizophrenia
Anthony Da Piazza, 129–172
Jennifer Ingram, 358
Seasonal affective disorder
Jennifer Ingram, 357

Social anxiety disorder (SAD)
Sophia Hastings, 303, 315
Social phobia
Sophia Hastings, 303
Somatoform disorders
Grace Jin, 387–389, 402, 416
Substance abuse. *See also* Alcohol
abuse
James Avery, 6–7, 10
Anthony Da Piazza, 130, 134, 135,
138–139, 167
Dorothy Ewing, 181–183
Stephen Franken, 223, 224,
225–232, 233–254
Amelia Gutierrez, 271
Sophia Hastings, 330
Jennifer Ingram, 343, 349
Grace Jin, 385
Suicidal ideation
James Avery, 1, 8, 9–14, 43–44
Amy Cahill, 93, 95, 103, 105, 107,
114–115, 117, 118–120, 125–126
Anthony Da Piazza, 160
Amelia Gutierrez, 261–264,
267–269, 287, 295
Jennifer Ingram, 347, 351

Terminal illness
Dorothy Ewing, 173–212

Unipolar mania
Jennifer Ingram, 349